MW00352716

FETAL MONITORING *Interpretation*

FETAL MONITORING

Interpretation

Micki L. Cabaniss, MD

Associate Professor, Department of Obstetrics and Gynecology
University of North Carolina at Chapel Hill
Chapel Hill, North Carolina

Director, Maternal-Fetal Medicine
Obstetrics-Gynecology Department
Mountain Area Health Education Center
Asheville, North Carolina

Dimitri Karetnikov

Medical Illustrator

J. B. Lippincott Company
Philadelphia

Sponsoring Editor: Lisa McAllister
Assistant Editor: Paula Callaghan
Indexer: Maria Coughlin
Interior Designer: Anne O'Donnell
Cover Designer: Anne O'Donnell
Production Manager: Lori J. Bainbridge
Production Service: Ruttle, Shaw & Wetherill, Inc.
Compositor: Compset Inc.
Printer/Binder: Arcata Graphics/Halliday

6   5   4   3   2   1

Library of Congress Cataloging-in-Publications Data

Cabaniss, Micki L.
     Fetal monitoring interpretation / Micki L. Cabaniss ; Dimitri
Karetnikov, medical illustrator.
          p.   cm.
     Includes bibliographical references and index.
     ISBN 0-397-50824-7
     1. Fetal heart rate monitoring—Interpretation.   I. Karetnikov,
Dimitri.   II. Title.
     [DNLM: 1. Fetal Monitoring.   WQ 210 C112f]
RG628.3.H42C33   1992
618.3'207543—dc20
DNLM/DLC
for Library of Congress   92-49157
                                                                                     CIP

The authors and publisher have exerted every effort to ensure that drug selection and dosage
set forth in this text are in accord with current recommendations and practice at the time of
publication. However, in view of ongoing research, changes in government regulations, and
the constant flow of information relating to drug therapy and drug reactions, the reader is urged
to check the package insert for each drug for any change in indications and dosage and for
added warnings and precautions. This is particularly important when the recommended agent
is a new or infrequently employed drug.

Dedicated to my family

Contributors

Co-author Section IV: Dysrhythmias

C. Daniel Cabaniss, MD
Consultant Cardiologist
Haywood County Hospital and
    Mountain Medical Associates
Clyde, North Carolina

Co-author Chapter 1: Classification of Fetal Monitoring Patterns

Patricia C. Wagner, MSN, RNC
Former Director, The Center for Women and Children
Mobile Infirmary
Mobile, Alabama

Consultants

Pediatric Cardiology

Walter Johnson, MD
Birmingham, Alabama

Legal

Morton Harris
Columbus, Georgia

Thomas Stennis*
Gulfport, Mississippi

*deceased

Publishing

Jesse Littleton, MD
Mobile Alabama

Rebecca Rinehart
Formerly at American College of Obstetrics and
Gynecology
Washington, DC

Lisa Biello
Philadelphia, Pennsylvania

Participants

Case Studies

Patricia C. Wagner, RNC, MSN
Roatan Bay Islands
Honduras, Central America

Jane Vaughn, RNC
Columbus, Georgia

Dorothy May, RNC, BSN
Mobile, Alabama

Manuscript Preparation

Judy Jasinski, New York, New York
Susan Price, Orlando, Florida
Marietta Harris, Pikeville, Tennessee
John M. Souma, Pensacola, Florida

Bibliography Preparation

Neva Rogers, RNC, MSN, Huntsville, Alabama
Peggy Chance, Mobile, Alabama
Tally Beard, RN, Pensacola, Florida
Florence Ruby, BS:ML Pensacola, Florida

Art Development

Frank Vogtner, Mobile, Alabama
Wendy Hill, Mobile, Alabama
Michele Souma, New Orleans, Louisiana

Foreword

*T*he clinical use of electronic fetal heart rate monitoring that began in the United States in the early 1970s was based on considerable background research but not on a wealth of clinical "field testing." This introduction was followed by a rush of using, learning, and teaching electronic fetal monitoring (EFM). In our enthusiasm for this new clinical tool, terms such as "fetal distress" and "fetal asphyxia" were misused and EFM was credited with more than it could deliver. The early wave of unnecessary cesarean deliveries based on faulty interpretation waned, but left the monitor suspect of bringing as much potential risk as benefit to obstetrics. Initially, EFM was faulted for inhibiting our patients' maternal experience, distracting our attention from our patients, and not clearly distinguishing between the well-oxygenated and oxygen-deprived fetus and newborn. Retrospective studies praising the monitor were eventually succeeded by controlled prospective studies demonstrating that frequent auscultation may be as beneficial as EFM in preventing newborn morbidity in the normal patient. Although EFM fell short of our ability to diagnose the distressed fetus to expedite delivery, the monitor brought a new dimension to obstetrics: growth in our understanding of the intrapartum fetal, maternal, and placental physiology. In the long run, EFM brought us back to the patient. More than ever before, many basic scientific concepts entered into the clinical arena of the labor room: placental oxygen transfer, placental reserves, fetal compensatory mechanisms, and uterine dysfunction. Information gained from the monitor further clarified these concepts. As we learned more about threats to the in utero environment, we learned new methods for improving uterine-umbilical blood flow and oxygenation. We not only became better scientists, we also became better clinicians.

The monitor has earned a place in the intrapartum validation of the 90% to 95% of fetuses who are well-oxygenated. EFM is now a guide for therapeutic intervention for the healthy but stressed fetus and for investigation of the potentially sick fetus. The value of EFM is in preventing clinically marked fetal asphyxia. In the future, EFM will be used to determine the point at which fetal oxygen deprivation exists. Such an advance will require continuing education and investigation.

This book is a labor of love. It contains a comprehensive presentation of recognized fetal heart rate and uterine activity patterns, considered within the context of possible clinical outcomes. The author is to be congratulated for her patience, persistence, and data collections; she presents new classifications and interpretations of the data without overstepping the bounds or making quantum leaps in conclusions. Electronic fetal heart rate monitoring must be used in relationship to new knowledge and interpretation of the data based on sound clinical judgment. This book ties together physiology and pathophysiology with clear and concise EFM patterns and contains a full explanation of interpretation and a wealth of background literature for easy reference.

Medicine is a mixture of art and science and as such is imperfect. We are not perfect in identifying the distressed fetus, but this book will allow us to travel the road that will lead us to a clearer understanding of electronic fetal heart rate patterns.

Robert C. Cefalo, MD, PhD
Professor, Obstetrics and Gynecology
Director, Maternal-Fetal Medicine
Assistant Dean, Head of the Office of
Graduate Medical Education
University of North Carolina School of
Medicine
Chapel Hill, North Carolina

Preface

The primary purpose of this book is to teach fetal monitoring interpretation through a pattern-oriented approach. Unlike books on fetal monitoring that present separate sections on technology, pathology, physiology, patient management, and so forth, such material is presented throughout this book as it directly relates to fetal monitoring patterns encountered during actual patient care. A classification of interpretations is introduced that is based on the type of clinical management that may be prompted by the pattern. The fetal heart rate patterns are organized in the book in a standard fashion, beginning with baseline findings and followed by periodic and nonperiodic changes from the baseline. Uterine activity and superimposed maternal/fetal movement are presented in a separate section. Many causes of multiple heart rate traces now exist in the field of fetal monitoring, including simultaneous maternal/fetal and twin monitoring as well as arrythmias and artifacts. These are presented together to foster an appreciation of dual monitoring and to enhance recognition of artifactual heart rate traces. Although dysrhythmias are presented throughout the book, the separate section on dysrhythmias enables further study of these unique fetal monitoring heart rate traces accompanied by electrocardiograms and echocardiograms.

Explanation of the Fetal Monitoring Tracings

All tracings used in this book are authentic and unretouched (unless specifically indicated because of damage, fading, or the removal of markings that identify the patient or her attendants). In a few cases, the only access to the original tracing is through microfilm, a photograph, or photocopied form. Words that were handwritten on the tracing were always placed there at the time of the original patient care. Tracings from early monitors are purposefully included because such monitors remain in use in some institutions, and the information derived from them may continue to be reviewed for years to come.

Explanation of Electrocardiograms and Echocardiograms

Many fetal ECGs were obtained by cable transmission from the fetal monitor to a separate electrocardiograph. Others were obtained directly through a machine feature (Litton): arrhythmia/artifact detector. One is obtained at the time of fetal echocardiogram, and one is presented using older abdominal ECG technology.

With no exceptions, every electrocardiogram and echocardiogram in this text is the actual fetal or newborn tracing that was obtained from the same patient as the monitoring tracing.

Several fetal electrocardiograms in the book do not permit the degree of interpretation possible at the patient's bedside. In some of these cases, enhancement is used and is so specified. In all cases, the information from the refined electrocardiogram may be derived from the accompanying diagrammatic teaching rendition.

Explanation of Inserts

Occasionally, with permission, a previously published tracing of other investigators is used in this volume for comparison with the tracing presented. These are in the form of text inserts. Additional examples of a particular pattern are also presented in this fashion. Interpretation and outcome of the inserts is not provided.

Explanation of Interpretations

Interpretations, including classification of the patterns, were prepared by review of the authentic tracing segment (not just the diagrammed portion) as though there were no information available about the clinical setting of the pattern. This allows the sample tracing to be used for *teaching* beyond the implications of the circumstances of the individual case. In *actual patient care*, the clinician usually reviews a larger segment of fetal heart rate monitoring tracing and simultaneously alters impressions based on such known clinical factors as gestation, status of labor, and anticipated time and mode of delivery. In addition, during actual patient care, the effect of therapeutic interventions is prospectively observed and not retrospectively extrapolated.

Explanation of Outcomes

All cases in this book are authentic and occurred between 1977 and 1988. Maternal and newborn courses are accurate and verifiable. Cases were selected to present a potential outcome that illustrates the teaching points being made by the monitoring pattern under study. However, they are not intended to represent the only or the most likely outcome possible with the pattern. Most of the cases represent the author's own patients, on whom bedside observations were made during actual recording, or cases in which review of the tracing was performed in a timely association with occurrence, with personnel available who cared for the patient and were able to clarify many details.

Explanation of the Art Diagrams

The diagrams used throughout this work were derived using a simple grid from sketches prepared from the authentic tracing. Alterations in spacing and other features of the original tracings were liberally used to present maximum teaching in a small space. The original tracing is always depicted to document actual time/space relationships. Gray shading is often used to enhance teaching.

Explanation of Terminology

The word "tracing" refers to the entire fetal monitoring data display, including fetal heart rate and uterine/maternal activity information. The word "trace" refers to an individual heart rate or uterine activity line on the tracing whether produced by fetal- or maternal-derived signals.

The terms "bradycardia" and "tachycardia" are reserved for true baseline changes (e.g., patterns of longer than 10 minutes in duration or otherwise reflecting the true basal heart rate of the fetus). Changes of shorter duration are termed accelerations and decelerations so that baseline trends may be distinguished from heart rate changes from the baseline.

When fetal monitoring findings appear magnified from the norm, the term "marked" is most consistently used (with "moderate" indicating an intermediate step from normal) except in the case of variability where "increased" is more popularly used than "marked" and in the case of variable decelerations where "severe" is more popularly used than "marked." The term "exaggerated" is reserved for erroneously or artifactually increased phenomena.

"Terminal" could mean just before death or just before delivery. Because this produces confusion, the term is herein reserved for patterns preceding death. Instead of being referred to as late labor, "terminal" is termed as such or as "end stage," "second stage," or "expulsion phenomena."

"Periodic" refers to recurrent changes in heart rate that are associated with uterine contractions and "nonperiodic" with any not associated with uterine contractions. "Sporadic" may be considered synonymous with nonperiodic but is herein reserved for very infrequently occurring fetal heart changes.

Variable decelerations are first classified by size[2] and then by presence or absence of atypia.[1] Krebs distinguishes pure variable decelerations from atypical decelerations. The word "pure" is replaced by "classical" within the pages of this book, as it provides a clearer contrast to the term "atypical." The term "initial" is replaced by "primary" as a clearer counterpart to "secondary" when referring to accelerative components of variable decelerations.

The fetal monitor cannot consistently diagnose fetal distress. Therefore, the term is not used in direct reference to a fetal monitoring pattern interpretation. More commonly, the terms "distress-like" and "high risk of low Apgar score/acidosis" are used when identifying the potentially distressed fetus based on fetal monitoring heart rate pattern data.

New terms introduced in this book are "slipping," "atypical accelerations," and "S" sign.

References

1. Krebs H-B, Petres RE, Dunn LJ: Intrapartum fetal heart rate monitoring. VIII. Atypical variable decelerations. Am J Obstet Gynecol 145:297, 1983.
2. Kubli FW, Hon EH, Khazin AF, et al: Observations on heart rate and pH in the human fetus during labor. Am J Obstet Gynecol 104:1190, 1969.

Acknowledgments

*T*his book evolved from material collected for purposes of teaching fetal monitoring to attending physicians, residents, nurses, and students by means of case-study exercises titled "Tracing of the Week." The teaching activity consisted of selecting a tracing and posting it without identifying information for participants to interpret. A formal teaching interpretation accompanied by supporting references from the medical literature was displayed the following week along with a new "unknown" tracing. "Tracing of the Week" was conducted at The Medical Center, Columbus, Georgia, during the late 1970s and early 1980s and at the University of South Alabama Medical Center Hospital, Mobile, Alabama, during the mid-1980s. During that time period, over 30,000 tracings were reviewed, from which the teaching cases were selected. I am thankful to those physicians, nurses, and students who inspired the original project, who supplied energy through their participation, and who assisted in the care and preservation of the tracings.

I am thankful to Hiram Mendenhall, MD, former Chairman of the Department of Obstetrics and Gynecology at the University of South Alabama, for his support of the initial decision to transform the "Tracing of the Week" material into a textbook. I also am grateful to Robert Boerth, MD, Chairman of the Department of Pediatrics at the University of South Alabama, for generously teaching me and sharing with me fetal echocardiography material. I greatly value the support and encouragement I received from the faculty and fellows of the Division of Maternal-Fetal Medicine and Obstetrics and Gynecology Department at the University of South Alabama throughout the development of this book.

I appreciate the fetal monitoring equipment provided through grants and loans. Support was given by all of the major manufacturers of fetal monitoring instruments. Helpful even beyond their assistance with the equipment was the encouragement regarding this book that the representatives of the monitoring industry gave me. For this I thank Tom Lewis, Ray Griffin, John Edwards, Susan Gregg, Pat Dwyer, Tom Fisher, and George Hojaiban.

I would also like to acknowledge the help provided by several additional people, without which the publication of this volume would have been impossible. Many cases were brought to my attention by the attending physicians and residents of the Obstetrical Service, The Medical Center, Columbus, Georgia, from 1973 to 1982 and the Obstetrical Service, University of South Alabama Medical Center Hospital, from 1982 to 1988.

Many individuals graciously gave me access to cases from their personal files. Used in this book are the cases of Everett Beguin, MD, Mo Fitzgerald, MD, Tim Johnson, MD, Earl Perrett, MD, Conrad Pierce, MD, and Sage Smith, MD.

Special case studies were supplied by Brian McWeier, MD, Mike Farrell, MD, Tom Miller, MD, Carol Porter, RN, and Lisa Dunning, MD.

The manuscript was carefully read and critiqued by William C. Brannon, MD, and Watson A. Bowes, MD.

I am thankful to Jack F. Huddleston, MD, for his role as a mentor in my development of the concepts of fetal stress and distress used in this book.

Secretarial assistance with the manuscript was provided by Anita Holder, Darcy Martin, Susan Gray, Lynda Kennedy, Diane Grover, and Heidi Boone.

I am very proud of the publisher that I selected, J. B. Lippincott Company. I have enjoyed working with the publication staff led by Lisa McAllister with Susan Hess Blaker and Lori Bainbridge. The publisher used superior judgment in procuring the help of Kathy Barrett and her coworkers Peg Markow, Janet Nuciforo, Barbara Lipson and Anne O'Donnell of Ruttle, Shaw & Wetherill. The unique tasks this book has required have been accomplished with untiring enthusiasm by the publishing team.

The work entailed in preparing this book, the rewriting, redrawing, and making of additions and deletions, has occupied many years. It has been very important to me that the book be comprehensive, current, accurate, and visually clear. I hope you will use and enjoy *Fetal Monitoring Interpretation*.

Contents

Section IV
UTERINE/MATERNAL/FETAL
ACTIVITY   333

15   Uterine Activity   335

USE AND LIMITATIONS
OF THE FETAL MONITOR

Section I

*T*erms used in connection with fetal monitoring such as "bradycardia," "deceleration," and "variability," may be seen as the basic language used in communicating fetal monitoring information (data base) (see Tables 1 and 2). However, the use of the fetal monitor in clinical management depends upon organization of that data into a refined diagnosis. It is upon this assessment or interpretation that a management plan is based. Such diagnoses may therefore be grouped or classified according to the nature of information derived about the fetal condition and the type of clinical responses it provokes (see Table 3). A functional classification of fetal monitoring patterns is as follows:

Class I: Normal Patterns

Class II: Stress Patterns

Class III: Nondiagnostic Patterns

Class IV: Patterns with Atypia

Class V: Distress-like Patterns

Class 0: Quality not suitable for interpretation

The criteria for inclusion in these categories and the subsequent clinical response are discussed in this section. The fetal monitor is used with high reliability to identify the healthy fetus—the very fetus for whom intervention to effect a positive outcome as a result of fetal monitoring is least frequently necessary. The monitor is perhaps best used in preventive care of the stressed fetus. Highly diagnostic patterns demonstrating the fetal use of compensatory mechanisms to maintain homeostasis may be observed for positive change in response to early intervention. The monitor provides the least useful information about fetal condition with nondiagnostic patterns, but in such cases it serves as a screening tool to direct the acquisition of other information.

When the clinician encounters patterns with atypia, he or she has the greatest challenge. Widely variable monitoring data are combined with the clinical background and course in order to make individualized decisions. The monitor is limited in its ability to predict the sick fetus, but certain patterns indicate sufficient risk of an abnormal outcome to permit monitoring data to be used in selecting fetuses for prompt delivery.

Also reviewed in this section are limitations of the monitor in fulfilling these roles, including Class 0, technically uninterpretable patterns.

Table 1-1. Classification of Fetal Heart Pattern Monitoring Features: An Overview

Baseline Features	Periodic and Nonperiodic Change		
Heartrate	**Accelerations**		
Normal (120–160 bpm)	Uniform		
Bradycardia	Variable		
Moderate (100–120 bpm)	Special patterns:		
Marked (<100 bpm)	Periodic		
Tachycardia	Lambda		
Moderate (160–180 bpm)	Prolonged		
Marked (>180 bpm)	Atypical		
	Marked		
Variability	**Decelerations**		
Short-term/Long-term	Uniform: Early		
Average (normal)	Late		
Increased (>25 bpm)	Variable: Classic	Atypical features:	
Decreased (<6 bpm), Absent (flat line)	Mild (V)	Loss of primary acceleration	
Sinusoidal (2–5 cycles/min, 5–15 bpm)	Moderate	Loss of secondary acceleration	
Marked (>15 bpm)	Severe	Prolonged secondary acceleration	
		Continuation of the baseline at	
Baseline Stability		a lower level	
Trends/Shifts		Slow recovery	
Instability		Biphasic (W)	
Obscured		Loss of variability (U)	
	Late/variable (S)		
Dysrhythmias	Unusual Findings: Asystole,		
	arrhythmias, overlap		
Bradyarrhythmias	Combined: Variable and late decelerations		
Atrioventricular block	Mixed: Variable and early decelerations		
Nonconducted premature	Prolonged (>2–3 min): With full recovery		
supraventricular depolarizations in	Without full recovery		
bigeminy	Recurrent		
Tachyarrhythmias			
Supraventricular tachycardia			
Atrial flutter			
Premature depolarizations			
Supraventricular			
Ventricular			

Table 1-2. Classification of Pattern Features for Uterine Contractions and Maternal/Fetal Activity: An Overview

Uterine Activity			Maternal/Fetal Activity
Normal Absent Unrecorded	Hypoactive	Hyperactive Skewed Polysystole Tachysystole Paired Hypertonia Tetany	Movement Respirations Seizures

Table 1-3. Functional Classification of Fetal Heart Rate Patterns

Class I. Normal Patterns (fetal heart rate patterns of the unstressed healthy fetus)
    A. Classic normal (average variability with non-periodic accelerations)
    B. Baseline bradycardia with normal variability
    C. Early decelerations
    D. Mild classic variable decelerations
    E. Accelerations followed by brief decelerations (Lambda)
    Response: No Intervention

Class II. Stress Patterns (healthy fetus using compensatory mechanisms in response to hypoxia or other stresses)
    A. Increased variability
    B. Tachycardia with good variability
    C. Periodic accelerations and certain marked and prolonged accelerations
    D. Late decelerations with good variability
    E. Classic moderate to severe variable decelerations (without atypia)
    F. Prolonged deceleration with normal/full recovery
    Response: Revert to Class I If Possible

Class III. Nondiagnostic Patterns (associated with healthy or sick fetus)
    A. Absent variability (flat line)
    B. Long-term variability present, no short-term variability
    C. Short-term variability present, no long-term variability
    D. Sinusoidal pattern
    E. Tachyarrhythmias and bradyarrhythmias
    Response: Obtain Further Information

Class IV. Patterns with Atypia
    A. Mild and moderate variable decelerations with varying atypia and baseline changes
    B. Severe variable decelerations with atypia, normal baseline stability, rate, and variability
    C. Atypical accelerations
    Response: Individualize Case by Case

Class V. Distress-like Patterns
    A. Repetitive late decelerations with no variability
    B. Severe variable decelerations with atypia and baseline changes (loss of variability and tachycardia)
    C. The late/variable decelerations (S sign) associated with no baseline variability
    D. Prolonged decelerations without recovery (and certain prolonged decelerations with progressive recurrence)
    E. Marked sinusoidal pattern
    F. Agonal patterns
    Response: Delivery Planning

Functional Classification
of Fetal Monitoring Patterns

Chapter 1

Class I: Normal Patterns

Class II: Stress Patterns

Class III: Nondiagnostic Patterns

Class IV: Patterns with Atypia

Class V: Distress-like Patterns

Class I. Normal Patterns

*T*he fetal monitor is a highly sensitive indicator of good fetal condition.[2] A normal fetal heart rate pattern has a 95% or better correlation with a fetus (were it to be delivered) that is nonhypoxic and nonacidotic.[48] A classic normal tracing is defined as a stable baseline at a normal rate, with normal short- and long-term variability and accelerations present.[17] Routine intermittent maternal and fetal assessments throughout labor are appropriate for patients with a classic normal tracing when in a clinical setting without accompanying risk factors.[1,23,28,37] In addition to this pattern, other fetal heart rate patterns that are demonstrated in an unstressed, healthy fetus include:

Baseline bradycardia (with normal variability and reactivity)

Early decelerations

Mild classic variable decelerations

Accelerations followed by brief decelerations (Lambda pattern)

These display reflex responses to nonthreatening stimuli. These are also associated with good fetal outcome but are appropriately reassessed, at least intermittently, for transition to other less reassuring patterns.

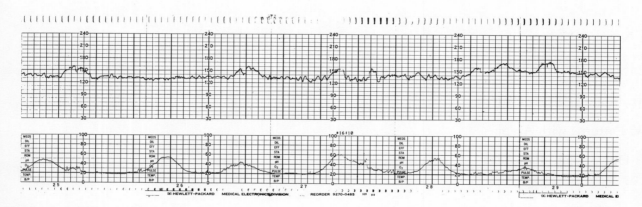

CASE INTERPRETATION: Class I

Baseline Information: normal rate, average variability, stable baseline.

Periodic or Nonperiodic Changes: nonperiodic uniform and variable accelerations.

Uterine Activity: regular contractions with normal waveform, rare skewing.

Significance: good fetal condition, favorable immediate newborn outcome anticipated.

CASE OUTCOME: Thirty-four-year-old gravida 2, para 1001, at 38 weeks' gestation, delivered vaginally with epidural anesthesia a living female, 7 pounds, 6 ounces (3345 grams); Apgar score 8/9. Uncomplicated newborn course.

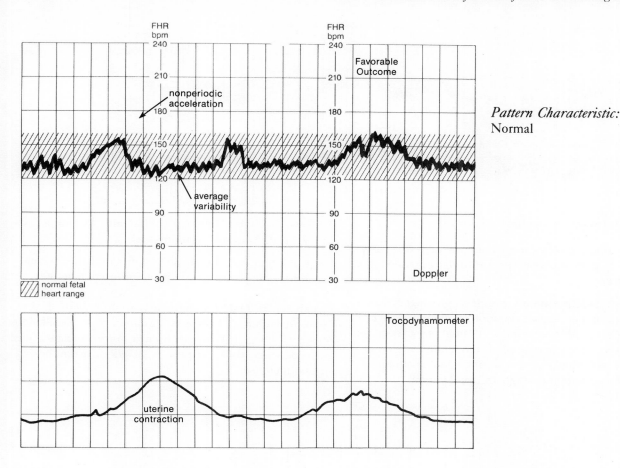

Pattern Characteristic:
Normal

Class II. Stress Patterns

*S*tress patterns are indicative of a fetus who is demonstrating healthy protective responses to such stimuli as hypoxemia, hypovolemia and sinus node suppression. Examples of compensatory mechanisms in response to hypoxic stress are redistribution of blood flow, increased oxygen extraction at the placenta, and increased or decreased heart rate and escape rhythms.[7,30,33,36,42,45] Escape rhythms are unique lifesaving responses of the healthy fetus to abrupt reflex slowing of the heart. Under all circumstances, the excellent baseline variability with or without reactivity suggests a compensated state.[34,38] It has been demonstrated that pH studies are nonacidotic under these circumstances.[20] However, further stress may deplete compensatory mechanisms. The challenge in the management of these patterns is to diminish present stresses while producing optimum placental perfusion and fetal oxygenation. Measures that may be selected to do so include maternal oxygen administration, maternal repositioning, maternal hydration, discontinuation or reduction of oxytocin infusion, decreasing of maternal straining, tocolytic therapy, amnioinfusion, and reduction of maternal fever.[5,15,25,31,33] These therapeutic measures are individualized according to specific heart rate and uterine monitoring data as well as the clinical circumstances.[11,32] Fetal response varies with the basal condition and the nature and degree of stressful stimulus.[41] It is also appropriate, when possible, to minimize additional stress during subsequent labor and delivery.[5]

Stress patterns include:

Increased variability

Tachycardia with good variability

Periodic accelerations and some patterns of marked or prolonged accelerations

Late decelerations with good variability

Classic moderate or severe variable decelerations (without atypia)

Isolated prolonged decelerations with normal/full recovery

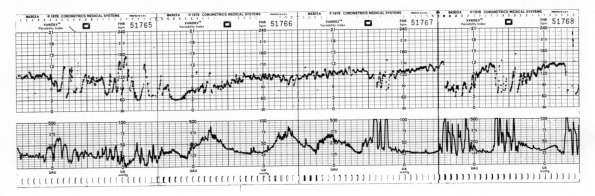

CASE INTERPRETATION: Class II

Baseline Information: normal rate, increased variability (saltatory pattern), associated with decelerations in a mixed pattern.

Periodic or Nonperiodic Changes: prolonged deceleration (seven minutes in duration) with full recovery, maintaining excellent variability throughout except for transient sinus node suppression, moderate variable decelerations with slow recovery during maternal straining, variability maintained throughout deceleration.

Uterine Activity: frequent contractions without a resting interval. Maternal straining.

Significance: stress of healthy fetus probably secondary to hypoxia produced by increased uterine activity.

CASE OUTCOME: Nineteen-year-old gravida 2, para 0010, delivered at 42 weeks' gestation an 8 pound, 9½ ounce (3898 gram) female from a vertex presentation with local anesthesia; Apgar score 9/9. Uncomplicated newborn course.

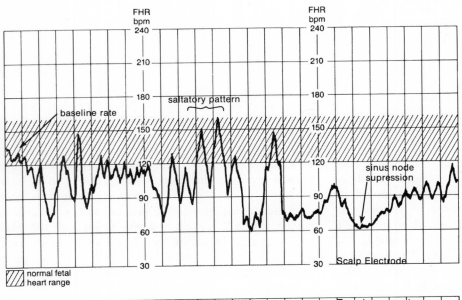

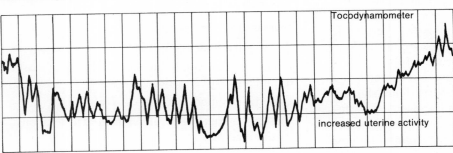

Pattern Characteristic:
Stress Pattern

Class III. Nondiagnostic Patterns

*N*ondiagnostic patterns have decreased or absent variability and no periodic changes to aid diagnosis. They may be associated with the entire spectrum from a healthy to a sick fetus. The patterns have insufficient information that is necessary for clarifying fetal status. Some other information must be sought, for example the fetal pH.[36,38] The incidence of acidosis when there is no other heart rate abnormality except decreased variability may be as low as 5%.[7] However, fetal acidosis may contribute to neurologic deficits in the fetus. When fetal scalp sampling is not possible or unavailable, delivery of the intrapartum fetus may be indicated, unless there is additional information that provides special knowledge about good fetal condition in selected case settings,[40] (e.g., reassuring fetal response to stimulation or a pre-vious normal tracing followed by response to drug administration). Nonintervention may in turn be selected when clinical information supports a diagnosis of fetal brain death.[26]

Nondiagnostic patterns include:

No short- and long-term variability (flat line patterns)

Long-term variability present, no short-term variability

Short-term variability present, no long-term variability

Sinusoidal pattern

Tachyarrhythmias and bradyarrhythmias

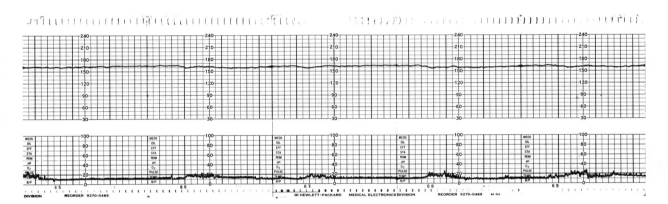

CASE INTERPRETATION: Class III

Baseline Information: upper limits of normal, decreased long- and short-term variability. Slight drifting (wandering) of baseline (possibly produced by shallow deceleration).

Periodic or Nonperiodic Changes: possible shallow decelerations coincidental with uterine contractions in onset but delayed recovery (late decelerations).

Uterine Activity: small contractions recorded every three minutes by external monitor.

Significance: nondiagnostic of the fetal condition. Information about fetal pH is needed unless the pattern immediately preceding or superceding demonstrates reassuring reactivity. Delivery may be indicated if a fetal pH is not feasible.

CASE OUTCOME: Twenty-five-year-old gravida 2, para 1001, delivered at 40 weeks' gestation, with general anesthesia by cesarean section for fetal acidosis, a 7 pound, 6 ounce (3345 gram) male, with a scalp pH of 7.19 11 minutes prior to delivery; Apgar score 1/3. There was thick meconium, and a cord pH 7.135 (arterial), 7.22 (venous). The newborn was hospitalized 11 days; his course was complicated by persistent fetal circulation.

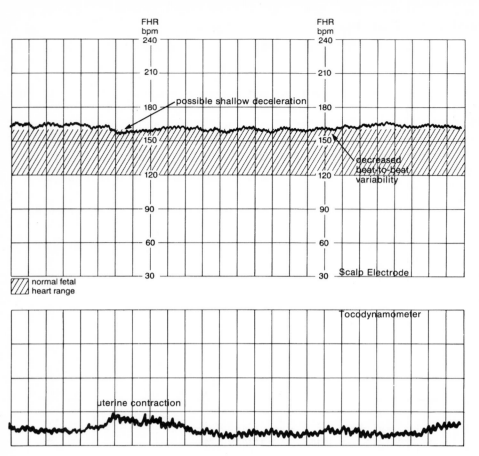

Pattern Characteristic:
Nondiagnostic Pattern

Class IV. Patterns with Atypia

*V*ariable decelerations with atypia have an increased risk of a low Apgar score and acidosis.[19,21] However, outcome varies widely, for example, the risk of a low Apgar score at five minutes ranges from 7% to 20%, depending on the number and type of atypical findings.[21] Management is based on consideration of three sets of factors. The first is the pattern itself—no two are alike. The specific atypical features, the number of atypical features, and the association with baseline alterations all are considered in predicting the degree of risk of a low Apgar score and acidosis.

The second group of factors are the clinical circumstances. Management must be individualized according to gestation; duration of the pattern; estimated duration to delivery; predicted ease of delivery; and the presence of other risk factors, especially intrauterine growth retardation, prematurity, postdate gestation, and thick meconium.[5,11,14,24,31]

The third set of factors are the responses of the fetus to measures used to produce optimal fetal oxygenation. These measures may include amnioinfusion when cir-

cumstances are appropriate as well as optimum maternal positioning, maternal hyperoxia and hydration, and reduction of uterine activity.[5,25] For those persistent atypical variable decelerations managed expectantly, availability of emergency cesarean section and close surveillance of the tracing for change are appropriate.

Accelerations may also, on occasion, vary from classical presentations. The range of outcomes for fetuses exhibiting atypical accelerations has not been studied and, therefore, each case is appropriately individualized.

Patterns with atypia include:

Mild and moderate variable decelerations, with varying atypia (such as loss of variability in the deceleration, biphasic features, slow recovery, and changes in the associated primary and secondary accelerations) and baseline changes

Severe variable decelerations, with atypia, normal baseline stability, rate, and variability

Atypical accelerations

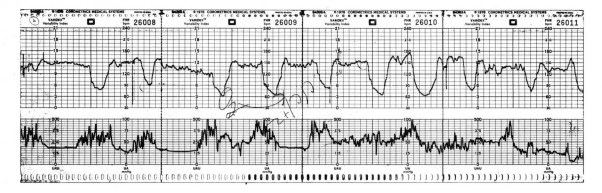

CASE INTERPRETATION: Class IV

Baseline Information: high normal rate, normal variability. Downward drift in baseline after some decelerations.

Periodic or Nonperiodic Changes: moderate variable decelerations with atypia characterized by loss of variability in decelerations and occasional loss of primary accelerations. Some of the decelerations have late occurrence.

Uterine Activity: frequent contractions by external monitor with some loss of resting interval.

Significance: presence of atypia in variable decelerations predicts an increased risk of low Apgar score and acidosis. Management is influenced by the individual clinical situation. While planning delivery, steps taken to reduce uterine activity and diminish cord impingement, while achieving maximum fetal oxygenation, are potentially beneficial.

CASE OUTCOME: Fifteen-year-old primigravida delivered vaginally at 39 weeks' gestation a 5 pound, 13 ounce (2637 gram) male, local/pudendal anesthesia; Apgar score 6/9. Nuchal cord. Newborn course complicated by mild hyperbilirubinemia.

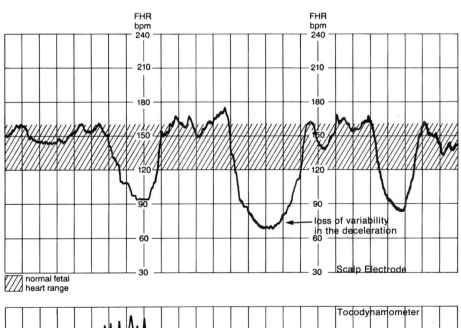

Pattern Characteristic:
Pattern with Atypia

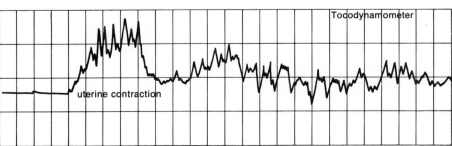

Class V. Distress-like Patterns

*T*he term "fetal distress" is reserved for situations of deterioration of fetal compensatory mechanisms in the face of hypoxia such that metabolic acidosis ensues.[3,26,39] Prediction of a sick newborn by fetal monitoring information is only 20% to 75% reliable.[6,8,9,10,13,44,46] This varies with the criteria used for monitoring interpretation, newborn assessment standards, and other study design features.[47] Although distress-like patterns do not predict a universally poor outcome, they are patterns that have been associated a significant number of times with the fetus who has experienced stress and is undergoing decompensation of its normal homeostatic mechanisms.[12,18,20] They are found with such a high incidence of fetal acidosis and low Apgar scores that if persistent, delivery by the most expeditious route is the usual clinical management.[4,16,22,28,34,35,46] In some circumstances, it is appropriate to not delay this management by doing fetal pH procedures (unless they are immediately available). Usual measures to improve fetal perfusion/oxygenation may be conducted throughout the emergency delivery preparations, with the hope of bringing about correction of the pattern, but even more so, for the purpose of producing an improvement in the newborn condition at birth. This may include tocolytic therapy when circumstances are appropriate.[5,25,29] It is important to note, however, that because of the underlying condition of some fetuses with certain distress-like monitoring patterns, they may not gain measurable benefit from either prompt or operative delivery.

Distress-like patterns include:

Recurrent late decelerations with no variability

Severe variable decelerations with atypia and baseline changes (i.e., loss of variability and tachycardia)

The late/variable deceleration associated with absent baseline variability (S sign)

Prolonged decelerations without recovery

Marked sinusoidal pattern

Agonal patterns

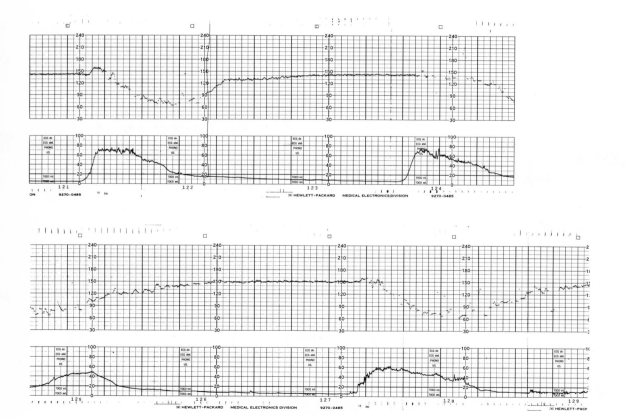

CASE INTERPRETATION: Class V

Baseline Information: normal rate, no variability.

Periodic or Nonperiodic Changes: late/variable decelerations with delayed return to baseline.

Uterine Activity: polysystolic, markedly skewed, infrequent contractions.

Significance: probable chronic and significant fetal jeopardy. Prompt delivery is an appropriate response if the fetus is viable, while simultaneously performing measures to improve fetal oxygenation.

CASE OUTCOME: Eighteen-year-old primigravida delivered at 44 weeks' gestation by cesarean section for possible fetal distress, a 9 pound, 2 ounce (4139 gram) male; Apgar score 2/4. The fetus was in a vertex presentation, in an occiput posterior position, and thick meconium was present. The maternal course was complicated by preeclampsia and wound infection. The newborn was dismissed with the mother at eight days of life.

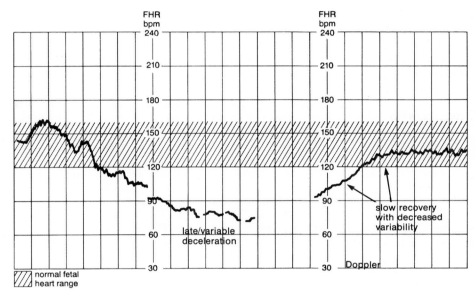

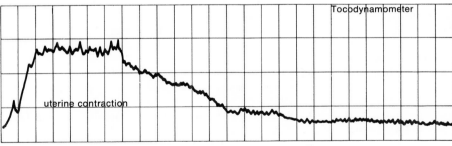

Pattern Characteristic:
Distress-like Pattern

References

1. ACOG Newsletter Committee Comments in EFM Controversy, May 1979.
2. ACOG Newsletter: Electronic fetal monitoring-state-of-the-art opinions, p. 5, June 1988.
3. Assessment of fetal and newborn acid base status. *ACOG Technical Bulletin* no. 127, April 1989.
4. Beard RW, Brudenhall JM, Feroze RM, et al: Intensive care of the high risk fetus in labor. *J Obstet Gynaecol, British Commonwealth* 78:882, 1971.
5. Campbell WA, Ventzileos AM, Nochinson DJ: Intrauterine versus extrauterine management/resuscitation of the fetus/neonate. *Clinical Obstet Gynecol* 29:33, 1986.
6. Chik L, Sokol RJ, Rosen MG: "Prediction" of the one-minute Apgar score from fetal heart rate data. *Obstet Gynecol* 48:452, 1976.
7. Clark SL, Miller FC: Scalp blood sampling-FHR patterns tell you when to do it. *Contemporary OB/GYN* p. 47, January 1984.

8. Curzen P, Bekir JS, McLintock DG, et al: Reliability of cardiotocography in predicting baby's condition at birth. *Brit Med J* 289:1345, 1984.

9. Fleischer A, Schulman H, Jagani N, et al: The development of fetal acidosis in the presence of an abnormal fetal heart rate tracing. I. The average for gestational age fetus. *Am J Obstet Gynecol* 144:55, 1982.

10. Gilstrap LC, Hauth JC, Hankins GDV, et al: Second-stage fetal heart rate abnormalities and type of neonatal acidemia. *Obstet Gynecol* 70:191, 1987.

11. Gimovsky ML, Bruce SL: Aspects of FHR tracings as warning signals. *Clinical Obstet Gynecol* 29:51, 1986.

12. Goodlin RC: Fetal cardiovascular responses to distress. *Obstet Gynecol* 49:371, 1977.

13. Haesslein HC, Niswander DR: Fetal distress in term pregnancies. *Am J Obstet Gynecol* 137:245, 1980.

14. Hon EH, Zannini D, Quilligan EJ: The neonatal value of fetal monitoring. *Am J Obstet Gynecol* 122:508, 1975.

15. Huddleston JF: *Intrapartum Fetal Distress in Diagnosis and Management of Obstetric Emergencies.* Hossam E, Fadel MD (eds). Addison-Wesley Publishing Co., Menlo Park, CA, 1982, p. 144.

16. Intrapartum fetal heart rate monitoring. *ACOG Technical Bulletin* no. 132, September 1989.

17. Intrapartum fetal monitoring. *ACOG Technical Bulletin* no. 44, January 1977.

18. Keegan KA, Waffarn F, Quilligan EF: Obstetric characteristics and fetal heart rate patterns of infants who convulse during the newborn period. *Am J Obstet Gynecol* 153:732, 1985.

19. Krebs HB, Jordaan HVF, Petres RE, et al: I. Classification and prognosis of fetal heart rate patterns in labor. *Am J Obstet Gynecol* 133:762, 1979.

20. Krebs HB, Jordaan HVF, Petres RE, et al: II. Multifactorial analysis of intrapartum fetal heart tracings. *Am J Obstet Gynecol* 133:773, 1979.

21. Krebs HB, Petres RE, Dunn LJ: Intrapartum fetal heart rate monitoring. VIII. Atypical variable decelerations. *Am J Obstet Gynecol* 145:297, 1983.

22. Kubli FW, Hon EH, Khazin AF, et al: Observations on heart rate and pH in the human fetus during labor. *Am J Obstet Gynecol* 104:1190, 1969.

23. Leveno KJ, Cunningham FG, Nelson S, et al: A prospective comparison of selective and universal electronic fetal monitoring in 34,995 pregnancies. *N Engl J Med* 315:615, 1986.

24. Lin C-C, Moawad AH, Rosenow PJ, et al: Acid-base characteristics of fetuses with intrauterine growth retardation during labor and delivery. *Am J Obstet Gynecol* 137:553, 1980.

25. Lipshitz J: Use of a β_2-sympathomimetic drug as a temporizing measure in the treatment of acute fetal distress. *Am J Obstet Gynecol* 129:31, 1977.

26. Low JA: The role of blood gas and acid-base assessment in the diagnosis of intrapartum fetal asphyxia. *Am J Obstet Gynecol* 159:1235, 1988.

27. Luthy DA, Shy KK, Van Belle G, et al: A randomized trial of electronic fetal monitoring in preterm labor. *Obstet Gynecol* 69:687, 1987.

28. Mendez-Bauer C, Arnt IC, Gulin L, et al: Relationship between blood pH and heart rate in the human fetus during labor. *Am J Obstet Gynecol* 97:530, 1967.

29. Mendez-Bauer C, Shekarloo A, Cook V, et al: Treatment of acute fetal distress by β_2-sympathomimetics. *Am J Obstet Gynecol* 156:638, 1987.

30. Meschia G: Placental respiratory gas exchange and fetal oxygenation, in Creasy RK, Resnick R (eds): *Maternal-Fetal Medicine. Principles and Practice.* Philadelphia, W.B. Saunders, 1984.

31. Mitchell J, Schulman H, Fleischer A, et al: Meconium aspiration and fetal acidosis. *Obstet Gynecol* 65:352, 1985.

32. Miyazaki FS, Nevarez F: Saline amnioinfusion for relief of repetitive variable decelerations: A prospective randomized study. *Am J Obstet Gynecol* 153:301, 1985.

33. Nijhuis JG, Crevels AJ, Van Dongen PWJ: Fetal brain death: The definition of a fetal heart rate pattern and its clinical consequences. *Obstet Gynecol Surv* 45:229, 1990.

34. O'Gureck JE, Roux JF, Neuman MR: Neonatal depression and fetal heart rate patterns during labor. *Obstet Gynecol* 40:347, 1972.

35. Painter MJ, Depp R, O'Donoghue PD: Fetal heart rate patterns and development in the first year of life. *Am J Obstet Gynecol* 132:271, 1978.

36. Parer JT: Fetal acid-base balance, in Creasy RK, Resnick R (eds): *Maternal-Fetal Medicine. Principles and Practice.* Philadelphia: W.B. Saunders, 1984.

37. Parer JT: FHR monitoring: Answering the critics. *Contemp Obstet Gynecol* 17:163, 1981.

38. Paul RH, Suidan AK, Yeh S-Y, et al: Clinical fetal monitoring. VII. The evaluation and significance of intrapartum baseline FHR variability. *Am J Obstet Gynecol* 206:123, 1975.

39. Pearson JF: Maternal and fetal acid-base balance, in Beard RW, Nathanielsz PW (eds): *Fetal Philosophy and Medicine. The Basis of Perinatology.* Philadelphia, W.B. Saunders, 1976.

40. Perkins RP: Perinatal observations in a high-risk population managed without intrapartum fetal pH studies. *Am J Obstet Gynecol* 149:327, 1984.

41. Reece EA, Antoine C, Montgomery J: The fetus as the final arbiter of intrauterine stress/distress. *Clinical Obstet Gynecol* 29:23, 1986.

42. Rudolph AB, Itskovitz J, Iwamoto HJ, et al: Fetal cardiovascular responses to stress. *Seminars in Perinatology* 5:109, 1981.

43. Schifrin BS: Fetal heart rate monitoring during labor. *JAMA* 222:196, 1972.

44. Schifrin BS, Dame L: Fetal heart rate patterns. Prediction of Apgar score. *JAMA* 219:1322, 1972.

45. Sureau C: The stress of labor, in Aladjem S, Brown AK (eds): *Clinical Perinatology,* 1st ed. St. Louis, C.V. Mosby, 1974.

46. Sykes GS, Molloy PM, Johnson P, et al: Fetal distress and the condition of newborn infants. *Brit Med J* 287:943, 1983.

47. Wood C: Difficulties in fetal heart rate monitoring. *Int J of Gynaecol Obstet* 10:176, 1972.

48. Zuspan FP, Quilligan EJ, Iams JD, et al: NICHD Consensus Development Task Force Report. Predictors of intrapartum fetal distress: The role of electronic fetal monitoring. *J Reprod Med* 23:207, 1979.

Limitations of Fetal Monitoring

Chapter 2

Normal Pattern—Unfavorable Outcome

Distress-like Pattern—Favorable Outcome

Similar Patterns with High Risk of Low Apgar
Score/Acidosis—Dissimilar Outcomes

Class O: Uninterpretable Pattern—
Unsatisfactory Fetal Heart Trace

Class O: Uninterpretable Pattern—
No Uterine Trace

Normal Pattern—Unfavorable Outcome

*T*here are multiple explanations for the rare occasion when a fetus with a low Apgar score or acidosis is delivered after obtaining a normal tracing. There is growing evidence that the majority of neurologic deficits may occur as a result of factors preceding the intrapartum course.[16,17,19] Full understanding of such events and their sequelae awaits further study.

Intrapartum events that may be associated with unheralded poor infant health include:[1,8,14,21]

A passage of time from the fetal monitoring segment to delivery

Stressful delivery events

In utero meconium aspiration

Anesthesia or drug effects

Genetic/metabolic disease

Infection

Extreme prematurity

Neonatal resuscitation events

Early neonatal problems such as hypoglycemia or hypoxia

Inaccurate interpretation of monitoring data may also be implicated at times.[11,22]

Obtaining the umbilical cord pH may be an adjunct to assessment of the fetus with a normal tracing who has other risk factors for a low Apgar score such as the presence of thick meconium that requires tracheal suctioning or extreme prematurity.[7,9,10,27]

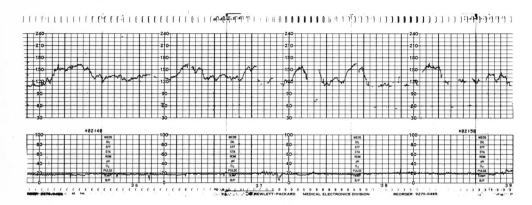

CASE INTERPRETATION: Class I

Baseline Information: normal rate, average variability.

Periodic or Nonperiodic Changes: nonperiodic accelerations, some marked, no decelerations.

Uterine Activity: none displayed.

Significance: pattern has high correlation with healthy vigorous newborn.

CASE OUTCOME: Twenty-four-year-old gravida 2, para 1001, delivered vaginally, with epidural anesthesia, at 37½ weeks' gestation, a 6 pound, 4½ ounce (2849 gram) male; Apgar score 2/1. A nuchal cord was present. The newborn expired in the delivery room secondary to renal agenesis.

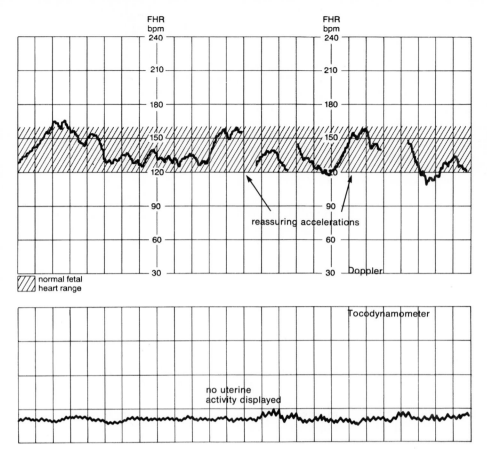

Pattern Characteristic:
Normal Pattern–Unfavorable
Outcome

Distress-like Pattern—Favorable Outcome

*T*he fetal monitor is not able to consistently predict an abnormal fetus when the heart rate pattern is not "normal."[3,32] In fact, a fetus with an unfavorable outcome can be predicted only 20% to 75% of the time, depending on the criteria used to define an abnormal tracing and an abnormal newborn outcome (see page 12).[31]

Good beat-to-beat variability is a prerequisite of a tracing that may be used to predict, with high reliability, a normal outcome. When variability is absent, the fetus still may be in no jeopardy because the mechanism for loss of variability may be due to a cause as unthreatening as fetal sleep or a drug effect. Another cause for "false positive" monitor information is a transient acidosis from which the fetus recovers by in utero compensatory mechanisms.[28] The cause in some cases of persistent, but apparently insignificant, lack of short- and long-term variability remains unexplained. Because a fetus who does not demonstrate beat-to-beat variability cannot be distinguished from the sick fetus on the basis of the intrapartum fetal monitoring pattern alone, other information such as fetal pH or fetal response to stimulation is an adjunct to diagnosis.[18,29] By careful analysis of the fetal heart tracing, one may glean information about the preceding fetal condition that may obviate the need for pH testing in some clinical settings.[20,30]

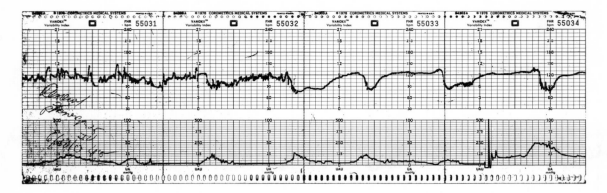

CASE INTERPRETATION: Class IV/V

Baseline Information: unstable, low normal rate, absent variability, beginning abruptly.

Periodic or Nonperiodic Changes: mild and moderate variable decelerations with atypia, including loss of variability, loss of some primary and secondary accelerations, slow return to baseline.

Uterine Activity: contractions every two to three minutes, not well recorded by tocodynamometer, which appear brief with a resting phase present.

Significance: atypical variable decelerations plus baseline loss of variability predicts an increased risk of a low Apgar score and fetal acidosis. However, normal variability at the beginning of the fetal trace is inconsistent with a sick fetus. A fetal pH may clarify the fetus's condition.

CASE OUTCOME: Thirty-year-old gravida 5, para 4004 (1 set of term twins and 1 neonatal death), at 39 weeks' gestation, delivered vaginally with no anesthesia, a 7 pound, 12 ounce (3515 gram) male; Apgar score 8/8. The fetus was in a vertex presentation, in an occiput anterior position. The infant followed a normal newborn course. Reassuring scalp pHs (average 7.35) suggested that loss of variability was secondary to narcotic analgesia administration. The patient's last pregnancy was complicated by neonatal demise secondary to severe meconium aspiration.

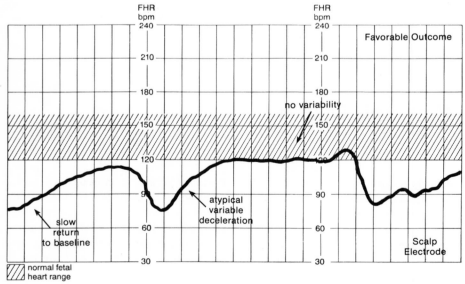

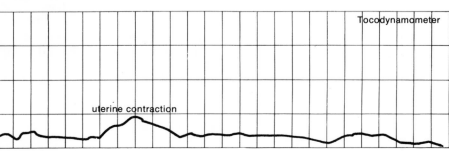

Pattern Characteristic:
Pattern with High Risk of Low Apgar/Acidosis. Favorable Outcome

Similar Patterns with High Risk of Low Apgar Score/Acidosis—Dissimilar Outcomes

Although the monitor has high sensitivity in predicting the normal fetus, the fetal monitor is not able to accurately and consistently predict a sick newborn.[2,23] To emphasize the limitations of the fetal monitor, two tracings that have almost indistinguishable features and which thus have a similar interpretation outside of the context of clinical information are presented here. The outcomes were markedly different. The pattern has been associated with severe fetal asphyxia, cerebral palsy, and fetal or neonatal death.[5,24] Yet one fetus was healthy except for the effects of prematurity.

Clinical decisions are influenced by previous information obtained by study of the preceding fetal monitoring tracing, response to measures to produce optimum uterine blood flow and placenta oxygen exchange, fetal pH studies, and other clinical information. Prompt delivery is usually appropriate with a persistent pattern that is associated with high risk of a low Apgar score or fetal acidosis.

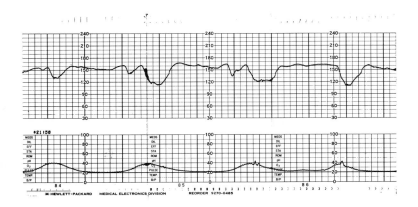

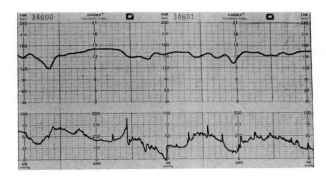

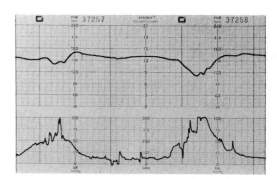

CASE INTERPRETATION (A and B): Class V

Baseline Information: unstable (wandering), high normal rate, absent short-term (beat-to-beat) variability, irregular, undulating long-term variability.

Periodic or Nonperiodic Changes: atypical variable decelerations with slow return to baseline, prolonged or absent secondary accelerations, biphasic pattern: W sign. Also late occurrence.

Uterine Activity: contraction frequency consistent with active labor. Superimposed maternal activity obscures waveform. Case A: little interval relaxation.

Significance: high risk of fetal acidosis and a low newborn Apgar score. Delivery is usually indicated; fetal pH studies may be an adjunct to diagnosis if a normal tracing with excellent variability preceded medication administration, but it may delay care unless it is immediately available.

CASE A OUTCOME: Twenty-nine-year-old gravida 3, para 1011, delivered vaginally with pudendal anesthesia at 33½ weeks' gestation, a 3 pound, 10½ ounce (1655 gram) female; Apgar score 8/8. The newborn course was complicated by hyperbilirubinemia, which responded to phototherapy. The newborn was dismissed well on the twenty-third day of life, gaining weight on oral feedings.

CASE B OUTCOME: Nineteen-year-old primigravida delivered at 40 weeks' gestation by cesarean section due to possible fetal distress and failure to progress, under general anesthesia from a vertex presentation, a 5 pound, 15½ ounce (2710 gram) female; Apgar score 1/2. The newborn died on the day of birth. An autopsy revealed a partly liquefied brain.

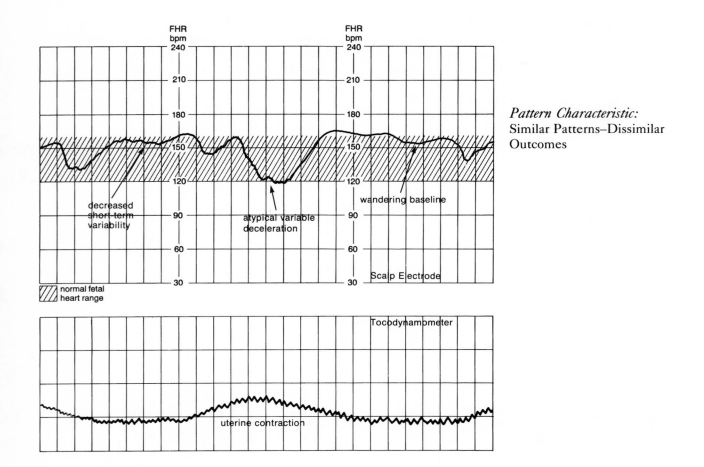

Pattern Characteristic:
Similar Patterns–Dissimilar
Outcomes

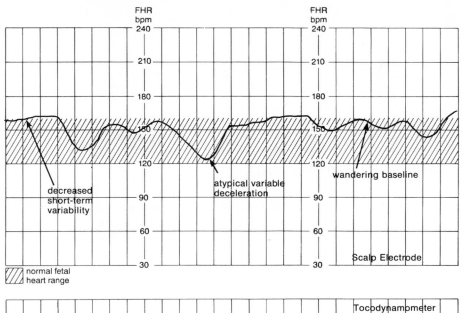

Pattern Characteristic:
Similar Patterns–Dissimilar
Outcomes

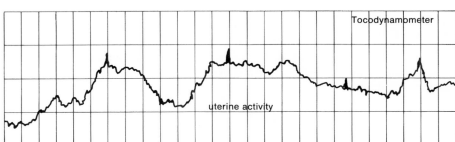

Class 0: Uninterpretable Pattern—Unsatisfactory Fetal Heart Trace

*F*actors that may negatively influence the ability to obtain a fetal heart rate trace that is satisfactory for interpretation include maternal obesity, fetal position, quality of instrumentation, and instrument application.

A diagnosis of the fetal condition based on visual criteria may not be possible in some cases if there is an unsatisfactory fetal heart rate recording.

Manipulating maternal position, replacing the Doppler transducer, or changing instruments, if feasible, are alternatives for the patient who is not a candidate for internal fetal monitoring. Scalp electrode placement, when safe and feasible, is an ideal response to an unsatisfactory external monitoring tracing. In the low risk patient, auscultation of the fetal heart rate at regular intervals by skilled professionals has been accepted as a safe alternative.[6,12,15] In high risk patients also, frequent skilled auscultation may be comparable to continuous electronic fetal monitoring in directing appropriate intrapartum management.[26]

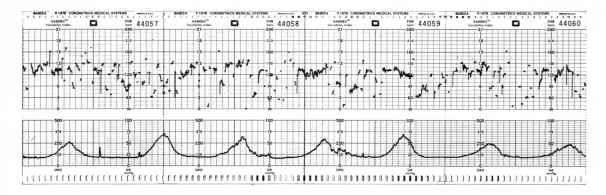

CASE INTERPRETATION: Class 0

Baseline Information: only transiently able to identify baseline and variability.

Periodic or Nonperiodic Changes: decelerations or accelerations might be present but are unable to be identified amid the artifact.

Uterine Activity: contractions of normal configuration every two minutes by tocodynamometer.

Significance: reassurance of good fetal welfare is not established during this fetal monitor segment. The Dop-

pler transducer may be repositioned or a monitor using autocorrelation may be used. Frequent skilled auscultation is an appropriate response if one is unable to monitor electronically. A scalp electrode trace usually produces an interpretable trace if its application is safe and feasible.

CASE OUTCOME: Twenty-year-old gravida 2, para 1001, at 36 weeks' gestation delivered vaginally with local/pudendal anesthesia a 6 pound, 1½ ounce (2764 gram) male; Apgar score 8/10. The infant followed a normal newborn course.

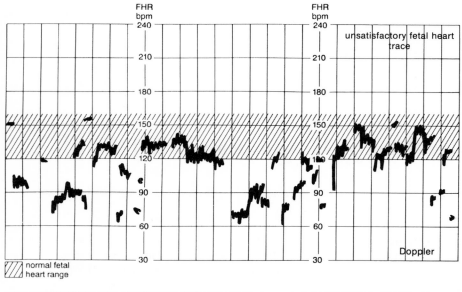

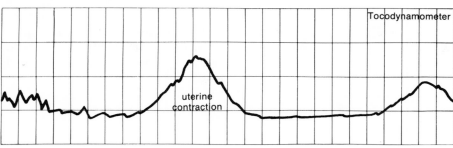

Pattern Characteristic:
Uninterpretable Pattern

Class 0: Uninterpretable Pattern—No Uterine Trace

*F*etal heart rate data cannot be assessed at as high a level of interpretation as possible if a uterine activity trace is not displayed. The major reason for this is that changes in the fetal heart trace are best interpreted in association with the presence of stimuli such as uterine contractions.

Even in the presence of normal variability and accelerations, decelerations that are present may be so subtle as to be mistaken for negligible variations in the baseline, unless attention is directed by a near-simultaneous occurrence of a similarly shaped uterine contraction. Decelerations under such conditions suggest an early point in the potential continuum from mild hypoxia to asphyxia.[4]

Even documentation of the absence of detectable uterine activity is useful information, as are varying types of maternal and fetal activity that may be superimposed on the uterine trace. It is rare for the uterine trace to produce an absolutely flat line, unless the transducer is disengaged or the baseline is set at or below zero. Obesity and a small uterus of a premature gestation may be factors interfering with a clear uterine contraction waveform, but usually various maternal movements cause deflections on the uterine trace.[13]

At times it may be desirable to remove the tocodynamometer, such as during epidural anesthesia administration or abdominal antiseptic skin preparation or for patient comfort. In such cases, uterine activity information is extrapolated from other portions of the tracing where more complete data have been collected.

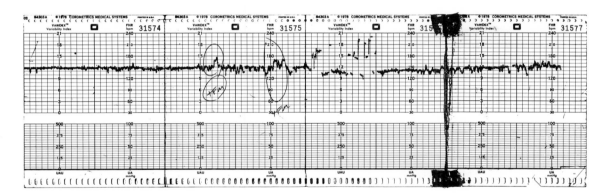

CASE INTERPRETATION: Class 0

Baseline Information: normal rate, decreased variability even with external monitoring.

Periodic or Nonperiodic Changes: small increases in fetal heart rate do not meet criteria for accelerations, possible prolonged shallow deceleration with rebound tachycardia.

Uterine Activity: apparently unrecorded.

Significance: nonreactive baseline (no 15 second by 15 bpm accelerations). Possible shallow deceleration may indicate a fetus with a hypoxic environment if the deceleration is associated with an antecedent uterine contraction.

CASE OUTCOME: Thirty-two-year-old gravida 3, para 2002, delivered vaginally at 28 weeks' gestation a stillborn 3 pound, 10 ounce (1644 gram) female from a frank breech presentation. There was a premature rupture of her membranes for 2½ weeks preceding delivery. Chorioamnionitis was suspected. Fetal heart tones disappeared 29 hours after the tracing was obtained. An autopsy confirmed chorioamnionitis and revealed acute bronchopneumonia.

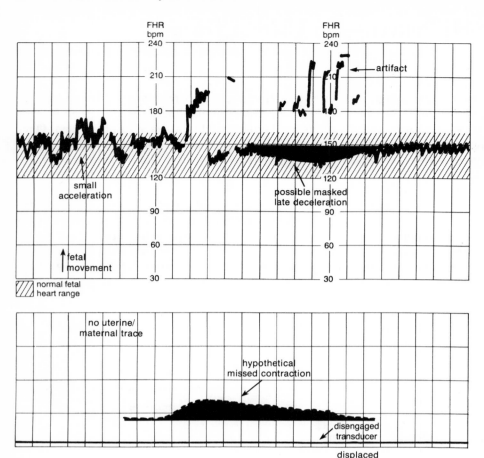

Pattern Characteristic:
Uninterpretable Pattern

References

1. Apgar scores as a predictor of fetal outcome. State-of-the-art opinions. *ACOG Newsletter* p. 5, June 1988.
2. Use and misuse of the Apgar score. *ACOG Newsletter* p. 8, Jan. 1987.
3. Benson RC, Shubeck R, Deutschberger J, et al: Fetal heart rate as a predictor of fetal distress. *Obstet Gynecol* 32:36, 1968.
4. Braly P, Freeman R: The significance of fetal heart rate reactivity with a positive oxytocin challenge test. *Obstet Gynecol* 50:689, 1977.
5. Cetrulo CL, Schifrin BS: Fetal heart rate patterns preceding death in utero. *Obstet Gynecol* 48:521, 1976.
6. Cohen WB, Schifrin BS: Diagnosis and treatment of fetal distress, in Bolognese JL, Schwarz RH, Schneider J (eds): *Perinatal Medicine: Management of the High Risk Fetus and Neonate,* 2d ed. Baltimore, Williams & Wilkins, 1982.
7. Crawford JS: Apgar score and neonatal asphyxia. *Lancet* 1:684, 1982.
8. Curzen P, Bekir JS, McLintock DG, et al: Reliability of cardiotocography in predicting baby's condition at birth. *Brit Med J* 289:1345, 1984.
9. Fields LM, Entman SS, Boehm FH: Correlation of the one-minute Apgar score and the pH value of umbilical arterial blood. *Southern Med J* 76:1477, 1983.
10. Goldenberg RL, Huddleston JF, Nelson KG: Apgar scores and umbilical arterial pH in preterm newborn infants. *Am J Obstet Gynecol* 651:149, 1984.
11. Goodlin RC: Electronic fetal monitoring as seen through

the looking glass (letter). *Am J Obstet Gynecol* 155:454, 1986.

12. Haverkamp AD, Thompson HE, McFee JG, et al: The evaluation of continuous fetal heart rate monitoring in high risk pregnancy. *Am J Obstet Gynecol* 125:310, 1976.

13. Hutson JM, Petrie RH: Possible limitations of fetal monitoring. *Clinical Obstet Gynecol* 29:104, 1986.

14. Krebs HB, Petres RE, Dunn LJ, et al: Intrapartum fetal heart rate monitoring. III. Association of meconium with abnormal fetal heart rate patterns. *Am J Obstet Gynecol* 137:936, 1980.

15. Levenco KJ, Cunningham FG, Nelson S, et al: A prospective comparison of selective and universal electronic fetal monitoring in 34,995 pregnancies. *N Engl J Med* 315:615, 1986.

16. Naeye RL, Peters EC: Antenatal hypoxia and low IQ values. *Am J Dis Children* 141:50, 1987.

17. Nelson KB, Ellenberg JH: Antecedents of cerebral palsy multivariate analysis of risk. *N Engl J Med* 315:81, 1986.

18. Page FO, Martin JN, Palmer SM, et al: Correlation of neonatal acid-base status with Apgar scores and fetal heart rate tracings. *Am J Obstet Gynecol* 154:1306, 1986.

19. Painter MJ, Depp R, O'Donoghue PD: Fetal heart rate patterns and development in the first year of life. *Am J Obstet Gynecol* 132:271, 1978.

20. Paul RH, Yonekura ML, Cantrell CJ, et al: Fetal injury prior to labor: Does it happen? *Am J Obstet Gynecol* 154:1187, 1986.

21. Perkins RP: Perinatal observations in a high risk population managed without intrapartum fetal pH studies. *Am J Obstet Gynecol* 149:327, 1984.

22. Rayburn WF, Anderson CW, O'Shaughnessy RW, et al: Predictability of the distressed term infant. *Am J Obstet Gynecol* 140:489, 1981.

23. Roux JF: Pitfalls in FHR monitoring. *Contemp OB/GYN* 5:51, 1975.

24. Schifrin BS: The case against the fetal monitor. *Southern Med J* 71:1058, 1978.

25. Serafini PC, Amsial PA, Murgalo JA, et al: Unusual fetal heart rate pattern associated with neonatal asphyxia and death. *Am J Obstet Gynecol* 140:715, 1985.

26. Shy KK, Luthy DA, Bennett FC, et al: *N Engl J Med* 322:588, 1990.

27. Silverman F, Suidan J, Wasserman J, et al: The Apgar score: Is it enough? *Obstet Gynecol* 66:331, 1985.

28. Suidan JS, Young BK: Acidosis in the vigorous newborn. *Obstet Gynecol* 65:361, 1985.

29. Tejani N, Mann LI, Bhakthavathsalan A: Correlation of fetal heart rate patterns and fetal pH with neonatal outcome. *Obstet Gynecol* 48:460, 1976.

30. Wible JL, Petrie RH, Koons A, et al: The clinical use of umbilical cord acid-base determination in perinatal surveillance and management. *Clinics in Perinatology* 9:387, 1982.

31. Wood C: Difficulties in fetal heart rate monitoring. *Int J Gynaecol Obstet* 10:176, 1972.

32. Zuspan FP, Quillipan EJ, Iams JD, et al: NICHD Consensus Development Task Force Report. Predictors of intrapartum fetal distress: The role of electronic fetal monitoring. *J Reprod Med* 23:207, 1979.

BASELINE INFORMATION

Section II

*T*he baseline fetal heart rate is determined by observation of the fetal heart rate between (or in the absence of) uterine contractions. It is also described as the fetal heart rate observed in the absence of periodic fetal heart rate changes.

A change in fetal heart rate must exceed 10 minutes in duration to be considered a new fetal heart rate baseline. Baseline changes are thus differentiated from prolonged accelerations and decelerations, which are not true baseline changes.

The baseline fetal heart rate is assessed as a rate and by variability and stability.

The number of beats per minute (bpm) of the baseline fetal heart rate is, under normal circumstances, controlled by the sinoatrial pacemaker, modulated by primarily parasympathetic and, to a much lesser degree, sympathetic factors. These factors are affected by stimuli triggering chemoreceptors and baroreceptors and by fetal respiration, wakefulness, and body movements. The accepted normal range of the fetal heart rate is 120–160 bpm. However, most normal fetal heart rates fall between 110 and 150 bpm. Although rapid and slow fetal heart rates demand careful assessment for fetal jeopardy, baseline rates outside of normal range but accompanied by normal variability may be displayed by a healthy fetus in certain conditions. On the other hand, a sick fetus may maintain a heart rate in the normal range until just before death.

Fetal heart rate variability is the irregularity of the fetal heart rate. The parasympathetic system is the major control of beat-to-beat variability in the fetus. Variability is measured in the amplitude of change from beat to beat (short-term variability) and in the range and frequency of oscillations per minute (long-term variability). Short-term variability or beat-to-beat variability reflects R wave–interval differences in successive cardiac cycles and thus requires an electrocardiogram signal. Less reliable, but markedly improved by modern methodology, are measurements from successive mechanical events in the cardiac cycle through Doppler fetal heart rate monitoring. The normal range of beat-to-beat difference is 6 to 10 bpm. The presence of short-term variability is the most significant indicator of fetal homeostasis, particularly when accompanied by accelerations. It reflects a normal autonomic nervous system as well as intact circulatory system responses.

Changes in long-term variability usually accompany similar changes in short-term variability. Long-term variability is less useful as a predictor of good fetal condition and therefore receives less attention in modern fetal monitoring classifications. In fact, there are certain fetal heart rate patterns with a decrease in short-term variability with preservation of long-term variability that are associated with an increased risk of poor fetal outcome. On the other hand, patterns with short-term variability without long-term variability are less reassuring than patterns with the presence of both. The normal frequency of long-term fluctuations is 2 to 6 cycles or oscillations per minute. The normal amplitude of change is 6 to 10 bpm, with a usual range of 5 to 20 bpm. Sinusoidal patterns are an unusual variant of regular long-term variability without short-term variability. These must be distinguished from other undulating fetal heart rate patterns.

The baseline stability itself may serve as an indicator of fetal condition. Both upward and downward trends may reflect maternal temperature changes. Less commonly, hypoxia may produce upward baseline trends. Progressive parasympathetic effects of head compression may gradually lower the heart rate. Unstable wandering baselines may denote loss of nervous regulation of the heart but must be distinguished from patterns of the normal fetus.

Bradycardia

Chapter 3

Moderate Sinus Bradycardia

*M*oderate fetal bradycardia is defined as a fetal heart baseline rate of 100 to 119 bpm.[8] It has also been called mild bradycardia. When accompanied by normal variability, especially with the presence of accelerations, this pattern is not indicative of fetal distress.[9,11,12,25] The pattern is most often seen as a second stage gradual fall from a normal or low normal baseline heart rate occurring earlier in labor.[19,20] A proposed mechanism for the bradycardia is a parasympathetic response to continuous head compression. Therefore, it is not surprising to note an association with primigravid labors, large babies, and relative cephalopelvic disproportion secondary to occiput posterior or transverse positions.[40] Disappearance of

moderate bradycardia after spontaneous rotation of the vertex from occiput posterior to occiput anterior has been reported (see page 157). The bradycardia is not relieved by oxygen administration or a change in maternal position. Fetal scalp blood pH, continuous tissue pH, and umbilical artery pH at delivery have been demonstrated to be normal in the presence of this pattern.[41,42]

Drug therapy (such as beta blocking agents) may produce moderate bradycardia without eradicating variability.[12] Bradycardia secondary to arrhythmia is usually in a lower range and is not accompanied by normal variability.

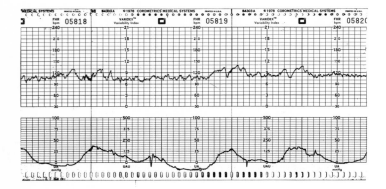

CASE INTERPRETATION: Class I

Baseline Information: good variability, moderate bradycardia.

Periodic or Nonperiodic Changes: reassuring nonperiodic accelerations.

Significance: normal fetal condition predicted, without hypoxia or acidosis; exclude the maternal signal.

CASE OUTCOME: Nineteen-year-old primigravida delivered vaginally at 39½ weeks' gestation, with epidural anesthesia, from an occiput posterior position, a 7 pound, 6½ ounce (3360 gram) male, Apgar score 8/9. The infant followed a normal newborn course.

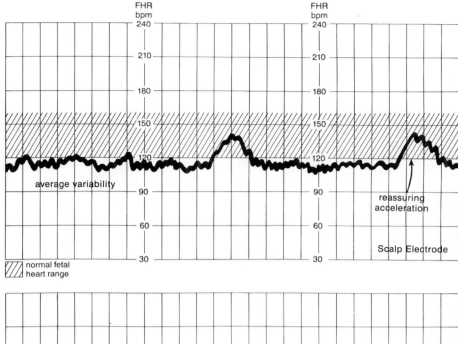

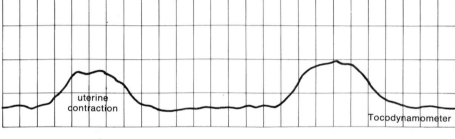

Pattern Characteristic:
Moderate Sinus Bradycardia

Marked Sinus Bradycardia

*M*arked sinus bradycardia is defined as a fetal heart rate of 99 or less bpm.[8] It has also been called severe bradycardia. The latter form infers a more ominous connotation to the pattern than is deserved in its pure form.

A baseline bradycardia associated with good baseline variability is usually not indicative of fetal distress even at rates of 80 to 100 bpm. Just as with moderate bradycardia, this pattern is believed to reflect a parasympathetic response to such a situation as continuous head compression. The clinician is alerted to an increased possibility of relative or absolute cephalopelvic disproportion.[40] Although a fetus may eventually suffer deterioration through inadequate cardiac output at the markedly low heart rate, it would be expected that this would be heralded by signs of hypoxia. The two important steps in assessing a fetal heart rate of less than 100 are: (1) distinguishing a low baseline heart rate from a prolonged deceleration[17] and (2) excluding artifact (e.g., maternal heart rate) or arrhythmia.

Prolonged decelerations are distinguished from baseline bradycardia by the presence of a previous higher baseline rate.[14] If the low rate is encountered at the initiation of monitoring, a prolonged deceleration is suspected when there is reduced or absent variability, as may be caused by sinuatrial node suppression or acidosis.[3] However, with placental abruption variability may be preserved amid severe fetal jeopardy. Clinical findings assist in distinguishing this from benign bradycardias. Bradycardias secondary to arrhythmia such as complete atrioventricular block are usually 70 bpm or less and do not have normal variability. Maternal heart rate artifact is excluded by simultaneous maternal heart rate recording. Bradycardia secondary to maternal hypothermia, an uncommon occurrence, has been seen to revert to normal with the return of the maternal temperature to normal (see page 155).

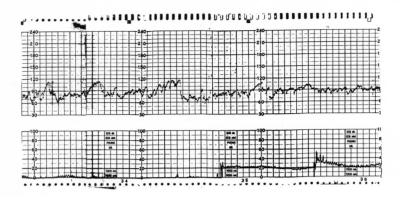

CASE INTERPRETATION: Class I

Baseline Information: good variability, marked bradycardia.

Periodic or Nonperiodic Changes: reassuring nonperiodic accelerations.

Uterine Activity: recording not satisfactory for interpretation.

Significance: normal fetal condition predicted, without hypoxia or acidosis; exclude the maternal signal.

CASE OUTCOME: Twenty-four-year-old primigravida delivered at 43 weeks' gestation by cesarean section due to cephalopelvic disproportion, with an epidural anesthesia, a 10 pound, 11½ ounce (4862 gram) male; Apgar score 9/10. The infant followed a normal newborn course.

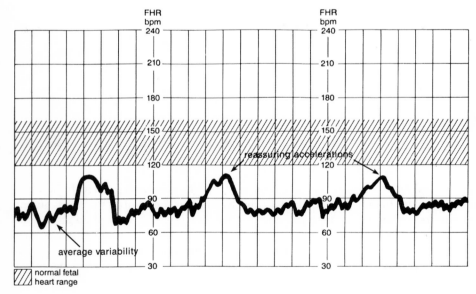

Pattern Characteristic:
Marked Sinus Bradycardia

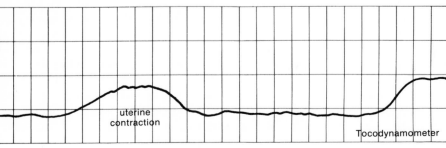

Marked Sinus Bradycardia Associated with Hypothermia

Marked to moderate bradycardia secondary to hypothermia is an uncommon occurrence.[5] Examples of clinical conditions that may produce hypothermia are endotoxic shock and hypoglycemic shock as well as direct exposure to low temperatures.[22] The pattern may be accompanied by normal variability. It has been shown to revert to normal with the correction of hypothermia. (See page 155 for a demonstration of the normalization of fetal heart rate with the correction of hypothermia secondary to hypoglycemia.

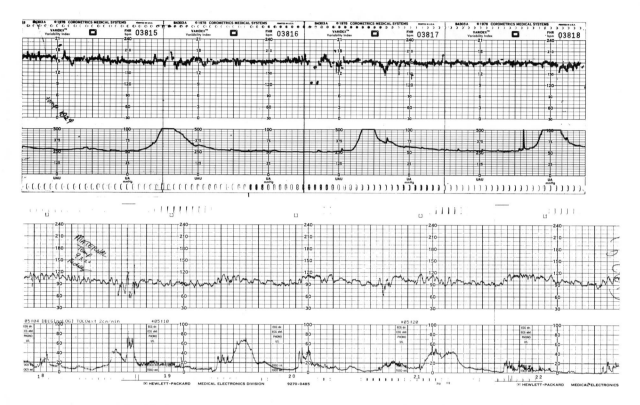

CASE INTERPRETATION: Class I–II

Baseline Information: marked bradycardia during temperature recording of 93.2°F, normal variability but monitor speed is two centimeters per minute; moderate to marked tachycardia with decreased variability when the temperature is recorded at 102.4°F on a different monitor. There is some instability of the baseline.

Periodic or Nonperiodic Changes: nonperiodic accelerations, mild multiphasic variable decelerations while at bradycardic rate.

Uterine Activity: irregular polysystolic contractions recorded by external monitoring.

Significance: bradycardia may be attributable to low maternal temperature. Good variability and reactivity suggests that there is no immediate fetal jeopardy. Readjust paper speed to three centimeters per minute.

CASE OUTCOME: Twenty-nine-year-old gravida 5, para 4004, with known adenocorticotropic hormone (ACTH) deficiency and hypothyroidism, developed maternal hypothermia after antibiotic treatment for pyelonephritis. The bradycardia resolved with the normalization of maternal temperature. The patient later underwent cesarean section for possible fetal distress with the delivery of a 5 pound, 5½ ounce (2424 gram) female, from a vertex presentation; Apgar score 4/6. The newborn was dismissed from the hospital after 11 days.

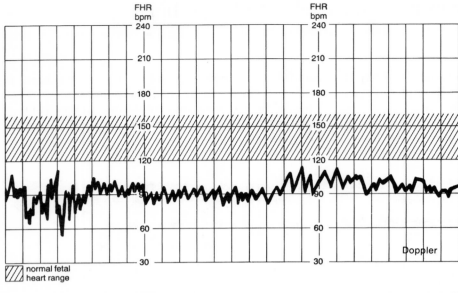

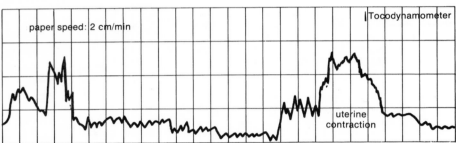

Pattern Characteristic:
Sinus Bradycardia Marked.
Hypothermia

Sinus Bradycardia with Increased Variability: Mixed Pattern

*M*oderate or severe baseline bradycardia is often seen in a mixed pattern with increased variability. This is not surprising since both baseline bradycardia and increased variability are believed to be responses to increased parasympathetic tone, the capability for which increases with gestational age.

This mixed pattern is most often seen in second stage labor. The pattern is also seen commonly with uterine hypertonus and postdate pregnancy, both of which are associated with increased variability.

If delivery were to occur promptly after such a pattern, a healthy newborn is predicted. The increased variability indicates that the fetus is able to compensate for hypoxic stress at present and is *not in immediate* jeopardy. If oxytocin is being infused, it is appropriate to diminish the dosage. If the increased variability is secondary to spontaneous uterine hyperactivity, pharmacologic treatment is an option used to reduce uterine activity. If delivery does not occur within a reasonable period of time *or* if the hypoxia-inducing events are not resolved, the compensatory response of the fetus may eventually be depleted, and fetal distress may ensue. Increased variability in the presence of thick meconium has been associated with an increased incidence of meconium aspiration (see page 71).

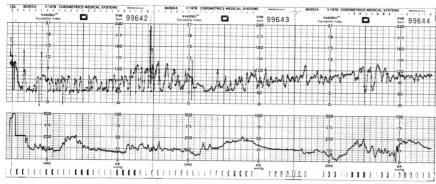

Recreation of original tracing

CASE INTERPRETATION: Class II

Baseline Information: increased variability, marked bradycardia.

Periodic or Nonperiodic Changes: pattern may obscure mild variable decelerations.

Uterine Activity: skewed contractions, poorly recorded.

Significance: the fetus who exhibits this pattern is usually vigorous at delivery. The fetus is not in immediate jeopardy and is presently compensating for stressful stimuli. Reduction of stress is the appropriate management.

CASE OUTCOME: Twenty-two-year-old primigravida at 41 weeks' gestation delivered by cesarean section for a diagnosis of possible fetal distress, with general anesthesia, a 6 pound, 6 ounce (2892 gram) male; Apgar score 8/9. The nuchal cord was times 2 and cord pH 7.30. The infant followed a normal newborn course.

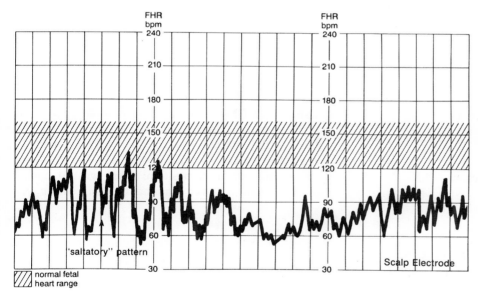

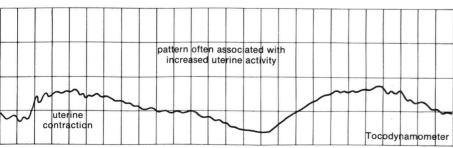

Pattern Characteristic:
Sinus Bradycardia with Increased Variability. Mixed Pattern

Sinus Bradycardia with Decelerations: Mixed Pattern

*W*hen baseline bradycardia is accompanied by normal variability, it is rarely associated with a depressed newborn. An exception to this could theoretically occur when the pattern is mixed with that of marked decelerations. When periodic changes occur in the presence of baseline bradycardia, standard interpretation based on the shape and timing of the decelerations is used. The nadir of the deceleration should be assessed based on the depth from the lowered baseline and not solely on the numerical heart rate at the nadir. In other words, a variable deceleration that falls to 70 from a reactive baseline of 150 is of more concern than a variable deceleration that falls to 70 from a reactive baseline of 100.

When a deceleration occurs from an already significantly low baseline, however, (e.g., a fall of only 50 bpm, but from a baseline of 90 bpm) the fetus may not receive adequate perfusion of vital structures during the deceleration. This would be expected to be evidenced by progressive development of hypoxic changes.[11] Both baseline bradycardia and variable decelerations have been associated with an output posterior position.[18,40]

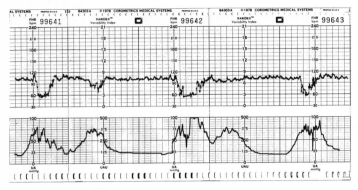

Recreation of original tracing

CASE INTERPRETATION: Class I–II

Baseline Information: moderate bradycardia, good beat-to-beat variability, stable.

Periodic and Nonperiodic Changes: mild and moderate variable decelerations, some atypia characterized by a minor degree of slow return to baseline.

Uterine Activity: polysystole.

Significance: mildly stressed fetus at this time, observation for hypoxic changes in the pattern is appropriate, as is reduction of stress.

CASE OUTCOME: Twenty-nine-year-old gravida 4, para 2012, at 40 weeks' gestation. Spontaneous vaginal delivery with local/pudendal anesthesia of a 5 pound, 14 ounce (2665 gram) male; Apgar score 9/9. The fetus was in an occiput posterior position; there was no nuchal cord. The infant followed a normal newborn course.

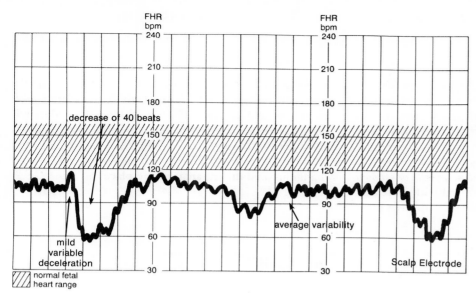

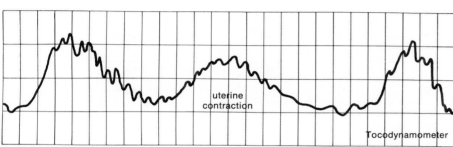

Pattern Characteristic:
Sinus Bradycardia with
Deceleration. Mixed Pattern

Marked Bradycardia Associated with Placental Abruption

A change in fetal heart rate secondary to extensive placental abruption may take many forms. Examples are tachycardia, prolonged decelerations, and erratic undulating decelerations, sometimes with a falsely reassuring intermittent return to an apparently normal baseline. Baseline bradycardia originating as a deceleration but lasting more than 10 minutes may be seen *with or without* loss of variability. Bradycardia associated with increased uterine activity on the basis of placental abruption must be distinguished by individual clinical findings from that produced by increased uterine activity associated with other causes. See page 317 for a prolonged deceleration that is associated with placental abruption, which demonstrates the presence of variability. A rationale for its preservation is the increased efficiency of oxygen exchange in unabrupted areas of the placenta.

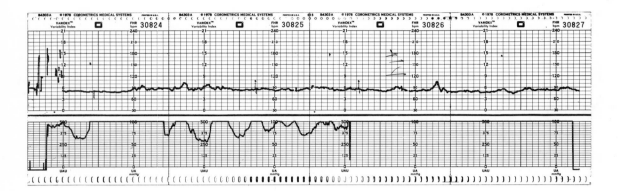

CASE INTERPRETATION: Class III

Baseline Information: marked bradycardia; short-term variability recorded by scalp electrode is diminished but present. Mostly a flat line pattern, but some areas of long-term variability are present.

Periodic or Nonperiodic Changes: small, sporadic accelerations.

Uterine Activity: tocodynamometer records increased uterine activity with frequent skewed and tachysystolic contractions. There are large segments in which uterine activity is unidentified because of the tocodynamometer setting.

Significance: because this heart rate of 80 to 90 bpm lasts more than 10 minutes, it qualifies as a true bradycardia, as opposed to a prolonged deceleration, even though the fetus may have had a normal baseline previously. The excessive uterine activity suggests that the bradycardia is a fetal response to an abnormal environment. Prompt delivery or cessation of uterine activity are options that depend upon the clinical circumstances.

CASE OUTCOME: Twenty-seven-year-old gravida 3, para 2002, at 43 weeks' gestation delivered by primary cesarean section with general anesthesia performed for possible fetal distress and clinical diagnosis of placental abruption, a 6 pound, 4 ounce (2835 gram) female; Apgar score 2/7. There was a cord pH of 6.9 and a total placental abruption. There was a first newborn pH of 7.1. The newborn followed an uncomplicated nursery course.

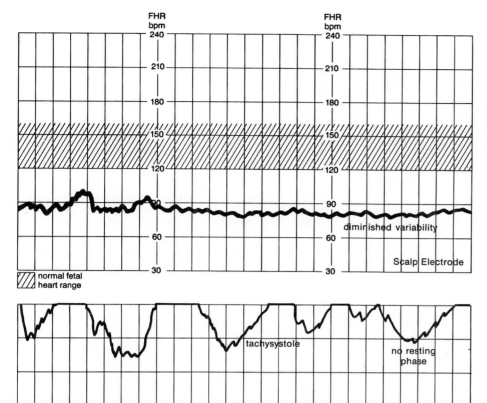

Pattern Characteristic:
Marked Bradycardia. Placental Abruption

Agonal Bradycardia

A severe bradycardia is a common terminal event preceding intrapartum fetal death.[20] Under most circumstances, the fetus at one time had a fetal heart rate in the normal range with normal variability and has subsequently undergone a progression through periodic hypoxic changes and loss of variability and often tachycardia preceding the terminal bradycardia.[3,4,16] The fetal monitor may not have been applied during the time of those progressive changes, making distinction from other types of bradycardia difficult. Such a terminal bradycardia is always accompanied by loss of variability and often, but not always, a wandering baseline.[6,14,26,27] The fetal heart may no longer be capable of periodic changes related to uterine contractions because of severe myocardial or central nervous system depression.[23,26] Even in the face of severe asphyxia the fetal heart rate may remain in a normal range until moments before fetal death.[15,37]

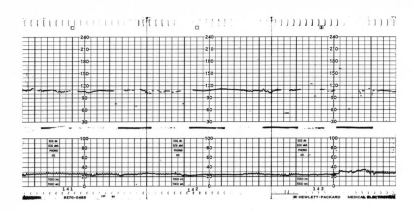

CASE INTERPRETATION: Class III/V

Baseline Information: absent variability, moderate bradycardia, unstable baseline.

Periodic or Nonperiodic Changes: shallow decelerations may be present.

Uterine Activity: appears normal.

Significance: there may be severe fetal distress.

CASE OUTCOME: Twenty-one-year-old primigravida at 35 weeks' gestation, with severe preeclampsia, delivered vaginally with general anesthesia a 2 pound, 8½ ounce (1148 gram) stillborn female, with a 60% placental abruption and the umbilical cord looped around the extremities.

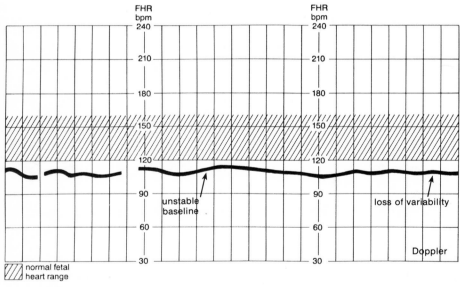

Pattern Characteristic:
Agonal Bradycardia

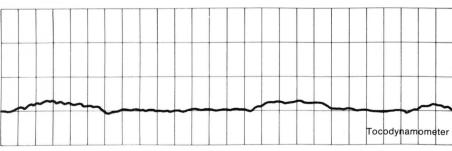

Bradycardia Secondary to Complete Atrioventricular Block: Arrhythmia

A bradyarrhythmia is suspected when the baseline fetal heart rate is below 90 bpm, with a loss of normal variability. Because of absent variability, it must be distinguished from a prolonged deceleration already in process at the initiation of the electronic monitoring or from an agonal bradycardia.

The most common persistent bradyarrhythmia in the fetus is complete atrioventricular block. An electrocardiogram-derived fetal monitor tracing shows a relatively fixed rate due to an escape rhythm (which could be junctional or ventricular). Because of the atrioventricular dissociation there is relatively little if any variability of the ventricular rate.

A fetal electrocardiogram or echocardiogram is helpful for diagnosis.[35] The latter also enables evaluation of the fetal heart for structural defects, which is important because the associated incidence of congenital heart disease is approximately 30%.[33]

There is a high incidence of co-existing maternal collagen vascular disease. Even the asymptomatic mother may have positive test results. Because of close correlation in the mother with the presence of the autoantibody SS-A/Ro, it is postulated the IgG antibodies crossing to the fetus disturb the developing conduction system by forming immune complexes.[35] Immunoglobulin has, in fact, been demonstrated through use of a immunofluorescence technique in the cardiac tissue of an infant with fatal complete atrioventricular block.[24]

Viral disease of the fetus such as cytomegalic inclusion disease has also been associated with complete atrioventricular block.

Although this bradycardia does not necessarily produce hypoxia, the decreased cardiac output over a prolonged duration may result in fetal cardiac decompensation.[30] Therefore, serial evaluation with ultrasonography of the fetus for edema and ascites is appropriate. Early delivery may be necessary if fetal hydrops is developing. However, fetal hydropic changes have been shown to resolve in utero with steroid therapy.[31]

Determining fetal pH during labor is recommended because the absence of beat-to-beat variability of the ventricular activity limits fetal assessment. Atrial variability may be monitored, however, by a strategically placed Doppler (external fetal heart rate monitoring) or by calculations from electrocardiogram (ECG) P waves. It is appropriate for the newborn to be evaluated for a pacemaker at delivery.

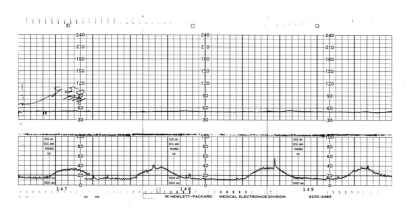

CASE INTERPRETATION: Class III

Baseline Information: absent variability, marked bradycardia.

Periodic or Nonperiodic Changes: none seen.

Uterine Activity: appears normal.

Significance: probable complete atrioventricular block; confirm with echocardiogram or ECG, assess fetus with ultrasonography. Monitoring atrial activity and the scalp pH may permit a course of labor. Preparation for a newborn cardiology evaluation and maternal assessment for autoantibodies are appropriate.

CASE OUTCOME: Eighteen-year-old, gravida 4, para 3003, at 40 weeks' gestation delivered vaginally, with low forceps and epidural anesthesia, a 7 pound, 13 ounce (3544 gram) female; Apgar score 9/9. The newborn heart rate was less than 70 bpm. The infant did not require a pacemaker. The maternal evaluation for collagen vascular disease was negative.

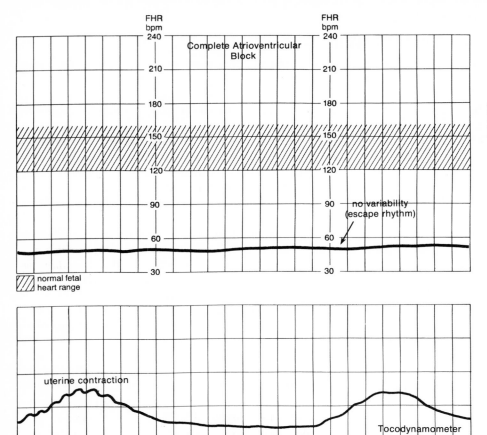

Pattern Characteristic:
Bradycardia Arrhythmia. Heart
Block

Bradycardia Secondary to Nonconducted Premature Supraventricular Depolarizations in Bigeminal Pattern: Arrhythmia

A bradyarrhythmia is suspected when the baseline fetal heart rate is below 90 bpm, especially when there is loss of normal variability.

A rare bradyarrhythmia is nonconducted premature bigeminal supraventricular depolarizations. All reported cases diagnosed antenatally have been associated with surviving newborns who did not have significant structural cardiac defects.[1,6,29,38] Fetal blood sampling has consistently failed to show acidosis.

A fetal electrocardiogram or fetal echocardiogram is helpful for diagnosis to distinguish this from bradyarrhythmias secondary to atrioventricular block. The diagnosis may be suspected when the bradyarrhythmia is found to be mixed, with areas of normal variability (sinus rhythm), particularly during contractions, or areas compatible with conducted premature beats. In the adult, this entity is well recognized. It is thought to be due to an alteration in cardiac milieu such as an electrolyte im-

balance, acid-base disturbance, or drug effect (including caffeine, nicotine, and alcohol).

Because the bradycardic rate is one half the usual rate, half counting may be suspected. However, half counting usually occurs at baseline heart rates greater than the normal fetal heart rate. Careful auscultation, as well as maternal heart rate recording, should exclude this artifact.

The pattern must also be differentiated from a prolonged deceleration with junctional rhythm or an agonal bradycardia preceding fetal death.

There is an artifactual fetal heart rate pattern produced by a fetal arrhythmia that is indistinguishable from this pattern by external monitoring. That is *conducted* premature atrial depolarization in bigeminy when the monitor "counts" every other beat. The premature beat occurs so close to the sinus node beat that it is discarded by the logic of the monitor.[39]

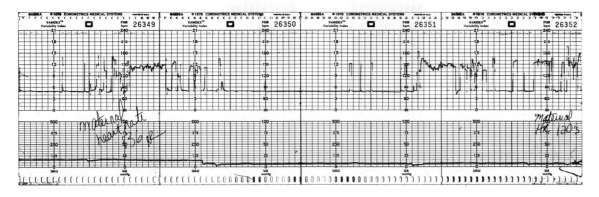

CASE INTERPRETATION: Class III

Baseline Information: two baselines are present, one within a normal fetal heart range and one with marked bradycardia. The higher baseline has good variability; the lower baseline has absent variability.

Periodic or Nonperiodic Changes: none seen.

Uterine Activity: this is not a satisfactory recording for interpretation.

Significance: possible artifact or arrhythmia. Artifact is determined by auscultation, with attention to the maternal heart rate.

CASE OUTCOME: Thirty-seven-year-old gravida 4, para 3003, at 34 weeks' gestation delivered by cesarean hysterectomy for maternal carcinoma of the cervix uteri, with general anesthesia, a 4 pound, 4 ounce (1928 gram) female; Apgar score 2/8. During the newborn course, an electrocardiogram confirmed that there were blocked premature supraventricular beats. This gradually resolved. The newborn had features of fetal alcohol syndrome. (See page 484 for a discussion of this arrhythmia accompanied by the newborn electrocardiogram.)

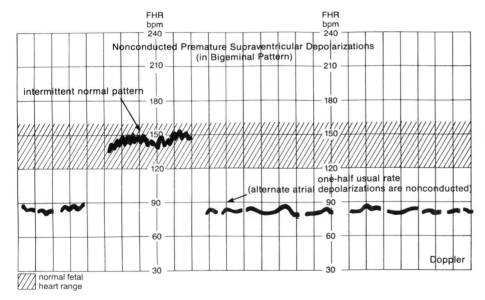

Pattern Characteristic:
Bradycardia Arrhythmia. Atrial Bigeminy Nonconducted

Bradycardia Secondary to Maternal Heart Rate, External Monitoring: Artifact

*T*he site where the Doppler transducer is placed or the movement of the fetus may result in recording of the maternal heart rate rather than the fetal heart rate.

The Doppler transducer contains a transmitter that continuously sends out an ultrasonic beam. It also contains a receiver to which the transmitted signal returns after being reflected by an interface of increased density. If that interface is moving, a frequency change occurs in the signal. This is sensed by the fetal monitor and converted to an electronic signal both as a sound and as a mark on the tracing.

The fetal monitor is therefore able to detect movement of maternal blood vessels and record the resulting signal. The monitor is less likely to reject the maternal signals if they approximate the normal fetal heart rate.

The most rapid method of identifying that the recorded heart rate is maternal is simultaneous palpation of the mother's pulse. The most precise method of differentiation is simultaneous monitoring of maternal and fetal electrocardiogram-derived signals.

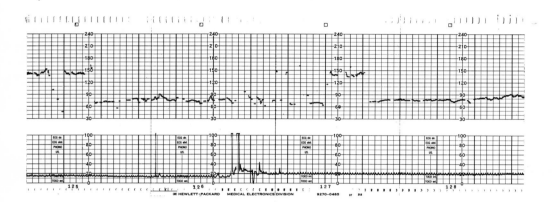

CASE INTERPRETATION: Class III/0

Baseline Information: two baselines are present, one in a normal fetal heart range and one with marked bradycardia. The higher rate is of insufficient duration to interpret variability, and results are unreliable with the external monitoring of this machine. The lower rate appears to have decreased variability.

Periodic or Nonperiodic Changes: none seen.

Significance: it is unlikely that this is half counting. A distinction should be made between arrhythmia versus maternal heart recording.

CASE OUTCOME: Forty-one-year-old, gravida 4, para 3003, was admitted in premature labor at 24½ weeks' gestation. She was treated with intravenous ritodrine. The maternal pulse coincided with the lower heart rate on the tracing. The patient was dismissed undelivered. She was readmitted at 37½ weeks' gestation. By spontaneous vaginal delivery, with epidural anesthesia, she gave birth to a 6 pound, 3 ounce (2807 gram) female; Apgar score 8/9. A nuchal cord was noted at delivery. The infant followed a normal newborn course.

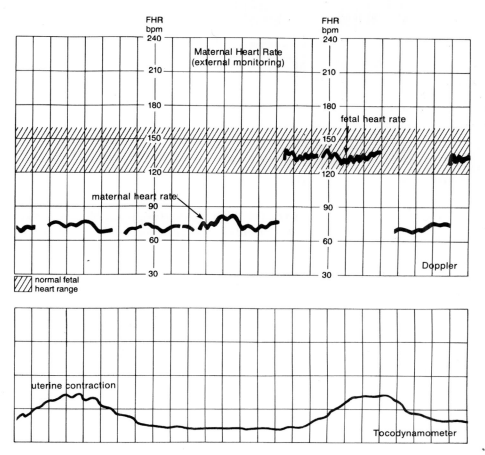

FHR
bpm

FHR
bpm

Maternal Heart Rate
(external monitoring)

fetal heart rate

maternal heart rate

normal fetal
heart range

Doppler

uterine contraction

Tocodynamometer

Pattern Characteristic:
Artifactual Bradycardia

Bradycardia Secondary to Maternal Heart Rate, Internal Monitoring: Artifact

*W*hen the scalp electrode is used to monitor a fetus that is alive, the mother's poorly conducted electrocardiographic signal is masked by the more directly derived fetal electrocardiogram. When the fetus dies, a system in fetal monitors called the Automatic Gain Control may amplify the maternal signals and cause them to be displayed on the tracing.[32,36] This may cause the maternal heart rate to be mistaken for fetal bradycardia. Maternal tachycardia may be mistaken for a normal fetal rate. The transmitted maternal heart rate may show good variability (sinus arrhythmia) and often demonstrates accelerations[19] and occasionally decelerations with contractions.[21]

There are numerous ways to distinguish whether the recorded heart rate is fetal or maternal. The most precise method is simultaneous recording of fetal and maternal heart rates.[2] This is conveniently accomplished with modern monitors with dual-channel capabilities. This, coupled with real time ultrasonography for intrauterine fetal cardiac activity, should clarify the situation. Simultaneous maternal and fetal electrocardiograms enable the distinction between fetal and maternal signals to be made by duration of the QRS. The mother's (0.08–0.10 second) is usually twice as long as that of the fetus (0.04–0.06 second).

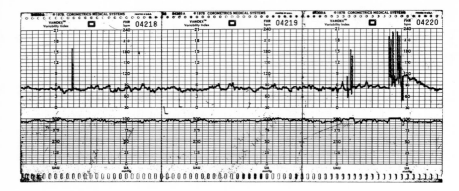

CASE INTERPRETATION: Class I (artifactual)

Baseline Information: fair variability, marked brady-cardia.

Periodic or Nonperiodic Changes: single accelera-tion seen.

Uterine Activity: tocodynamometer reading is set high on the graph.

Significance: the pattern is reassuring if there is a live fetus, but in cases of bradycardia, detecting a maternally derived signal may be important.

CASE OUTCOME: Thirty-seven-year-old gravida 10, para 9009, at 40 weeks' gestation, delivered vaginally, with no anesthesia, a stillborn 7 pound, 6½ ounce (3360 gram) male. Intrauterine fetal demise was confirmed by real time ultrasonography. The fact that the scalp electrode was recording the maternal heart rate was detected by simultaneous timing of the maternal pulse. Personnel encountered difficulty in setting the tocodynamometer loosely on the abdomen of this markedly obese patient.

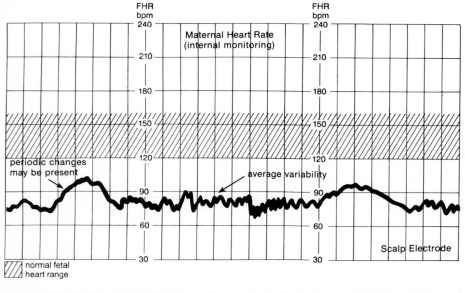

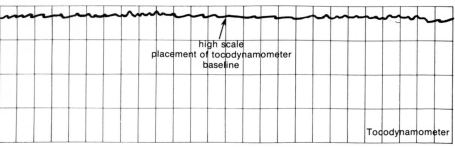

Pattern Characteristic:
Artifactual Bradycardia

Bradycardia Secondary to Half Counting Maternal Heart Rate: Artifact

Not only is the maternal heart rate a potential source of artifact with external or internal monitoring but with Doppler-derived signals the fetal monitor may half count or double count the artifactual maternal heart rate.[27] This is seen with newer monitors that use autocorrelation as well as with older monitors.

Half counting smooths variability because the heart rate information is compressed on a smaller scale. Likewise, double counting exaggerates variability, as heart rate information is spread over a larger scale.

Maternal heart rate artifact is suspected when parallel double lines appear while monitoring a fetus with no audible arrhythmia. Half counting of the maternal heart rate is implicated by a mathematical association between the marked bradycardia rate and the maternal heart rate, the latter verified by simultaneous carotid artery palpation or by comparison to a maternal electrocardiogram-derived monitor signal.

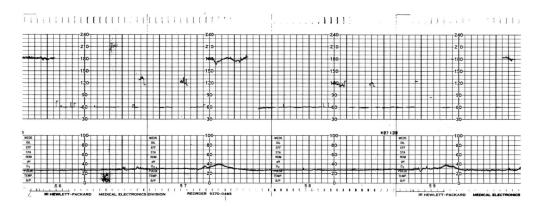

CASE INTERPRETATION: Class III/0

Baseline Information: three rates are seen. One, with moderate to marked tachycardia and reduced short-term variability. A second, at low normal to moderate bradycardia, with insufficient segments for diagnosis. A third, at severe bradycardia of 60 bpm, with absent (flat line) short- and long-term variability.

Periodic or Nonperiodic Changes: none seen.

Uterine Activity: small infrequent contractions of a normal configuration.

Significance: a pattern is seen with the maternal heart rate artifact half counting the maternal heart rate. This may be distinguished from intermittent arrhythmia by doing bedside auscultation of the true fetal heart rate.

CASE OUTCOME: Thirty-year-old gravida 3, para 2002, at 40 weeks' gestation, delivered vaginally, with local anesthesia, an 8 pound, 1 ounce (3657 gram) female; Apgar score 8/8. The fetus was in a vertex presentation. There was an uncomplicated newborn course.

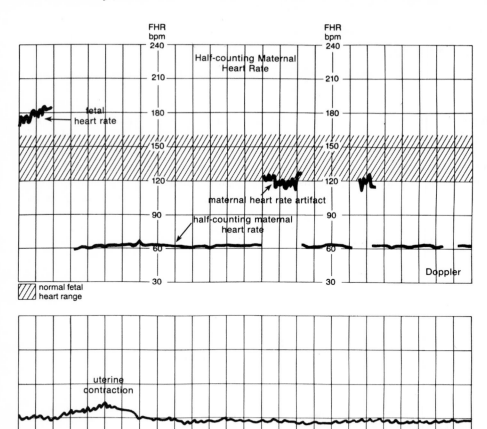

Pattern Characteristic:
Artifactual Bradycardia

References

1. Abinader EG, Klein A, Eibschitz I, et al: The significance of fetal electrocardiography in the diagnosis of intrauterine bradyarrhythmia. *Am J Obstet Gynecol* 128:266, 1976.
2. Barrett JM, Boehm FH: Documentation of recent fetal demise with simultaneous maternal and fetal heart rate monitoring. *Obstet Gynecol* 55:288, 1980.
3. Cetrulo CL, Schifrin BS: Fetal heart rate patterns preceding death in utero. *Obstet Gynecol* 48:521, 1978.
4. Cibils LA: Clinical significance of fetal heart rate patterns during labor. IV. Agonal patterns. *Am J Obstet Gynecol* 129:833, 1977.
5. Cunningham FG, MacDonald PC, Gant NF: Techniques to evaluate fetal heart, in *Williams Obstetrics*, 18th ed. Norwalk, CT, Appleton and Lange, 1989, p. 299.
6. Dgani R, Borenstein R, Levavi E, et al: Prenatally diagnosed blocked atrial premature beats. *Obstet Gynecol* 51:507, 1978.
7. Emmen L, Huisjes HJ, Aarnoudse JE, et al: Antepartum diagnosis of the "terminal" fetal state by cardiotocography. *Brit J Obstet Gynaecol* 82:353, 1975.
8. Fetal heart rate monitoring. Guidelines for monitoring. Terminology and instrumentation. *ACOG Technical Bulletin* no. 32, June 1975.
9. Garite TJ, Freeman RK: Bradycardias with normal variability usually benign. *Contemp Obstet Gynecol* 19:29, 1982.
10. Gaziano EP: A study of variable decelerations in association with other heart rate patterns during monitored labor. *Am J Obstet Gynecol* 135:360, 1979.
11. Gaziano EP, Freeman DW, Bendel RP: FHR variability and other heart rate observations during second state labor. *Obstet Gynecol* 58:42, 1980.
12. Gilstrap L, Hauth JC, Toussaint S: Second state fetal heart rate abnormalities and neonatal acidosis. *Obstet Gynecol* 62:209, 1984.

13. Gleicher N, Elkayam U: Intrauterine dysrhythmias, in *Cardiac Problems in Pregnancy.* New York, Alan R. Liss, 1982, p. 535.

14. Goodlin RC, Haesslein HC: Fetal reacting bradycardia. *Am J Obstet Gynecol* 129:845, 1977.

15. Hon EH: The fetal heart rate patterns preceding death in utero. *Clin Obstet Gynecol* 78:47, 1959.

16. Hon EH, Lee ST: Electronic evaluation of the fetal heart rate. VIII. Patterns preceding fetal death, further observations. *Am J Obstet Gynecol* 87:814, 1963.

17. Hon EH, Quilligan EJ: Electronic evaluation of fetal heart rate. IX. Further observations on "pathologic" fetal bradycardia. *Clin Obstet Gynecol* 11:151, 1968.

18. Ingemarsson E, Ingemarsson I, Solum T, et al: Influence of occiput posterior position on the fetal heart rate pattern interpretation. *Obstet Gynecol* 55:301, 1980.

19. Klapholz H, Schifrin BS, et al: Role of maternal artifact in fetal heart rate pattern interpretation. *Obstet Gynecol* 44:373, 1974.

20. Krebs HB, Petres RE, Dunn LJ: Intrapartum fetal heart rate monitoring. V. Fetal heart rate patterns in the second state of labor. *Am J Obstet Gynecol* 140:435, 1981.

21. Lackritz R, Schiff I, Gibson M, Safon L: Decelerations on fetal electrocardiography with fetal demise. *Obstet Gynecol* 51:367, 1978.

22. Langer O, Cohen WR: Persistent fetal bradycardia during maternal hypoglycemia. *Am J Obstet Gynecol* 149:688, 1984.

23. LaSala AP, Strassner HT: Fetal death. *Clinical Obstet Gynecol* 29:95, 1986.

24. Litsey SE, Noonan JA, O'Connor WN, et al: Maternal connective tissue disease and congenital heart block. Demonstration of immunoglobulin in cardiac tissue. *N Engl J Med* 312:98, 1985.

25. Low JA, Cox MJ, Karchmar EJ, et al: The prediction of intrapartum fetal metabolic acidosis by fetal heart rate monitoring. *Am J Obstet Gynecol* 139:299, 1981.

26. Martin CB: Regulation of the fetal heart rate and genesis of FHR patterns. *Seminars in Perinatology* 2:131, 1978.

27. Parer JT: The fetal heart rate monitor, in *Handbook of Fetal Heart Rate Monitoring.* Philadelphia, W.B. Saunders, 1983, p. 59.

28. Parer JT: Fetal heart rate patterns preceding death in utero, in *Handbook of Fetal Heart Rate Monitoring.* Philadelphia, W.B. Saunders, 1983, p. 147.

29. Redman RG: The significance of some unusual foetal cardiac arrhythmias. *J Obstet Gynaecol Br Empire* 65:314, 1958.

30. Reid RL, Pancham BR, Kean WF, et al: Maternal and neonatal implications of congenital complete heart block in the fetus. *Obstet Gynecol* 54:470, 1979.

31. Richards DS, Wagman AJ, Cabaniss ML: Fetal ascites not due to congestive heart failure in a fetus with lupus induced heart block. *Obstet Gynecol* 76:957, 1990.

32. Schneiderman CI, Waxman B, Goodman CJ: Maternal-fetal electrocardiogram conduction with intrapartum fetal death. *Am J Obstet Gynecol* 113:1130, 1972.

33. Shenker L: Fetal cardiac arrhythmias. *Obstet Gynecol Surv* 34:561, 1979.

34. Singsen BH, Akhter JE, Weinstin MM, et al: Congenital complete heart block and SSA antibodies: Obstetric implications. *Am J Obstet Gynecol* 152:655, 1985.

35. Smith JJ, Schwartz ED, Blatman S: Fetal bradycardia—fetal distress or cardiac abnormality? *Obstet Gynecol* 15:761, 1960.

36. Timor-Tritsch I, Gergely Z, Abramovici H, et al: Misleading information from fetal monitoring in a case of intrapartum fetal death. *Obstet Gynecol* 43:713, 1974.

37. Tushuizen PBT, Stoot JEGM, Obachs JMH: Fetal heart rate monitoring of the dying fetus. *Am J Obstet Gynecol* vol. 120:922, 1974.

38. Webster RD, Cudmors DW, Gray J: Fetal bradycardia without fetal distress. *Obstet Gynecol* 50:50s, 1977.

39. Wright AJ: Fetal arrhythmia masquerading as fetal distress. *J Repr Med* 34:301, 1989.

40. Young BK, Weinstein HM: Moderate fetal bradycardia. *Am J Obstet Gynecol* 126:271, 1976.

41. Young BK, Katz M, Klein SH: The relationship of heart rate patterns and tissue pH in the human fetus. *Am J Obstet Gynecol* 134:685, 1979.

42. Young BK, Katz M, Klein SA, et al: Fetal blood and tissue pH with moderate bradycardia. *Am J Obstet Gynecol* 135:45, 1979.

Tachycardia

Chapter 4

Moderate Sinus Tachycardia

*M*oderate fetal tachycardia is defined as a fetal heart baseline rate of 160 to 179 bpm.[7] It has also been called mild tachycardia.

The most common etiology of moderate fetal tachycardia is maternal fever. The fetus, dependent upon the mother for heat exchange, cannot escape increased metabolic demands in the presence of maternal fever.[21,29] If the etiology is noninfectious or secondary to extrauterine infection, the fetal heart rate returns to a normal range as the maternal hyperpyrexia resolves. Chorioamnionitis must always be suspected as an etiology. Fetal tachycardia may also be secondary to a drug effect, as in cases in which beta sympathomimetic agents are used to arrest premature labor. Beat-to-beat variability is usually preserved, although diminished. Other agents that have been reported to produce fetal tachycardia are atropine and hydroxyzine operating through a parasympatholytic mechanism.

Less common causes of moderate fetal tachycardia are maternal hyperthyroidism, maternal tachycardia or anxiety state, and mild fetal anemia.[11,17]

The fetal heart rate is said to gradually decline with gestational age. Therefore, the preterm fetus may have a slightly higher rate than the term or post-term fetus. However, both are usually within the normal fetal heart range.[6] Tachycardia should not be assumed to be solely caused by prematurity without consideration of other etiologies.

Although moderate tachycardia in the presence of normal variability and in the absence of hypoxic periodic changes is usually associated with a well fetus, a systematic evaluation for an etiology may be rewarding.[13]

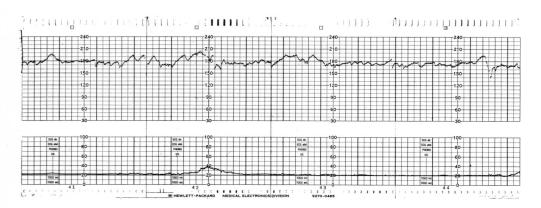

CASE INTERPRETATION: Class II

Baseline Information: moderate sinus tachycardia, normal variability.

Periodic or Nonperiodic Changes: sporadic accelerations present.

Uterine Activity: rare contraction displayed.

Significance: fetal tachycardia in the presence of normal variability with accelerations suggests a healthy fetus. It is appropriate to evaluate for maternal fever and drug effect.

CASE OUTCOME: Twenty-one-year-old gravida 4, para 2012, at 32 weeks' gestation. The maternal temperature was 101.6°F secondary to pyelonephritis, which responded to intravenous ampicillin. The fetal heart rate reverted to a normal range with treatment of the maternal hyperpyrexia. The patient later delivered at term a 7 pound, 10 ounce (3459 gram) male; Apgar score 8/9. The infant followed an uncomplicated newborn course.

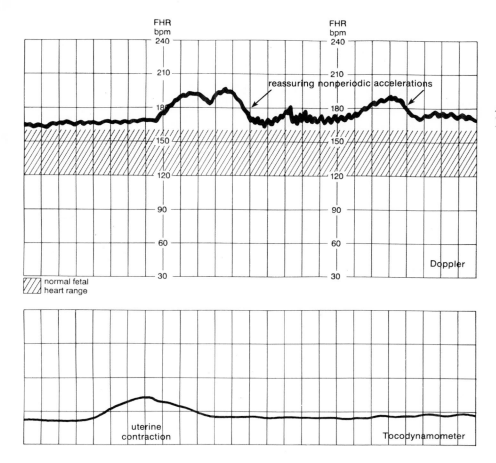

FHR bpm

normal fetal heart range

reassuring nonperiodic accelerations

Doppler

uterine contraction

Tocodynamometer

Pattern Characteristic:
Moderate Sinus Tachycardia

Marked Sinus Tachycardia

*M*arked fetal tachycardia is defined as a fetal heart baseline rate of 180 bpm or more.[7] It has also been called severe tachycardia.

With a heart rate of greater than 180 bpm, beat-to-beat variability is diminished even in the normal fetus because of relatively increased sympathetic activity in relationship to parasympathetic activity. This makes it difficult to distinguish between marked tachycardia that is due to fetal hypoxia and that which is due to other causes. The absence of periodic decelerative changes, the presence of accelerations, and the preservation of some degree of beat-to-beat variability are reassuring.

The etiologies of marked fetal tachycardia are similar to those of moderate fetal tachycardia but suggest a more intense degree. Maternal fever and drug effect (e.g., that of beta sympathomimetic agents) again lead the list of possible causes if variability is preserved and there are no periodic hypoxic changes.[26] Nevertheless chorioamnionitis must always be considered and excluded.[17,24] Fetal hypovolemia secondary to blood loss should be suspected, especially if there is vaginal bleeding or if it occurs following trauma.[8,9]

Fetal thyrotoxicosis secondary to placental transfer of thyroid stimulating antibody is a rare cause of marked fetal tachycardia.[20,28]

It is important to distinguish between marked fetal tachycardia and an arrhythmia, especially when the heart rate is 200 bpm or greater. A sinus tachycardia is more likely to have developed gradually from a slower baseline, as opposed to the usual abrupt onset of an arrhythmia. Fetal electrocardiography or echocardiography is helpful for diagnosis of specific arrhythmias.

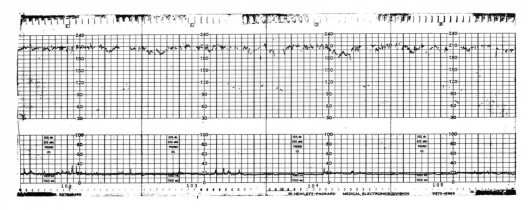

CASE INTERPRETATION: Class III

Baseline Information: marked tachycardia, apparent reduced beat-to-beat variability by external monitor.

Periodic or Nonperiodic Changes: possible shallow accelerations.

Uterine Activity: no contractions recorded.

Significance: nondiagnostic pattern. It is an appropriate response to exclude chorioamnionitis, evaluate for maternal fever and drug effect, and consider fetal anemia and maternal or fetal hyperthyroidism.

CASE OUTCOME: Twenty-five-year-old gravida 4, para 0212, in premature labor at 36 weeks' gestation was receiving intravenous isoxsuprine therapy for tocolysis. The contractions ceased, and the patient was dismissed undelivered. She later delivered at term a 7 pound, 2 ounce (3232 gram) female; Apgar score 5/9. The infant followed an uncomplicated newborn course.

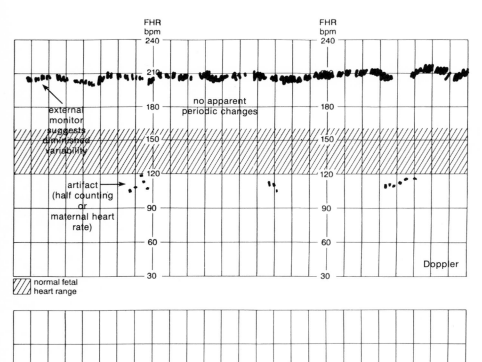

Pattern Characteristic:
Marked Sinus Tachycardia

Sinus Tachycardia with Decelerations: Mixed Pattern

As a general rule, tachycardia *per se* is not an indication of fetal distress.[13] Tachycardia in the presence of good variability implies a fetus appropriately compensating for changes in the environment.

When periodic changes are present, the decelerations themselves become a further indicator of the particular type and degree of stresses to which the fetus may be currently subjected, for example, hypoxia or a reflex response to cord compression. The basal condition of the fetus, however, is largely assessed by the presence or absence of good beat-to-beat variability. In the presence of good variability and a stable baseline with brief periodic changes, emergency cesarean section for possible fetal distress is rarely indicated. The pattern should continue to be observed for deterioration of variability or increas-ing atypia or duration of periodic changes because the combination of tachycardia and variable decelerations increases the risk of a low Apgar score or acidosis.[1,10] Reducing stresses (e.g., by decreasing excessive uterine activity, decreasing maternal pushing, decreasing maternal fever) may improve the pattern.

Occasionally, a fetus who is normally oxygenated when the heart is beating at a normal rate, demonstrates late decelerations at a faster heart rate. This is presumed to be secondary to the hypoxia associated with increasing metabolic demands. When the etiology of the tachycardia is maternal fever, the elevated temperature decreases fetal blood oxygen affinity as a further cause of hypoxemia. Tachycardia may then unmask a borderline compensated lack of oxygen reserve.[5,21]

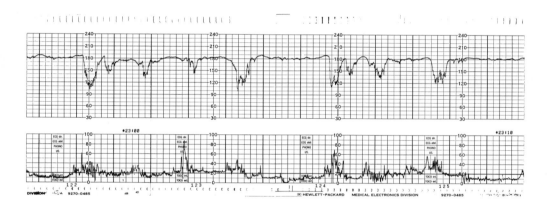

CASE INTERPRETATION: Class IV

Baseline Information: moderate to marked tachycardia, decreased variability in some areas, average variability in others.

Periodic or Nonperiodic Changes: mild to moderate variable decelerations with jagged features. Minimal atypia characterized by a rare loss of primary acceleration.

Uterine Activity: poorly recorded contractions with superimposed maternal activity.

Significance: jagged appearance of the variable decelerations is reassuring. There is minimal atypia present in the variable decelerations. However, a smoothing of the baseline as well as tachycardia are not reassuring, especially if they exist in combination. A decision as to when to deliver and by what route is based on gestation, underlying clinical factors, the estimated time to delivery and ease of delivery, and the response to measures taken to optimize the fetal condition in utero.

CASE OUTCOME: Eighteen-year-old primigravida delivered by low transverse cesarean section at 29½ weeks' gestation a 3 pound, 7½ ounce (1574 gram) male; Apgar score 7/9. The fetus was in a vertex presentation. Cesarean section was indicated by chorioamnionitis and possible fetal distress. (The fetal monitoring pattern progressed to severe variable decelerations with increased atypia.) The maternal course was complicated by the rupture of her membranes 38 hours before delivery, the lack of prenatal care, and a previously undiagnosed case of syphilis. The newborn was dismissed at one month of life.

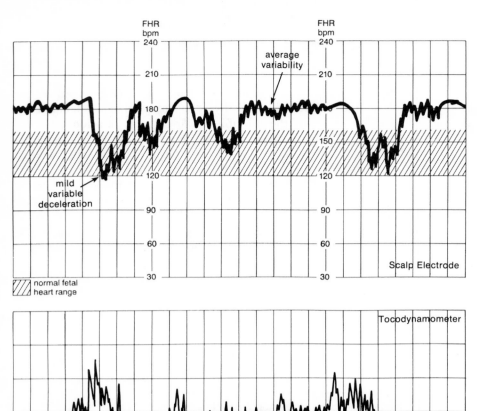

Pattern Characteristic:
Sinus Tachycardia and
Decelerations Mixed Pattern

Sinus Tachycardia with No Variability: Mixed Pattern

Sinus tachycardia is normally accompanied by a reduction, but not a complete loss, of variability.[8] When variability is markedly reduced or absent, the presence of fetal acidosis or fetal sepsis is a possibility.[17,22]

A scalp pH or fetal stimulation, when feasible, may be adjuncts to the fetal monitoring information in the presence of sinus tachycardia with no variability. The presence of fetal tachycardia, absent variability, and late decelerations or severe or atypical variable decelerations predicts a high incidence of acidosis or a low Apgar score (see Chap. 12). The absence of obvious periodic changes with contractions does not exclude fetal distress because with the presence of severe hypoxia with fetal acidosis, late decelerations may be very shallow.

With the absence of variability at rapid heart rates (>200 bpm), arrhythmia should also be considered, especially if the onset of the pattern was abrupt. Fetal electrocardiography and echocardiography may be adjuncts to the fetal monitor for diagnosis in such cases.

Sinus tachycardia with a loss of variability must be distinguished from reassuring prolonged nonperiodic accelerations. The predominance of sympathetic activity, in comparison to parasympathetic activity, accounts for the smoothing of the heart rate during accelerations. In cases of prolonged accelerations, review of the tracing usually reveals an intermittent return of the heart rate to a normal baseline with normal variability.

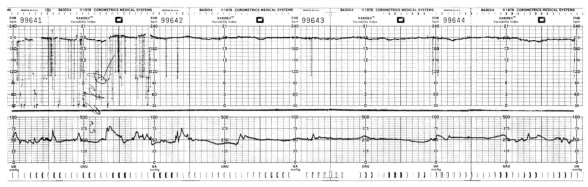

Recreation of original tracing

CASE INTERPRETATION: Class III

Baseline Information: marked tachycardia, absent beat-to-beat variability. Unstable wandering baseline.

Periodic or Nonperiodic Changes: possible shallow decelerations.

Uterine Activity: brief contractions every two minutes.

Significance: possible fetal distress. A fetal pH may assist in fetal assessment.

CASE OUTCOME: Twenty-year-old gravida 2, para 1001, at 40 weeks' gestation, delivered by primary cesarean section performed under general anesthesia for cephalopelvic disproportion, an 8 pound, 3 ounce (3714 gram) female; Apgar score 8/8. The mother was given oxytocin for ruptured membranes; she had a fever of 100.9°F. The fetal scalp pHs intrapartum were 7.28 and 7.30. The mother had insulin-dependent diabetes. Group B beta hemolytic *streptococcus* grew in the placental culture. The newborn received prophylactic antibiotics and was dismissed after four days.

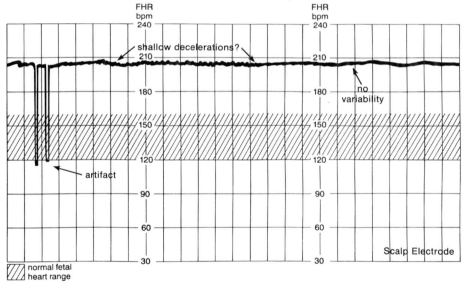

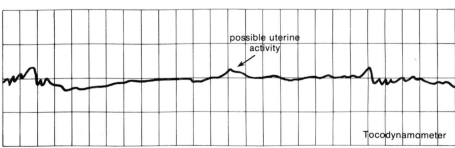

Pattern Characteristic:
Sinus Tachycardia with No Variability: Mixed Pattern

Sinus Tachycardia with Decelerations and No Variability: Mixed Pattern

*T*he presence of sinus tachycardia with decreased variability and periodic changes (specifically late decelerations or atypical severe variable decelerations) predicts a high incidence of fetal acidosis and/or a low Apgar score.[1,10,12,14]

If the pattern does not improve by position change, oxygen administration, and other appropriate measures of in utero resuscitation, delivery may be preferable to continued in utero management.

A decrease, but not absence, of variability in the presence of tachycardia with periodic decelerations with only minor atypia is a combination of findings in which fetal pH determination may be a useful adjunct. A progressive diminution of variability normally accompanies a rising baseline secondary to increasing sympathetic system activity, but loss of variability should not be presumed to be solely on this basis, especially in a mixed pattern with periodic changes.

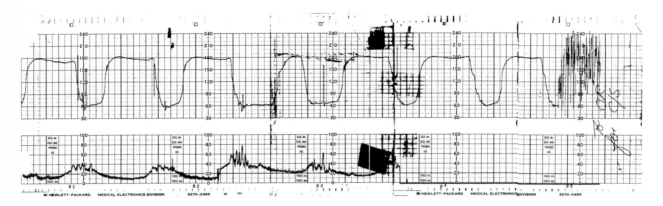

CASE INTERPRETATION: Class V

Baseline Information: moderate tachycardia, absent beat-to-beat variability.

Periodic or Nonperiodic Changes: severe variable decelerations with excessive depth and duration, abnormal primary and secondary accelerations, smoothing of contour.

Uterine Activity: skewed contractions with no resting interval.

Significance: high risk of compromised fetus, prompt delivery is appropriate.

CASE OUTCOME: Thirty-one-year-old gravida 2, para 1001, at 41 weeks' gestation, underwent cesarean section, with general anesthesia, at 9 centimeters cervical dilatation for possible fetal distress and cephalopelvic disproportion. The patient had received meperidine and propiomazine hydrochloride intrapartum. She delivered an 8 pound, 9½ ounce (3898 gram) female; Apgar score 1/5. The fetus was in a vertex presentation; there was thick meconium present; the location of the cord was not noted. The maternal course was complicated by mild hypertension and wound dehiscence. The newborn, who survived meconium aspiration pneumonitis, was dismissed after 10 days.

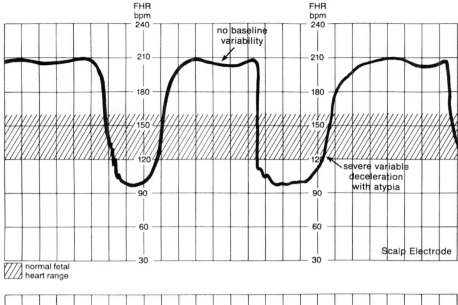

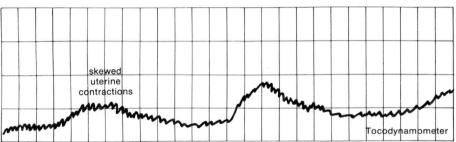

Pattern Characteristic:
Sinus Tachycardia with
Decelerations and No
Variability: Mixed Pattern

Rebound Tachycardia

*R*ebound tachycardia often occurs during the recovery phase of a prolonged deceleration.[3] It has also been termed "compensatory tachycardia." It is typically associated with a concurrent decrease in variability. Rebound tachycardia is more likely to be seen if the antecedent deceleration lasts more than two to three minutes. It is speculated that the mechanism producing the pattern is a combination of fetal epinephrine release and central nervous system depression. The belief is that during the recovery phase of a prolonged deceleration, the placenta is resuscitating the fetus in utero. During the deceleration, the fetus redistributes blood flow to protect coronary and cerebral vessels, resulting in peripheral vasoconstriction and a fall in oxygen partial pressure (PO_2) in certain tissue beds such as those of striated muscles. This is accompanied by an increase in local lactic acid

production. With recovery there is tachycardia, increased PO_2, and clearance of lactic acid with the correction of acidemia.[26] Serial pH determinations, should they be done in this time period, would be transiently low, followed by a progressive rise.[15,27] Periodic late decelerations may appear briefly during the recovery phase (see page 222).

With full recovery, the baseline fetal heart rate eventually returns to predeceleration levels, and the transiently diminished beat-to-beat variability is replaced by the pre-existing level.

It is important not to confuse the phenomenon of rebound tachycardia with the secondary acceleration (also termed "overshoot") associated with variable decelerations. The overshoot is a rebound acceleration, not a rebound tachycardia.[4]

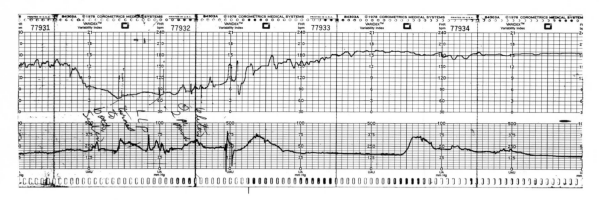

CASE INTERPRETATION: Class II

Baseline Changes: marked tachycardia upon recovery from a prolonged deceleration, accompanied by initial increase then decrease in previously normal variability.

Periodic or Nonperiodic Changes: prolonged deceleration with transient sinus node suppression.

Uterine Activity: possibly increased during the deceleration but repositioning of the patient is also taking place, making uterine activity unclear.

Significance: acute fetal stress with recovery.

CASE OUTCOME: Twenty-five-year-old primigravida at 36 weeks' gestation delivered vaginally a 4 pound, 9 ounce (2070 gram) (small for gestational age) female; Apgar score 9/10. Scalp pHs after recovery from the prolonged deceleration were 7.28, 7.36, and 7.36. The newborn was dismissed after three days.

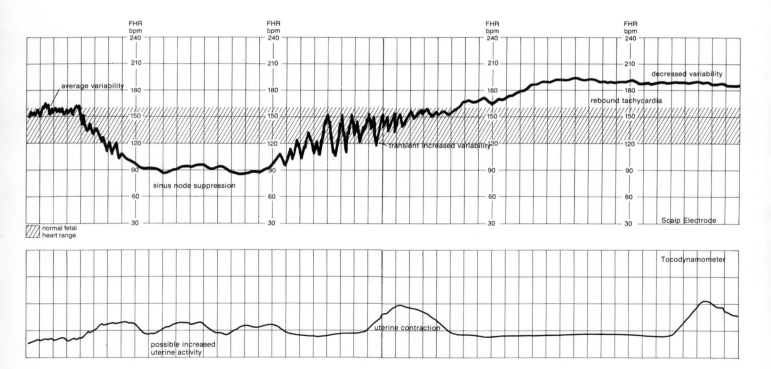

Pattern Characteristic:
Rebound Tachycardia

Tachycardia Produced by Supraventricular Tachyarrhythmia

*T*he recognition of tachyarrhythmias in the fetus has increased in frequency with the use of fetal monitoring. When supraventricular tachycardia occurs, it is usually at a rate of 200 to 240 bpm in the fetus.[2] There is an associated decrease in beat-to-beat variability. The fetal monitoring tracing does not distinguish between atrial flutter and other supraventricular tachycardias. Fetal electrocardiography may not be conclusive because of limitations demonstrating P waves. Echocardiography is most conclusive in differentiating between atrial flutter and other varieties of supraventricular tachycardia.

Digoxin has been the most commonly used initial drug for cardioversion, often necessitating higher than the usual dosage for adult therapy. Successful cardioversion after digoxin has failed has been reported with the use of verapamil, quinidine, propranolol, and procainamide.[2,11] The conversion of supraventricular tachyarrhythmia to a normal heart rate has been documented with umbilical cord compression under real time ultrasound observation.[18]

The diagnosis of fetal supraventricular tachycardia is an indication for evaluation of the fetal heart for structural abnormality. The incidence of congenital heart disease is 5% to 10%.[25] If the tachycardia persists, fetal hydrops and death secondary to heart failure may ensue. Serial ultrasonography is thus important in the management of the patient in whom delivery is not undertaken because of extreme prematurity.

This arrhythmia may occur abruptly during normal labor. It has also been reported secondary to ritodrine usage.

As with atrial flutter, half counting by the fetal monitor of rates greater than 200 bpm is common. This has been documented even with scalp electrode monitoring. Modern monitors may not print a fetal heart trace at all, neither half counting nor printing the rapid rate. See page 489 for further discussion of this pattern.

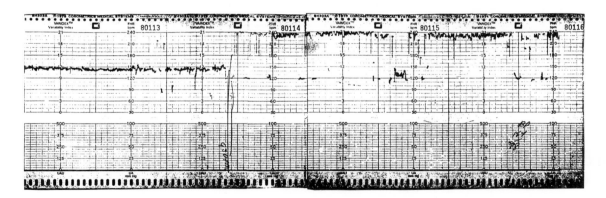

CASE INTERPRETATION: Class 0/III

Baseline Information: two heart rates are seen. The upper is either marked tachycardia, as seen with tachyarrhythmia, or double counting. The lower rate is either half counting, a true fetal heart rate, or the maternal heart rate. There is no reactivity. Variability appears decreased despite external monitoring.

Periodic or Nonperiodic Changes: none documented.

Uterine Activity: not recorded.

Significance: auscultation is essential to identify which rate is the true fetal heart rate. With tachyarrhythmia, echocardiography enables the distinction to be made between atrial flutter and other supraventricular tachycardias.

CASE OUTCOME: Twenty-year-old primigravida at 32 weeks' gestation. Echocardiogram had diagnosed supraventricular tachycardia present in a hydropic fetus. Successful in utero conversion to sinus rhythm at a normal heart rate occurred with maternal digoxin administration, and the newborn was delivered by cesarean section, performed for preeclampsia, the same day.

The newborn was a 5 pound, 3 ounce (2353 gram) male; Apgar score 1/7. The infant was treated for neonatal hydrops and respiratory distress syndrome. An echocardiogram found no structural heart disease. The newborn was dismissed after 26 days.

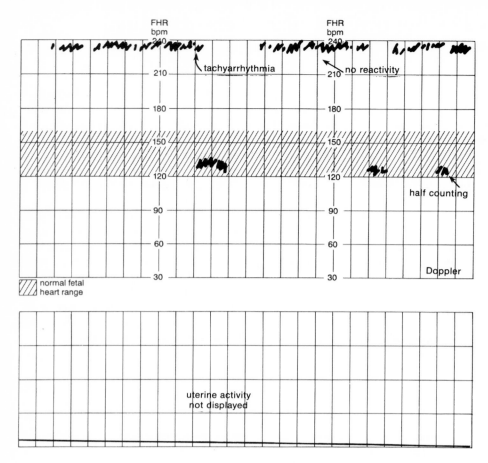

Pattern Characteristic:
Supraventricular Tachycardia

Tachycardia Produced by Atrial Flutter: Arrhythmia

Atrial flutter is a rare cause of fetal tachycardia. The fetal monitoring tracing is indistinguishable from that of supraventricular tachycardia. The distinction between atrial flutter and supraventricular tachycardia may be important in selecting pharmacologic therapy, assigning a fetal prognosis, and planning newborn care. Fetal electrocardiography has been used for in utero diagnosis of atrial flutter despite the difficulty in seeing flutter waves.[11] Echocardiography or electrocardiography, demonstrating a separate atrial and ventricular rate, determines the degree of block and documents whether it is fixed or variable.[16] It is theoretically possible for atrial flutter to go undetected by fetal monitoring alone if the degree of atrioventricular block places the ventricular rate in the normal fetal heart range (see page 97).

When an in utero diagnosis of atrial flutter is made, evaluation of the fetal heart for structural anomalies by echocardiography is important because congenital heart disease is reported to be as high as 20%.[25] The fetus is also evaluated ultrasonographically for polyhydramnios, hydrops and ascites, and evidence of congestive heart failure.

Agents that have been reported to be successful in treatment of tachyarrhythmias by pharmacocardioversion are: digoxin, propranolol, procainamide, verapamil, and quinidine. See page 492 for further discussion of this pattern.

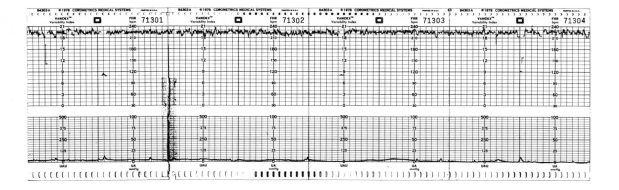

CASE INTERPRETATION: Class III

Baseline Information: marked tachycardia with a suggestion of decreased variability by external monitoring, as seen with tachyarrhythmia.

Periodic or Nonperiodic Changes: no reactivity or decelerations.

Uterine Activity: none recorded.

Significance: fetal arrhythmia. Needs echocardiogram (or scalp electrode electrocardiogram) for diagnosis of atrial flutter versus other supraventricular tachycardias.

CASE OUTCOME: Twenty-seven-year-old gravida 3, para 1011, at 32 weeks' gestation. Echocardiography diagnosis of atrial flutter with 2:1 atrioventricular block in the fetus with ascites. Treatment of the mother with digoxin and verapamil was unsuccessful in accomplishing fetal cardioversion. A hydropic 6 pound, 9 ounce (2420 gram) stillborn male was delivered by repeat cesarean section. The fetus was in a breech presentation and had trisomy 13 syndrome and multiple cardiac anomalies, including an atrioventricular (A-V) canal.

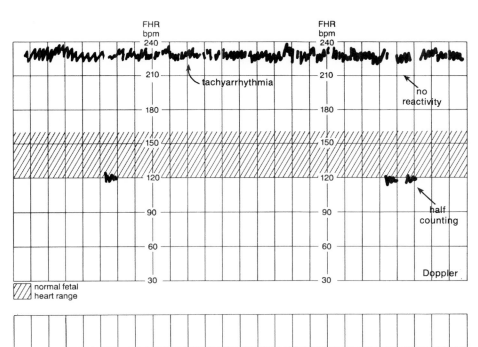

Pattern Characteristic:
Atrial Flutter

Tachycardia Produced by Double Counting Artifact

*D*oubling is usually considered a phenomenon of external monitoring. When using the Doppler method of fetal heart rate detection, a very slow rate may allow the second cardiac movement to fall outside the refractory window especially of the early fetal monitors. This results in double counting.[23] It is seen most often when the fetal heart rate falls below the normal range.

When the possibility of double counting is encountered, auscultation excludes intermittent tachycardia. If one mathematically halves the tachycardic rate and draws the resulting rate on the tracing, the subsequent line should fall into a continuous pattern with the printed areas of true fetal heart rate.

Double counting produces exaggerated variability because the resulting rate is spread over increased space (e.g., when 110–120 is doubled, a span of 10 beats is printed as 220–240, a span of 20 beats).

Double counting is not expected to occur with internal monitoring. An exception occurs when the monitor, programmed to be triggered by the R signal, encounters an unusually tall peaked T wave. If the R wave and T wave each trigger the monitor, the resulting printed heart rate is artifactually doubled.

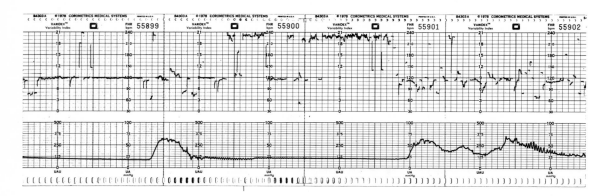

CASE INTERPRETATION: Class 0

Baseline Information: two rates, 115–120 and 220–240. Variability is diminished by the external monitor at the slower rate in comparison to the faster rate.

Periodic or Nonperiodic Changes: none clearly recorded.

Uterine Activity: skewed and polysystolic contractions present.

Significance: possible tachyarrhythmia versus double counting. Careful auscultation is needed for clarification.

CASE OUTCOME: Twenty-year-old primigravida at 35 weeks' gestation delivered vaginally a 4 pound, 3½ ounce (1920 gram) female; Apgar score 8/9. The fetus was in a vertex presentation. The pregnancy was complicated by mild preeclampsia. The newborn was dismissed after seven days.

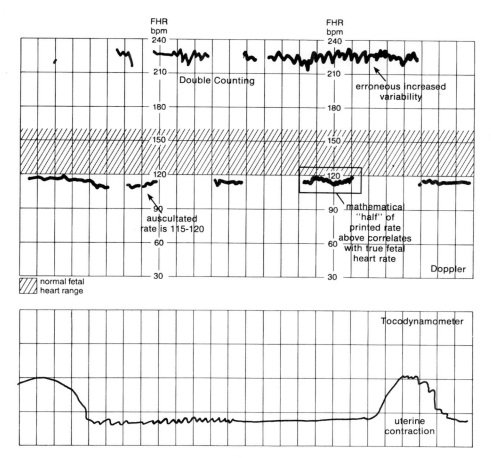

Pattern Characteristic:
Tachycardia Produced by
Artifact

Tachycardia Produced by Paper Insertion: Artifact

With older fetal monitors, it is possible to insert the recording paper reversed. When this occurs, the normal fetal heart trace is located on the uterine pressure portion of the paper and the uterine activity recording is usually located in the tachycardia range of the fetal heart rate graph. Uterine contractions become depicted as decelerations, and maternal respiratory motions may simulate beat-to-beat variability.

Retrospective interpretation of the printed tracing could lead to an inaccurate diagnosis of fetal tachycardia.

Most types of fetal monitoring paper have visible indications such as red or black lines marking the end of the strip. This reduces the possibility of paper insertion error, as does attention to the paper perforations.

Newer monitors periodically add printed information to the tracing such as date and time, establishing unequivocally the orientation of the paper in the machine.

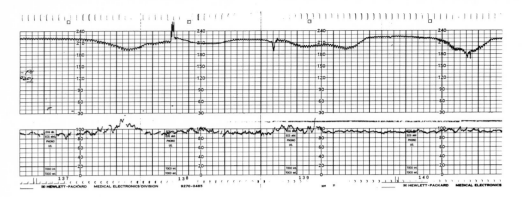

CASE INTERPRETATION: Class V (artifactual)

Baseline Information: marked sinus tachycardia (spurious), beat-to-beat variability is present, there is a spurious unstable wandering baseline.

Periodic or Nonperiodic Changes: prolonged accelerations or intermittent decelerations (spurious).

Uterine Activity: no distinct waveform, trace appears at top of the graph.

Significance: appearance is that which is produced by upside down paper insertion.

CASE OUTCOME: Twenty-eight-year-old gravida 3, para 2002, at 41 weeks' gestation delivered vaginally, with outlet forceps under epidural anesthesia, a 7 pound, 8 ounce (3402 gram) male; Apgar score 8/9. The fetus was in a vertex presentation. The infant followed a normal newborn course. The fetal monitor paper was inserted upside down.

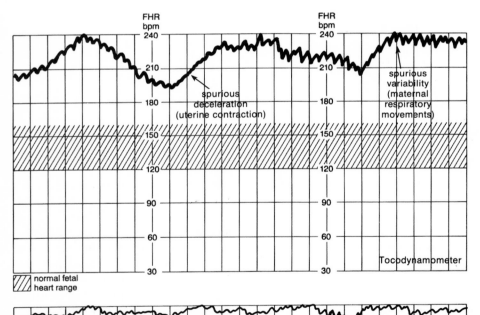

Pattern Characteristic:
Tachycardia Produced by Paper Insertion Artifact

References

1. Beard RW, Filshie GM, Knight CA, et al: The significance of the changes in the continuous fetal heart rate in the first stage of labour. *J Obstet Gynaecol Br Commonwealth* 78:865, 1971.
2. Bergmans MGM, Jonker GJ, Kock HCLV: Fetal supraventricular tachycardia. Review of the literature. *Obstet Gynecol Surv* 40:61, 1985.
3. Cibils LA: Clinical significance of fetal heart rate patterns during labor. *Am J Obstet Gynecol* 123:473, 1975.
4. Cohen WR, Schifrin BS: Diagnosis and treatment of fetal distress, in *Perinatal Medicine*, 1st ed. Baltimore, Williams & Wilkins, 1977, p. 141.
5. Cunningham FG, MacDonald PC, Gant NF: The morphologic and functional development of the fetus, in *Williams Obstetrics*, 18th ed. Norwalk, CT, Appleton and Lange, 1989, p. 102.
6. Druzin ML, Hutson JM, Edersheim TG: Relationship of baseline fetal heart rate to gestational age and fetal sex. *Am J Obstet Gynecol* 154:1102, 1986.
7. Fetal heart rate monitoring. Guideline for monitoring, terminology and instrumentation. *ACOG Technical Bulletin*. no. 32, June 1975.
8. Freeman RK, Garite TJ: *Basic Pattern Recognition in Fetal Heart Rate Monitoring.* Baltimore, Williams & Wilkins, 1981, pp. 63, 78.
9. Gabbe SG, Nelson LM, Paul RH: Fetal heart rate response to acute hemorrhage. *Obstet Gynecol* 49:247, 1977.
10. Gaziano EP: A study of variable decelerations in association with other heart rate patterns during monitored labor. *Am J Obstet Gynecol* 135:360, 1979.
11. Gleicher N, Elkayam U: *Intrauterine Dysrhythmias in Cardiac Problems in Pregnancy*, New York, Alan R. Liss, 1982.
12. Hager WD, Pauly TH: Fetal tachycardia as an indicator of maternal and neonatal morbidity. *Obstet Gynecol* 66:191, 1985.
13. Hobel CJ: Intrapartum clinical assessment of fetal distress. *Am J Obstet Gynecol* 110:336, 1971.
14. Krebs HB, Petres RE, Dunn LG, et al: Intrapartum fetal heart rate monitoring. I. Classification and prognosis of fetal heart rate patterns. *Am J Obstet Gynecol* 133:762, 1979.
15. Kubli FW, Hon EH, Khazin AF, et al: Observations on heart rate and pH in the human fetus during labor. *Am J Obstet Gynecol* 104:1190, 1969.
16. Losure TA, Roberts NS: In utero diagnosis of atrial flutter by means of real-time-directed M-mode echocardiography. *Am J Obstet Gynecol* 149:903, 1984.
17. Martin CB: Regulation of the fetal heart rate and genesis of FHR patterns. *Seminars in Perinatology* 2:131, 1978.
18. Martin CB, Nijhus JG, Weijer AA: Correction of fetal supraventricular tachycardia by compression of the umbilical cord: Report of a case. *Am J Obstet Gynecol* 150:326, 1984.
19. Maxwell KD, Kearney KK, Johnson JWC, et al: Fetal tachycardia associated with intrauterine fetal thyrotoxicosis. *Obstet Gynecol* 55:188, 1980.
20. Mueller-Heubach E, Myers RE, Adamsons K: Maternal factors affecting fetal condition during labor and delivery. *OB/GYN Digest*, Oct. 1974, p. 11.
21. Odendaal HJ, Kotze TJvW: The significance of tachycardia during antenatal fetal heart rate monitoring. *S Afr Med J* 58:881, 1980.
22. Parer JT: The fetal heart rate monitor, in *Handbook of Fetal Heart Rate Monitoring.* Philadelphia, W.B. Saunders, 1983, p. 59.
23. Pritchard JA, MacDonald PC, Gant NF: The morphologic and functional development of the fetus, in *Williams Obstetrics*. Norwalk, CT, Appleton-Century-Crofts, 1985, p. 152.
24. Schiano MA, Hauth JC, Gilstrap LC: Second-stage fetal tachycardia and neonatal infection. *Am J Obstet Gynecol* 148:779, 1984.
25. Shenker L: Fetal cardiac arrhythmias. *Obstet Gynecol Surv* 34:561, 1979.
26. Sureau C: The stress of labor, in *Clinical Perinatology*. St. Louis, C.V. Mosby, 1974, p. 320.
27. Tejani N, Mann LI, Bhakthavathsalan A, et al: Prolonged fetal bradycardia with recovery—its significance and outcome. *Am J Obstet Gynecol* 122:975, 1975.
28. Volpe R, Ehrlich R, Steiner G, et al: Graves' disease in pregnancy years after hypothyroidism with recurrent passive-transfer neonatal Graves' disease in offspring. *Am J Med* 77:572, 1984.
29. Walker DW, Wood C: Temperature relationship of the mother and fetus during labor. *Am J Obstet Gynecol* 107:83, 1970.

Increased Variability—Saltatory Pattern

Chapter 5

Increased Variability

*I*ncreased variability, excessive variability, marked variability, exaggerated variability, and saltatory pattern are all terms referring to rapid fluctuations of fetal heart rate of greater than 25 bpm in amplitude.[11] Webster's Dictionary defines saltatory as "characterized by leaping or dancing, proceeding by abrupt movements or changing by sudden variation."[21,24] The pattern is induced by fetal hypoxemia.[18,21]

Variability (or sinus arrhythmia) is generally believed to be produced by stimulation alternating with withdrawal of parasympathetic activity. Increased variability is therefore presumed to be a reflection of excessive vagal activity.[10,14] This concept is consistent with the frequent association of increased variability with bradycardia, believed to be secondary to increased parasympathetic tone during fetal head compression, and with the mature or postdate fetus with its fully developed parasympathetic system.

The saltatory pattern is distinguished from a sinusoidal pattern by its sharp oscillatory features (as opposed to the smooth, undulating features).[11] It has been noted during periods of increased fetal activity.[1,22] An association with hypertonic labor, postdate pregnancy meconium aspiration, ephedrine administration, bradycardia, and deceleration patterns is discussed in this chapter.

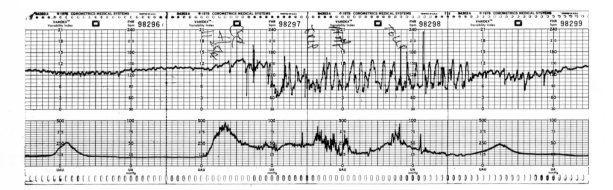

CASE INTERPRETATION: Class II

Baseline Information: normal heart rate and average variability followed by a six minute segment of increased variability at a lower heart rate.

Periodic or Nonperiodic Changes: accelerations present.

Uterine Activity: increased uterine activity is evidenced by an increased baseline tone and a polysystole lack of resting phase that is associated with the increased variability.

Significance: a healthy term or postdate fetus is meeting the hypoxic stress of increased uterine activity with compensatory responses.

CASE OUTCOME: Twenty-one-year-old primigravida, who received epidural anesthesia, delivered vaginally, with elective low forceps, at 40 weeks' gestation a 7 pound, 14 ounce (3572 gram) female; Apgar score 8/9. The fetus was in a vertex presentation. Oxytocin was infused during labor. The infant followed an uncomplicated newborn course.

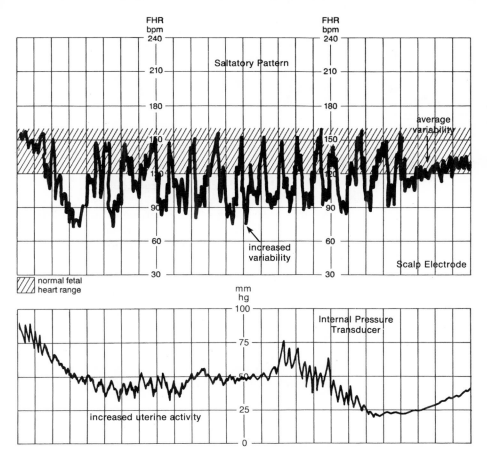

Pattern Characteristic:
Saltatory

Increased Variability Associated with Hypertonic Labor

*T*ypically, variability increases with advancing labor.[12] It is not surprising therefore, that increased variability is almost exclusively a fetal heart rate pattern of the laboring patient. Clinical experience shows a high association with hypertonic labor experienced by a healthy fetus.

The pattern is presumed to be an acute response of the fetus to the mild hypoxemia induced by the increased uterine activity as well as the vagal effects of head compression.[5,18,23] Because it is in a compensated state, it is not surprising that a fetus delivered while demonstrating a heart rate pattern of increased variability is usually vigorous.[4,19] Therefore, an alternative to untimely emergency delivery is removal of the hypoxic stress, (i.e., diminishing the tetanic labor through reduction or discontinuation of oxytocin or through tocolytic therapy). Oxygen administration to the mother, im-

proved uterine perfusion through assumption of a lateral position by the maternal patient, hydration and correction of hypotension, and an attempt to improve the umbilical cord perfusion through a position change are further measures that may allow continued conservative management while awaiting vaginal delivery. Failure to effect a change, however, may ultimately lead to an asphyxiated fetus as oxygen is depleted in spite of compensatory measures.[18]

In the presence of thick meconium, this pattern is associated with an increased risk of meconium aspiration.[6,9] This is in contrast to the decreased risk of meconium aspiration in severely distressed fetuses.[6] The role of delivery timing, delivery route, and pharmacologic therapy in such circumstances awaits clarification.

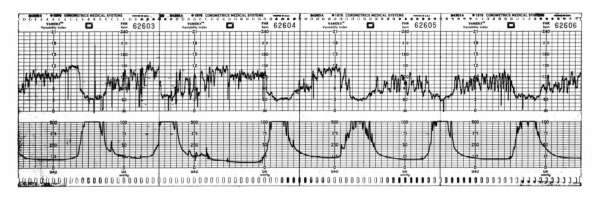

CASE INTERPRETATION: Class II

Baseline Information: increased variability, saltatory pattern. Fluctuating baseline heart rate in the range of low normal to moderate bradycardia.

Periodic or Nonperiodic Changes: moderate variable decelerations may be mixed with the saltatory pattern.

Uterine Activity: excess baseline tone; skewed, prolonged, intense contractions.

Significance: stress pattern of a healthy fetus. An appropriate response is to reduce uterine activity by, for example, decreasing oxytocin infusion if it is in process and administering oxygen to the mother. There may be an increased risk of meconium aspiration if thick meconium is present.

CASE OUTCOME: Twenty-four-year-old gravida 2, para 1001, delivered vaginally soon after the tracing segment, at 38 weeks' gestation, precipitously with no anesthesia, a 6 pound, 5 ounce (2863 gram) male; Apgar score 5/8. No oxytocin was infused intrapartum. A nuchal cord was present. There was no meconium. The infant followed a normal newborn course.

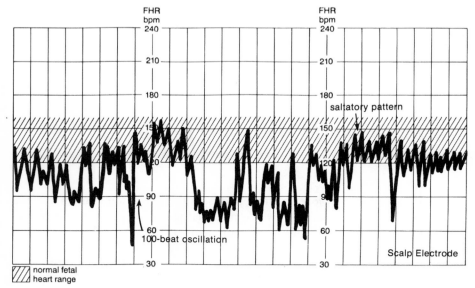

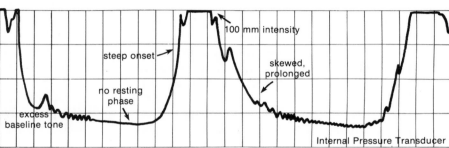

Pattern Characteristic:
Increased Variability Associated with Hypertonic Labor

Increased Variability Associated with Baseline Bradycardia

*T*he combined pattern of baseline bradycardia and increased variability is most commonly seen in late labor, a time of both increased uterine tone and head compression.[4] Both patterns reflect parasympathetic activity and thus are associated in increased frequency with advancing gestation.[2,10]

Good variability is the most important indicator of a healthy fetal condition. The fetus must have an intact and well-functioning autonomic nervous system to produce the fetal heart fluctuations seen. It follows that increased variability also implies a healthy fetus, but the question must be asked: Why is this organism being called upon to produce such marked shifts of heart rate response to maintain homeostasis? Uterine hypertonus is usually the answer.

Control of excessive labor by diminishing oxytocin, using tocolytic therapy, or even decreasing maternal pushing efforts while administering oxygen to the mother may improve the pattern and allow continued conservative management.

Although the presence of increased variability predicts a compensated fetus, a low Apgar score may accompany the pattern when it is associated with thick meconium in the postdate fetus.[9] In such cases, tracheal cleansing techniques and the problems of meconium aspiration may affect the newborn performance. The answer to whether earlier delivery or pharmacologic therapy in such a case would alter the outcome awaits further study.

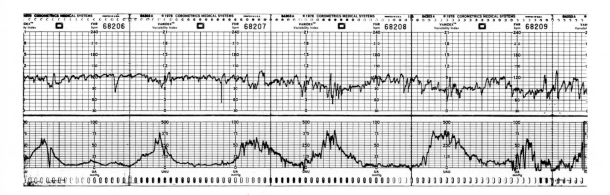

CASE INTERPRETATION: Class II

Baseline Information: moderate to marked bradycardia, increased variability (saltatory pattern).

Periodic or Nonperiodic Changes: possible mild variable decelerations, none are well defined.

Uterine Activity: prolonged, skewed contractions.

Significance: stress pattern of a healthy fetus. Attempts made to reduce uterine activity, if feasible, are in order. If delivery is imminent, continuation of expectant management is appropriate.

CASE OUTCOME: Nineteen-year-old primigravida at 40 weeks' gestation underwent primary cesarean section at 8 centimeters dilatation for cephalopelvic disproportion. She delivered a 7 pound, 8 ounce (3402 gram) male; Apgar score 8/9. The infant followed an uncomplicated newborn course.

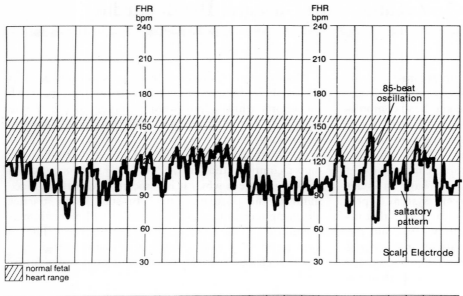

Pattern Characteristic:
Increased Variability Associated
with Baseline Bradycardia

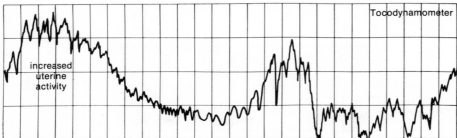

Increased Variability Produced by Ephedrine

*I*ncreased variability has been reported in sheep during increased alpha adrenergic activity that was activated by acute hypoxia.[19] This sympathetic system activity is a response that results in vasoconstriction of nonvital vascular beds. In the human fetus, increased variability is generally accepted as a parasympathetic system response to hypoxia. However, in support of the theory that the adrenergic system has a role in producing this pattern in human fetuses, is the occurrence of increased variability with ephedrine usage, as occurs in the treatment of maternal hypotension during usage of epidural anesthesia.[25] Whatever the mechanisms at play with this pattern, it denotes an intact autonomic nervous system of a fetus successfully using compensatory mechanisms to maintain homeostasis.

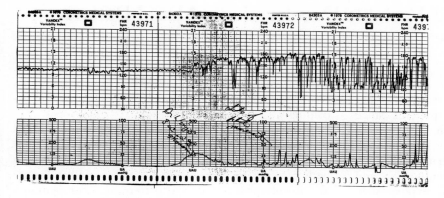

CASE INTERPRETATION: Class II

Baseline Information: normal rate and variability followed by the abrupt onset of increased variability and mild tachycardia after injection of ephedrine in a patient with epidural anesthesia.

Periodic or Nonperiodic Changes: none noted.

Uterine Activity: small contractions. Trace somewhat obscured by apparent spikes of fetal activity.

Significance: response of a healthy fetus to sudden change in the environment that is associated with increased fetal activity.

CASE OUTCOME: Thirty-six-year-old primigravida delivered at 41 weeks' gestation, with epidural anesthesia, a 7 pound, 14 ounce (3572 gram) female; Apgar score 9/9. Elective outlet forceps were used. There was heavy meconium staining. Increased variability occurred with the injection of ephedrine for hypotension associated with epidural administration. The infant followed a normal newborn course.

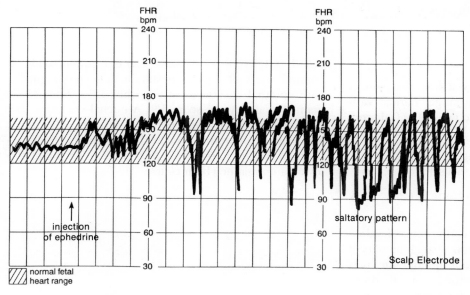

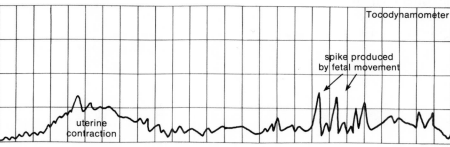

Pattern Characteristic:
Increased Variability Produced by Ephedrine

Increased Variability and Variable Decelerations: Mixed Pattern

*I*ncreased variability is often mixed with mild to moderate variable decelerations. In fact, it is at times not possible to demarcate the respective patterns since abrupt shifts in heart rate occur with both.

It is not surprising to find the two fetal monitoring patterns mixed when it is recognized that variable decelerations often denote umbilical cord compression, and increased variability is a response to mild hypoxia such as can occur with transient cord compression.[11,18] Both patterns are features more common to late labor.

Attempts to improve cord perfusion by altering maternal position and decreasing maternal pushing efforts may improve the pattern. It is important to be alert for a component of hypertonic labor and treat the patient accordingly.

Just as with increased variability alone, the fetus is presumed to be healthy and responding to stressful stimuli. There is an increased risk of a low Apgar score when both patterns are seen together.[15] Sharp oscillations are key to interpretation of the pattern as a compensated state. Smoothing of the features of either the increased variability or the variable decelerations is less reassuring.[8]

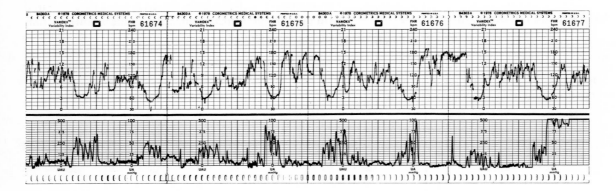

CASE INTERPRETATION: Class II

Baseline Information: unstable baseline, heart rate is often in the moderate bradycardia range, normal variability is interspersed with increased variability (saltatory pattern).

Periodic or Nonperiodic Changes: mild to severe variable decelerations are mixed with a saltatory pattern.

Uterine Activity: contraction waveform is replaced by maternal straining.

Significance: stress pattern of a healthy fetus. Evaluation of uterine activity and reduction of such activity if it is excessive and feasible to do so is appropriate, as is administration of oxygen to the mother. Continued expectant management is in order if the pattern improves and delivery is imminent. Further fetal stress is ideally avoided. There is an increased risk of meconium aspiration if thick meconium is present.

CASE OUTCOME: Fifteen-year-old primigravida at approximately 40 weeks' gestation delivered vaginally, with epidural anesthesia, a 6 pound, 12½ ounce (3076 gram) female; Apgar score 3/9. A nuchal cord and 10% placental abruption were noted at delivery. Meconium was present, requiring tracheal suctioning, which accounted for the initial low Apgar score. The infant followed a normal newborn course.

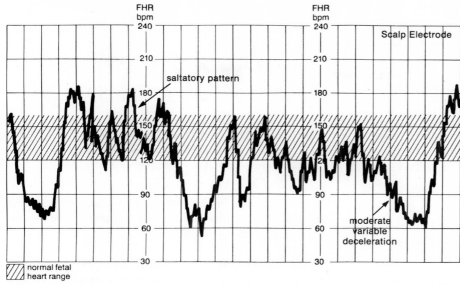

saltatory pattern

Pattern Characteristic:
Increased Variability and
Variable Decelerations: Mixed
Pattern

moderate
variable
deceleration

normal fetal
heart range

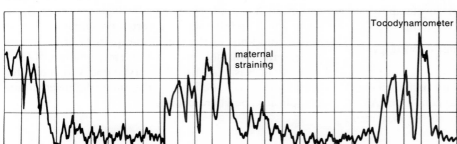

maternal
straining

Increased Variability Associated with Prolonged Deceleration: Mixed Pattern

*I*t is common to encounter increased variability at the onset of a prolonged deceleration and upon recovery.

When seen with prolonged decelerations, the preceding increased variability may reflect an acute compensatory fetal response to the onset of hypoxia until sinus node suppression occurs.[3,23] The etiology of the hypoxia is usually increased uterine activity. Because it reflects a compensated state, fetal pH is expected to be normal during the presence of the increased variability.

When increased variability is again encountered during the recovery phase, it usually denotes a healthy fetus, although the pattern is often followed by transient diminished variability.[13,18] See page 110 for a discussion of decreased variability upon recovery from a prolonged deceleration.

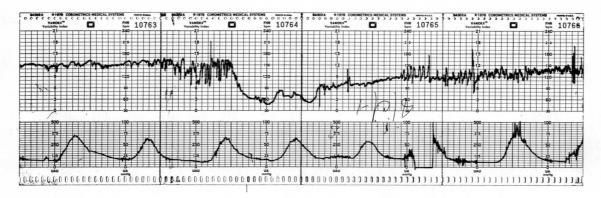

CASE INTERPRETATION: Class II

Baseline Information: normal rate and variability followed by transient saltatory pattern upon entry into and recovery from a prolonged deceleration.

Periodic or Nonperiodic Changes: two minutes of sinus node suppression in a prolonged deceleration with incomplete recovery in the depicted segment.

Uterine Activity: elevated basal tone; skewed, peaked contractions.

Significance: transient fetal stress with partial recovery depicted. Good basic underlying fetal condition. An attempt to reduce uterine activity, if feasible, may result in improvement in the pattern. Expectant management in a lateral decubitus position is appropriate if full recovery occurs with no recurrence.

CASE OUTCOME: Sixteen-year-old primigravida delivered vaginally, with local anesthesia, at 41 weeks' gestation an 8 pound, 9 ounce (3884 gram) male; Apgar score 7/9. The fetus was in a vertex presentation. There was a true knot in the cord. The pattern of prolonged deceleration did not recur. A moderate amount of fresh meconium was noted at delivery; none was recovered with DeLee trap suctioning. The infant followed an uncomplicated newborn course.

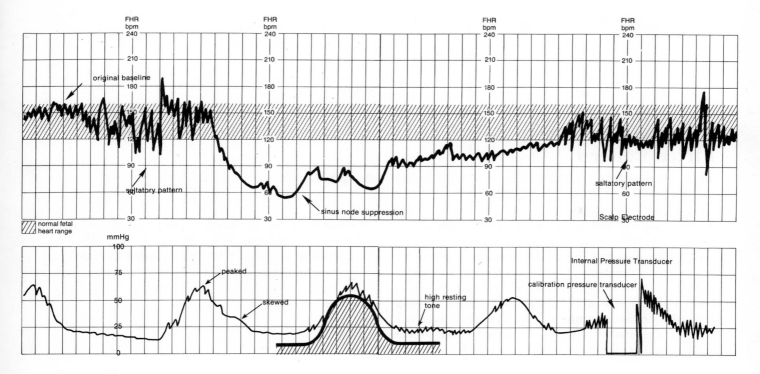

Pattern Characteristic:
Increased Variability Associated with Prolonged Deceleration

Increased Variability—Periodic, Late

*L*ate increased variability, a similar pattern to late decelerations with normal variability, signifies mild hypoxia.[19] As with other examples of increased variability, increased uterine activity is the most common cause of the mild hypoxia in an intrapartum setting.

Although it is a healthy fetus who responds to mild hypoxia with increased variability, in an antepartum set-

ting, this pattern, obtained during fetal assessment by fetal monitoring, is not as reassuring as a nonstress test demonstrating normal variability. See page 223 for further discussion of this pattern.

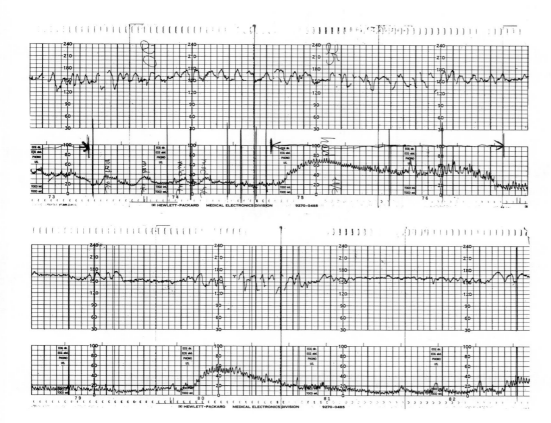

CASE INTERPRETATION: Class II

Baseline Information: high normal rate to moderate tachycardia, normal variability. Episodes of increased variability occur late, in association with uterine contractions.

Periodic or Nonperiodic Changes: variable nonperiodic accelerations.

Uterine Activity: prolonged, skewed contractions.

Significance: healthy but stressed fetus. When encountered during antepartum testing, an appropriate response is to manage the fetus as though late decelerations were encountered.

CASE OUTCOME: Twenty-four-year-old primigravida, with gestational onset diet-controlled diabetes, delivered at 41 weeks' gestation, with midforceps rotation and epidural anesthesia, an 8 pound, 13½ ounce (4011 gram) stillborn male. The placenta culture showed *Escherichia coli* and *Providencia stuartii*. This tracing was obtained during antepartum monitoring three days prior to the intrauterine fetal death.

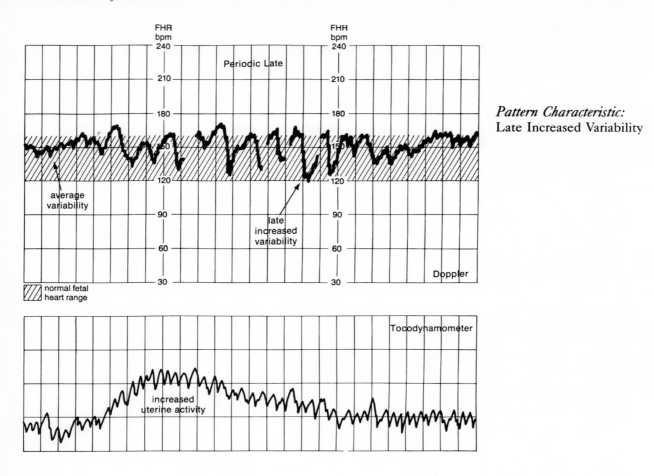

Pattern Characteristic:
Late Increased Variability

Exaggerated Variability Produced by Paper Speed: Artifact

*I*n the United States, 3 cm/min paper speed is used as the basis for fetal monitoring interpretation. In Europe, 1 or 2 cm/min paper speed is used. For prolonged monitoring of a single patient, use of one centimeter paper speed is an economical step, but the change in appearance makes interpretation more difficult.[22] Fetal monitoring interpretation is largely a visual skill, although quantitative methods of variability assessment have been developed to minimize observer bias.[5,16,20,26] Those trained in the use of one or two centimeter paper speed have learned to recognize variations from normal variability at the slower speed.

Failure to note the difference in speed could alter interpretation by either subjective or quantitative methods of evaluation. In addition to exaggerating apparent variability, uterine contractions appear to be peaked, with an increased frequency and a decreased resting phase. Periodic decelerations are altered in character, so that subtle fetal distress may be masked.[7]

The manufacturers of most U.S. fetal monitors have deleted the paper speed options because 3 cm/min has evolved as the speed most commonly used.

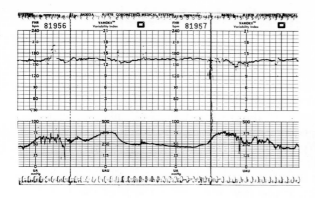
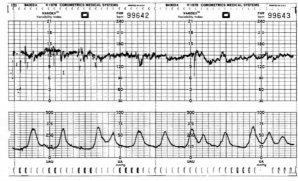

Recreation of original tracing

CASE INTERPRETATION: Class I/III

Comparable segments for the same patient, used in a different hospital, with a different monitor and different paper speed.

Baseline Information: the first segment is of a normal heart rate; the right hand segment shows very mild tachycardia. The variability in the left hand segment appears greater than would be explained solely by the difference in heart rate.

Periodic or Nonperiodic Changes: the small variable deceleration seen on the left may actually be masked late deceleration, as suggested on the right.

Uterine Activity: tachysystole appears in both segments, with a greatly altered appearance.

Significance: there is a slower paper speed in the first segment. Review of a larger segment of tracing for possible fetal distress at 3 cm/min is indicated, unless the clinician is skilled in visual interpretation of a slower paper speed.

CASE OUTCOME: Eighteen-year-old primigravida delivered vaginally at 32 weeks' gestation, with local anesthesia, a 3 pound, 15 ounce (1786 gram) male; Apgar score 9/9. A marginal placental abruption was noted at delivery. The newborn course was uncomplicated except for mild hyperbilirubinemia; the infant was hospitalized for 15 days. The mother had been transferred from another hospital, where the one centimeter paper speed was used.

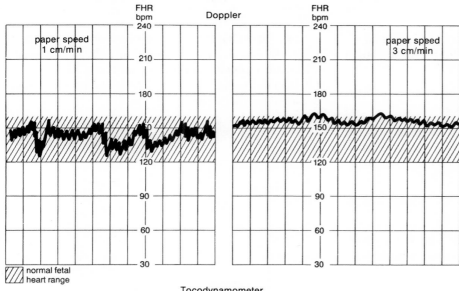

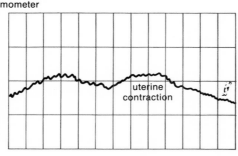

Pattern Characteristic:
Exaggerated Variability. Paper
Speed Artifact

Exaggerated Variability Produced by Paper Scale: Artifact

A paper (Hewlett Packard) with a fetal monitoring scale of 50 to 210 bpm instead of 30 to 240 bpm is in use in Europe and has received trial usage in the United States.

Because the fetal heart seldom is recorded below 50 or above 210 bpm, using the space available on the monitoring paper for the fetal heart trace for a scale limited to 50 to 210 bpm, rarely results in loss of fetal heart rate data. By thus enlarging the space for the normal fetal heart range from one and one-third centimeters to two centimeters, variability is in a sense "blown up" like a photographic enlargement, allowing a better look at it. Due to the importance of beat-to-beat variability in fetal assessment, this could be seen as an advantage. However, transition from the standard paper scale to this scale requires visual retraining. Otherwise, an interpretation of exaggerated variability may lead to a false sense of security about fetal welfare. The reverse occurs when a scale is used that reduces the normal fetal heart range to less than one and one-third centimeters on the monitor paper, as occurs with the second scale on the dual channel of certain machines (Litton). This artifactually compresses variability (see Chap. 17) and, again, requires visual retraining for interpretation.[22]

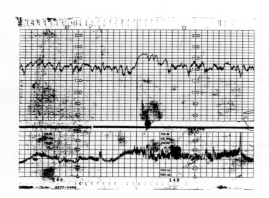 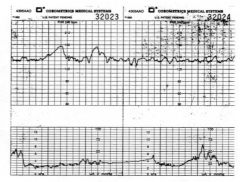

CASE INTERPRETATION: Class I/II (artifactual)

Comparable segments were used for the same patient but with different monitor paper.

Baseline Information: normal heart rate, variability appears greater in the right hand tracing.

Periodic or Nonperiodic Changes: accelerations are present, demonstrating smoothing of variability; acceleration appears taller in the right hand tracing (is actually of less amplitude).

Uterine Activity: small contractions are somewhat obscured by maternal activity/respirations.

Significance: different paper scale. The left is traditional, the right is European. Both denote a healthy fetus.

CASE OUTCOME: Twenty-two-year-old gravida 3, para 1011, at 37 weeks' gestation delivered vaginally, with local/pudendal anesthesia, an 8 pound, 7½ ounce (3841 gram) male; Apgar score 8/9. The infant followed a normal newborn course.

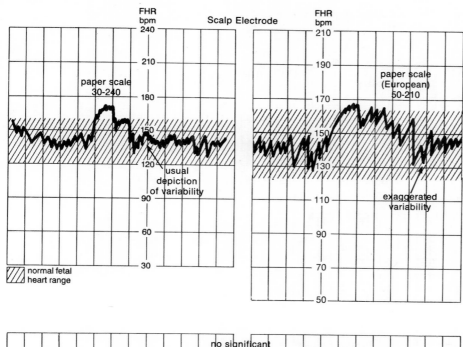

Pattern Characteristic:
Exaggerated Variability. Paper
Speed Artifact

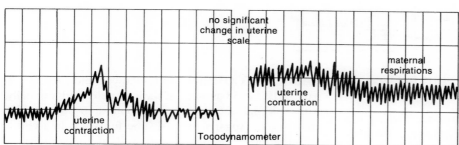

Exaggerated Variability Produced by Doppler Signal Processing—Clarified by Autocorrelation: Artifact

*T*he Doppler signal interpretation of older fetal monitors involves identifying the peak of each waveform produced by the motion-derived fetal heart signal. Each peak triggers the machine to record the beat. To reduce the artifact, some averaging is also used. Because the waveform of a moving fetus and a moving heart is a diffuse nonreproducible signal, the machine may "pick" a different place on the cardiac cycle for each new beat, thus creating exaggerated variability.[19,22,25] Also, cardiac waveforms are all different. When exaggerated variability is displayed, only a scalp-electrode derived signal or obvious acceleration can verify that the fetus is well.

Newer fetal monitors have a markedly improved fetal heart rate signal detection and recording. The Doppler signal for one beat is stored by computer and is sliced into numerous points. The waveform of the next beat, also sliced into numerous points, is overlaid on the first. The computer then matches the corresponding points and more accurately "picks" the same place on each cardiac cycle. This makes the external monitoring of modern machines essentially comparable to the quality of scalp electrode monitoring.[17] However, if the fetus moves away from the Doppler, the monitor may lose the signal.

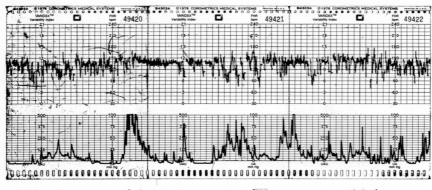

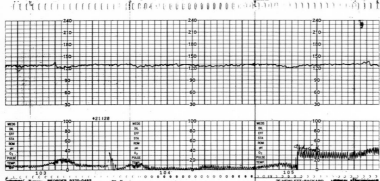

CASE INTERPRETATION: *Segment 1*—Class II (artifactual)/III

Baseline Information: normal heart rate. Tracing has the appearance of increased variability, but the first generation external monitor may exaggerate variability.

Periodic or Nonperiodic Changes: none identifiable.

Uterine Activity: much maternal activity is recorded; contractions appear irregular and skewed.

CASE INTERPRETATION: *Segment 2*—Class III

Baseline Information: normal heart rate, low normal beat-to-beat variability, absent long-term variability.

Periodic or Nonperiodic Changes: none noted.

Uterine Activity: maternal respirations and small uterine contractions.

Significance: the first segment is uninterpretable because of artifactual-increased variability. The second segment demonstrates sufficient reduction in beat-to-beat variability to warrant review of the entire tracing for accelerations or areas of improved variability. Internal monitoring, fetal pH, or continued observation with external monitoring may be in order.

CASE OUTCOME: Twenty-one-year-old gravida 2, para 0010, at 38 weeks' gestation, delivered vaginally, with epidural anesthesia, an 8 pound, 6 ounce (3799 gram) male; Apgar score 9/9. The fetus was in a vertex presentation. The infant followed an uncomplicated newborn course.

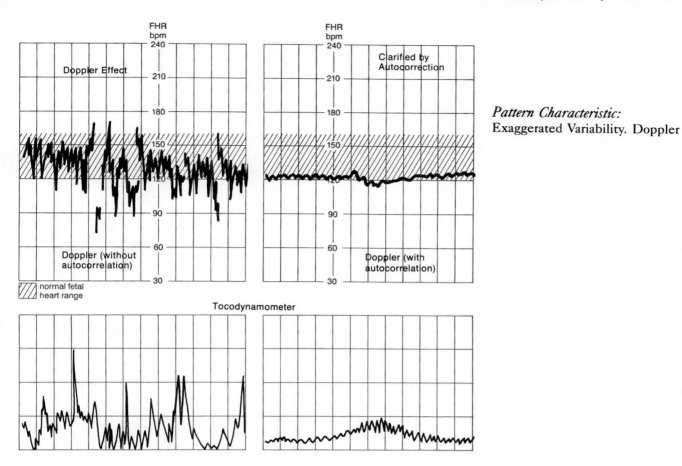

Pattern Characteristic:
Exaggerated Variability. Doppler

Exaggerated Variability Produced by Doppler Signal Processing—Clarified by Internal Monitor: Artifact

*T*he external Doppler transducer, particularly of early fetal monitors, may transmit erroneous variability.[19,25]

The reason for the artifactual variability is because the Doppler signal is derived from the movement of the fetal heart. This is a diffuse signal with systolic and diastolic components, making it impossible for a comparable moment to be selected in each cardiac cycle.[22] The scalp electrode enables transmission of the more precise signal of the fetal QRS. If reassuring reactivity is not observed with external fetal monitoring, a scalp electrode may assist fetal assessment, even in the presence of what appears to be good variability. When variability appears adequate with external monitoring, it may be actually diminished by internal heart rate monitoring. When variability appears decreased by external monitoring, it usually proves to be decreased by scalp electrode monitoring. This problem of erroneous variability, as displayed by external monitoring, is minimized by newer fetal monitors through the improved technology of autocorrelation.

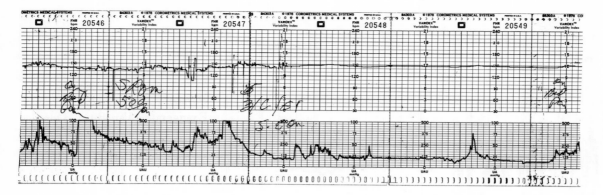

CASE INTERPRETATION: Class III

Baseline Information: normal fetal heart rate. Variability, although diminished, appears to be present until the scalp electrode is placed.

Periodic or Nonperiodic Changes: single, mild variable deceleration.

Uterine Activity: not well recorded, possible polysystole.

Significance: nondiagnostic pattern. Obtaining fetal pH is one option in response to this pattern.

CASE OUTCOME: Eighteen-year-old primigravida at 35 weeks' gestation delivered vaginally, with pudendal anesthesia, a 6 pound, 5 ounce (2863 gram) female; Apgar score 2/4. Scalp pHs in labor were 7.30 to 7.34. The pregnancy was complicated by preeclampsia. The mother was given magnesium sulfate and oxytocin. She also received meperidine and promethazine while in labor. The newborn was dismissed from the hospital at four days of life.

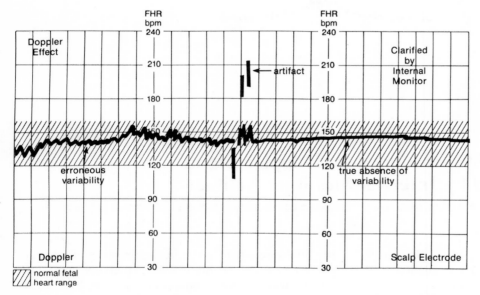

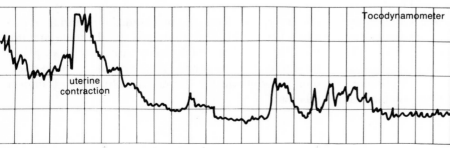

Pattern Characteristic:
Exaggerated Variability. Doppler

References

1. Brotanek V, Scheffs J: The pathogenesis and significance of saltatory patterns in the fetal heart rate. *Int J Gynaecol Obstet* 11:223, 1973.
2. Cibils LA: *Saltatory Pattern in Electronic Fetal-Maternal Monitoring: Antepartum, Intrapartum.* Boston, PSG Publishing, 1981, p. 274.
3. Dalton KJ, Dawes GS, Patrick JE: Diurnal, respiratory, and other rhythms of fetal heart rate in lambs. *Am J Obstet Gynecol* 127:414, 1977.
4. Divon MY, Muskat Y, Platt LD, et al: Increased beat-to-beat variability during uterine contractions: A common association in uncomplicated labor. *Am J Obstet Gynecol* 149:893, 1984.
5. Divon MY, Platt LD, Miskat Y, et al: Quantification of changes in fetal heart rate and beat-to-beat variability during labor. *Am J Perinatology* 3:63, 1986.
6. Dooley SL, Pesavento DJ, Depp R, et al: Meconium below the vocal cords at delivery: Correlation with intrapartum events. *Am J Obstet Gynecol* 153:767, 1985.
7. Floyd JS: Paper speed in electronic fetal heart rate monitoring (letter). *Am J Obstet Gynecol* 156:212, 1987.
8. Gaziano EP: A study of variable decelerations in association with other heart rate patterns during monitored labor. *Am J Obstet Gynecol* 135:360, 1979.
9. Goodlin RC: Fetal cardiovascular response to distress. *Obstet Gynecol* 49:371, 1977.
10. Goodlin RC: Detrimental perinatal associations with increased fetal reactivity. *Am J Obstet Gynecol* 149:801, 1984.
11. Hammacher K, Huter KA, Bokelmann J, et al: Foetal heart frequency and perinatal condition of the foetus and newborn. *Gynaecologia* 166:319, 1968.
12. Huey JR, Paul RH, Hadjiev AA, et al: Fetal heart rate variability: An approach to automated assessment. *Am J Obstet Gynecol* 134:691, 1979.
13. Hutson JM, Mueller-Heubach E: Diagnosis and management of intrapartum reflex fetal heart rate changes. *Clinics in Perinatology* 9:325, 1982.
14. Ikenoue T, Martin CB, Murata Y, et al: Effect of acute hypoxemia and respiratory acidosis on the fetal heart rate in monkeys. *Am J Obstet Gynecol* 141:797, 1981.
15. Krebs HB, Petres RE, Dunn LJ, et al: Intrapartum fetal heart rate monitoring. I. Classification and prognosis of fetal heart rate patterns. *Am J Obstet Gynecol* 133:762, 1979.
16. Laros RK, Wong WS, Heilbron DC, et al: A comparison of methods for quantitating fetal heart rate variability. *Am J Obstet Gynecol* 128:381, 1977.
17. Lawson GW, Belcher R, Dawes GS, et al: A comparison of ultrasound (with autocorrelation) and direct electrocardiogram fetal heart rate detector systems. *Am J Obstet Gynecol* 147:721, 1983.
18. Martin CB: Physiology and clinical use of fetal heart rate variability. *Clinics in Perinatology* 9:339, 1982.
19. Parer JT: The fetal heart rate monitor, in *Handbook of Fetal Heart Rate Monitoring.* Philadelphia, W.B. Saunders, 1983, pp. 60ff., 141ff.
20. Parer WJ, Parer JT, Holbrook RH, et al: Validity of mathematical methods of quantitating fetal heart rate variability. *Am J Obstet Gynecol* 153:402, 1985.
21. Petrie RH, Yeh S-Y, Murata Y, et al: The effect of drugs on fetal heart rate variability. *Am J Obstet Gynecol* 130:294, 1978.
22. Paul RH, Suidan AK, Yeh S, et al: Clinical fetal monitoring. VII. The evaluation and significance of intrapartum baseline FHR variability. *Am J Obstet Gynecol* 123:206, 1975.
23. Stange L, Rosen KG, Hokegard KH, et al: Quantification of fetal heart rate variability in relation to oxygenation in the sheep fetus. *Acta Obstet Gynecol Scand* 56:205, 1977.
24. Webster's New World Dictionary, Second College Edition. New York, Simon and Schuster, 1980, p. 1257.
25. Wright RG, Shnider SM, Levinson G, et al: The effect of maternal administration of ephedrine on fetal heart rate and variability. *Obstet Gynecol* 57:734, 1981.
26. Yeh S-Y, Forsythe A, Hon EH: Quantification of fetal heart beat-to-beat interval differences. *Obstet Gynecol* 41:355, 1973.

Decreased Variability

Chapter 6

No Variability, Flat Line—Unfavorable Outcome

No Variability, Flat Line—Favorable Outcome

Decreased Variability Associated with Extreme Prematurity

No Variability Associated with Fetal Neurologic Disease

No Variability, Transient: As with Fetal Sleep

No Variability, Transient, Produced by Half Counting Paroxysmal Tachycardia: Arrhythmia and Artifact

No Variability, Transient, Produced by Stylus Malfunction: Artifact

No Variability: Agonal

No Long-Term Variability, Short-Term Variability Present

No Short-Term Variability, Long-Term Variability Present

No Variability, Accelerations Present: Mixed Pattern

No Variability with Decelerations: Mixed Pattern

No Variability in Accelerations

No Variability During Recovery from a Prolonged Deceleration

No Variability Secondary to Sinus Node Suppression

No Variability Secondary to Bradyarrhythmia

No Variability Secondary to Tachyarrhythmia

No Variability Produced by Disengaged Transducer: Artifact

No Variability, Flat Line—Unfavorable Outcome

*E*xcellent beat-to-beat variability of the fetal heart is the best fetal monitoring indicator for predicting good fetal condition, especially when accompanied by accelerations.[14,24,31] A fetal heart trace derived from the R wave of an electrocardiogram signal provides the most accurate assessment of beat-to-beat variability. Absent variability, whether or not it is in combination with baseline tachycardia, causes concern about fetal welfare. When variability is absent, even if the fetal heart rate is in the normal range and even if there are no periodic changes, there is a lack of ability in using the monitor to determine whether the fetus is well. This is not a pattern *diagnostic* of fetal distress. One simply cannot exclude fetal distress.[20]

The causes of absent variability include:

fetal metabolic acidosis[32,39]

neurologic abnormality[48]

marked prematurity[12]

cardiac arrhythmia[32]

drug effect[2,41]

fetal sleep[27,51]

fetal inactivity[23,33]

variant of unknown cause seen in a normal fetus

A decrease in variability also accompanies a progressive increase in the baseline rate (see page 148).[42]

With such a wide range of causes of absent variability, which runs the gamut from signaling a healthy fetus to a dying fetus, additional information that assures one of the fetus's well-being must be obtained (such as by fetal pH determination) for conservative management of the viable fetus to be continued. The inability to obtain fetal pH studies (or acquire other reassuring information, for example, from fetal stimulation) usually warrants delivery. A pattern of no variability and an elevated baseline rate has been associated with fetal brain death and inevitable neonatal death.[36] The ability to make such a diagnosis in utero consistently enough to avoid cesarean section for nonviable fetuses awaits further study.

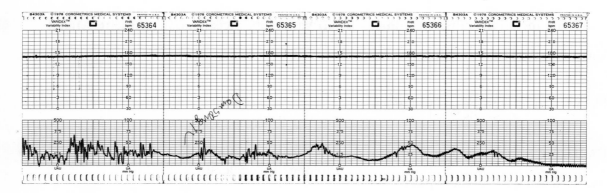

CASE INTERPRETATION: Class III

Baseline Information: moderate tachycardia, fixed rate, absent variability.

Periodic or Nonperiodic Changes: none.

Uterine Activity: frequent, prolonged contractions.

Significance: not diagnostic of the fetal condition. Appropriate management is exclusion of fetal acidosis if the pattern persists.

CASE OUTCOME: Nineteen-year-old primigravida at 34½ weeks' gestation delivered vaginally, more than 75 minutes after the displayed segment, a 5 pound, 4 ounce (2381 gram) female, from a vertex presentation, in an occiput posterior position; Apgar score 2/3. The mother was given pudendal/local anesthesia. The mean of four

nonacidotic intrapartum capillary pHs was 7.27, two and a half hours prior to delivery. Meperidine was administered one hour prior to this segment. The pregnancy was complicated by chorioamnionitis and maternal pyelonephritis. The newborn required endotracheal intubation for apnea. The infant survived and was dismissed at nine days of age.

COMMENT: At no time did the fetal heart trace revert to a pattern with normal variability. The normal pHs suggest that the low Apgar score was based on a cause other than metabolic acidosis. The fetal monitor provided no help in clarifying the fetal condition or predicting the newborn course. In actuality, when compared to fetal brain death, which is associated with a pattern identical to that displayed here, this case represents a favorable outcome.

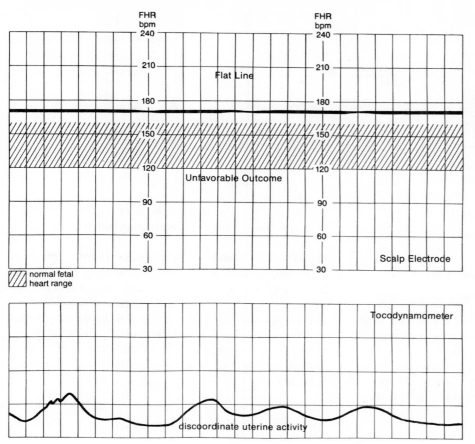

FHR
bpm

Flat Line

Pattern Characteristic:
No Variability. Unfavorable
Outcome

Unfavorable Outcome

normal fetal
heart range

Scalp Electrode

Tocodynamometer

discoordinate uterine activity

No Variability, Flat Line—Favorable Outcome

*T*he presence of excellent beat-to-beat variability provides the best fetal monitoring reassurance of good fetal condition, especially when accompanied by accelerations. Absence of variability limits the usefulness of the heart rate monitor to predict fetal outcome. The fetus may be normal, but the information present on the fetal heart trace is insufficient to exclude a sick fetus.[44] The fact that the heart rate is in a normal range is not reassuring because a normal rate may be maintained in a terminally ill fetus until moments before death. The fact that there are no periodic changes, particularly hypoxic in type (late decelerations or atypical variable decelerations), is not reassuring because with severe asphyxia, myocardial depression may be so marked that the fetal heart is unable to respond to further hypoxia changes by decelerating. Hypoxia may be so prolonged and severe

that contractions fail to elicit further changes.[19] The presence of accelerations is not consistently reassuring because in the very sick fetus only the prolonged secondary acceleration component of an atypical variable deceleration may be preserved and misdiagnosed as an acceleration (see page 160). The fact that the patient received drugs cannot be assumed to be the cause of the absent variability, unless fetal acidosis has been excluded or excellent variability was documented prior to administration of the drug, and no hypoxic periodic fetal heart rate changes have intervened.[34]

The fact that a fetus is premature should not be assumed to be the cause of absent variability, unless fetal acidosis is excluded. Variability may be reduced but is seldom absent on the basis of prematurity alone (see page 93).

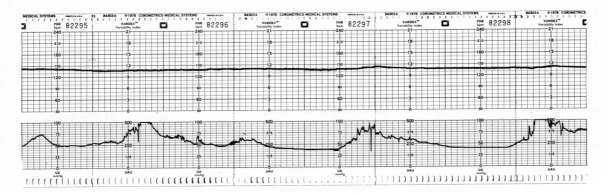

CASE INTERPRETATION: Class III

Baseline Information: normal rate, fixed. Absent variability.

Periodic or Nonperiodic Changes: none.

Uterine Activity: prolonged, skewed contractions.

Significance: nondiagnostic of fetal condition. If the pattern persists, management involves determination of a fetal pH that demonstrates the absence of fetal acidosis or delivery, unless other reassuring information is obtained, for example, from fetal stimulation, or study of the entire tracing. A good fetal condition prior to admin-istration of the narcotic, without any ensuing hypoxic changes, is an example of reassuring information.

CASE OUTCOME: Eighteen-year-old primigravida at 40 weeks' gestation delivered vaginally, with pudendal anesthesia, a 6 pound, 9 ounce (2977 gram) female; Apgar score 8/8. The fetus was in a vertex presentation. No pH studies were done. The mother received meperidine and promethazine intrapartum. Subsequent to this segment, accelerations and mild variable decelerations were displayed. The infant followed an uncomplicated newborn course.

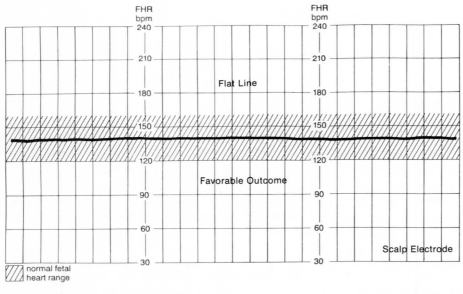

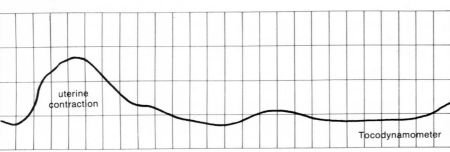

Pattern Characteristic:
No Variability. Favorable Outcome

Decreased Variability Associated with Extreme Prematurity

*B*eat-to-beat variability is governed by the parasympathetic nervous system. This system matures with advancing gestational age.[1,3,13] In fact, an association between decreased beat-to-beat variability and respiratory distress syndrome in the neonate has been noted.[6,35] It is not surprising, therefore, that the second-trimester and early-third-trimester healthy fetus does not consistently demonstrate normal or average variability.[30] A wandering baseline often reflects the developing long-term variability. (See pages 160–164 for other examples of a wandering baseline.) The finding of cyclic variation between patterns of no variability and variability in the fetus who may be too preterm for accelerations is somewhat reassuring.[48]

Without variability, the single best predictor of good fetal condition, fetal monitoring tracings are difficult to interpret at gestations occurring at the onset of viability.[5,45] The diminished variability should not be assumed to be solely on the basis of prematurity. When antepartum monitoring is used for interpretation in these fetuses, adjuncts to monitoring are frequently necessary for fetal assessment, for example, a biophysical profile and, when not contraindicated, contraction stress testing.

A biophysical profile and contraction stress testing are not consistently helpful in predicting the fetal outcome of the intrapartum patient.[19,43] In labor, a fetal pH or monitoring of the fetal heart rate response to stimulation is more useful for fetal assessment.

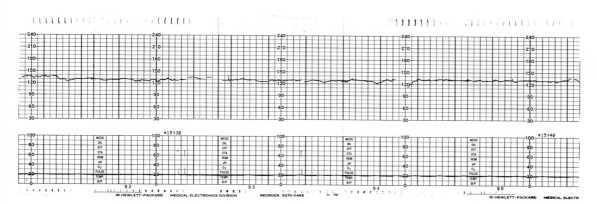

CASE INTERPRETATION: Class III

Baseline Information: normal heart rate; diminished short-term, minimal long-term variability; and a wandering baseline.

Periodic or Nonperiodic Changes: absent.

Uterine Activity: none recorded.

Significance: nondiagnostic pattern. This pattern is seen with an immature fetus. Good fetal welfare should be documented if this is a viable fetus. Appropriate management of the intrapartum patient of a viable gestation may include a fetal pH or fetal stimulation. If hypoxia is suspected and the gestation is viable, appropriate management of the antepartum patient is stress testing, a biophysical profile, or other fetal welfare assessment.

CASE OUTCOME: Twenty-two-year-old gravida 4, para 3003, delivered vaginally, with local anesthesia, at 40 weeks' gestation a 6 pound, 13 ounce (3090 gram) male; Apgar score 9/9. The infant followed a normal newborn course. The patient had been evaluated at 25 weeks' gestation (at the time of the displayed tracing) for a urinary tract infection and anemia.

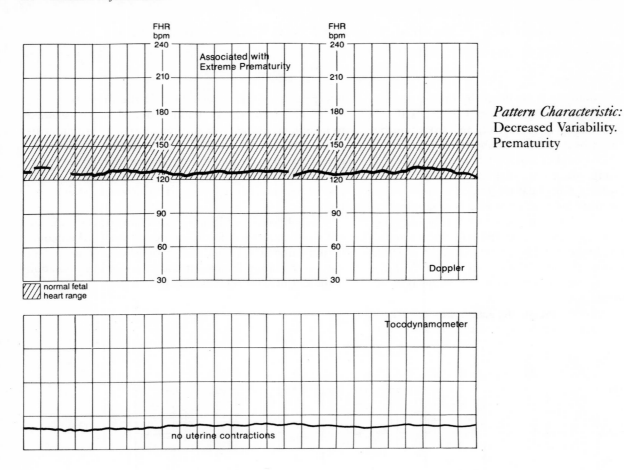

Pattern Characteristic:
Decreased Variability.
Prematurity

No Variability Associated with Fetal Neurologic Disease

*B*ecause variability is an end product of a well-functioning nervous system,[53] it is not surprising that abnormalities seen in the monitoring records of some fetuses with certain neurologic disorders such as anencephaly and hydrocephaly include the absence of variability. The majority of anencephalic fetuses demonstrate a diminution or complete loss of variability.[7,40,47] When beat-to-beat variability is present in the anencephalic fetus, it usually indicates that some degree of cerebral cortex is present. When decreased variability is encountered in cases with severe hydrocephalus, increased intracranial pressure is postulated as a contributing factor (see page 162).

The fetus with severe neurologic disease often suffers hypoxia and acidosis in labor, providing another potential etiology of the absent variability.

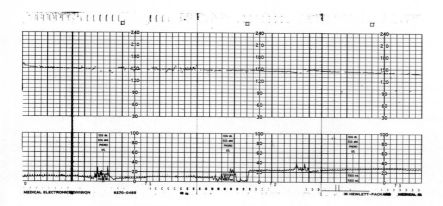

CASE INTERPRETATION: Class III

Baseline Information: high normal rate, absent variability, drifting baseline.

Periodic or Nonperiodic Changes: atypical variable deceleration with absent primary acceleration, prolonged secondary acceleration.

Uterine Activity: not recorded.

Significance: a nondiagnostic pattern. Further fetal assessment is indicated.

CASE OUTCOME: Seventeen-year-old primigravida at 34 weeks' gestation delivered vaginally a 3 pound, 1 ounce (1389 gram) anencephalic male stillborn. Other segments of the fetal monitoring intrapartum tracing demonstrated severe variable decelerations with atypia. In this case, the absent variability may be based on either hypoxia/acidosis or a neurologic problem.

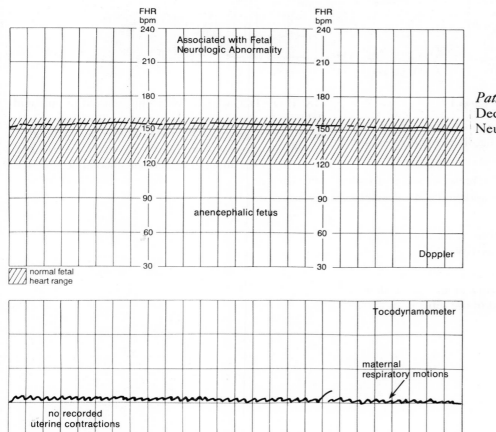

Pattern Characteristic:
Decreased Variability.
Neurologic Disease

No Variability, Transient: As with Fetal Sleep

*V*ariability in the fetus indicates autonomic nervous system responsiveness, particularly in the parasympathetic system, to varying stimuli. This responsiveness is diminished during fetal sleep cycles. These usually last 15 to 30 minutes at a time but not more than 60 minutes.[4,33,36,51] The fetus can ordinarily be aroused by manipulation such as scalp stimulation. During sleep, the fetal heart rate trace may demonstrate sufficient reduction in short- and long-term variability to produce a flat-line (fixed heart rate) pattern. When brief sleep segments are bracketed by areas of normal variability and reactivity, the flat-line traces should not bear an ominous connotation.[33] The fetal heart tracing cannot typically undergo a transition from normal variability and reactivity to a flat-line pattern *on the basis of hypoxia-induced acidosis* without traversing through a segment of hypoxic periodic or nonperiodic changes. On the other hand, if no areas of normal variability with reactivity bracket a flat-line segment, it cannot be assumed to be on the basis of fetal sleep.

Regular transition from fetal sleep to awake states and back is termed cyclic variation. Noting the presence of cyclic variation is especially useful in assessing the health of the preterm fetus when the ability to display accelerations may not yet be developed.[50] Cyclic variation is a pattern that persists in the healthy newborn.[51]

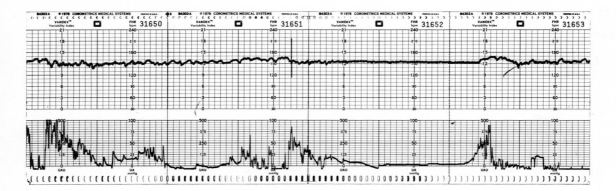

CASE INTERPRETATION: Class I

Baseline Information: high normal rate, normal variability with several minutes of flat-line absent short- and long-term variability.

Periodic or Nonperiodic Changes: accelerations present at the time of normal variability, no decelerations.

Uterine Activity: erratic pattern by tocodynamometer appears distorted by maternal activity.

Significance: a healthy fetus is denoted by the areas of good variability in close proximity to an area of diminished variability. A sleep period of the fetus is an explanation offered for this pattern.

CASE OUTCOME: Twenty-one-year-old primigravida delivered vaginally, with local and pudendal anesthesia, at 41 weeks' gestation an 8 pound, 8 ounce (3856 gram) female; Apgar score 8/9. The fetus was in a vertex presentation. The infant followed an uncomplicated newborn course.

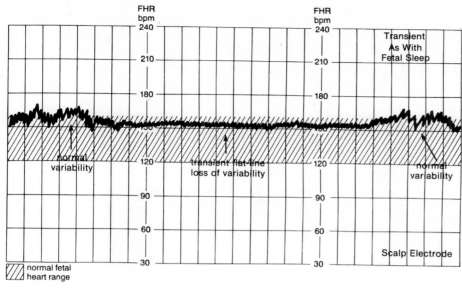

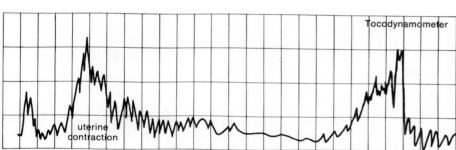

Pattern Characteristic:
No Variability. Fetal Sleep

No Variability, Transient, Produced by Half Counting Paroxysmal Tachycardia: Arrhythmia and Artifact

When an abrupt change occurs from normal variability to a flat-line pattern (absent short- and long-term variability), an arrhythmia or artifact is suspected. Loss of variability on the basis of acidosis, drug effect, or sleep is not abrupt and, in the former situation, there is typically interspersed a pattern of progressive hypoxia.

Most arrhythmias would also result in a heart rate change such as to a bradycardia or tachycardia range. An arrhythmia that at onset would produce an abrupt change in variability with an unchanged heart rate is a rare oc-

currence. Theoretically, atrial flutter with block that resulted in a ventricular rate in the normal fetal heart range could produce such an unusual event.

Double counting or half counting of a bradyarrhythmia or tachyarrhythmia, respectively, are mechanisms by which machine characteristics may serve to maintain a fetal heart rate artifactually in a normal range while displaying the altered variability of the arrhythmia.

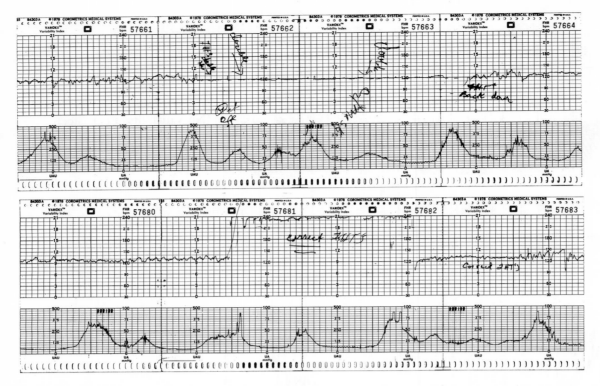

CASE INTERPRETATION: Class I (Class III during arrhythmia)

Baseline Information: 7 to 8 minute segment with no short- or long-term variability, bracketed by average variability.

Periodic or Nonperiodic Changes: accelerations present in segments with average variability.

Uterine Activity: discoordinated uterine activity, rising resting tone, no resting interval.

Significance: this pattern is similar to that seen with fetal sleep periods but abrupt onset and "recovery" is more typical of that seen with monitor malfunction. A tachyarrhythmia with block could also produce such a pattern, as could half counting of a tachyarrhythmia.

CASE OUTCOME: Twenty-year-old white primigravida delivered vaginally, with low elective forceps and epidural anesthesia, at 38½ weeks' gestation a 7 pound, 7 ounce (3374 gram) female; Apgar score 8/8. A paroxysmal tacchyarrhythmia occurred intrapartum. No arrhythmia was noted after birth. The newborn followed an uncomplicated newborn course.

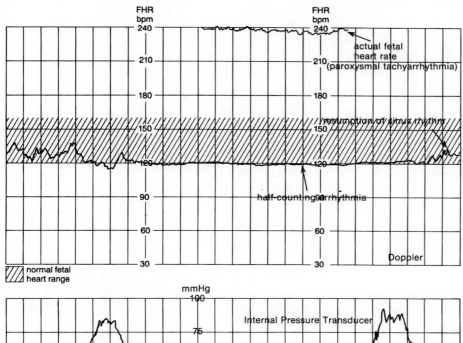

Pattern Characteristic:
No Variability–Produced by Artifactual Processing of Arrhythmia

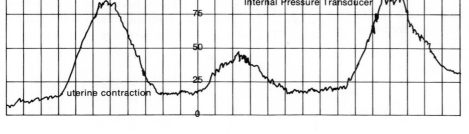

No Variability, Transient, Produced by Stylus Malfunction: Artifact

A malfunctioning stylus of older monitors must be considered in the etiology of flat-line traces, particularly when such traces are interspersed with abrupt changes from a normal reactive baseline that remains in the normal heart rate range.

It is not typical for the fetal heart rate to change from good beat-to-beat variability to sudden flat-line absence of variability unless it does so on the basis of either arrhythmia or artifact. Drug, sleep, or acidosis as causes of loss of variability would be expected to present a gradual change to a flat-line, the latter accompanied first by periodic or nonperiodic hypoxic changes. Arrhythmias with a loss of variability usually are accompanied by a change of the heart rate to a marked tachycardia or marked bradycardia range. An example of an arrhythmia that could rarely produce an abrupt appearance of a flat-line in the normal heart rate range is atrial flutter with block. The preceding case illustrates a similar pattern that was produced by a combination of arrhythmia and artifact.

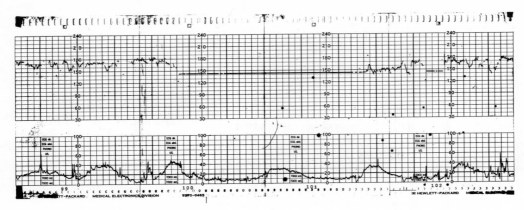

CASE INTERPRETATION: Class I/III

Baseline Information: baseline moderate tachycardia, normal variability; four to five minute segment of flat trace.

Periodic or Nonperiodic Changes: nonperiodic accelerations and small v-shaped variable decelerations.

Uterine Activity: regular contractions with a configuration that is within normal limits recorded by tocodynamometer.

Significance: artifact produced by a problem with the stylus, (tachyarrhythmia with block resulting in a normal heart rate is unlikely).

CASE OUTCOME: Sixteen-year-old primigravida at 44 weeks' gestation delivered vaginally, with local and pudendal anesthesia, a 7 pound, 8¼ ounce (3409 gram) female; Apgar score 9/9. The fetus was in a vertex presentation. The stylus stuck intermittently during monitoring. The infant followed a normal newborn course.

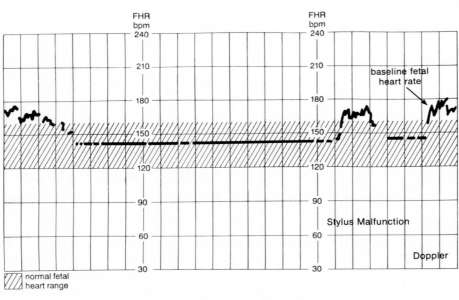

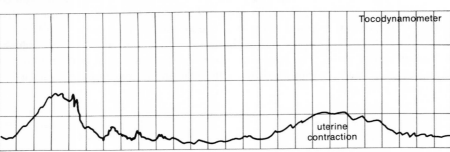

Pattern Characteristic:
No Variability. Artifact

No Variability: Agonal

A dying fetus may maintain a heart rate in the normal range until moments before death. However, short-term variability is always reduced before death in the fetus subjected to prolonged hypoxia and acidosis.[8,37,38] Absence of periodic changes is not reassuring. Late decelerations associated with contractions may be so shallow as to be missed or may be absent because of progressive myocardial depression and because hypoxia is so prolonged and severe that contractions fail to elicit further changes.[15,19,26] The baseline is often, but not always, wandering in appearance.

The administration of narcotic drugs or tranquilizers prior to documenting the fetal condition by fetal monitoring may, unfortunately, contribute to misinterpretation of the significance of the absent variability. External monitoring without autocorrelation may misrepresent the degree of variability. In the absence of periodic changes, which assist diagnosis, fetal pH studies may assist diagnosis. See page 39 for a similar pattern.

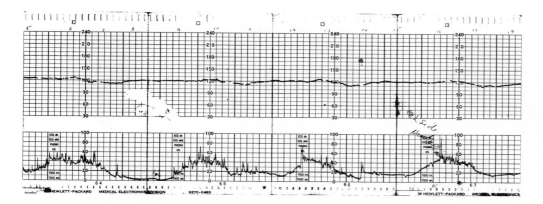

CASE INTERPRETATION: Class III/V

Baseline Information: low normal rate, absent variability, unstable (wandering) baseline.

Periodic or Nonperiodic Changes: shallow late decelerations.

Uterine Activity: regular contractions with configurations within normal limits.

Significance: possible severe fetal distress.

CASE OUTCOME: Fifteen-year-old primigravida delivered at 38 weeks' gestation by emergency cesarean section, with general anesthesia for possible fetal distress, 15 minutes after onset of a sudden prolonged deceleration without recovery, a 9 pound, 1 ounce (4111 gram) female; Apgar score 0/0, but the newborn was resuscitated. The infant expired 14 hours later. The infant was in a vertex presentation. There was "marked" meconium present. The mother received diazepam analgesia. The autopsy revealed perinatal anoxia.

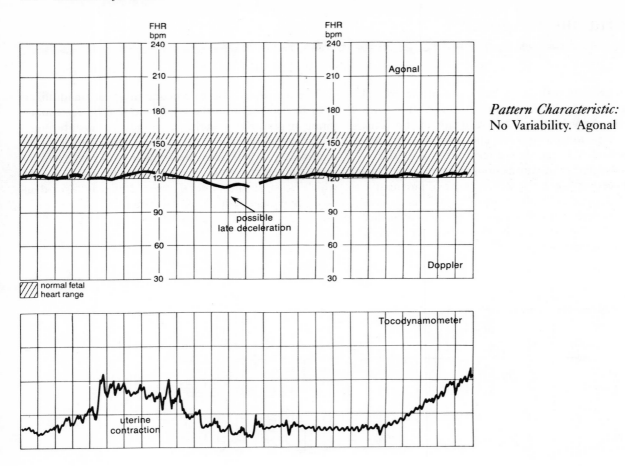

Pattern Characteristic:
No Variability. Agonal

No Long-Term Variability, Short-Term Variability Present

*T*he presence of normal or average (6–10 bpm) short-term (beat-to-beat) variability is a better predictor of fetal condition than is long-term variability.[4,16] Normal long-term variability is defined as fluctuations of 2 to 6 cycles per minute, with an amplitude of 6 to 10 bpm.[16] It may be preserved in a moribund fetus demonstrating no beat-to-beat variability. In such cases, in the absence of the "sharp," jagged effect of short-term variability, the long-term variability often has undulating features. In contrast, when long-term variability is absent, the preservation of short-term variability, albeit diminished (less than 6 bpm) is more reassuring than absent short-term variability. This is the pattern often seen, for example, in a healthy fetus during a sleep cycle (see page 96). However, when such a pattern persists, for example, for longer than 30 minutes, it should be approached with a similar degree of concern as would be applied to other flat-line patterns. It is not *diagnostic* of good fetal condition and has been reported preceding intrapartum fetal

death.[22] Therapy with magnesium sulfate has been demonstrated to reduce variability without obliterating it but may also be associated with an increase in variability or no change, so alterations cannot be *assumed* to be on that basis.[3,9,41,45] Confirmation of normal pH status may be an adjunct in fetal assessment, unless a positive response to fetal stimulation is elicited or excellent reactivity and variability preceded the pattern without intervening hypoxic patterns.

The length of gestation is a factor to be considered when interpreting the pattern.[12] Long-term variability and beat-to-beat variability typically increase with advancing gestation, as the parasympathetic system matures.[17] Therefore, diminished variability increases in significance with progressive gestational age.

Such a rare pattern may be better studied by electrocardiogram-derived beat-to-beat monitoring, even when using instrumentation employing autocorrelation.

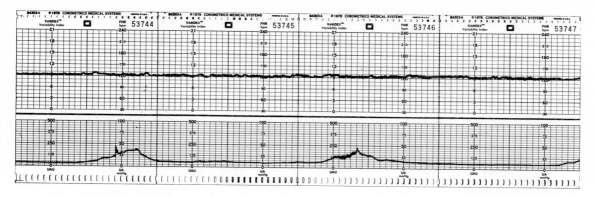

CASE INTERPRETATION: Class III

Baseline Information: absent long-term variability, diminished but present short-term variability with scalp electrode, stable baseline.

Periodic or Nonperiodic Changes: absent.

Uterine Activity: infrequent, prolonged contractions recorded with tocodynamometer.

Significance: more reassuring than absent short-term variability, but fetal pH study may be appropriate unless recent normal variability or reactivity has been documented.

CASE OUTCOME: Seventeen-year-old primigravida delivered at 43 weeks' gestation by primary cesarean section, with general anesthesia, performed for cephalopelvic disproportion, a 7 pound, 10 ounce (3459 gram) female; Apgar score 1/3. The mother had a fever of 102°F prior to delivery. The presence of meconium was noted at delivery. The patient received oxytocin augmentation for chorioamnionitis. Her membranes were ruptured for 15 hours. The mother received magnesium sulfate for preeclampsia. No fetal pH was obtained. The newborn was hospitalized for 10 days. Transient respiratory depression complicated the infant's course. Studies done for sepsis were negative. The newborn received antibiotics for seven days.

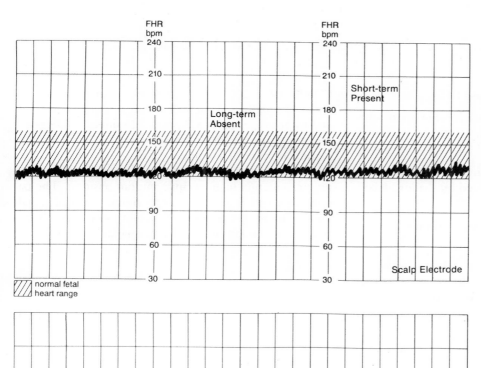

Pattern Characteristic:
No Long-Term Variability

No Short-Term Variability, Long-Term Variability Present

When short-term (beat-to-beat) variability is absent, the fetal monitor is failing to display the major determinant for use in predicting good fetal condition even if long-term variability is present.[4] Although such a pattern is commonly seen after narcotic administration, the presence of long-term variability is not in itself sufficiently reassuring and when undulating or erratic (as is often the case with the absence of short-term variability) can at times present a more ominous connotation than certain flat-line patterns. Long-term variability, unlike short-term variability, may be present, albeit abnormal, in the dying fetus.

The loss of short-term variability with the preservation of long-term variability is commonly seen with the administration of narcotic analgesic agents. One cannot be assured that the loss of variability is based on the drug effect unless a segment of tracing with normal variability is observed preceding administration of the drug. If there is no clear explanation for the absence of short-term variability, management should be the same as for other nondiagnostic patterns. This may include performing measures to improve fetal oxygenation, fetal pH testing or stimulation, and timely delivery if the pattern is not clarified or improved. See pages 160–164 for similar patterns with varying outcomes. See also page 123 for a discussion of "blunting," which is characterized by rounding of the long-term variability complexes associated with anemia.

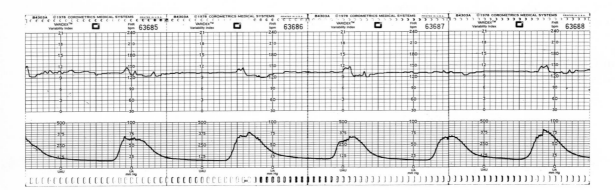

CASE INTERPRETATION: Class III

Baseline Information: normal rate, absent short-term variability, present long-term variability. Some instability (wandering) of the baseline.

Periodic or Nonperiodic Changes: there may be small accelerations, some are followed by shallow decelerations.

Uterine Activity: skewed, frequent uterine contractions recorded by tocodynamometer.

Significance: less reassuring than when short-term variability is present. Good fetal welfare is not verified. Fetal pH may be an adjunct to interpretation.

CASE OUTCOME: Thirty-five-year-old gravida 3, para 1011, delivered vaginally, with epidural anesthesia, at 39 weeks' gestation a 7 pound, 15 ounce (3600 gram) female; Apgar score 8/9. Labor was induced for premature rupture of membranes. Delivery occurred after 32 hours of ruptured membranes. The fetus was in a vertex presentation in an occiput anterior position. The patient received intravenous meperidine one and a half hours prior to this segment. Variability subsequently improved. The infant followed a normal newborn course.

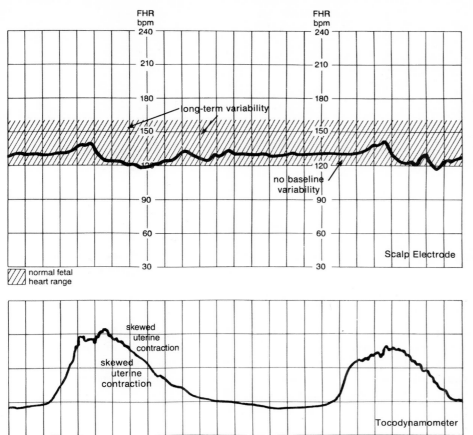

Pattern Characteristic:
No Short-Term Variability

No Variability, Accelerations Present: Mixed Pattern

*W*hen intrapartum drugs are administered to a mother with a healthy fetus, it is not unusual to see a pattern of absent short-term (beat-to-beat) variability.[41] Accelerations may or may not be preserved, reflecting the degree of sympathetic system suppression.[10] Particularly when excellent variability preceded the drug administration, these accelerations serve as useful indicators of continued evidence of good fetal condition.

This pattern must be viewed with caution however. A wandering, unstable baseline may give the erroneous appearance of accelerations. Also, a moribund fetus may display only the prolonged secondary acceleration component of an atypical variable deceleration, which also produces false reassurance. This emphasizes the value of making a basal fetal condition assessment through electronic fetal monitoring prior to administration of pharmacologic agents. See page 160 for a similar pattern with a dissimilar outcome.

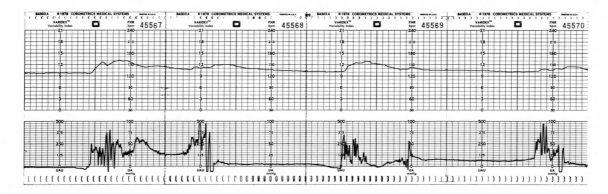

CASE INTERPRETATION: Class I/III

Baseline Information: normal rate, absent variability.

Periodic or Nonperiodic Changes: accelerations are present and prolonged.

Uterine Activity: irregular contractions are distorted by maternal activity, as recorded by tocodynamometer.

Significance: more reassuring than with no accelerations present, but assurance of good fetal condition is not verified because of absent variability. This pattern may be seen with narcotic analgesic administration, but loss of variability may not be assumed to be on that basis unless good variability was documented prior to the drug's administration.

CASE OUTCOME: Eighteen-year-old primigravida delivered vaginally, with low elective forceps and epidural anesthesia, a 9 pound, 2 ounce (4139 gram) male; Apgar score 7/9. The fetus was in a vertex presentation in an occiput anterior position. Meperidine and promethazine had been administered 44 minutes prior to the displayed segment. The narcotic administration was preceded by a fetal heart trace with average baseline variability. The infant followed a normal newborn course.

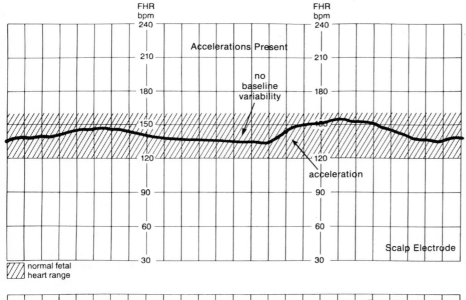

Pattern Characteristic:
No Variability: with
Accelerations

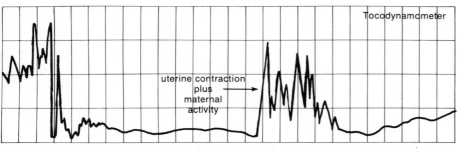

No Variability with Decelerations: Mixed Pattern

*W*hen variability is absent, with periodic decelerations present, more information is conveyed about the fetus than is derived from a flat-line tracing. When such a mixed pattern displays changes that have been seen with hypoxia, there is sufficient risk of acidosis and a low Apgar score to warrant delivery upon failure to demonstrate improvement promptly with maternal oxygen therapy and other measures aimed at improving fetal oxygena-

tion. A combined pattern of atypical variable deceleration and late decelerations with loss of baseline variability is such a pattern.[18,29] In using fetal pH studies for further assessment of such a pattern, one weighs the time required to perform the study against the likelihood of its altering management. Not all newborns are depressed, but this is a pattern demonstrated by certain compromised fetuses.[35]

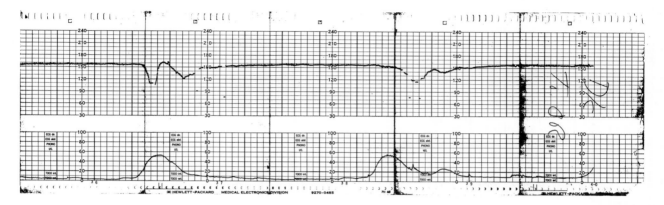

CASE INTERPRETATION: Class V

Baseline Information: high normal rate, absent variability, prolonged delay in return to baseline after decelerations.

Periodic or Nonperiodic Changes: the combination of atypical variable decelerations and late decelerations are similar to that seen with the "W sign."

Uterine Activity: skewed and polysystolic contractions.

Significance: a nonreassuring pattern. Management is dictated by clinical circumstances. Prompt delivery of a viable fetus with this pattern is usually the appropriate response.

CASE OUTCOME: Twenty-nine-year-old gravida 5, para 4004, at 40 weeks' gestation delivered by primary cesarean section, performed under general anesthesia for fetal distress, a 6 pound, 9 ounce (2977 gram) female; Apgar score 3/6. Meconium was present. The fetus was in a vertex presentation. The newborn was dismissed at eight days of life.

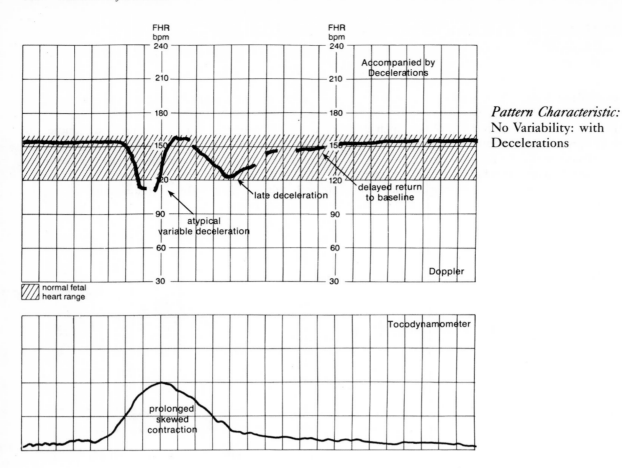

Pattern Characteristic:
No Variability: with
Decelerations

No Variability in Accelerations

*B*eat-to-beat variability is believed to be produced by parasympathetic system activity alternating with withdrawal. During accelerations, while the sympathetic system dominates, variability typically disappears.[34] Variability resumes upon return to the baseline. It is common for the acceleration to be followed by a transient deceleration, often with transiently increased variability with the return of parasympathetic system activation (Lambda pattern, see page 188). When accelerations are prolonged or continuous, the pattern may be confused with a tachycardia with reduced variability. Such a pattern would have a potentially ominous connotation—the loss of variability denoting obliteration of autonomic nervous system response of the fetus to stimuli in its environment—as compared to loss of variability with accelerations, a physiologic response to stimuli in a healthy fetus. Careful study of the entire tracing for identification of the baseline and then interpretation of the fetal condition based on the true baseline variability is usually of help in making a diagnosis.

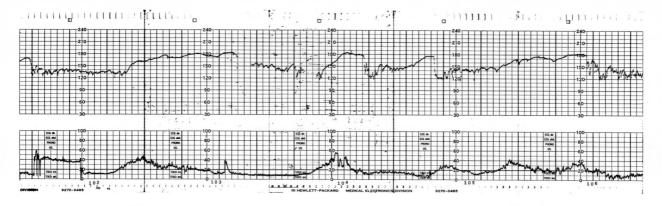

CASE INTERPRETATION: Class I

Baseline Information: normal rate, normal variability.

Periodic or Nonperiodic Changes: variable periodic accelerations (with loss of beat-to-beat variability during accelerations). Postacceleration decelerations.

Uterine Activity: irregular contractions of normal duration were recorded.

Significance: a healthy fetus is predicted.

CASE OUTCOME: Twenty-four-year-old primigravida at 42 weeks' gestation delivered by cesarean section for cephalopelvic disproportion, with general anesthesia, a 7 pound, 3½ ounce (3274 gram) male; Apgar score 8/8. The fetus was in a vertex presentation. The infant followed a normal newborn course.

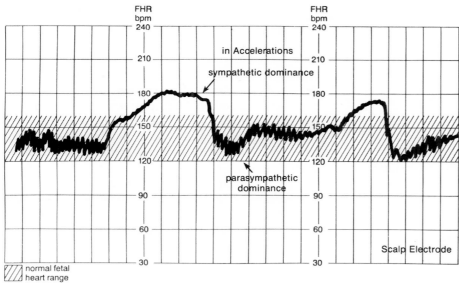

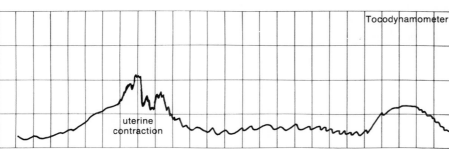

Pattern Characteristic:
No Variability in Accelerations

No Variability During Recovery from a Prolonged Deceleration

*T*ransient loss of variability often occurs upon recovery from a prolonged deceleration. It usually represents a predictable step in a physiologic process of response in a healthy fetus to hypoxic stress. Increased variability often precedes the loss of variability during the recovery process (see page 78), and tachycardia usually accompanies the transient loss of variability (see page 60).

During a transient hypoxic insult, the fetus is capable of maintaining oxygen delivery to vital organs such as the nervous system and cardiac muscle by vasoconstriction of less vital tissue beds. Upon recovery from the hypoxic episode, the vascular beds "reopen." During the transient decreased perfusion, local metabolic acidosis occurs as a result of anaerobic metabolism. Upon recovery, metabolites enter the general circulation, producing a transient lowering of pH in a fetus who is no longer hypoxic. Capillary and tissue pH results may vary in these circumstances because of differences in the reflection of general circulatory versus local changes. The persistent loss of variability after recovery from a prolonged deceleration may indicate continued fetal hypoxia.[28] See Chap. 14 for further discussion of these physiologic phenomena.

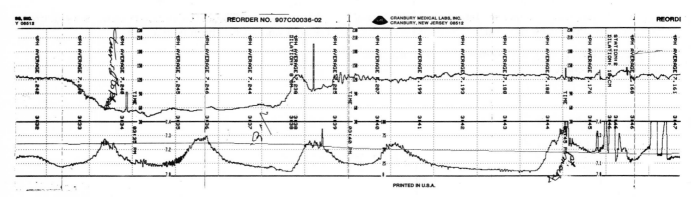

CASE INTERPRETATION: Class II

Baseline Information: low normal rate, average variability, transient increased variability followed by decreased variability upon recovery from prolonged decelerations.

Periodic or Nonperiodic Changes: six-minute prolonged transient deceleration associated with increased baseline uterine tone.

Uterine Activity: skewed contractions, increased baseline tone, areas without a resting phase.

Significance: stress of a healthy fetus presumed to be using escape rhythm and constriction of nonvital vascular beds (diving seal reflex) to respond to the stress of heart rate deceleration associated with increased uterine activity. Full recovery. Management is influenced by such factors as frequency of occurrence, gestation, estimated time to and ease of delivery, and the presence or absence of thick meconium.

CASE OUTCOME: Twenty-four-year-old primigravida delivered vaginally at 42 weeks' gestation an 8 pound, 5 ounce (3770 gram) female; Apgar score 6/8. Intrapartum course was complicated by recurring prolonged decelerations. Magnesium sulfate was administered for uterine hypertonus. Thick meconium was present. Continuous tissue (capillary) pH was recorded on the tracing. Scalp pHs were 7.35 to 7.40 prior to the episode. The infant was delivered 72 minutes later. The umbilical artery and vein pH were 7.28, 7.31, respectively. The infant followed an uncomplicated newborn course.

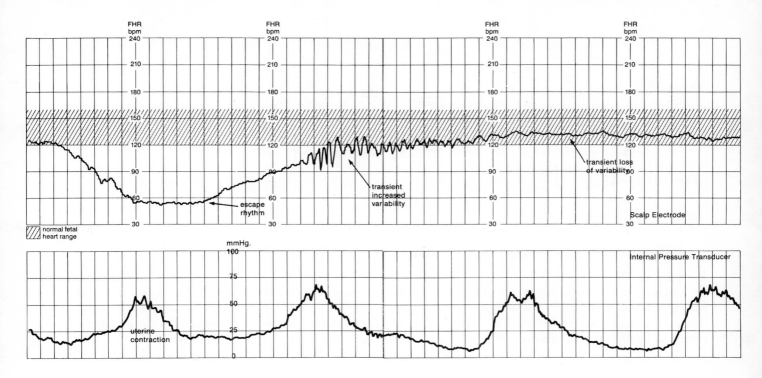

Pattern Characteristic:
No Variability During Recovery from Prolonged Deceleration

No Variability Secondary to Sinus Node Suppression

*A*s a lifesaving phenomenon, lower pacemaker centers in the conduction system of the heart assume control when the sinus node is suppressed. Examples of stimuli that can suppress the sinus node are a reflex burst of parasympathetic activity, as may occur from cord impingement by a uterine contraction; insertion of a scalp electrode; or acute hypoxia. During the ensuing escape rhythm, there may be no beat-to-beat variability because there is no responsiveness by the new pacemaker to sympathetic and parasympathetic stimuli.

Upon recovery, sinus arrhythmia resumes, often with transient increased variability followed by transient decreased variability (see pages 60, 78).

Sinus node suppression is also demonstrated in variable decelerations that exhibit a flat-line in the bottom of the deceleration, the flat-line denoting the transient escape rhythm. An electrocardiogram obtained during these patterns may demonstrate loss of P waves or P waves following the QRS complex.

Absent "variability" in these situations has a different significance than loss of baseline variability as a result of asphyxia. Here, a healthy fetus is using protective cardiac mechanisms during the stressful stimulus of sinus node suppression. In contrast, loss of baseline variability as a result of hypoxia leading to acidosis denotes a potentially unhealthy fetus whose compensatory mechanisms have been surpassed.[34] Fetal pH is an adjunct in determining which smooth baseline patterns are the result of acidosis versus other causes such as sleep or drugs. Fetal pH studies are not necessary during the smooth/flat-line portion of a prolonged deceleration or variable deceleration. Failure to recover prompts intervention. If recovery occurs, the nature of the recovery process itself, as depicted on the fetal monitoring tracing, may be analyzed for information about fetal health in response to stress in lieu of pH studies.

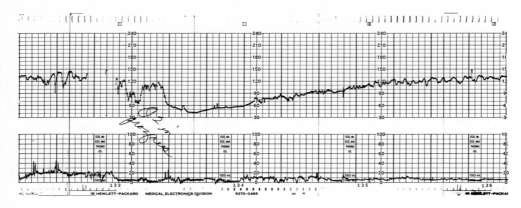

CASE INTERPRETATION: Class II

Baseline Information: normal rate, normal variability.

Periodic or Nonperiodic Changes: prolonged non-periodic deceleration with suppression of sinus node, resulting in a two to two and a half minute escape rhythm followed by sinus node recovery. The trace has not returned to baseline in this segment.

Uterine Activity: none recorded.

Significance: response of a healthy fetus to an environmental stimulus with recovery.

CASE OUTCOME: Twenty-four-year-old gravida 2, para 0010, at 41½ weeks' gestation delivered vaginally, with outlet forceps and general anesthesia, a 9 pound, 8 ounce (4309 gram) female; Apgar score 5/9. The fetus was in a vertex presentation. The delivery was complicated by shoulder dystocia. Meconium was present. The infant followed an uncomplicated newborn course.

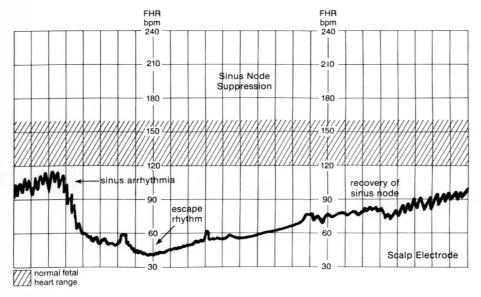

Pattern Characteristic:
No Variability Arrhythmia. Sinus Node Suppression

No Variability Secondary to Bradyarrhythmia

*L*oss of variability secondary to a bradyarrhythmia implies a cardiac focus originating in other than the sinus node and, therefore, one that is unresponsive to the autonomic nervous system. Junctional and ventricular rhythm have little or no variability (see page 42). Bradycardia secondary to nonconducted premature beats in a bigeminal pattern has a decreased variability because only every other cardiac cycle is represented; the effect is similar to that of machine averaging.

Bradyarrhythmias can be confused with a prolonged deceleration from a higher baseline if the monitor recording began after the deceleration occurred and recovery has not taken place. Absent variability in such a situation may be from escape rhythm secondary to sinus node suppression or from actual acidosis. Therefore, the clinical situation must be carefully assessed. Fetal pH studies are an adjunct to the intrapartum monitoring in the case of complete atrioventricular block, unless atrial activity can be mapped with a Doppler-derived signal as an indicator of autonomic nervous system health.

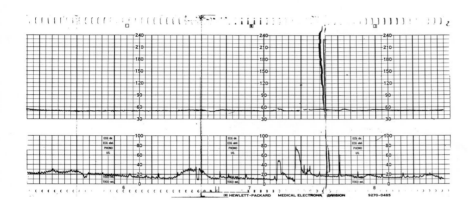

CASE INTERPRETATION: Class III

Baseline Information: marked bradycardia, absent variability.

Periodic or Nonperiodic Changes: none.

Uterine Activity: infrequent contractions.

Significance: probable bradyarrhythmia as opposed to a bradycardia resulting from prolonged deceleration from a higher baseline, without recovery.

CASE OUTCOME: Eighteen-year-old gravida 4, para 3003, at 40 weeks' gestation delivered vaginally, with low forceps and epidural anesthesia, a 7 pound, 13 ounce (3544 gram) female; Apgar score 9/9. The newborn's heart rate was greater than 70 bpm. The infant did not require a pacemaker. Maternal evaluation for collagen vascular disease was negative. The infant followed a normal newborn course.

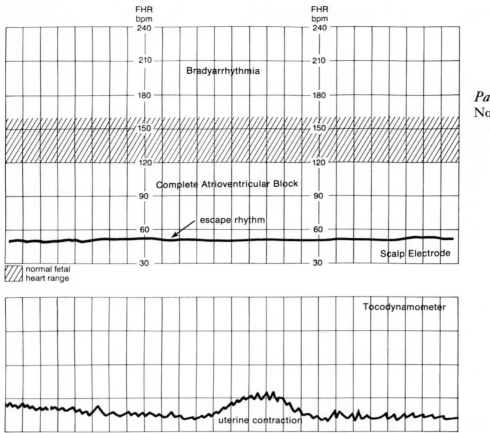

Pattern Characteristic:
No Variability. Bradyarrhythmia

No Variability Secondary to Tachyarrhythmia

A tachyarrhythmia has little or no variability because the ectopic pacemaker is not under autonomic nervous system control, unlike the sinus node pacemaker. Sinus tachycardias have decreased variability because of sympathetic system dominance, but the fetal heart rate is usually not fixed (unless by drug effect, acidosis, or rarely, decerebration). Echocardiography (or electrocardiography) is helpful for diagnosis of the particular tachyarrhythmia and to determine if, along with atrial flutter, block exists (see pages 61 and 62).

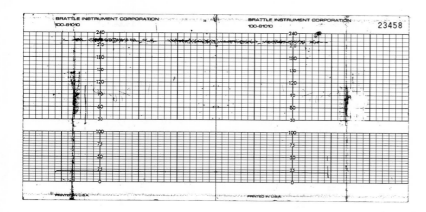

CASE INTERPRETATION: Class III

Baseline Information: marked tachycardia, absent variability.

Periodic or Nonperiodic Changes: none.

Uterine Activity: none recorded.

Significance: probable tachyarrhythmia, needs further assessment such as echocardiography for diagnosis.

CASE OUTCOME: Twenty-seven-year-old gravida 3, para 1011, at 32 weeks' gestation. Echocardiographic diagnosis was of atrial flutter with 2:1 atrioventricular block in the fetus with ascites. Maternal treatment with digoxin and verapamil was unsuccessful in accomplishing fetal cardioversion. A hydropic 5 pound, 5½ ounce (2420 gram) stillborn male was delivered by repeat cesarean section. The fetus had trisomy 13 syndrome. Multiple cardiac anomalies were present, including an atrioventricular canal.

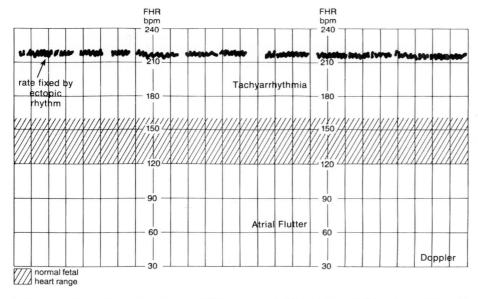

Pattern Characteristic:
No Variability. Tachyarrhythmia

No Variability Produced by Disengaged Transducer: Artifact

*T*he fetus with absent long- and short-term variability produced by various causes may display a fetal heart trace that is ruler-flat. Such a pattern has been called "flat,"[36] "fixed," or "silent" or one with "no irregular-ity."[21,25,52] Knowledge of the clinical circumstances excludes or establishes artifact in any given case. It may be indistinguishable from an artifactually produced trace such as occurs with a disengaged transducer.

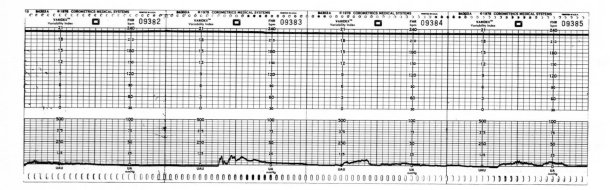

CLASS INTERPRETATION: Class III (artifactual)

Baseline Information: marked tachycardia, absent variability.

Periodic or Nonperiodic Changes: none present.

Uterine Activity: maternal respirations recorded by tocodynamometer, possible irregular uterine contractions.

Significance: differential diagnosis of this pattern is tachyarrhythmia versus mechanical artifact. The latter is more likely because of the difficulty for the fetal monitor to record very rapid heart rates in an uninterrupted fashion.

CASE OUTCOME: Thirty-five-year-old gravida 2, para 1001, delivered vaginally, with no anesthesia, a 7 ounce (196 gram) stillborn fetus of indeterminant sex from a breech presentation at 30 weeks' gestation. An autopsy revealed severe intrauterine growth retardation of approximately 21 weeks' gestation and multiple congenital anomalies suggestive of an associated abnormal chromosomal pattern. There was a disengaged fetal heart rate transducer.

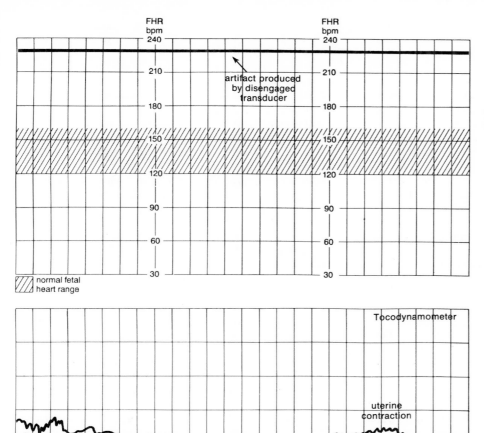

Pattern Characteristic:
No Variability. Artifact

References

1. Assali NS, Brinkman CR, Woods JR, et al: Development of neurohumoral control of fetal, neonatal, and adult cardiovascular functions. *Am J Obstet Gynecol* 129:748, 1977.

2. Ayromlooi J, Tobias M, Berg P: The effects of scopolamine and ancillary analgesics upon the fetal heart rate recording. *J Reprod Med* 25:323, 1980.

3. Babaknia A, Neibyl JR: The effect of magnesium sulfate on fetal heart rate baseline variability. *Obstet Gynecol* 51:25, 1978.

4. Boehm FH: FHR variability: Key to fetal well-being. *Contemp Obstet Gynecol* 9:57, 1977.

5. Braithwaite NDJ, Milligan JE, Shennan AT: Fetal heart rate monitoring and neonatal mortality in the very preterm infant. *Am J Obstet Gynecol* 154:250, 1986.

6. Cabal LA, Siassi B, Zanini B, et al: Factors affecting heart rate variability in preterm infants. *Pediatrics* 65:50, 1980.

7. Caldeyro-Barcia R, Mendez-Bauer C, Poseiro JJ, et al: Control of human fetal heart rate during labor, in *The Heart and Circulation of the Newborn and Infant*, Cassels DE (ed). New York, Grune and Stratton, 1966, p. 7.

8. Cetrulo CL, Schifrin BS: Fetal heart rate patterns preceding death in utero. *Obstet Gynecol* 48:521, 1976.

9. Cibils LA: Clinical significance of fetal heart rate patterns during labor. VII. Hypertensive conditions. *J Reprod Med* 26:471, 1981.

10. Dalton KJ, Phil D, Dawes GS, et al: The autonomic nervous system and fetal heart rate variability. *Am J Obstet Gynecol* 146:456, 1983.

11. Dawes GS, Houghton CRS, Redman CWG, et al: Pattern of the normal human fetal heart rate. *Brit J Obstet Gynaecol* 89:276, 1982.

12. Devoe L: Antepartum fetal heart rate testing in preterm pregnancy. *Obstet Gynecol* 60:431, 1982.

13. Druzin ML, Fox A, Kogut E, et al: The relationship of the nonstress test to gestational age. *Am J Obstet Gynecol* 153:386, 1985.

14. Earn AA: A proposed international scoring system for predicting fetal status derived from fetal heart rate patterns: Compatible with current tests. (The fetal heart rate response as an aid in predicting perinatal status.) *Obstet Gynecol Surv* 35:265, 1980.

15. Emmen L, Huisjes HJ, Aarnoudse JG, et al: Antepartum diagnosis of the "terminal" fetal state by cardiotocography. *Brit J Obstet Gynaecol* 82:353, 1975.

16. Fetal heart rate monitoring. Guidelines for monitoring, terminology and instrumentation. *ACOG Technical Bulletin,* no. 32, June 1975.

17. Gagnon R, Campbell K, Hunse C, et al: Patterns of human fetal accelerations from 26 weeks to term. *Am J Obstet Gynecol* 157:743, 1987.

18. Gaziano EP: A study of variable decelerations in association with other heart rate patterns during monitored labor. *Am J Obstet Gynecol* 135:360, 1979.

19. Gaziano EP, Freeman DW: Analysis of heart rate patterns preceding fetal death. *Obstet Gynecol* 50:578, 1977.

20. Gimovsky ML, Caritis SN: Diagnosis and management of hypoxic fetal heart rate patterns. *Clinics in Perinatology* 9:313, 1982.

21. Hammacher K, Huter KA, Bokelmann J, et al: Foetal heart frequency and perinatal condition of the foetus and newborn. *Gynaecologia* 166:349, 1968.

22. Hayashi RH, Fox ME: Unforeseen sudden intrapartum fetal death in a monitored labor. *Am J Obstet Gynecol* 122:786, 1975.

23. Hensen G, Dawes GS, Redman CWG: Characterization of the reduced heart rate variation in Growth-Retarded fetuses. *Brit J Obstet Gynaecol* 91:751, 1984.

24. Hon EH: Detection of asphyxia in utero—fetal heart rate, in Gluck L (ed): *Intrauterine Asphyxia and the Developing Fetal Brain.* Chicago, Yearbook Medical Publishers, 1977:167.

25. Hon EH: *An Introduction to Fetal Heart Rate Monitoring.* Los Angeles, Postgraduate Division University of Southern California School of Medicine, 1973.

26. Hon EH, Lee ST: Electronic evaluation of the fetal heart rate. VIII. Patterns preceding fetal death, further observations. *Am J Obstet Gynecol* 87:814, 1963.

27. Hoppenbrouwers T, Combs D, Ugargechea JC, et al: Fetal heart rates during maternal wakefulness and sleep. *Obstet Gynecol* 57:301, 1981.

28. Hutson JM, Mueller-Heubach E: Diagnosis and management of intrapartum fetal heart rate changes. *Clinics in Perinatology* 9:325, 1982.

29. Krebs H-B, Petres RE, Dunn LJ: Intrapartum fetal heart rate monitorings. VIII. Atypical variable decelerations. *Am J Obstet Gynecol* 145:297, 1983.

30. Lavin JP, Miodovnik M, Barden TP: Relationship of non-stress test reactivity and gestational age. *Obstet Gynecol* 63:338, 1984.

31. Leveno KJ, Williams ML, Depalma RT, et al: Perinatal outcome in the absence of antepartum fetal heart rate acceleration. *Obstet Gynecol* 61:347, 1983.

32. Martin CB: Regulation of the fetal heart rate and genesis of FHR patterns. *Seminars in Perinatology* 2:131, 1978.

33. Martin CB: Behavioral states in the human fetus. *J Reprod Med* 26:425, 1981.

34. Martin CB: Physiology and clinical use of fetal heart rate variability. *Clinics in Perinatology* 9:339, 1982.

35. Martin CB, Siassi B, Hon EH: Fetal heart rate patterns and neonatal death in low birthweight infants. *Obstet Gynecol* 44:503, 1974.

36. Nijhuis JG, Crevels AJ, Van Dongen PWJ: *Obstet Gynecol Surv* 45:229, 1990.

37. Parer JT: Basic patterns, their classification and in utero treatment, in *Handbook of Fetal Heart Rate Monitoring.* Philadelphia, W.B. Saunders, 1983, p. 88.

38. Parer JT: Fetal heart rate patterns preceding death in utero, in *Handbook of Fetal Heart Rate Monitoring.* Philadelphia, W.B. Saunders, 1983, p. 147.

39. Paul RH, Suidan AK, Yeh S, et al: Clinical fetal monitoring. VII. The evaluation and significance of intrapartum baseline FHR variability. *Am J Obstet Gynecol* 123:206, 1975.

40. Peleg D, Goldman JA: Fetal heart patterns: A study of the anencephalic fetus. *Obstet Gynecol* 53:530, 1979.

41. Petrie RH, Yeh S, Surata Y, et al: The effect of drugs on fetal heart rate variability. *Am J Obstet Gynecol* 130:294, 1978.

42. Roemer VM, Heinzl S, Peters FD, et al: Oscillation-frequency and baseline fetal heart rate in the last 30 minutes of labour. *Brit J Obstet Gynaecol* 86:472, 1979.

43. Sassoon DA, Castro LC, Davis JL, et al: The biophysical profile in labor. *Obstet Gynecol* 76:360, 1990.

44. Smith JH, Dawes GS, Redman CWG: Low human heart rate variation in normal pregnancy. *Br J Obstet Gynaecol* 94:656, 1987.

45. Sorokin Y, Dierkin LJ, Pillay SK, et al: The association between fetal heart rate patterns and fetal movements in pregnancies between 20 and 30 weeks' gestation. *Am J Obstet Gynecol* 143:243, 1982.

46. Stallworth JC, Yeh S, Petrie RH: The effect of magnesium sulfate on fetal heart rate variability and uterine activity. *Am J Obstet Gynecol* 140:702, 1981.

47. Terao T, Kawashima Y, Noto H, et al: Neurological control of fetal heart rate in 20 cases of anencephalic fetuses. *Am J Obstet Gynecol* 149:201, 1984.

48. van der Moer PE, Gerretsen G, Vuisser GHA: Fixed fetal heart rate pattern after intrauterine accidental decerebration. *Obstet Gynecol* 65:125, 1985.

49. van Geijn HP, Jongsma HW, de Haan J, et al: Heart rate as an indicator of the behavioral state. Studies in the newborn infant and prospects for fetal heart rate monitoring. *Am J Obstet Gynecol* 136:1061, 1980.

50. Vintzileos AM, Campbell WA, Bors-Koefoed R, et al: The relationship between cyclic variation of fetal heart rate (FHR) patterns and fetal acidosis in very preterm gestations, no. 2. *Proceedings of the Society of Perinatal Obstetricians Eighth Annual Meeting,* 1988.

51. Visser GHA, Goodman JDS, Levine DH, et al: Diurnal and other cyclic variations in human fetal heart rate near term. *Am J Obstet Gynecol* 142:535, 1982.

52. Young BK, Weinstein HN, Hochberg HM, et al: Observations in perinatal heart rate monitoring. I. A quantitative method of describing baseline variability of the fetal heart rate. *J Reprod Med* 20:205, 1978.

53. Zugaib M, Dorsythe AB, Muwayhid B, et al: Mechanisms of beat-to-beat variability in the heart rate of the neonatal lamb. I. Influence of the autonomic nervous system. *Am J Obstet Gynecol* 138:444, 1980.

Sinusoidal and Other Undulating Patterns

Chapter 7

Sinusoidal Pattern

A fetal monitoring pattern that has been associated with much confusion and conflicting published information is the sinusoidal fetal heart pattern. One reason is because, as with "flat-line" absent variability, it may accompany extremes of fetal conditions, that is, well or moribund. Also contributing to the conflicting reports in the past, was a lack of standardization of the criteria for sinusoidal patterns.[3,52,65] This was rectified in 1982 by Modanlou and Freeman, who reviewed the existing literature on sinusoidal patterns and found that only 27 of 41 cases that were accompanied by figures of actual tracings portrayed a true sinusoidal pattern. The criteria that this classic paper established for diagnosis are:[39]

Stable baseline heart rate of 120 to 160 bpm with regular oscillations

Amplitude of five to 15 bpm, rarely greater

Frequency of two to five cycles per minute (as long-term variability)

Fixed or flat short-term variability

Oscillation of the sinusoidal wave from above and below a baseline (sine wave)

No areas of normal fetal heart rate variability or reactivity

Most instances of true sinusoidal pattern (also termed minor sinusoidal pattern when amplitude is restricted to five to 15 bpm), reflect a benign fetal response secondary to a drug effect. Other causes are severe fetal anemia (such as that caused by severe isoimmunization, fetal-maternal transfusion, placental abruption) or perinatal asphyxia.[8,13,14,52,62,63] In the latter group of cases, the pattern is an ominous one, usually predicting severe fetal or neonatal jeopardy.[2,8,34,62] A transient appearance and reversal of a sinusoidal pattern have each been demonstrated with the transfusion of the fetus or the neonate when associated with fetal anemia.[8,26,34,41,62]

When associated with the administration of narcotic agents, alphaprodine, a centrally acting synthetic narcotic, has received most of the attention although other agents have been implicated.[23,25,50,55,59] In this situation, the pattern has been found to be usually transient. It has also been reported with gastroschisis and amnionitis.[22,29]

The presence of a true sinusoidal pattern does not preclude a decelerative fetal heart rate response.[2,21,63] In fact, a pattern of periodic late decelerations has been described as a common forerunner of nonbenign types of sinusoidal patterns, with the decelerative response to contractions diminishing and sinusoidal pattern persisting as the fetal condition worsens.

The insert displays an example of a true sinusoidal pattern associated with erythroblastosis fetalis.

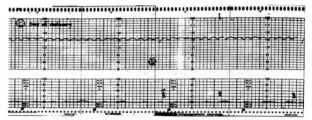

Reprinted with permission from the American College of Obstetricians and Gynecologists. *Am J Obstet Gynecol* 142: 1036,1982.

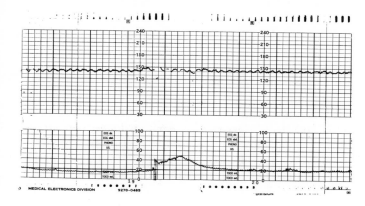

CASE INTERPRETATION: Class III

Baseline Information: normal rate, absent short-term variability, undulating long-term variability with sine wave configuration.

Periodic or Nonperiodic Changes: absent.

Uterine Activity: infrequent contractions, normal in appearance, as recorded by a tocodynamometer.

Significance: a sinusoidal pattern may be associated with a fetus with anemia, narcotic administration, or hypoxia.

CASE OUTCOME: Twenty-eight-year-old gravida 5, para 4004, delivered vaginally, with ketamine anesthesia, at 39½ weeks' gestation a 7 pound, 8¼ ounce (3409 gram) male; Apgar score 9/10. Meperidine and propiomazine were received intrapartum. The fetus was in a vertex presentation, with the cord around the neck. The maternal blood type was O positive, without antibodies. The infant followed a normal newborn course.

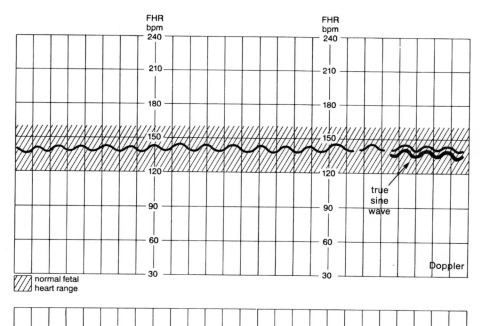

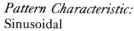

Pattern Characteristic:
Sinusoidal

Marked Sinusoidal Pattern

*T*he classical definition of sinusoidal pattern is "an amplitude of five to 15 bpm, rarely greater." Therefore, a pattern that meets criteria of a sinusoidal pattern except for an amplitude that is greater than 15 bpm is appropriately named a "marked" sinusoidal pattern.[39] It has also been called a major sinusoidal pattern.[31] The pattern is thought to be produced by hypoxia acting at the medullary center, which produces a derangement in cardiac regulatory mechanisms.[5] Marked sinusoidal patterns, unlike classic sinusoidal patterns, do not *always* have a perfect sine wave configuration but often have a V-shape to the inferior undulations.[5,57]

When encountering this pattern, as with a true sinusoidal pattern, the possibility of severe fetal anemia, placental abruption, and severe fetal hypoxia must all be entertained. Other clinical features that have been reported to be associated at times with the pattern include: postdate pregnancy, meconium aspiration, diabetes, and preeclampsia.[12,24] Rarely, intrauterine growth retardation is observed as a cause of the fetal hypoxia.

Most published cases have been associated with poor fetal outcome.[5,19]

The management consists of correlating predisposing clinical features with other maternal/fetal assessment. Ultrasonography may be used to detect the presence of fetal hydrops. The role a biophysical profile may play as an adjunct for diagnosis awaits further study.[53] A Kleihauer-Betke determination on maternal venous or vaginal blood may be helpful in detecting the etiology of fetal anemia. Use of a scalp electrode for the intrapartum patient documents the presence or absence of variability.[38] A fetal pH and hematocrit may add valuable information, if they are feasible.[32] Prompt delivery is appropriate if evaluation supports the concern that there is perinatal jeopardy in a pregnancy with a viable fetus. A benign pattern that simulates a marked sinusoidal pattern should be excluded if possible (see page 134).

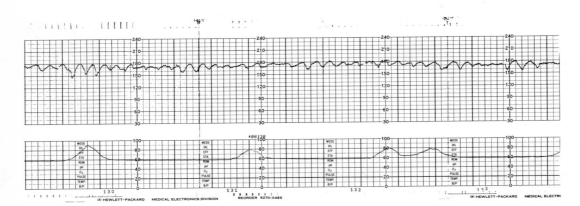

CASE INTERPRETATION: Class V

Baseline Information: absent short-term variability, undulating long-term variability with an amplitude of five to 30 bpm in a marked sinusoidal pattern.

Periodic or Nonperiodic Changes: none seen, some undulations, however, have the appearance of V-shaped variable decelerations.

Uterine Activity: bell-shaped, infrequent uterine contractions.

Significance: probable fetal jeopardy associated with severe fetal anemia, fetal hypoxia, placental abruption, and/or postdate pregnancy. A maternal Kleihauer-Betke determination and antibody screen may be helpful, as may a fetal pH and hematocrit, if they are feasible.

Prompt delivery is appropriate if the fetus is of a viable gestation, unless overriding reassuring information of good fetal condition is obtained. Normal variability interspersed on the tracing would disqualify this as a marked sinusoidal pattern.

CASE OUTCOME: Eighteen-year-old primigravida at 28 weeks' gestation delivered by cesarean section performed for high risk of fetal distress, with general anesthesia, a 2 pound, 2 ounce (960 gram) female; Apgar score 1/6. Neonatal death occurred at five days of life. The neonatal course was complicated by severe intrauterine growth retardation and marked intracerebral bleeding. The umbilical cord pHs were arterial 7.37 and venous 7.41.

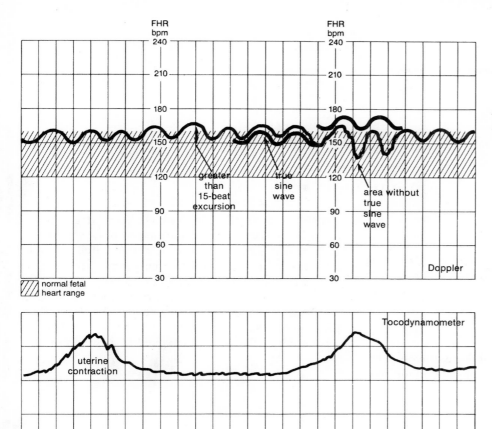

Pattern Characteristic:
Marked Sinusoidal

Sinusoidal Pattern Associated with Severe Fetal Anemia

*M*any true sinusoidal patterns have been diagnosed in the presence of fetal anemia. In addition to Rh sensitization, other associated causes of anemia include: massive fetal-maternal transfusion, vasa previa, placental chorioangioma, fetal blood loss associated with placental abruption, and chronic blood loss secondary to a true knot in the umbilical cord.[2,4,13,17,28,40,57]

A Kleihauer-Betke determination has proven to be useful in antepartum documentation of a fetal-maternal transfusion.[13] Ultrasonography may be used to demonstrate the presence or absence of fetal hydrops and/or ascites.

The typical appearance of the sinusoidal pattern when it is associated with severe anemia is that of low-amplitude, low-frequency, rounded smooth oscillations, in contrast to the true sinusoidal and nonsinusoidal patterns that are seen with narcotic administration.[21,30] Depending on the degree of hypoxia and acidosis, the pattern may co-exist with areas of no variability.[60] A transitional pattern characterized by "blunting" of the fetal heart rate variability complexes has been described, with an intermediate anemia in the fetus (hematocrit 20%–30%) who has erythroblastosis fetalis.[37] The pattern may reflect the relative oxygenation level as opposed to the hemoglobin deficit.[43]

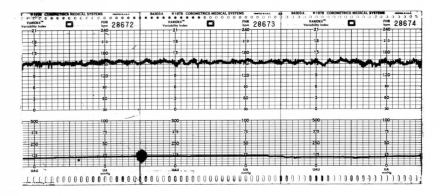

CASE INTERPRETATION: Class V

Baseline Information: high normal to moderate tachycardic rate, absent short-term variability, undulating long-term variability greater than 15 bpm in areas.

Periodic or Nonperiodic Changes: none present.

Uterine Activity: none recorded.

Significance: marked sinusoidal pattern. Evaluate the fetus for anemia, acidosis, and neurologic disease. This is a coarser pattern than is seen with narcotic administration.

CASE OUTCOME: Twenty-eight-year-old primigravida at 26 weeks' gestation delivered by primary cesarean section, with general anesthesia, performed for possible fetal distress in a patient with premature ruptured membranes a 2 pound, 5 ounce (1049 gram) male; Apgar score 1/1. The fetus was in a vertex presentation. The newborn had an unexplained hematocrit of 9 at birth. The Kleihauer-Betke determination on the maternal blood was negative. The newborn expired at six weeks of age.

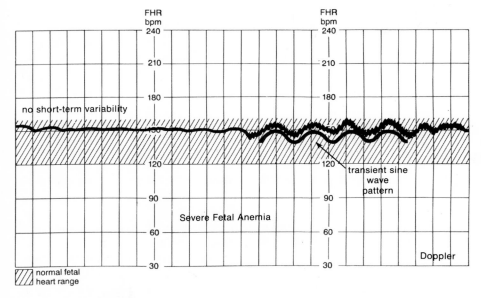

Pattern Characteristic:
Sinusoidal Pattern with Anemia

Sinusoidal Pattern Associated with Possible Hypoxia

A sinusoidal pattern may be seen intermittently or continuously in the evolution of patterns associated with an asphyxiated fetus.[11,12,18,46,49,61] Asphyxia in this text is defined as the presence of metabolic acidosis induced by hypoxia. When produced by this cause, the pattern may fluctuate with a fixed (flat) baseline with absent short- and long-term variability. This may be an agonal pattern in the postdate fetus (see page 320).

The mechanism for a sinusoidal pattern is not fully elucidated. It is postulated to be an absence of central control of heart regulation. In decerebrate adults such patterns have been seen, the oscillations correlating with respirations. An association with periodic agonal respiratory activity has been suggested but not confirmed in the neonate. A sinusoidal pattern in the fetus has been detected in association with both respiratory sinus arrhythmia and fetal sucking.[6,44,48] Alteration of the pattern with atropine suggests some central nervous system responsiveness.[7,42] The pattern is most generally accepted to be a result of tissue hypoxia at the cardiac center of the medulla. Such being the case, it need not be accompanied by fetal acidosis in all situations.[32]

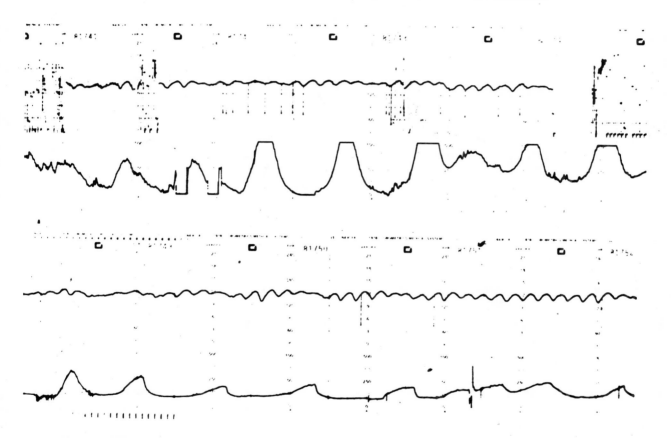

CASE INTERPRETATION: Class V

Baseline Information: normal rate, absent short-term variability, regular undulating long-term variability of greater than 15 bpm, interspersed with areas of fixed baseline.

Periodic or Nonperiodic Changes: none present.

Uterine Activity: skewed, regular contractions.

Significance: a marked sinusoidal pattern. This pattern may be associated with severe fetal anemia or hypoxia of various causes.

CASE OUTCOME: Nineteen-year-old primigravida delivered vaginally at term, with a history of no prenatal problems but with intrapartum findings of preeclampsia, a 5 pound, 2½ ounce (2340 gram) newborn; Apgar score 1/4. The newborn course was complicated by neonatal seizures that required phenobarbital therapy. There was no evidence of anemia or blood loss in the neonate.

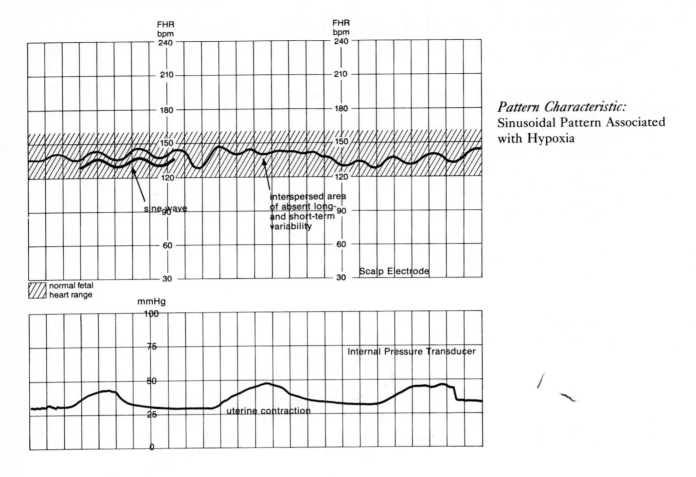

Pattern Characteristic:
Sinusoidal Pattern Associated
with Hypoxia

Marked Sinusoidal Pattern Associated with Anencephaly

*T*he intrapartum course of an anencephalic fetus provides an opportunity to observe many patterns seen in the moribund fetus. Abnormal patterns are probably a combination of the effects of the underlying central nervous system disease and intrapartum hypoxia. Although beat-to-beat variability is usually absent unless there is some degree of cortical tissue present, an anencephalic fetus may demonstrate a sinusoidal pattern because long-term variability may be produced with only a medulla oblongata or midbrain.[58] A sinusoidal fetal heart rate pattern has also been reported in association with congenital hydrocephalus.[45]

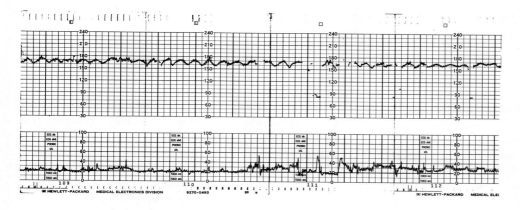

CASE INTERPRETATION: Class V

Baseline Information: moderate tachycardia, absent short-term variability, undulating long-term variability with sine wave configuration, greater than 15 bpm in amplitude.

Periodic or Nonperiodic Changes: none present.

Uterine Activity: maternal respirations and possible contractions recorded by a signal from a tocodynamometer transducer.

Significance: a marked sinusoidal pattern, coarser than that seen with narcotic administration. It is appropriate to evaluate the fetus for causes of anemia or for neurologic disease. There is a high risk of a low Apgar score.

CASE OUTCOME: Twenty-year-old primigravida at 34 weeks' gestation delivered by primary cesarean section for premature breech a 4 pound, 6 ounce (1984 gram) female with undiagnosed anencephaly; Apgar score 1/0. Spina bifida was also noted. The mother received ritodrine and diazepam while in labor. Polyhydramnios was present.

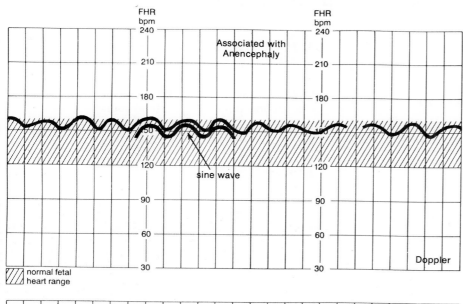

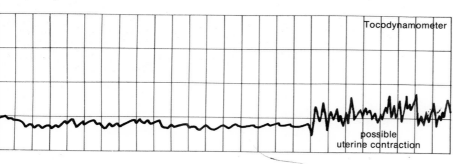

Pattern Characteristic:
Sinusoidal Pattern.
Anencephaly

Nonsinusoidal Undulating Pattern Produced by Regular Long-Term Variability

*I*t is possible for normal fetal sinus arrhythmia to be sufficiently regular in its irregularity to produce a pattern similar to a sinusoidal pattern. This nonsinusoidal pattern, formerly called "pseudosinusoidal," "sinuslike," or "sinuform," meets several criteria of the sinusoidal pattern: It has regular oscillations of the proper frequency and proper amplitude at the proper stable baseline rate.[20,27] However, it is not a sine wave. For example, it is not unusual for peaked oscillations to occur above the baseline but not to an equal degree below the baseline (sawtooth pattern). There are usually interspersed areas of normal baseline with normal variability. It is common for fetal activity accelerations to be present. It is possible at times to convert the pattern to normal by stimulation of the fetus.[33] This is a variant of normal short- and long-term variability, with the usual good prognosis.[56]

This pattern has been associated with the administration of butorphanol, with promethazine and meperidine, with promethazine alone, with nalbuphine hydrochloride, and with alphaprodine.[1,9,15,16,27,29,64]

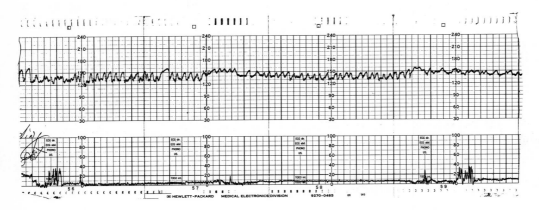

CASE INTERPRETATION: Class I

Baseline Information: normal rate, normal short- and long-term variability. There is an undulating configuration to the long-term variability in areas, but not that of a sine wave.

Periodic or Nonperiodic Changes: small accelerations, no decelerations.

Uterine Activity: maternal respirations recorded by tocodynamometer, no contractions recorded.

Significance: nonsinusoidal pattern, a variant of normal variability. A healthy fetus is predicted.

CASE OUTCOME: Twenty-two-year-old gravida 4, para 1112, at 34 weeks' gestation, delivered vaginally a 4 pound, 8 ounce (2041 gram) male; Apgar score 9/10. The fetus was in a vertex presentation. The infant followed an uncomplicated newborn course.

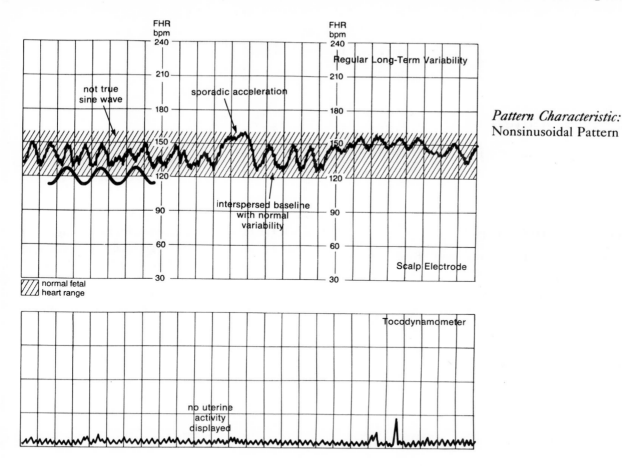

Pattern Characteristic:
Nonsinusoidal Pattern

Nonsinusoidal Undulating Pattern Produced by Rhythmic Accelerations

*W*hen brief accelerations occur with rhythmic regularity, the resulting pattern may be confused with a sinusoidal pattern. Decreased short-term variability is a normal finding, with accelerations believed to be a result of sympathetic system dominance.

When a normal interspersed baseline with average variability is visible, the pattern is quickly disqualified as a sinusoidal pattern. Fetal prognosis is excellent, predicted both by normal baseline variability and the reassuring presence of accelerations.

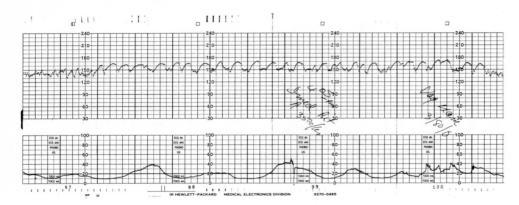

CASE INTERPRETATION: Class I

Baseline Information: high normal rate. Brief segments of normal short-term variability.

Periodic or Nonperiodic Changes: an undulating pattern of accelerations, resembling, but not meeting the criteria for, a sine wave configuration.

Uterine Activity: frequent uterine contractions of varying configuration, with little resting phase.

Significance: the presence of accelerations denotes a healthy fetal response to various stimuli.

CASE OUTCOME: Seventeen-year-old primigravida delivered vaginally at 44 weeks' gestation, with epidural anesthesia by midforceps rotation from the right occiput posterior to the right occiput anterior, a 6 pound, 11¾ ounce (3055 gram) female; Apgar score 9/10. Labor was induced. The infant followed a normal newborn course.

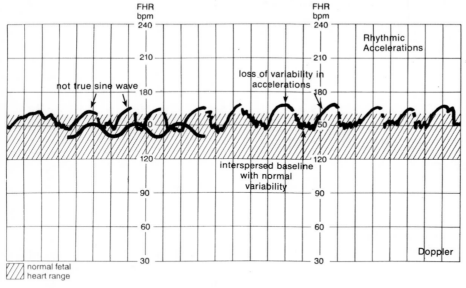

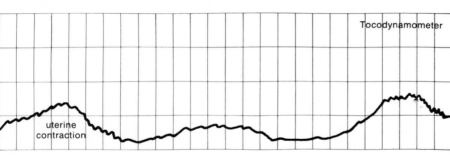

Pattern Characteristic:
Nonsinusoidal Pattern

Nonsinusoidal Undulating Pattern Produced by Rhythmic Accelerations: Baseline Obscured

*R*hythmic accelerations may be confused with a sinusoidal pattern. The distinction is extremely important because of the ominous nature of sinusoidal patterns in the absence of drug administration and the reassuring nature of the presence of accelerations.

The differentiation is most difficult if there are no areas of baseline with normal variability to exclude a sinusoidal pattern. The appearance of the rhythmic accelerations may simulate a sine wave, with the valleys between the accelerations mistaken for undulations below a baseline.

Because accelerations are associated with fetal activity, real time ultrasound documentation of rhythmic fetal movements would support the diagnosis of accelerations but does not exclude a true sinusoidal pattern.[51] Complete absence of fetal movements has been observed in some fetuses with sinusoidal pattern, but extensive study of the range of fetal behavior associated with sinusoidal patterns is awaited.

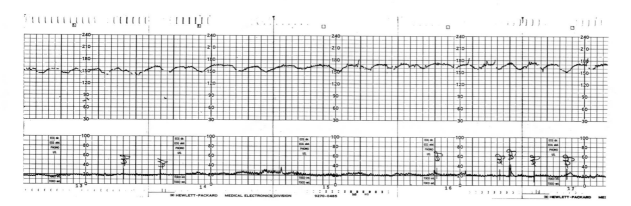

CASE INTERPRETATION: Class I

Baseline Information: high normal rate to moderate tachycardia, absent variability. Appearance of undulating long-term variability.

Periodic or Nonperiodic Changes: a diagnosis of rhythmic accelerations with an obscured baseline is made possible in this case only through review of other portions of the tracing for baseline information supported by the associated fetal activity.

Uterine Activity: fetal activity spikes are noted, there are no contractions.

Significance: a nonsinusoidal pattern that is produced by recurrent accelerations, even without an interspersed baseline, when associated with fetal activity, is most reassuring.

CASE OUTCOME: Twenty-three-year-old gravida 2, para 1001, at term delivered vaginally, with local and pudendal anesthesia, a 6 pound, 8½ ounce (2962 gram) male; Apgar score 9/10. The infant followed an uncomplicated newborn course. This tracing was obtained antepartum at 37 weeks' gestation because of an interval of maternally perceived decreased fetal movement. This pattern persisted with each subsequent weekly study.

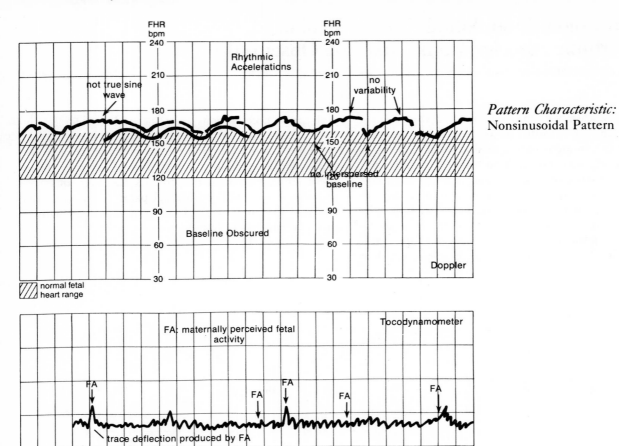

Pattern Characteristic:
Nonsinusoidal Pattern

Nonsinusoidal Undulating Pattern Produced by Regular Accelerations: Evolution and Resolution

*O*bserving the evolution of a rhythmic acceleration pattern and its return to a normal baseline facilitates understanding of the pattern, one which needs careful distinction from a sinusoidal pattern.

A search of the fetal monitoring trace for areas of stable baseline with normal variability and intermittent accelerations assists in distinguishing an intermittent coarse undulating pattern from a true sinusoidal pattern.

This is of particular help when there are no areas of interspersed variability during the undulations. An undulating pattern should persist for at least 10 minutes before being considered as a possible sinusoidal pattern.[65] Assessment of fetal status with ultrasonography may differentiate a rhythmically moving fetus from a moribund inert fetus but is not in itself consistently reliable in excluding all sinusoidal patterns.[51,53]

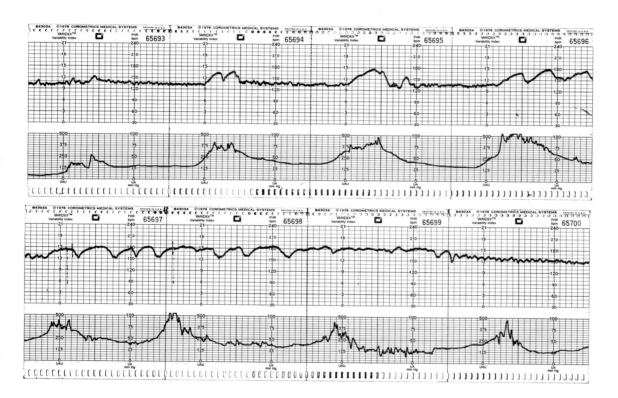

CASE INTERPRETATION: Class I-II

Baseline Information: normal rate, average variability.

Periodic or Nonperiodic Changes: variable accelerations that are initially periodic, become continuous then disappear at the end of the segment.

Uterine Activity: prolonged, skewed contractions with no resting phase.

Significance: a healthy fetus who may be responding to a variety of stimuli, including mild hypoxia. If persistent, the pattern is appropriately observed for progression to other stress patterns.

CASE OUTCOME: Twenty-one-year-old primigravida at 42½ weeks' gestation delivered vaginally, with pudendal anesthesia, a 9 pound, 3½ ounce (4172 gram) female; low one minute Apgar score of 4 was associated with the tracheal suctioning of thick meconium, the five minute Apgar score was 9. The fetus was in a vertex presentation, in an occiput anterior position. No abnormal cord position was noted. The infant followed a normal newborn course.

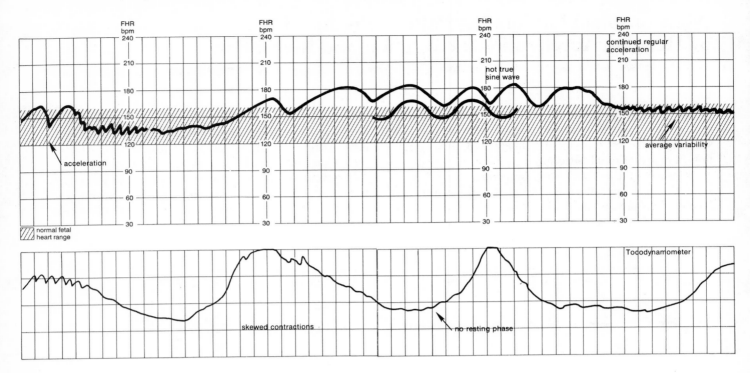

Pattern Characteristic:
Nonsinusoidal Undulating Pattern Evolution and Resolution

Nonsinusoidal Undulating Pattern Simulating Marked Sinusoidal Pattern

*R*arely, a heart rate pattern of a normal fetus may simulate a marked sinusoidal pattern. It appears to occur in situations of fetal stimulation.[35] Fetal tachycardia is a recognized fetal heart rate response to a maternal anxiety state. The pattern depicted here may also be encountered during maternal anxiety states.[10] It has also been detected during cases of ultrasound-observed fetal sucking behavior.[44,48] The presence of normal variability within, or bracketing, the undulating portion of the trace excludes the ominous marked sinusoidal pattern.

Because of the diagnostic challenge presented by this pattern, it is appropriate to assess the clinical situation for risk factors of fetal jeopardy such as hypovolemia or hypoxia as well as to meticulously study the tracing.

An insert is provided here of a true marked sinusoidal pattern that is almost indistinguishable from this case illustration that simulates it.

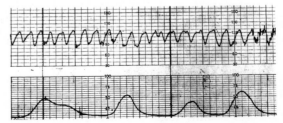

Reprinted with permission from the American College of Obstetricians and Gynecologists. *Obstet Gynecol* 44: 380, 1974.

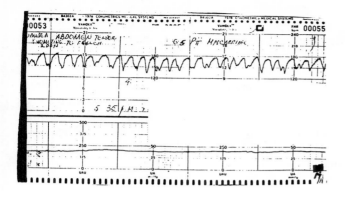

CASE INTERPRETATION: Class I (Class II during rhythmic accelerations)

Baseline Information: normal rate, baseline obscured, absent short-term variability, undulating long-term variability. Resembles marked sinusoidal pattern, including V-shaped inferior undulations and rounded superior undulations. Amplitude is greater than 15 bpm in areas. There was a normal baseline rate and variability in a subsequent segment.

Periodic or Nonperiodic Changes: none identified. Accelerations were present on a subsequent segment.

Uterine Activity: none recorded.

Significance: although not strictly a sine wave, this pattern is very similar to published patterns identified as marked sinusoidal. Evaluation for causes of fetal jeopardy such as anemia is appropriate.

CASE OUTCOME: Thirty-one-year-old gravida 5, para 2022, at 36 weeks' gestation had an antepartum tracing transmitted on xerox telecopier because of abdominal pain, a tender uterus, and vomiting. The pattern reverted to normal (see the segment) before further fetal evaluation was initiated. There was no recurrence. Eight days later, the mother went into spontaneous labor, and a normal intrapartum pattern was recorded. She delivered vaginally a 7 pound, 5 ounce (3317 gram) female; Apgar score 7/8. The infant followed a normal newborn course.

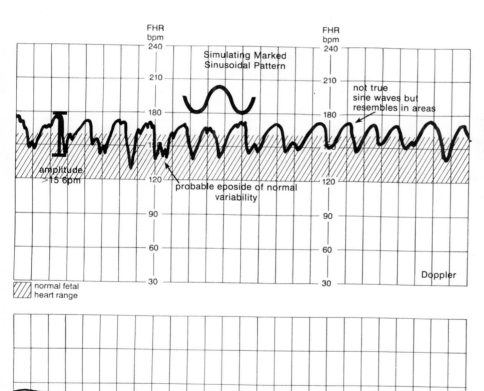

Pattern Characteristic:
Nonsinusoidal Undulating Pattern

Nonsinusoidal Premortem Pattern

*U*ndulating fetal heart rate patterns of the moribund fetus may simulate sinusoidal patterns. These have been termed "premortem."[40] Features that frequently disqualify the pattern from being truly sinusoidal are: less than two cycles per minute, lack of regularity of oscillations, and/or lack of a stable baseline of 120 to 160 bpm.

The pattern is appropriately termed premortem because of the poor perinatal outcomes reported.[49,54,55] Associated clinical problems include severe placental abruption and fetal bleeding.

The undulating appearance is attributed to a failure to establish a baseline between frequent decelerations, smoothed by loss of variability. The overshoot occurring after the ascending limb of one deceleration becomes continuous with the descending limb of the next deceleration.

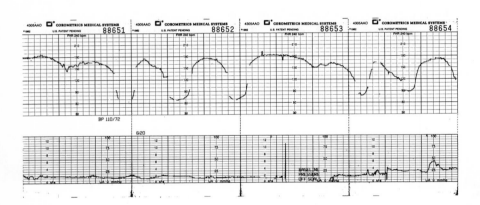

CASE INTERPRETATION: Class V

Baseline Information: moderate tachycardia, decreased variability, an unstable or obscured baseline.

Periodic or Nonperiodic Changes: moderate and severe variable decelerations with atypia: loss of primary accelerations, loss of variability in decelerations, prolonged secondary accelerations.

Uterine Activity: poorly recorded.

Significance: high risk of fetal acidosis. Prompt delivery is usually indicated if the fetus is viable.

CASE OUTCOME: Thirty-two-year-old primigravida was evaluated for vaginal bleeding at 25 weeks' gestation. In utero fetal death occurred, presumably secondary to placental abruption. The patient subsequently delivered vaginally a 1 pound (569 gram) male stillborn.

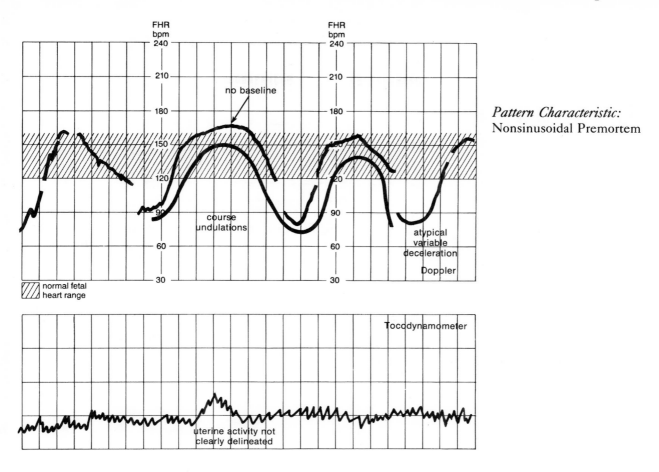

Pattern Characteristic:
Nonsinusoidal Premortem

Nonsinusoidal Premortem Undulating Pattern Associated with Anencephaly

The anencephalic fetus may demonstrate various fetal heart rate patterns that are seen with severe fetal distress. This may be due to a combination of two factors: severe hypoxia permitted to progress without intervention in the nonviable fetus and changes resulting from the neurologic abnormalities. A coarse, undulating pattern with decreased short-term variability is an example of a pattern that may be seen in the anencephalic fetus as well as in the moribund fetus without anencephaly.[39,47] See page 126 for a true sinusoidal pattern associated with fetal anencephaly.

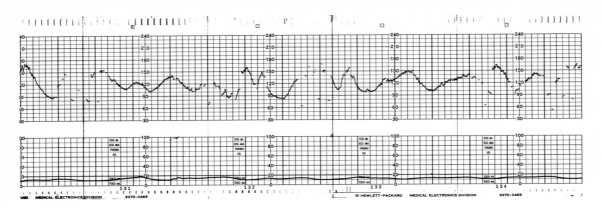

CASE INTERPRETATION: Class V

Baseline Information: obscured by periodic changes. Decreased variability.

Periodic or Nonperiodic Changes: late decelerations with absent variability, which are occurring so frequently that each begins before there is complete recovery of the previous one.

Uterine Activity: poorly recorded, but the wavering trace suggests that contractions precede many of the decelerations.

Significance: this pattern is predictive of a high incidence of poor newborn outcome. It usually warrants prompt delivery if the fetus is viable.

CASE OUTCOME: Forty-year-old gravida 2, para 1001, delivered vaginally at 34 weeks' gestation an anencephalic 3 pound, 3¾ ounce (1467 gram) female stillborn. The postpartum course was complicated by group B beta-hemolytic streptococcal endometritis.

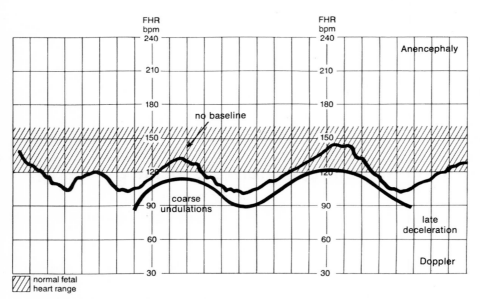

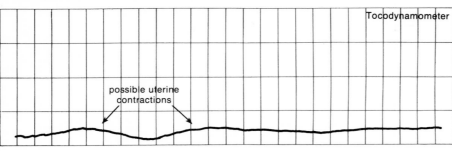

Pattern Characteristic:
Nonsinusoidal Premortem.
Anencephaly

Nonsinusoidal Undulating Pattern Associated with Unfavorable Outcome

*W*hen an undulating pattern is seen in combination with periodic hypoxic decelerations (for example periodic late decelerations, late/variable decelerations, or atypical variable decelerations) there is an increased risk of fetal jeopardy, even if the baseline pattern does not meet the precise criteria for a sinusoidal pattern.[54]

Considering the undulating pattern to be a variant of a baseline variability in which there is diminished short-term variability with preservation of long-term variability makes interpretation on which to base management clearer. If the pattern is intermittent, it is appropriate to pay critical attention to the quality of the baseline variability to which the pattern reverts. The pattern may be approached as one would approach other patterns of decreased beat-to-beat variability in combination with hypoxic decelerations, that is by observing for prompt improvement with such measures as maternal oxygen administration, position change, reducing uterine activity, and hydration. If there is no response, delivery by cesarean section, unless the patient is in the process of delivering vaginally, is usually appropriate, especially if fetal bleeding or a placental abruption are suspected. Using a scalp electrode-derived signal to document beat-to-beat variability, if feasible, and obtaining a fetal pH if the variability is equivocal are adjuncts in management.

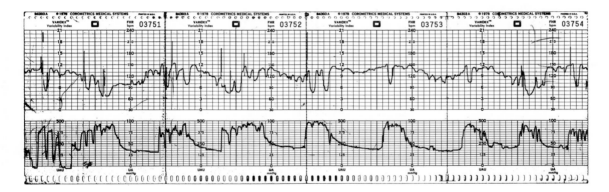

CASE INTERPRETATION: Class III/IV

Baseline Information: unstable but normal rate, decreased short-term variability, long-term variability present. There are areas of undulating features.

Periodic or Nonperiodic Changes: mild variable decelerations with atypia.

Uterine Activity: prolonged, skewed contractions with little resting phase.

Significance: nondiagnostic pattern. A fetal pH may be helpful if continued conservative management is proposed.

CASE OUTCOME: Eighteen-year-old primigravida at 40 weeks' gestation spontaneously delivered vaginally, with pudendal anesthesia, a 6 pound, 12 ounce (3062 gram) male; Apgar score 1/5. Thick meconium was present during labor. Successive scalp pHs were: 7.20, 7.26, and 7.40, repeated at 30-minute intervals in late labor. None were obtained in the last two hours prior to delivery. Neonatal demise occurred on the first day of life; the newborn course was complicated by persistent fetal circulation.

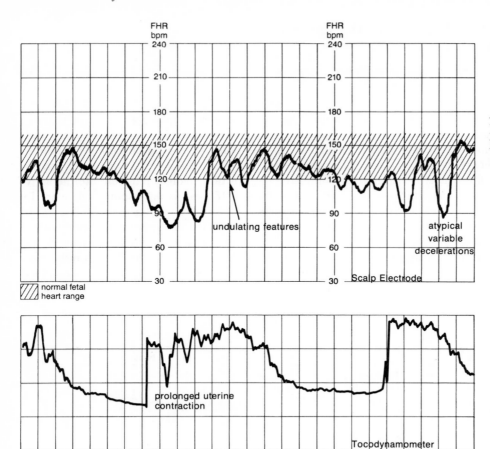

Pattern Characteristic:
Nonsinusoidal Undulating
Pattern–Unfavorable Outcome

Undulating Pattern in Late Labor: Evolution

*A*ny pattern that has smoothing of short-term variability with marked long-term variability gives an undulating appearance. Such a pattern must have a duration of more than 10 minutes as well as meet the other criteria of a sinusoidal pattern before it can be so labeled. When an undulating pattern is of short duration, developing in late labor in a fetus with recent excellent short-term vari-ability, a favorable outcome is expected. However, fetal heart rate tracings in a postdate pregnancy may demon-strate a sinusoidal pattern produced by hypoxia followed by rapid deterioration, so clinical circumstances must be correlated with the pattern in order to exercise appropri-ate clinical judgment.[12]

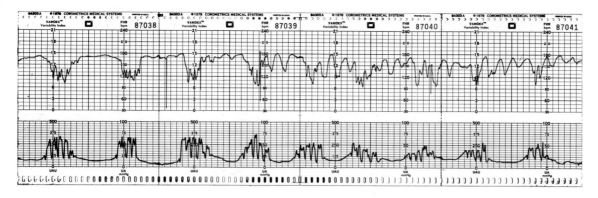

CASE INTERPRETATION: Class IV

Baseline Information: moderate tachycardia, decreased variability. Evolution of an undulating baseline with an absence of short-term variability, increased (marked) long-term variability.

Periodic or Nonperiodic Changes: multiphasic moderate variable decelerations with atypia: loss of primary and secondary accelerations, decreased variability within the decelerations.

Uterine Activity: frequent contractions with a configuration compatible with maternal straining (pushing).

Significance: increased risk of a low Apgar score and acidosis. The pattern is of short duration in a patient who is probably in late labor. The delivery decision is based on clinical factors, including gestation, anticipated time for vaginal delivery, and ease of vaginal delivery.

CASE OUTCOME: Nineteen-year-old primigravida spontaneously delivered vaginally at 42½ weeks' gestation a 7 pound, 12 ounce (3515 gram) female; Apgar score 8/9. No abnormal cord position was noted. The mother received epidural anesthesia in labor but pudendal and local anesthesia for delivery. She also received oxytocin augmentation in labor. Delivery occurred just a few minutes after the segment displayed. The newborn followed an uncomplicated newborn course.

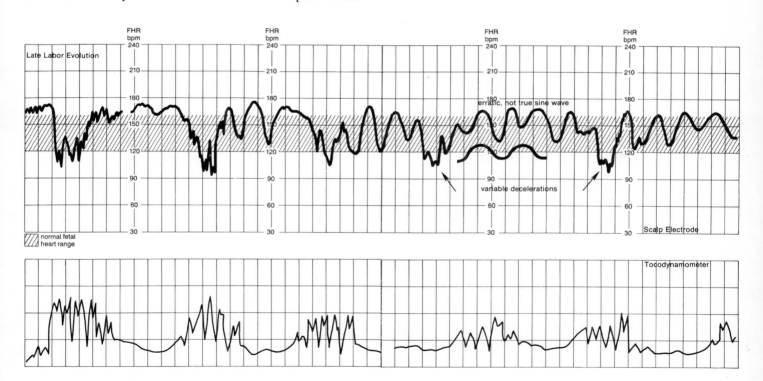

Pattern Characteristic:
Undulating Pattern in Late Labor Evolution

Undulating Pattern Associated with Obstetrical Forceps Usage

*U*ndulating patterns of varying appearance are seen during forceps application and/or traction.[66] This appears to be a rhythmic variant of long-term variability. Fetal condition is better predicted by the appearance of the tracing prior to the forceps application combined with the actual delivery events, rather than the bizarre pattern during the actual forceps procedure.[36] Two additional examples of erratic baseline changes during forceps application are included as inserts.

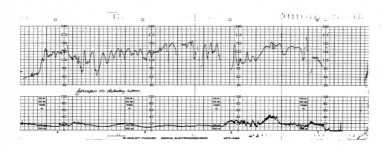

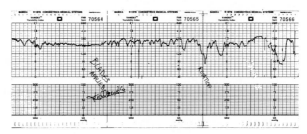

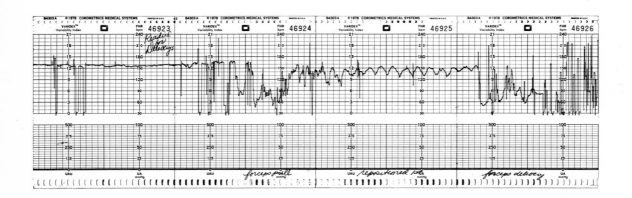

CASE INTERPRETATION: Class II

Baseline Information: high normal rate, normal variability changes to decreased short-term variability with undulating long-term variability in the baseline between episodes of forceps traction.

Periodic or Nonperiodic Changes: variable decelerations of two minute duration occur during each forceps pull.

Uterine Activity: not recorded.

Significance: there are undulating baseline changes during forceps application. The fetal condition is assessed by the preceding monitoring information and delivery events.

CASE OUTCOME: Thirty-four-year-old primigravida delivered vaginally, with epidural anesthesia, at 41 weeks' gestation an 8 pound, 8 ounce (3856 gram) male; Apgar score 9/10. The fetus was in a vertex presentation, in an occiput anterior position; outlet forceps were used. There was a probable maternal coccyx fracture. The infant followed an uncomplicated newborn course.

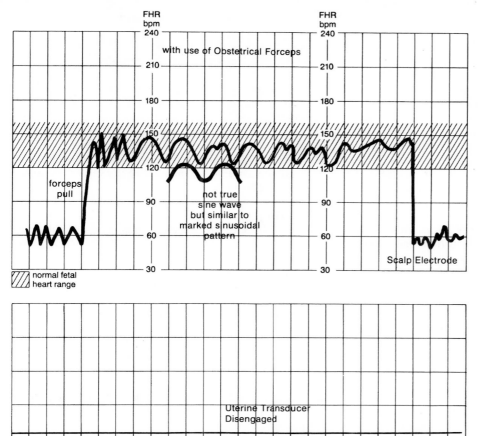

Pattern Characteristic:
Undulating Pattern with Forceps

References

1. Angel JL, Knuppel RA, Lake M: Sinusoidal fetal heart rate pattern associated with intravenous butorphanol administration: A case report. *Am J Obstet Gynecol* 149:465, 1984.
2. Antoine C, Young BK, Silverman F, et al: Sinusoidal fetal heart rate pattern with vasa previa in twin pregnancy. *J Reprod Med* 27:295, 1982.
3. Ayromlooi J, Berg P, Tobias M: The significance of sinusoidal fetal heart rate pattern during labor and its relation to fetal status and neonatal outcome. *Int J Gynaecol Obstet* 16:341, 1979.
4. Backes C, Cordero L, Warner R: Sinusoidal heart rate pattern and fetal distress secondary to severe anemia. *J Reprod Med* 24:167, 1980.
5. Baskett TF, Koh KS: Sinusoidal fetal heart pattern. A sign of fetal hypoxia. *Obstet Gynecol* 44:379, 1974.
6. Berestka JS, Johnson TRB, Hrushesky WJM: Sinusoidal fetal heart rate pattern during breathing is related to the respiratory sinus arrhythmia. A case report: *Am J Obstet Gynecol* 160:690, 1989.
7. Blanco CE, Krediet TG, Trimbos B: Neonatal sinusoidal heart rate pattern; changes after atropine administration. *Europ J Obstet Gynecol Reprod Biol* 11:39, 1980.
8. Boylan P: Sinusoidal-like tracing in fetus with rhesus-hemolytic anemia (letter). *Am J Obstet Gynecol* 145:892, 1983.
9. Busacca M, Sementi P, Ciralli I, et al: Sinusoidal fetal heart rate associated with maternal administration of me-

peridine and promethazine in labor. *J Perinat Med* 10:215, 1982.

10. Cabaniss ML: Personal observation. Unpublished data.

11. Cetrulo CL, Schifrin BS: Fetal heart rate patterns preceding death in utero. *Obstet Gynecol* 48:521, 1976.

12. Cibils LA: *Postterm Fetuses in Electronic Fetal-Maternal Monitoring: Antepartum, Intrapartum.* Chicago, John Wright PSG, 1981, p. 374ff.

13. Clark SL, Miller FD: Sinusoidal fetal heart rate pattern associated with massive fetomaternal transfusion. *Am J Obstet Gynecol* 149:97, 1984.

14. Elliott JP, Modanlou HDER, O'Keeffe DF, et al: Significance of fetal and neonatal sinusoidal heart rate pattern: Further clinical observations in Rh incompatibility. *Am J Obstet Gynecol* 138:227, 1980.

15. Epstein H, Waxman A, Gleicher N, et al: Meperidine-induced sinusoidal fetal heart rate pattern and reversal with naloxone. *Obstet Gynecol* 59:228, 1982.

16. Feinstein SJ, Lodeiro JG, Vintzileos AM, et al: Sinusoidal fetal heart rate pattern after administration of nalbuphine hydrochloride: A case report. *Am J Obstet Gynecol* 154:159, 1986.

17. Fitzsimons RB, Kearney PJ, Fenton DV: Sinusoidal fetal heart rate pattern (letter). *Am J Obstet Gynecol* 144:995, 1982.

18. Freeman RK, Garite TJ: *Basic Pattern Recognition in Fetal Heart Rate Monitoring.* Baltimore, William & Wilkins, 1981, p. 82.

19. Gal D, Jacobson LM, Ser H, et al: Sinusoidal pattern: An alarming sign of fetal distress. *Am J Obstet Gynecol* 132:903, 1978.

20. Garite TJ, Modanlou HD, Freeman RK: Sinusoidal fetal heart rate pattern (letter). *Am J Obstet Gynecol* 139:226, 1981.

21. Garite TJ: Sinusoidal pattern from anemia. *Contemporary OB/Gyn* May 1988, p. 42.

22. Gleicher N, Runowicz CD, Brown BL: Sinusoidal fetal heart rate pattern in association with amnionitis. *Obstet Gynecol* 56:109, 1980.

23. Gray JH, Cudmore DW, Luther ER, et al: Sinusoidal fetal heart rate pattern associated with alphaprodine administration. *Obstet Gynecol* 52:678, 1978.

24. Haswell GL: Management of abnormal fetal heart tracings. *Perinatology/Neonatology* Sept-Oct:25, 1978.

25. Hatjis CG, Meis PJ: Sinusoidal fetal heart rate pattern associated with butorphanol administration. *Obstet Gynecol* 67:377, 1986.

26. Hatjis CG, Mennuti MT, Sacks LM, et al: Resolution of a sinusoidal fetal heart rate pattern following intrauterine transfusion. *Am J Obstet Gynecol* 132:109, 1978.

27. Hofmeyr GJ, Sonnendecker EWW: Pseudosinusoidal fetal heart rate patterns. *Brit J Obstet Gynecol* 90:1193, 1983.

28. Hurwitz A, Milwidsky A, Yarkoni S, et al: Severe fetal distress with hydramnios due to chorioangioma. *Acta Obstet Gynecol Scand* 62:633, 1983.

29. Johnson TRB, Compton AA, Rotmenson J, et al: Significance of the sinusoidal fetal heart rate pattern. *Am J Obstet Gynecol* 139:446, 1981.

30. Kariniemi V: Fetal anemia and heart rate patterns. *J Perinat Med* 10:167, 1982.

31. Katz M, Meizner I, Shani N, et al: Clinical significance of sinusoidal fetal heart rate patterns. *Brit J Obstet Gynaecol* 90:832, 1983.

32. Katz M, Wilson SJ, Young BK: Sinusoidal fetal heart rate. II. Continuous tissue pH studies. *Am J Obstet Gynecol* 136:594, 1980.

33. Krebs H: Definition of sinusoidal fetal heart rate. *Am J Obstet Gynecol* 138:1231, 1980.

34. Lowe TW, Leveno KJ, Quirk JG, et al: Sinusoidal fetal heart rate pattern after intrauterine transfusion. *Obstet Gynecol* 64:218, 1984.

35. Martin CB: Regulation of the fetal heart rate and genesis of FHR patterns. *Seminars in Perinatology* 2:131, 1978.

36. Mega M, Cerutti R, Miccoli P, et al: Usefulness of cardiotocography in expulsion period. *Clin Exp Obst Gynecol* 8:3, 1981.

37. Milio LA, Arnold SA, Parer JT: The relationship between fetal heart rate variability and hematocrit in Rh isoimmunization. *Proceedings of the Society of Perinatal Obstetricians Eighth Annual Meeting*, San Francisco, 1988.

38. Modanlou HD: Guide to sinusoidal FHR patterns. *Contemporary OB/GYN* August:94, 1983.

39. Modanlou HD, Freeman RK: Sinusoidal fetal heart rate pattern: Its definition and clinical significance. *Am J Obstet Gynecol* 142:1033, 1982.

40. Modanlou HD, Freeman RK, Ortiz O, et al: Sinusoidal fetal heart rate patterns and severe fetal anemia. *Obstet Gynecol* 49:537, 1977.

41. Mueller-Heubach E, Caritis SN, Edelstone DI: Sinusoidal fetal heart rate pattern following intrauterine fetal transfusion. *Obstet Gynecol* 52:43, 1978.

42. Murata Y, Miyake Y, Yamamoto T, et al: Experimentally produced sinusoidal fetal heart rate pattern in the chronically instrumented fetal lamb. *Am J Obstet Gynecol* 153:693, 1985.

43. Nicolaides KH, Sadovsky G, Cetin E: Fetal heart rate patterns in red blood cell isoimmunized pregnancies. *Am J Obstet Gynecol* 161;351, 1989.

44. Nijhuis JG, Staisch KJ, Martin CB, et al: A sinusoidal-like fetal heart-rate pattern in association with fetal sucking—report of two cases. *Eur J Obstet Gynecol Reprod Biol* 16:353, 1984.

45. Ombelet W, Van Der Merwe JV: Sinusoidal fetal heart rate pattern associated with congenital hydrocephalus. A report of 2 cases. *S Afr Med J* 67:423, 1985.

46. Parer JT: Fetal heart rate patterns preceding death in utero, in *Handbook of Fetal Heart Rate Monitoring.* Philadelphia, W.B. Saunders, 1983, p. 147.

47. Peleg D, Goldman JA: Fetal heart patterns. A study of the anencephalic fetus. *Obstet Gynecol* 53:530, 1979.

48. Pillai M, James D: The development of fetal heart rate patterns during normal pregnancy. *Obstet Gynecol* 76:812, 1990.

49. Reid MM, Jenkins J, McClure G: Sinusoidal heart rate rhythms in severe neonatal hypoxia. *Archives of Disease in Childhood* 54:432, 1979.

50. Sacks DA, Bell KE, Schwimmer WB, et al: Sinusoidal fetal heart rate patterns with intrapartum fetal death. *J Reprod Med* 24:171, 1980.

51. Sadovsky E, Ohel T: Sinusoidal FHR patterns (letter). *Contemp Obstet Gynecol* January 1985, p. 15.

52. Sanchez-Ramos L, Robertson EG, Beydoun S: Importance of sinusoidal fetal heart rate pattern (letter). *Am J Obstet Gynecol* 144:863, 1982.

53. Schneider EP, Tropper PJ: Sinusoidal fetal heart rate. *Clin Obstet Gynecol* 29:70, 1986.

54. Serafini PC, Amisial PA, Murgalo JA, et al: Unusual fetal heart rate pattern associated with severe neonatal asphyxia and death. *Am J Obstet Gynecol* 140:715, 1981.

55. Sibai BM, Lipshitz J, Schneider JM, et al: Sinusoidal fetal heart rate pattern. *Obstet Gynecol* 55:637, 1980.

56. Souma ML: Sinusoidal fetal heart rate (letter). *Am J Obstet Gynecol* 139:320, 1981.

57. Stiller AG, Skafish FR: Placental chorioangioma: A rare cause of fetomaternal transfusion with maternal hemolysis and fetal distress. *Obstet Gynecol* 67:296, 1986.

58. Terao T, Kawashima Y, Noto H, et al: Neurological control of fetal heart rate in 20 cases of anencephalic fetuses. *Am J Obstet Gynecol* 149:201, 1984.

59. Theard JFC, Penney LL, Otterson WN: Sinusoidal fetal heart rate. Ominous or benign? *J Reprod Med* 29:265, 1984.

60. Thiessen P, Robinson K, Shennan AT: Intrapartum cardiac monitor abnormality associated with severe fetal anemia and hypoxia. *Am J Obstet Gynecol* 130:731, 1978.

61. Tushuizen PBT, Stoot JEGM, Ubachs JMH: Fetal heart rate monitoring of the dying fetus. *Am J Obstet Gynecol* 120:922, 1974.

62. Verma U, Tejani N, Weiss RR, et al: Sinusoidal fetal heart rate patterns in severe Rh disease. *Obstet Gynecol* 55:666, 1980.

63. Visser GHA: Antepartum sinusoidal and decelerative heart rate patterns in Rh disease. *Am J Obstet Gynecol* 143:538, 1982.

64. Welt SI: Sinusoidal fetal heart rate and butorphanol administration. *Am J Obstet Gynecol* 152:362, 1985.

65. Young BK, Katz M, Wilson SJ: Sinusoidal fetal heart rate. I. Clinical significance. *Am J Obstet Gynecol* 136:587, 1980.

66. Zilianti M, Cabello F, Estrada MA: Fetal heart rate patterns during forceps operation. *J Perinat Med* 6:80, 1978.

Baseline Shifts

Chapter 8

Increasing Baseline Rate

*B*oth gradual increases and decreases in baseline heart rate may reflect fetal response to maternal temperature changes.[4,5,23,30]

A gradual increase in maternal temperature during labor, accompanied as a rule by a simultaneous fetal heart rate increase, is seen with maternal infection such as pyelonephritis, with a healthy fetus. Usually, normal variability is displayed. Correction of maternal fever by antipyretic agents or treatment of the etiology of the infection is typically accompanied by normalization of the fetal heart rate. Fetal heart rate increase may parallel development of chorioamnionitis before or during labor.[2] When the fetus is sick with the infection, variability may be diminished. Occasionally, gradual increase in fetal heart rate accompanies the use of epidural anesthesia.[9,11,14,20] This mechanism may be secondary to maternal temperature changes.[7,9,14] The newborn may display transient increased temperature, which falls rapidly, as does the maternal fever, without therapy after delivery.[14]

An increasing baseline rate may reflect a healthy fetal response to mild hypoxia.[4] A fetus may demonstrate late decelerations at rapid heart rates that disappear with normalization of the fetal heart rate, suggesting a compensated hypoxia unveiled by the increased metabolic demands accompanying the faster heart rate. A slight decrease in variability typically accompanies an increase in heart rate because of increased sympathetic tone. It is important that this be distinguished from decreased variability produced by depletion of fetal compensatory mechanisms resulting in acidosis.

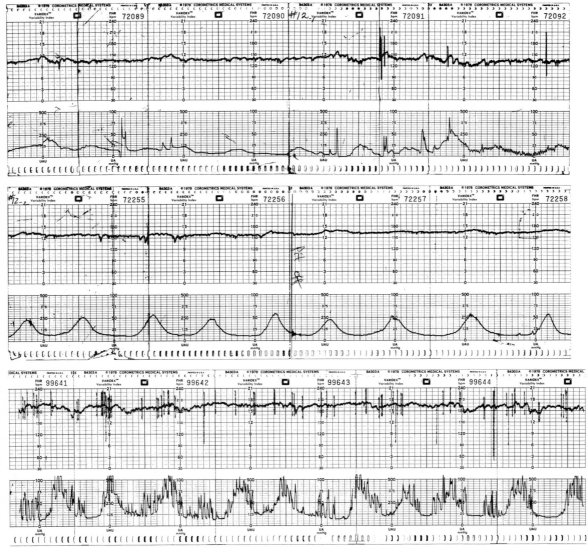

Recreation of original tracing

CASE INTERPRETATION: Class II

Baseline Information: rising baseline from the initial normal rate to marked tachycardia, average variability. Vertical spikes are probably produced by artifact.

Periodic or Nonperiodic Changes: accelerations present.

Uterine Activity: a progression from a small waveform as measured by a tocodynamometer, to peaked contractions to contractions reflecting probable maternal straining.

Significance: with good variability, in the absence of periodic changes, the most likely etiology is a healthy fetus subjected to maternal fever of various possible etiologies.

CASE OUTCOME: Twenty-one-year-old primigravida delivered vaginally at 43 weeks' gestation a 9 pound, 9 ounce (4337 gram) male; Apgar score 8/9. The mother received oxytocin augmentation; she had a 20-hour labor. The mother's temperature increased steadily following epidural anesthetic administration. She received cefamandole intrapartum for cystitis; urine cultures were negative. Placental cultures showed anaerobic, gram-negative and gram-positive organisms, which were unidentified. There followed both a normal-newborn and uncomplicated postpartum course.

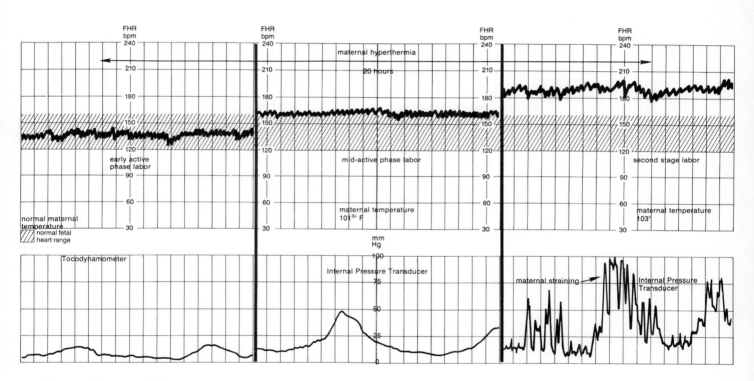

Pattern Characteristic:
Increasing Baseline Rate

Increasing Baseline Rate with Decelerations: Mixed Pattern

A gradual increase in the baseline rate over several hours may reflect a healthy fetal response to the stress of mild hypoxia (as well as maternal temperature changes), particularly when normal variability is preserved. When accompanied by decelerations, which may present clues that help in the diagnosis of the etiology of the hypoxic stress, the rise in baseline rate may indicate fetal stress.[12,13,25] Such a pattern is often seen in the last 30 minutes of labor, when variable decelerations occur with increased frequency secondary to cord impingement and expulsive efforts.[1]

Management of a stress pattern is focused on relieving stresses, for example, by changing maternal position, decreasing maternal straining, diminishing uterine hyperactivity, improving fetal oxygenation, and planning a delivery that minimizes avoidable additional stresses.

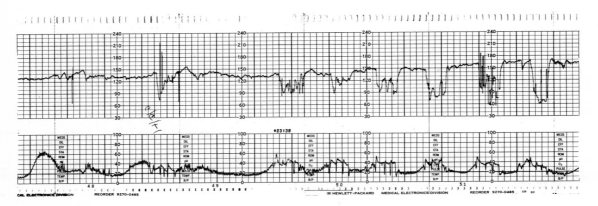

CASE INTERPRETATION: Class II

Baseline Information: a rising baseline from a normal rate to the upper limits of normal, bordering on moderate tachycardia. Average to decreased variability.

Periodic or Nonperiodic Changes: variable decelerations progress from mildly V-shaped to moderate multiphasic to severe by virtue of a depth of 60 bpm, while retaining classic features.

Uterine Activity: maternal straining appears at complete cervical dilatation with the increased frequency of contractions, and there is an eventual obliteration of the resting phase.

Significance: hypoxic stress of a healthy fetus, probably secondary to cord impingement. Appropriate management includes a change in maternal position and administration of oxygen. A healthy fetus is anticipated if delivery is imminent.

CASE OUTCOME: Twenty-three-year-old gravida 3, para 2012, at 37 weeks' gestation delivered vaginally, with epidural anesthesia, from an occiput anterior position, a 6 pound, 7 ounce (2920 gram) female; Apgar score 8/9. The infant followed an uncomplicated newborn course.

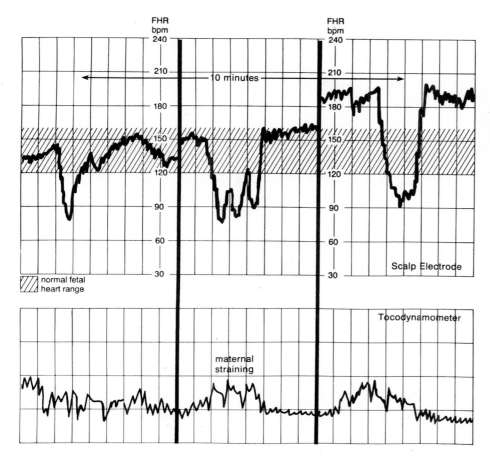

Pattern Characteristic:
Increasing Baseline Rate with
Decelerations: Mixed Pattern

Decreasing Baseline Rate

A gradual downward drift in the baseline rate from low normal range to moderate or marked bradycardia, when accompanied by normal variability and reactivity, is a typical pattern believed to be produced by the parasympathetic effects of chronic head compression.

This pattern (also discussed on pages 30 and 31) is associated with primigravid labor, a large fetus, a vertex presentation, an occiput posterior position, cephalopelvic disproportion, and ruptured membranes.[29] The pattern may also accompany maternal cooling.[17]

The preservation of normal variability and absence of hypoxia-induced stress patterns is in keeping with the clinical experience that this bears no pathologic connotation.[32] The pattern must be distinguished from other etiologies of bradycardia and observed for change. For example, should decelerations occur from an already slow rate (see page 36), a significantly reduced perfusion of the fetus might theoretically result.

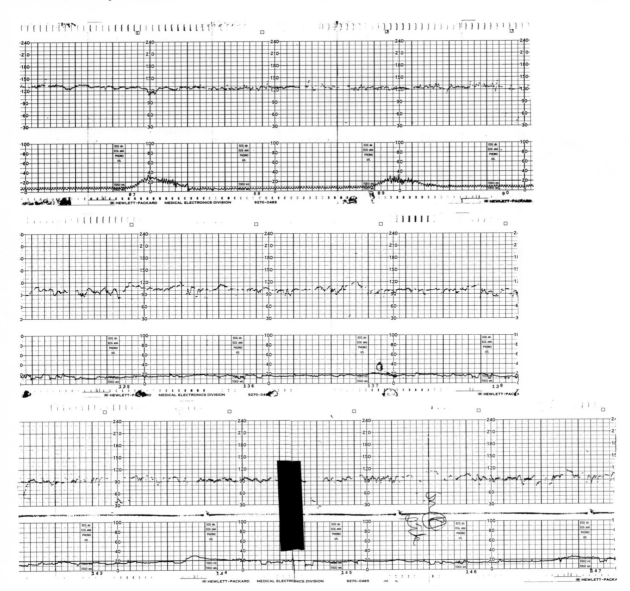

CASE INTERPRETATION: Class I

Baseline Information: a falling baseline, initially from a normal range to marked bradycardia. Average variability.

Periodic or Nonperiodic Changes: none.

Uterine Activity: initially infrequent contractions followed by poor recording versus diminution of uterine activity.

Significance: a pattern seen with the progressive compression of the fetal head with the progression of labor, which is often associated with an occiput posterior position.

CASE OUTCOME: Thirty-year-old primigravida delivered vaginally at 42 weeks' gestation, by low forceps from an occiput anterior position, with epidural anesthesia, an 8 pound, 9 ounce (3856 gram) male; Apgar score 10/10. Slight meconium was present. The infant followed a normal newborn course. The child has mild autism.

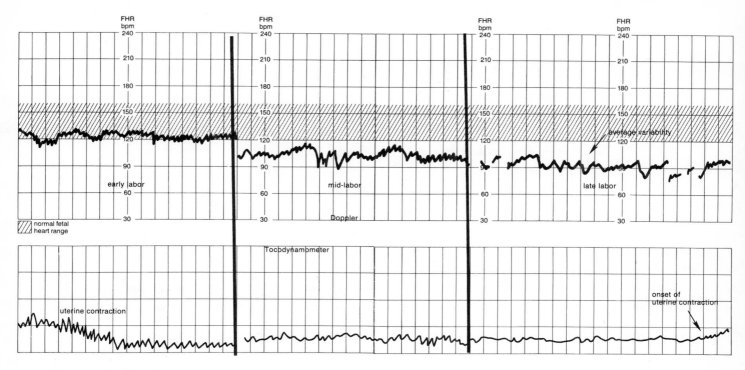

Pattern Characteristic:
Decreasing Baseline Rate

Decreasing Baseline Rate with Decelerations: Mixed Pattern

*C*ontinuation of the baseline at a lower level is one of the seven atypical variable decelerations, albeit rare (7.5% of atypical variable decelerations). As such, it predicts an increased risk of a low Apgar score, but only in the neighborhood of approximately 7% at five minutes (see page 248).[18]

Most likely, this pattern represents slow recovery from a variable deceleration in a situation in which the next deceleration occurs before the baseline is reached. Eventually, an overlap phenomenon (see page 277) may occur, with confluence of the nadirs of each deceleration simulating a bradycardia or prolonged deceleration.

Management is directed at reduction of uterine hyperactivity, if present, change in maternal position for reduction of cord impingement, and examination for a prolapsed cord. A decision regarding delivery is influenced by the response to these and other measures to maximize fetal oxygenation, a change in the pattern with the progress of labor, gestation, the basal condition of the fetus based on clinical data (e.g., growth, gestation), maternal clinical factors, and anticipated time to and ease of vaginal delivery.

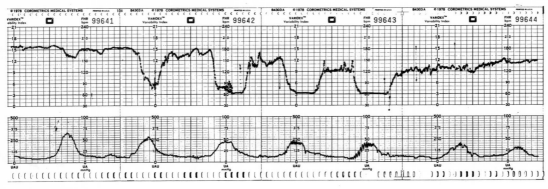

Recreation of original tracing

CASE INTERPRETATION: Class IV

Baseline Information: progressive lowering of the baseline after a deceleration from severe tachycardia, low normal range, good variability.

Periodic or Nonperiodic Changes: variable decelerations that are moderate to severe. Atypia characterized by continuation of the baseline at a lower level.

Uterine Activity: regular contractions, minimally skewed.

Significance: one of the "atypical" variable decelerations, denoting increased risk of an eventual low Apgar score. The presence of good variability excludes a possibility of significant acidosis at this time. Management is based on the clinical setting and response to measures to improve the fetal umbilical flow and oxygenation.

CASE OUTCOME: Twenty-five-year-old gravida 4, para 2012, at 32 weeks' gestation delivered vaginally, with pudendal anesthesia, a 4 pound (1814 gram) male; Apgar score 8/9. The pregnancy was complicated by illegal drug use. There were premature ruptured membranes for 24 hours before delivery. Chorioamnionitis was found, as were positive group B streptococcal amniotic fluid and placental cultures. The newborn had negative cultures, was treated with antibiotics, and followed a normal course. No abnormal cord position was noted. The fetal monitoring pattern appeared early in labor and was followed by improvement.

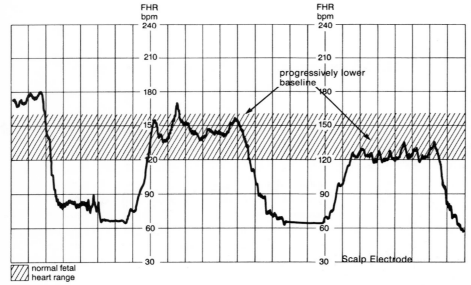

Pattern Characteristic:
Decreasing Baseline Rate–with Decelerations

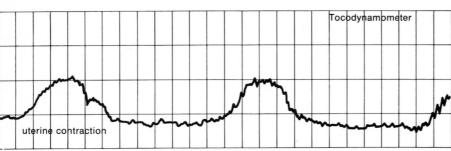

Normalization of Baseline Rate—Correction of Maternal Hypothermia

*G*radual baseline fetal heart rate shifts accompany the normalization of abnormal maternal temperature, whether the correction is for hyperthermia or hypothermia.[17]

The fetus has no heat exchange system save through the mother, so that maternal temperature changes are readily reflected in fetal metabolic performance and thus in the fetal cardiac rate.[23,30]

Causes of maternal hypothermia include severe hypoglycemia use of magnesium sulfate, and the post-treatment phase of severe sepsis.[26] An association between fetal bradycardia and maternal hypoglycemia has been noted without reference to low maternal temperature as an etiology.[19]

Beat-to-beat variability may also change, reflecting the "normalization" process from both high and low temperatures. See page 33 for further discussion of hypothermia-associated fetal bradycardia.

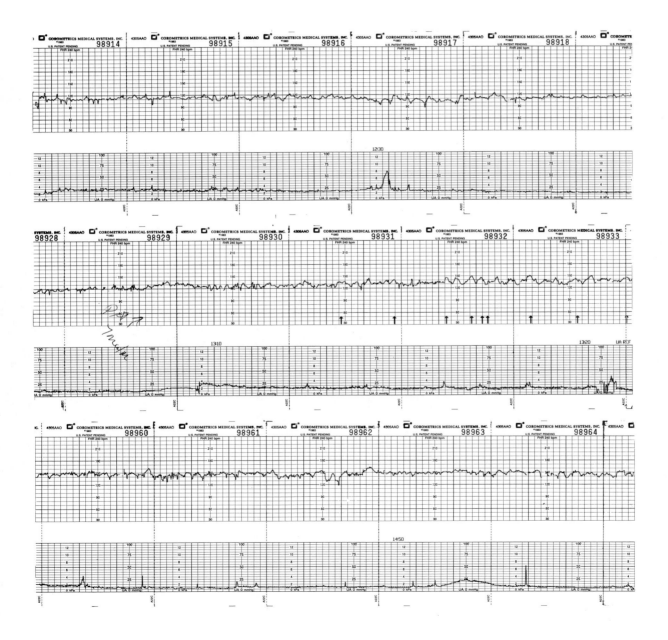

CASE INTERPRETATION: Class I

Baseline Information: heart rate increases from moderate bradycardia to the upper limits of the normal range; there is average variability throughout.

Periodic or Nonperiodic Changes: none seen.

Uterine Activity: uterine contractions are not displayed.

Significance: a good fetal condition most often accompanies a gradual rise in heart rate when associated with a temperature increase, especially in the absence of labor.

CASE OUTCOME: Thirty-seven-year-old primigravida, with type I diabetes mellitus, delivered vaginally, with epidural anesthesia and elective outlet forceps, a 6 pound, 3 ounce (2087 gram) female; Apgar score 8/9. The fetus was in a vertex presentation. The infant followed an uncomplicated newborn course.

This segment was obtained four days prior to delivery when the mother was admitted in severe insulin shock and associated hypothermia (94°F). She recovered with insulin therapy without any apparent maternal or fetal sequelae.

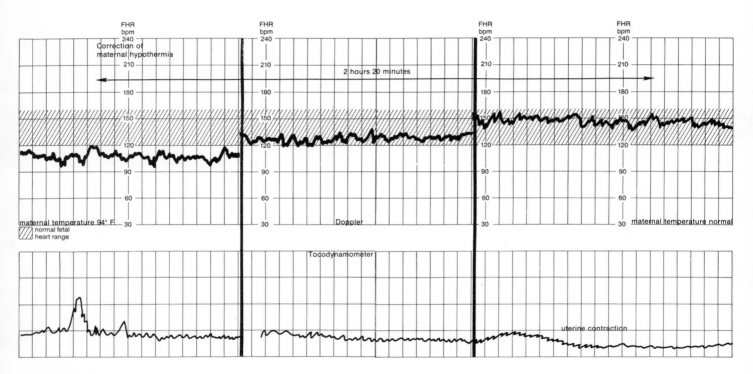

Pattern Characteristic:
Normalization of Baseline Rate

Upward Baseline Shift—Late Labor

A baseline moderate or marked bradycardia accompanied by normal or increased variability and reactivity may be associated with an occiput posterior position of a vertex presentation.[28] This is also most frequently a pattern of the primigravid labor with a large fetus.

Occasionally, an upward shift or "normalization" of the fetal heart rate accompanies rotation to an occiput anterior position.[31]

The bradycardia associated with an occiput posterior position is believed to reflect parasympathetic stimulation.[18]

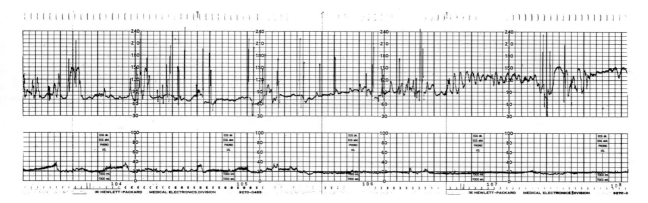

CASE INTERPRETATION: Class IV, II, I

Baseline Information: marked bradycardia with a change in the baseline to a normal rate, normal variability, and increased variability during resolution of the bradycardia.

Periodic or Nonperiodic Changes: atypical accelerations, single moderate variable deceleration with slight smoothing of secondary acceleration.

Uterine Activity: poorly recorded. Changing maternal breathing was noted.

Significance: a baseline change from bradycardia to normal is seen with rotation of an occiput posterior position to an occiput anterior position. The clinical setting and normal variability combine to predict a healthy fetus. It is critical to distinguish this pattern from a prolonged deceleration or bradycardia associated with placental abruption. See page 194 for a discussion of atypical accelerations.

CASE OUTCOME: Twenty-four-year-old primigravida delivered vaginally, with local anesthesia, at 40 weeks' gestation a 9 pound, 10 ounce (4366 gram) male; Apgar score 9/10. Baseline bradycardia with good variability was present throughout labor. Spontaneous rotation of the fetus from an occiput posterior to an anterior occiput position was accompanied by recovery to a normal fetal heart rate baseline just prior to delivery.

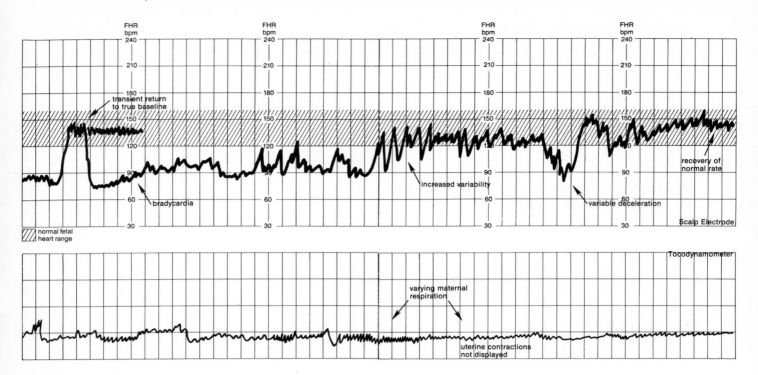

Pattern Characteristic:
Upward Baseline Shift—Rotation of Occiput Posterior

Downward Baseline Shift—Late Labor

A shift in the baseline fetal heart rate is identified when the new level persists for 10 or more minutes.[16] With parasympathetic responses to increased fetal head compression occurring in late labor, baseline bradycardia may abruptly appear as a baseline shift, initially suggesting a prolonged deceleration. However, baseline variability is preserved (no sinus node suppression), is often increased, and return to the previous baseline does not occur after 10 minutes or often throughout the remainder of the labor. As with most fetal monitoring interpreta-

tion, baseline variability is the major determinant of fetal condition and supports expectant management. The presence of decreased variability in decelerations heightens concern.[13] A baseline shift to marked bradycardia that precedes fetal death is typically void of beat-to-beat variability.[3,27] When variability is increased, reflecting hypoxia, usually secondary to uterine hyperactivity, measures are in order to improve fetal oxygenation and reduce uterine hyperactivity.

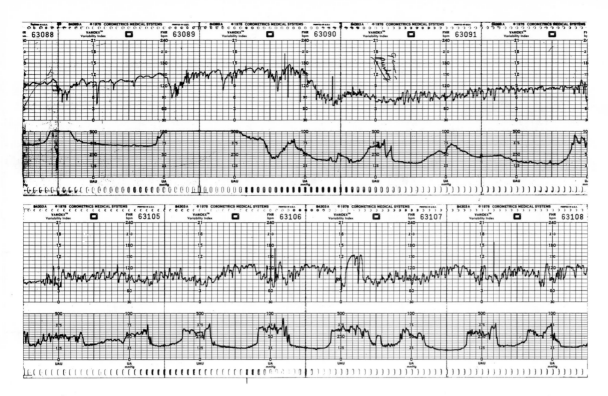

CASE INTERPRETATION: Class II

Baseline Information: normal baseline heart rate of approximately 130 bpm. This shifts with the onset of maternal pushing at nine centimeters dilatation to 90 to 120 bpm, which is associated with an increase in beat-to-beat variability.

Periodic or Nonperiodic Changes: a mixed pattern of accelerations and V-shaped variable decelerations precede the shift in association with a prolonged contraction. A single atypical acceleration occurs in the midst of the new baseline.

Uterine Activity: initially prolonged, skewed contractions are followed by frequent contractions with maternal straining.

Significance: The baseline instability may represent continuous decelerations, from which there is no return to baseline, or a true baseline shift. The latter designation is appropriate because more than 10 minutes pass at the new rate. In this case, either signifies a healthy stressed fetus.

CASE OUTCOME: Twenty-six-year-old primigravida delivered vaginally, with local anesthesia, at 41 weeks' gestation a 7 pound, 12 ounce (3515 gram) male; Apgar score 9/9. The fetus was in a vertex presentation. A tight nuchal cord was noted. Both the postpartum and newborn courses were uncomplicated.

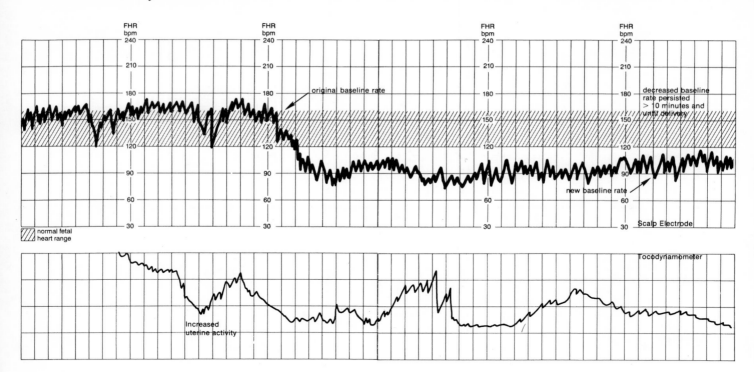

Pattern Characteristic:
Downward Baseline Shift Late Labor

Wandering Baseline—Unfavorable Outcome

A fetal monitoring pattern that displays no short-term variability, although sometimes seen in the patterns of a healthy fetus, is not diagnostic of a fetus in good condition. The presence of long-term variability is not consistently reassuring, nor are apparent accelerations (unless excellent variability and reactivity immediately preceded the administration of drugs known to obliterate variability).

A wandering baseline may reflect the lack of central nervous system regulation of cardiac responses due to immaturity, anomalous development, or terminal hypoxia; the pattern may be mistaken for a pattern with accelerations.[10]

A particularly confusing pattern is one in which only the prolonged secondary acceleration of an atypical variable deceleration may predominate. Variable decelerations, like late decelerations, may become shallower and blunted as contractions and further cord impingement fail to produce significant variations in the environment of the already severely compromised fetus.

Such a pattern may precede fetal death, therefore, it is appropriate to respond to such a pattern with fetal pH studies (or delivery if pH studies are not available), unless review of the entire tracing and knowledge of specific clinical circumstances including response to fetal stimulation, influence the decision otherwise.[3,10]

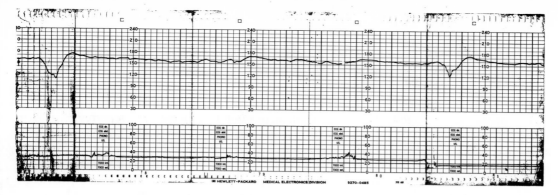

CASE INTERPRETATION: Class IV (Class III if observing diagrammed portion alone)

Baseline Information: high normal rate, absent short-term variability, wavering long-term variability that produces a wandering baseline.

Periodic or Nonperiodic Changes: typical mild to moderate variable decelerations with prolonged secondary accelerations and loss of variability in the decelerations produce a wandering baseline and give the appearance of shallow accelerations.

Uterine Activity: minimal tocodynamometer-derived deflections suggest contractions every three to four minutes.

Significance: the increased risk of a low Apgar score and acidosis is sufficient to warrant intervention if the fetus is viable unless there is other reassuring information.

CASE OUTCOME: Twenty-year-old gravida 4, para 1111, delivered by cesarean section for fetal distress at 29 weeks' gestation a 1 pound, 14 ounce (850 gram) female; Apgar score 1/2. The fetus was in a breech presentation. The membranes were ruptured for three days. Chorioamnionitis was diagnosed. The newborn survived despite having respiratory distress and possible necrotizing enterocolitis. The infant was dismissed at 80 days of life. The child was subsequently diagnosed as having cerebral palsy.

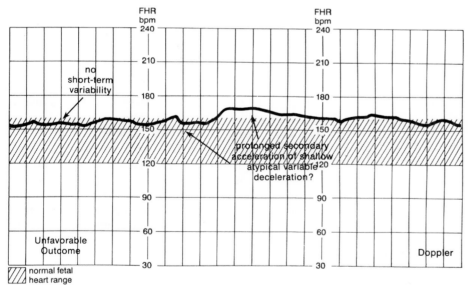

Pattern Characteristic:
Unstable Baseline. Unfavorable Outcome

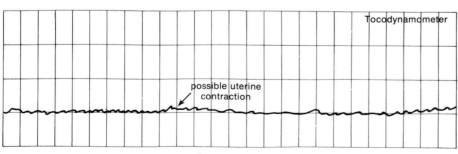

Wandering Baseline Associated with Fetal Neurologic Disease

*J*ust as a wandering baseline may be encountered when neurologic control of cardiac changes is obliterated by asphyxia, it is also reasonable that similar patterns may be encountered in the neurologically abnormal fetus.[3,10]

The presence of short-term variability in the anencephalic fetus has been demonstrated to require the presence of the fetal medulla and hypothalamus. Loss of beat-to-beat variability may be produced by the structural absence of these centers or by asphyxial decommission of these centers. Long-term variability in anencephalic fetuses correlates with the presence of the medulla and midbrain.

Hydrocephalic fetuses have been reported to demonstrate tachycardia and no variability, but no pathonomic pattern exists. In fact, possible patterns range from normal to sinusoidal.[8,22,24] The abnormalities may be caused by tissue hypoxia of the medullary centers that occurs as a result of pressure on brain centers produced by the intracerebral ventricular dilatation.[8] They also may be influenced by prematurity and intrapartum events.[22,24]

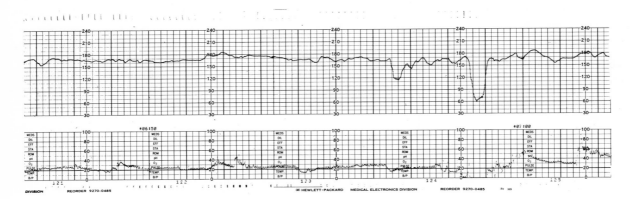

CASE INTERPRETATION: Class IV (Class III if observing diagrammed portion only)

Baseline Information: moderate tachycardia, absent beat-to-beat variability, wavering long-term variability that produces a wandering baseline.

Periodic or Nonperiodic Changes: atypical mild to severe variable decelerations with loss of variability in the decelerations and a delayed return to baseline, some preservation of classical primary and secondary accelerations. Long-term fluctuations have the appearance of accelerations.

Uterine Activity: small, poorly recorded contractions, some "reversed."

Significance: increased risk of a low Apgar score and acidosis. Management is influenced by gestation, estimated duration to delivery, and response to maternal position change and administration of oxygen. A fetal pH or fetal stimulation test may be an adjunct, depending upon previous information about fetal health, including the presence or absence of variability prior to any medication usage.

CASE OUTCOME: Twenty-seven-year-old gravida 2, para 0010, delivered vaginally, from a vertex presentation, at 27 weeks' gestation a 3 pound, 3 ounce (1446 gram) male; Apgar score 7/7. Local and pudendal anesthesia was administered. Hydrocephalus and meningomyelocele were diagnosed antepartum. The newborn underwent meningomyeloplasty on the fifth day of life and the procedure for a ventriculoperitoneal shunt at three weeks of life. A poor prognosis was made for normal neurologic function.

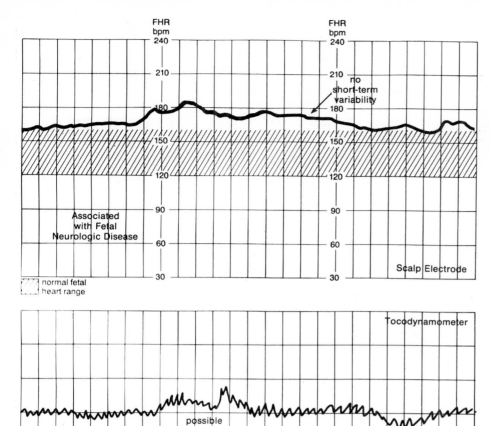

Pattern Characteristic:
Unstable Baseline. Neurologic Disease

Wandering Baseline—Favorable Outcome

*I*t is not possible for the fetal monitor to diagnose the fetal condition reliably in the absence of beat-to-beat variability. Nonreassuring fluctuations in long-term variability or blunted atypical variable decelerations may be mistaken for reassuring accelerations. Therefore, use of fetal pH may be helpful in patterns with absent short-term variability, even though long-term variability is present, just as with "flat-line" patterns.

Because diminished short-term variability with preservation of long-term variability that produces a wandering baseline is a pattern preceding fetal death, loss of beat-to-beat variability[2,10] should not be assumed to be on the basis of drug therapy, although such a pattern often results, unless normal variability and reactivity immediately preceded the drug therapy without any intervening hypoxic periodic changes.[6,21] See page 86 for a wandering baseline associated with prematurity in a healthy fetus.

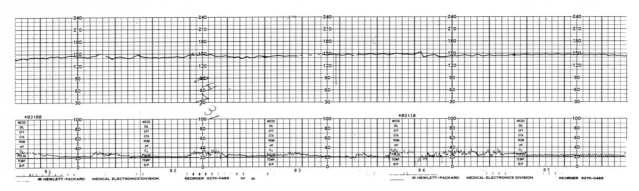

CASE INTERPRETATION: Class III

Baseline Information: normal rate, absent beat-to-beat variability, wavering long-term variability producing a wandering baseline.

Periodic or Nonperiodic Changes: fluctuations in long-term variability have the appearance of shallow accelerations followed by shallow decelerations.

Uterine Activity: poorly recorded contractions approximately every two minutes as measured by a tocodynamometer.

Significance: lack of diagnostic information about fetal welfare. Additional information such as fetal pH may be helpful to assure the safety of continuing conservative intrapartum management.

CASE OUTCOME: Thirty-five-year-old gravida 3, para 2002, delivered by cesarean section for cephalopelvic disproportion at 38 weeks' gestation a 12 pound, 10 ounce (5727 gram) male; Apgar score 8/9. The pregnancy was complicated by mild preeclampsia, insulin-dependent diabetes mellitus, and obesity greater than 300 pounds. The mother received magnesium sulfate and insulin infusions intrapartum. The scalp pH was 7.31 at the time of this segment. The newborn course was complicated by transient hypoglycemia. The patient had an average baseline variability earlier in labor prior to the administration of narcotic analgesics and magnesium sulfate.

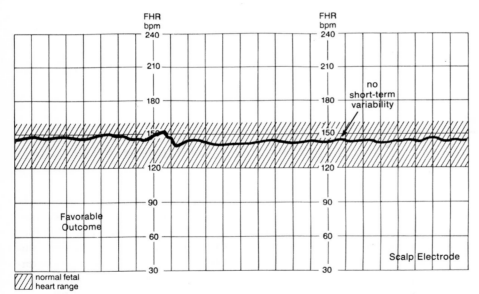

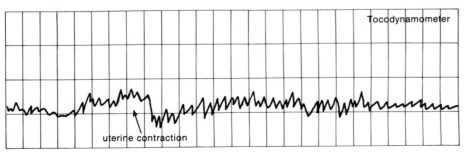

Pattern Characteristic:
Unstable Baseline. Favorable Outcome

Baseline Obscured by Increased Variability

*I*t is not uncommon when encountering increased variability, produced by the mildly hypoxic effects of increased uterine activity in late labor, to see a lowering of the fetal heart baseline rate accompanying the parasympathetic-dominated heart rate changes.

The wide fluctuations occurring with the saltatory pattern, however, may obscure identification of the baseline rate. With intermittent cessation of uterine activity, vestiges of the original baseline rate or the new lower baseline rate or both may appear between bursts of the saltatory pattern. The baseline rate is not as important in diagnosis of the fetal condition as is the variability. The saltatory pattern is displayed by a healthy stressed fetus responding to mild hypoxia, usually produced by increased uterine activity.[15,21]

Management of this, as is the case with other stress patterns, is directed at alleviating stress and planning that no additional avoidable stress be superimposed in the subsequent intrapartum and early neonatal course (see Chap. 5 for further discussion of stress patterns characterized by increased variability).

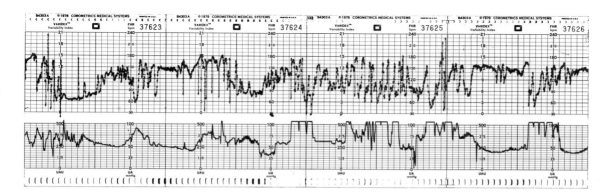

CASE INTERPRETATION: Class II

Baseline Information: unstable baseline, assigning a baseline rate is not possible because it is unstable and obscured by the increased variability. Transiently, a baseline rate of 140 to 150 bpm is suggested. Rates of 65 to 85 bpm probably represent partially obscured decelerations. Rates of 90 to 100 bpm could herald a downward true baseline shift if labor were to continue.

Periodic or Nonperiodic Changes: probable obscured, severe variable decelerations.

Uterine Activity: frequently skewed contractions with indications of maternal straining, suggesting the second stage of labor.

Significance: healthy, stressed fetus. Management may include reduction of uterine activity and straining, if feasible. There is an increased risk of meconium aspiration if thick meconium is present. There is no fetal acidosis at this time. The stress may eventually exhaust the fetal compensatory mechanisms if stress is not relieved.

CASE OUTCOME: Nineteen-year-old primigravida delivered vaginally, with epidural anesthesia, at 37½ weeks' gestation an 8 pound, 7 ounce (3827 gram) male; Apgar score 8/9. The amniotic fluid was clear. A nuchal cord was noted at delivery. The infant followed an uncomplicated newborn course.

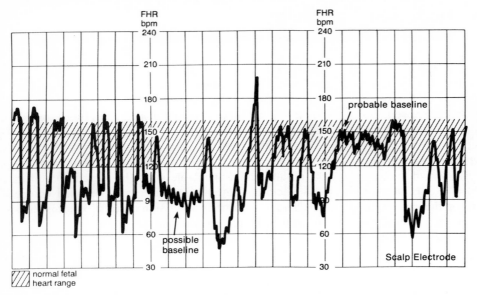

Pattern Characteristic:
Baseline Obscured by Increased Variability

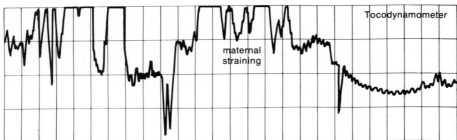

Baseline Obscured by Accelerations

When accelerations are prolonged and confluent, the true baseline heart rate may be obscured. The resulting pattern suggests tachycardia with loss of variability and even an undulating or unstable, wandering baseline.

To make a correct diagnosis of the fetal condition, attention must be given to clinical details such as the degree of uterine activity and the presence or absence of other hypoxic insults to the fetus. A study of the entire heart rate trace for clues regarding true baseline level and variability may also be helpful (see also pages 133 and 191 for a study of other prolonged acceleration patterns).

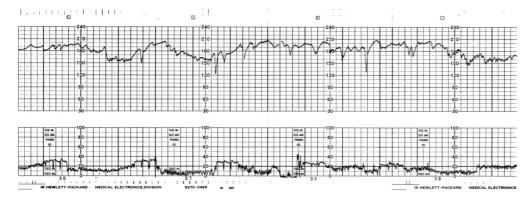

CASE INTERPRETATION: Class II

Baseline Information: the high normal rate of 150 to 160 bpm with average variability is obscured for most of the segment by accelerations, with an associated decrease in short-term variability.

Periodic or Nonperiodic Changes: prolonged and marked accelerations, small V-shaped variable decelerations within the accelerations.

Uterine Activity: contractions appear every three minutes, as measured by a tocodynamometer, and display a configuration seen with maternal straining.

Significance: a healthy fetus who is responding to the mild hypoxic stress of activity and/or labor. Cord impingement is predicted by the appearance of the small variable decelerations within the accelerations.

CASE OUTCOME: Twenty-three-year-old primigravida delivered vaginally, with epidural anesthesia and the use of midforceps, at 40 weeks' gestation a 7 pound, 1½ ounce (3218 gram) female; Apgar score 9/9. The fetus was in a persistent occiput posterior position. The infant followed an uncomplicated newborn course.

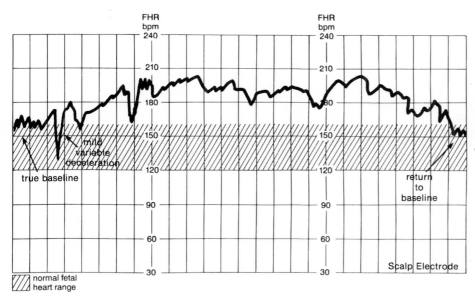

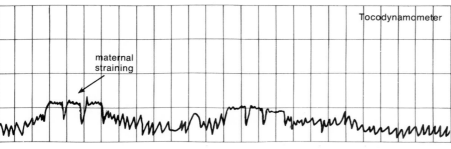

Pattern Characteristic:
Baseline Obscured by
Accelerations

Baseline Obscured by Decelerations

*O*n occasion, a fascinating pattern is seen in late labor in which the baseline heart rate appears to progressively rise accompanied by mild or moderate variable decelerations, while the nadir of the decelerations consistently resides at the level of the original baseline. When both "baselines" appear to have comparable variability, identification of the true baseline is confusing. The association of the decelerations with contractions, absence of typical features of accelerations, and analysis of the progression of the pattern may clarify that the more rapid baseline is the "new" baseline. The pattern of variable decelerations and tachycardia has been associated with increased risk of a low Apgar score; but in the presence of good baseline variability, the pattern suggests a healthy stressed fetus.[12] Usual measures to reduce present stresses and to not add future stress are appropriate.

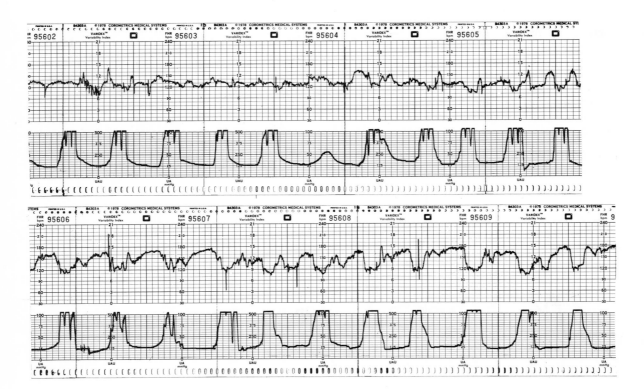

CASE INTERPRETATION: Class II

Baseline Information: unstable and obscured baseline. It is not clear whether the baseline rate is approximately 120 bpm with accelerations or 170 bpm with decelerations. There is average variability throughout.

Periodic or Nonperiodic Changes: it is not immediately clear whether variable decelerations are present with a delayed return to an elevated baseline or whether accelerations are present from a low normal baseline.

Uterine Activity: internal pressure transducer-monitored contractions with high baseline tone and an appearance of maternal straining.

Significance: probably a rising baseline with variable rounded appearance of accelerations. The lower rate coincides with contractions, suggesting the nadir of variable decelerations, which, occurring at the level of the previous baseline, causes confusion. This pattern suggests a healthy stressed fetus late in labor.

CASE OUTCOME: Fifteen-year-old gravida 2, para 0010, delivered spontaneously at 40 weeks' gestation, with epidural anesthesia, a 7 pound, 3 ounce (3260 gram) male; Apgar score 3/6. The fetus was in a vertex presentation. The newborn course was complicated by transient sinus tachycardia, mild acidosis, which responded to oxygen administered in a hood, and hyperbilirubinemia, which responded to phototherapy.

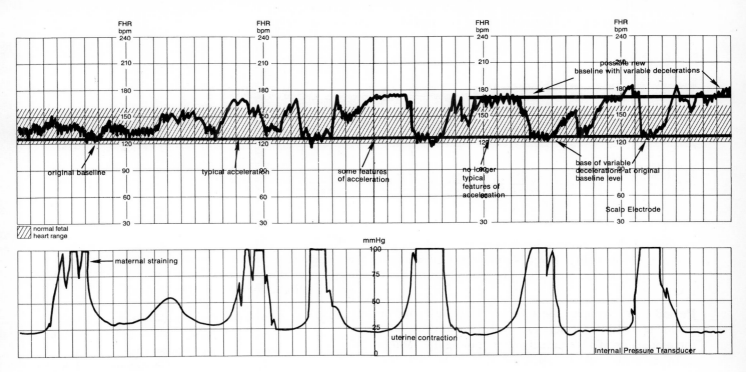

Pattern Characteristic:
Baseline Obscured by Decelerations

Baseline Obscured by Arrhythmia

When premature beats are the basis for a fetal heart arrhythmia, the baseline is usually identified by normal cardiac cycles interspersed between premature supraventricular or ventricular depolarizations and compensatory pauses (see pages 472, 482, and 500). Three horizontal parallel lines result. Baseline variability can be assessed to a limited degree by reading that of the middle line, which represents the normal cardiac cycles.

In the case of bigeminal patterns, it is not possible to identify an accurate baseline rate because the pattern is produced only by premature depolarizations (upper horizontal line) and compensatory pauses (lower horizontal line). No judgments can be thus made about baseline heart rate or variability. This pattern occurs most commonly at rates slightly below the usual fetal heart range, as though partial sinus node suppression has occurred. The pattern usually denotes a healthy fetus using protective cardiac mechanisms in response to a slowing of the heart rate, although similar patterns are reported as a preterminal event in some dying fetuses.[3] Fetal condition is assessed by studying the tracing for quality of variability in areas of normal fetal heart rate.

An electrocardiogram may assist in diagnosis of the site of the ectopic focus of the premature depolarizations.

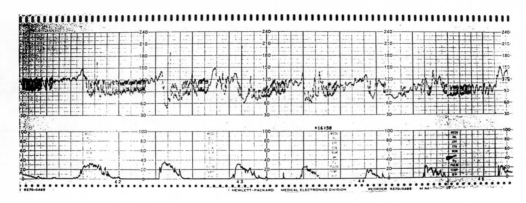

CASE INTERPRETATION: Class II

Baseline Information: normal heart rate and average to increased variability. There is a progressive downward shift in the baseline with recovery from each deceleration.

Periodic or Nonperiodic Changes: atypical mild to moderate variable decelerations with slow recovery with the production of a bigeminal pattern during the nadir or recovery phase, which appears to disappear each time the rate of approximately 120 bpm is achieved.

Uterine Activity: prolonged, skewed contractions with a progressive loss of information, except for apices of contractions, because of the tocodynamometer trace placement.

Significance: healthy stressed fetus with an ectopic focus outside the sinus node, which appears intermittently during episodes of decreased heart rate.

CASE OUTCOME: Thirty-two-year-old gravida 3, para 1011, delivered vaginally at 40 weeks' gestation a normal term weight female; Apgar score 9/9. The infant followed an uncomplicated newborn course. Labor was induced by amniotomy because of decreased fetal activity.

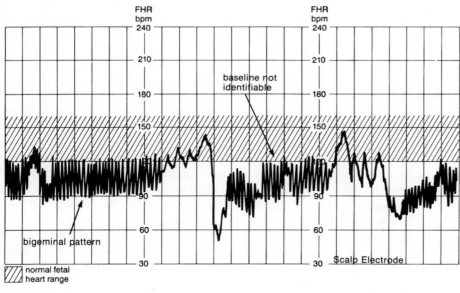

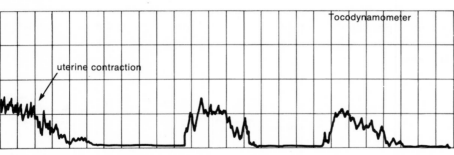

Pattern Characteristic:
Baseline Obscured by
Arrhythmia

References

1. Abbasi IA, Johnson T: Intrapartum fetal tachycardias. #178 *Proceedings of the Society of Perinatal Obstetricians Annual Meeting,* Las Vegas, 1985.
2. Bobbitt JR, Ledger WJ: Obstetric observations in eleven cases of neonatal sepsis due to the group B hemolytic streptococcus. *Obstet Gynecol* 47:439, 1976.
3. Cetrulo CL, Schifrin BS: Fetal heart rate patterns preceding death in utero. *Obstet Gynecol* 48:521, 1976.
4. Cibils L: *Fetal Heart Baseline Patterns in Electronic Fetal-Maternal Monitoring.* Chicago, John Wright, PSG, 1981, p. 278.
5. Cibils L: Clinical significance of fetal heart rate patterns during labor. I. Baseline patterns. *Am J Obstet Gynecol* 125:290, 1976.
6. Cohen WR, Yeh S: The abnormal fetal heart rate baseline. *Clin Obstet Gynecol* 29:73, 1986.
7. Cronje HS: Intra-uterine temperature measurements during fetal tachycardia. *S Afr Med J* 52:476, 1977.
8. Dicker D, Gingold A, Peleg D, et al: Effect of intracranial pressure changes on the fetal heart rate. Study of a hydrocephalic fetus. *Isr J Med Sci* 19:364, 1983.
9. Farrell JM, Souma ML, Evans JA: Unexplained fetal tachycardia associated with epidural anesthesia. Unpublished data presented at Family Practice Resident Research Day, April 24, 1981.
10. Freeman RK, Garite TJ: *The Clinical Management of Fetal Distress in Fetal Heart Rate Monitoring.* Baltimore, William & Wilkins, 1981, p. 100.
11. Fusi L, Steer PJ, Maresh MJA, et al: Maternal pyrexia associated with the use of epidural analgesia in labour. *Lancet,* June, p. 1250–252, 1989.
12. Gaziano EP: A study of variable decelerations in association with other heart rate patterns during monitored labor. *Am J Obstet Gynecol* 135:360, 1979.
13. Gimovsky ML, Caritis SN: Diagnosis and management of hypoxic fetal heart rate patterns. *Clinics in Perinatology* 9:313, 1982.
14. Goodlin RC, Chapin JW: Determinants of maternal temperature during labor. *Am J Obstet Gynecol* 143:97, 1982.
15. Hammacher K, Huter KA, Bokelmann JW, et al.: Foetal heart frequency and perinatal condition of foetus and newborn. *Gynaecologia* 166:349, 1968.
16. Hon EH: Baseline fetal heart rate, in *An Introduction to Fetal Heart Rate Monitoring.* Los Angeles, University of Southern California School of Medicine, 1973, pp. 37–41.
17. Jadhon ME, Main EK: Fetal bradycardia associated with maternal hypothermia. *Obstet Gynecol* 72:496, 1988.
18. Krebs HB, Petres RG, Dunn LJ: Intrapartum fetal heart rate monitoring. VIII. Atypical variable decelerations. *Am J Obstet Gynecol* 145:297, 1983.
19. Langer O, Cohen WR: Persistent fetal bradycardia during maternal hypoglycemia. *Am J Obstet Gynecol* 149:688, 1984.
20. Lavin JP: The effects of epidural anesthesia on electronic fetal heart rate monitoring. *Clinics in Perinatology* 9:55, 1982.
21. Martin CB: Physiology and clinical use of fetal heart rate variability. *Clinics in Perinatology* 9:339, 1982.
22. McCrann DJ, Schifrin BS: Heart rate patterns of the hydrocephalic fetus. *Am J Obstet Gynecol* 117:69, 1973.
23. Mueller-Heubach E, Myers RE, Adamsons K: Maternal factors affecting fetal condition during labor and delivery. *Obstet Gynecol Dig* Oct:11, 1974.
24. Ombelet W, Van Der Merve JV: Sinusoidal fetal heart rate pattern associated with congenital hydrocephalus. *South Afr Med J* 67:423, 1985.
25. Paul RH, Suidan AK, Yeh S, et al: Clinical fetal monitoring. VII. The evaluation and significance of intrapartum baseline FHR variability. *Am J Obstet Gynecol* 123:206, 1975.
26. Quirk JG, Miller FC: FHR tracing characteristics that jeopardize the diagnosis of fetal well-being. *Clin Obstet Gynecol* 29:12, 1986.
27. Rodis JF, Vintzileos AM, Campbell WA, et al: Maternal hypothermia: An unusual complication of magnesium sulfate therapy. *Am J Obstet Gynecol* 156:435, 1987.
28. Sokol RJ, Roux JF, McCarthy S: Computer diagnosis of labor progression. VI. Fetal stress and labor in the occipitoposterior position. *Am J Obstet Gynecol* 122:253, 1975.
29. Stewart KS, Philpott RH: Fetal response to cephalopelvic disproportion. *Br J Obstet Gynecol* 87:641, 1980.
30. Walker DW, Wood C: Temperature relationship of the mother and fetus during labor. *Am J Obstet Gynecol* 107:85, 1970.
31. Young BK, Weinstein HM: Moderate fetal bradycardia. *Am J Obstet Gynecol* 126:271, 1986.
32. Young BK, Katz M, Klein SA, et al: Fetal blood and tissue pH with moderate bradycardia. *Am J Obstet Gynecol* 45:135, 1979.

PERIODIC AND NONPERIODIC CHANGES

Section III

*P*eriodic and nonperiodic fetal heart rate changes are relatively abrupt heart rate alterations from the baseline heart rate that usually last at least 15 seconds. Most briefer alterations are considered fluctuations of long-term variability or, if consisting of only one or two beats, vertical deflections, as seen with arrhythmia or artifact. It is apparent that since alterations must occur in a direction of either increase or decrease in the heart rate, these changes consist of accelerations or decelerations, respectively. Changes are termed "periodic" when associated with uterine contractions and "nonperiodic" when not so associated.

Accelerations, with rare exceptions, provide reassuring evidence of good fetal condition, whether they are produced as a response to fetal stimulation or activity or by a baroreceptor response to partial cord impingement. Accelerations that are secondary components of variable decelerations when prolonged indicate varying degrees of fetal hypoxia, and are thus less reassuring.

Decelerations are first classified by shape, separating uniform (similar in shape with gradual onset and recovery) from variable (dissimilar from one deceleration to the next, usually with abrupt deceleration and recovery limbs).

Uniform decelerations are then subclassified, based on the timing in relationship to the uterine contraction. Early decelerations have simultaneous onset, nadir, and recovery with the contraction onset, peak, and resolution. These are relatively shallow. They are reflex mediated and thus carry no ominous significance but must be carefully distinguished from late decelerations and variable decelerations.

Late decelerations have onset, nadir, and/or recovery shifted to some degree to the right of onset, peak, and resolution, respectively, of the uterine contraction; are produced by hypoxia; and, when associated with good variability, are usually eradicated by maternal hyperoxia and improved uterine blood flow (improved placental oxygen exchange). When associated with decreased variability, regardless of depth, there is an increased association with fetal acidosis.

Variable decelerations vary in appearance, temporal relationship to contractions, and significance. Variable decelerations are first identified by relative "size," as

173

characterized by absolute depth and duration as well as distance of the nadir from the baseline. They are next classified according to the preservation of classic features versus the superimposition of various atypical features. Influenced by both a baroreceptor response to cord compression and a chemoreceptor response to a drop in fetal oxygenation, the significance of variable decelerations spans the gamut from healthy fetal responses to the heart rate changes of a moribund fetus. The late/variable deceleration is a unique deceleration, often seen in combination with late decelerations. The pattern is associated with an increased risk of chronic fetal hypoxia, often with chronic oligohydramnios as a contributing factor.

Prolonged decelerations may evolve from uniform or variable decelerations. These may occur as an isolated intrapartum event experienced by a healthy fetus, or they may reflect the progression of deterioration secondary to a compromised environmental or fetal condition.

When periodic changes accompany baseline fetal heart rate abnormalities, the additional information derived may be useful for diagnosis of fetal status. For example, the periodic changes may reflect the type of intermittent stimulus to which the fetus is subjected, leading to changes eventually reflected on the basal condition.

Accelerations

Chapter 9

Nonperiodic Accelerations: Uniform and Variable

*A*ccelerations are increases of fetal heart rate of at least 15 bpm that last 15 seconds or more but do not exceed 10 minutes in duration.

Accelerations shorter in duration, for example, 10 seconds, are sometimes described as small. These may not be distinguishable from fluctuations of long-term variability. Accelerations that are not associated with uterine contractions are termed "nonperiodic," or "sporadic," the latter implying an infrequent occurrence.[14,17]

Nonperiodic accelerations may be produced by direct or indirect stimulation of the fetus.[4,13] They are usually accompanied by fetal movement, whether maternally perceived or not, as demonstrated by ultrasonography.

Nonperiodic accelerations are consistent indicators of good fetal condition when associated with good baseline beat-to-beat variability.[18,19,20,27] During the accelerations themselves, however, variability is typically lost, as the sympathetic system transiently dominates.

The reassuring connotation of accelerations has been supported by statistical analysis of newborn outcome as well as fetal pH determinations. Frequency, duration, and amplitude of accelerations also correlate positively with the fetal condition.[16,5]

The size and frequency of occurrence of accelerations increases with advancing gestation.[50,53] Accelerations typically diminish as labor progresses. Accelerations are reassuring indicators of fetal condition intrapartum as well as antepartum.

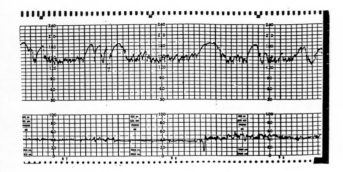

CASE INTERPRETATION: Class I

Baseline Information: normal rate and variability.

Periodic and Nonperiodic Changes: nonperiodic accelerations that are variable and uniform.

Uterine Activity: none clearly recorded.

Significance: a healthy fetus is predicted.

CASE OUTCOME: Twenty-eight-year-old gravida 3, para 2002, at 40 weeks' gestation delivered vaginally, with epidural anesthesia and low forceps from a vertex presentation, a 9 pound, 12½ ounce (4437 gram) female; Apgar score 9/9. The infant followed an uncomplicated newborn course. The accelerations throughout the intrapartum course showed no association with the uterine contractions.

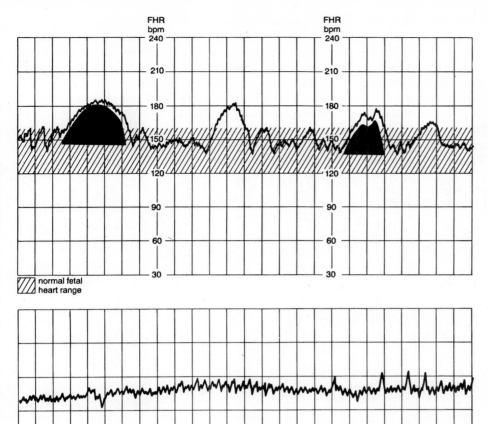

Pattern Characteristic:
Nonperiodic Accelerations—
Uniform and Variable

Nonperiodic Accelerations Associated with Fetal Activity

*B*oth fetal movement and accelerations are positive indicators of the fetal condition. It is a particularly reassuring sign for both to occur together. Accelerations with fetal movement begin simultaneously with the onset of the fetal activity, suggesting a coordinated cortical control.[52]

The term "periodic" is reserved for changes from the baseline heart rate, which occur repeatedly in association with uterine contractions. Therefore fetal-activity accelerations are nonperiodic, even though they often represent a recurring, at times even rhythmic, response to an intermittent stimulus.

There is a general increase in the frequency of activity-induced accelerations with advancing gestational age.[29,31,45] Accelerations are most reliably predictive of good fetal condition if variability is also present.[28]

Fetal activity accelerations provide the basis for nonstressed antepartum monitoring.[20,44] The presence of accelerations (such as two of greater than 15 seconds duration and amplitude occurring in 20 minutes) is indicative of fetal well-being. Spikes may be seen on the uterine trace as the fetal movement displaces the tocodynamometer. Such accelerations are reassuring, even if the occurrence is not documented to be associated with spontaneous fetal movement.[53]

Many accelerations not associated with fetal movement are, in actuality, a response to fetal movement that is not perceived by the mother.[42] Under ultrasonographic surveillance, most are documented to be associated with fetal movement, but spontaneous accelerations also occur without fetal movement,[53] the frequency diminishing with fetal maturation.[30]

On the contrary, the absence of acceleration of the fetal heart rate with fetal movement is *not* diagnostic of fetal distress. The frequency of movement-associated accelerations vary widely in normal fetuses.[6,30] It is, therefore, simply an absence of reassuring information. One must look further for evidence of good fetal condition.

However, absence of accelerations persisting for more than 80 minutes has a high correlation with eventual neonatal morbidity.[22,38]

Accelerations may coexist with late decelerations.[7,25] Although they still provide reassurance of a currently responsive fetus, the combination in antepartum monitoring may indicate early hypoxemia. Such a pattern is to be distinguished from decelerations following accelerations, a common reflex-triggered complex occurring in the healthy fetus (see page 188).

Accelerations induced by acoustic stimulation are believed to be secondary to fetal movement (startle) produced during the change from sleep to wakefulness.[20]

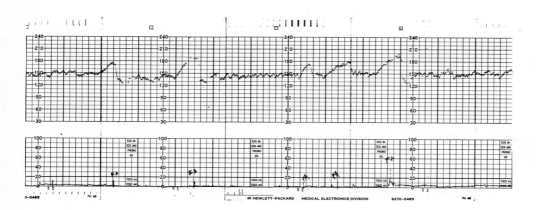

CASE INTERPRETATION: Class I

Baseline Information: normal rate, fair variability.

Periodic or Nonperiodic Changes: accelerations occurring in association with the handwritten data entries that denote fetal activity.

Uterine Activity: none recorded.

Significance: a healthy fetus is predicted.

CASE OUTCOME: Twenty-eight-year-old gravida 3, para 2002, at 36 weeks' gestation at the time of a nonstress test performed for Class A diabetes. At 40 weeks' gestation she delivered by cesarean section performed for a failed serial induction of labor, under general anesthesia, an 8 pound, 6½ ounce (3813 gram) male; Apgar score 8/10. The infant followed a normal newborn course.

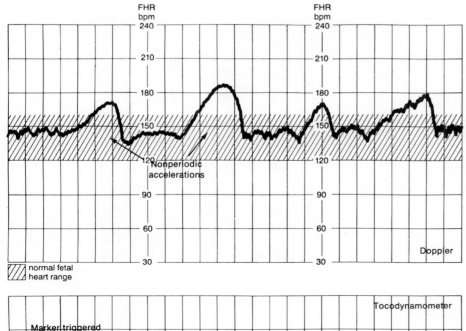

Pattern Characteristic:
Nonperiodic Accelerations
Associated with Fetal Activity

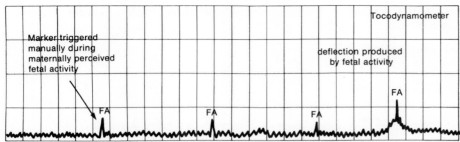

Nonperiodic Accelerations Produced by Fetal Stimulation

Accelerations of the fetal heart may be produced by stimulation of the fetus by such means as palpation, noise, or light stimuli.[10,26,40] Even accelerations with uterine contractions (periodic accelerations) may reflect fetal arousal.[5,13]

Fetal scalp stimulation has been demonstrated to frequently induce an acceleration in fetal heart rate in the healthy fetus, predicting a normal pH, as demonstrated by fetal scalp sampling.[3,4,43]

Documentation of the accelerations produced by fetal acoustic stimulation has provided an attractive alternative to nonstress monitoring because testing time is reduced since it is not delayed by periods of fetal quiescence.[10,49]

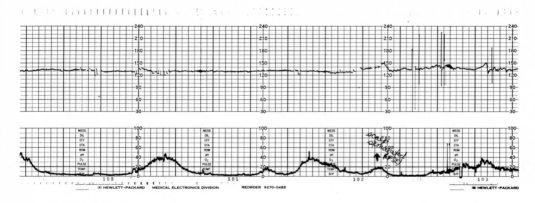

CASE INTERPRETATION: Class I

Baseline Information: normal heart rate, absent short-term variability, minimal long-term variability, flat-line pattern.

Periodic or Nonperiodic Changes: sporadic acceleration (rate increase of 20 bpm, lasting more than 15 seconds) is simultaneous with fetal scalp stimulation.

Uterine Activity: irregular, skewed contractions as measured by tocodynamometer.

Significance: this is a reassuring response by a healthy fetus to scalp stimulation.

CASE OUTCOME: Thirty-five-year-old gravida 2, para 0010, delivered vaginally, with epidural anesthesia, at 38 weeks' gestation a 5 pound, 8 ounce (2495 gram) female; Apgar score 8/9. The fetus was in a vertex presentation. The infant followed an uncomplicated newborn course. The tracing segment was obtained by stimulating the fetal head while attaching a scalp electrode.

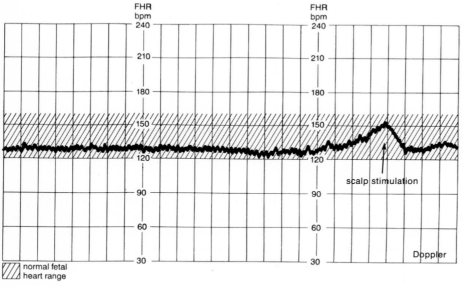

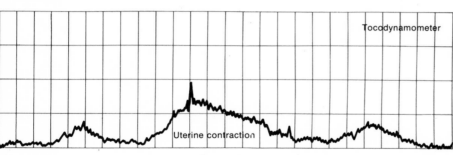

Pattern Characteristic:
Nonperiodic Acceleration(s)
Produced by Fetal Scalp
Stimulation

Periodic Accelerations: Uniform, Single Form

*P*eriodic accelerations occur simultaneously and repeatedly with uterine contractions. The fetal monitoring pattern is believed to denote partial umbilical cord compression. The proposed basis for this pattern is a baroreceptor-induced transient increase in fetal heart rate, which occurs as a result of fetal hypotension that is produced by compression of the umbilical vein without compression of the thicker-wall higher-pressure umbilical arteries.[8] This pattern frequently progresses through double form periodic accelerations to variable decelerations.

The pattern has a high association with a breech presentation, probably because of the increased cord vulner-ability. As with other accelerations, this denotes a response of a healthy fetus to cardiovascular stimuli in contrast to a sign of fetal distress. However, the pattern may progress to more ominous changes induced by the cord compression. It is considered to be a very early phase in a continuum of fetal heart response that may eventually progress to significant hypoxia and an associated low Apgar score. Therefore, the pattern is not as reassuring as nonperiodic accelerations.[11] Fetal movements commonly accompany the contractions with which periodic accelerations are associated.[46]

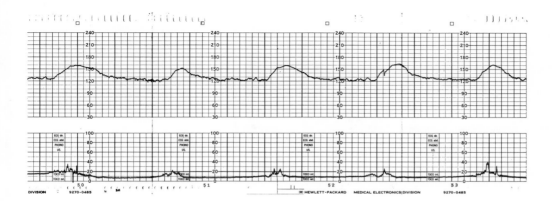

CASE INTERPRETATION: Class II

Baseline Information: normal rate, reduced variability.

Periodic or Nonperiodic Changes: periodic single form, uniform accelerations. The notching seen in the last acceleration denotes a transition to a double form acceleration.

Uterine Activity: regular contractions with small deflections as measured by the tocodynamometer.

Significance: periodic accelerations suggest partial cord impingement. A vulnerable cord such as with breech presentation or a velamentous insertion is possible. Such a pattern typically progresses to variable decelerations.

CASE OUTCOME: Nineteen year-old gravida 2, para 0010, delivered, vaginally, with local and pudendal anesthesia a 7 pound, 8 ounce (3402 gram) female; Apgar score 9/10. The fetus was in a vertex presentation. No unusual cord location was noted. The infant followed a normal newborn course.

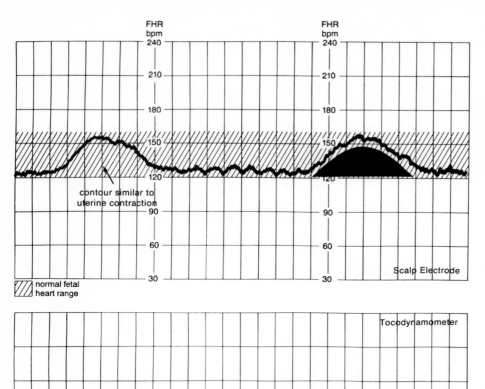

Pattern Characteristic:
Periodic Accelerations: Uniform, Single Form

Periodic Accelerations: Uniform, Double Form

A striking fetal monitoring pattern that is usually indicative of partial cord compression is double form periodic accelerations. The appearance is that of the single form uniform acceleration with the addition of a notch that is central or eccentric in location. The notch does not fall below the original baseline. The notch is believed to represent very transient umbilical artery impingement, flanked by the tachycardic response that is produced by isolated umbilical vein impingement.

The pattern typically converts to variable decelerations as the notch progressively deepens.[21]

The cord compression may be "occult," that is the umbilical cord is not always found in a vulnerable location at vaginal delivery. The pattern is frequently associated with a breech presentation, probably because of the high incidence of umbilical cord vulnerability. A velamentous cord insertion is another clinical situation of "cord vulnerability" that may be associated with periodic accelerations.

The pattern is increased in preterm fetuses, and is believed to be secondary to incomplete development of the parasympathetic nervous system.

Sympathetic blockade with propranolol has been demonstrated to abolish this pattern in baboons and rhesus monkeys.[15] It is increased with atropine administration.

Although periodic accelerations may herald fetal compromise because of the hypoxemic effects of cord compression, it is a well fetus who produces this pattern that employs protective reflexes. The asphyxiated fetus may show no fetal heart changes or only decelerations during partial cord occlusion.[15]

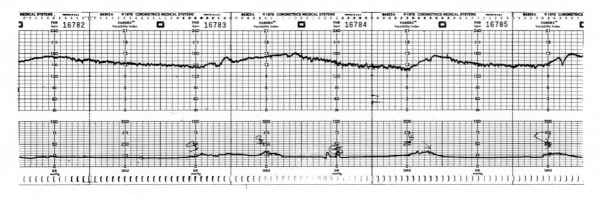

CASE INTERPRETATION: Class II

Baseline Information: normal heart rate and variability.

Periodic or Nonperiodic Changes: periodic accelerations, single and double form.

Uterine Activity: regular contractions with a small deflection of the tocodynamometer.

Significance: this is a healthy fetal response to probable partial cord compression. There is an increased incidence of breech presentation.

CASE OUTCOME: Twenty-four-year-old gravida 3, para 2002, delivered vaginally at 40 weeks' gestation a 7 pound, 4 ounce (3289 gram) female; Apgar score 8/9. The fetus was in a breech presentation. The infant followed an uncomplicated newborn course.

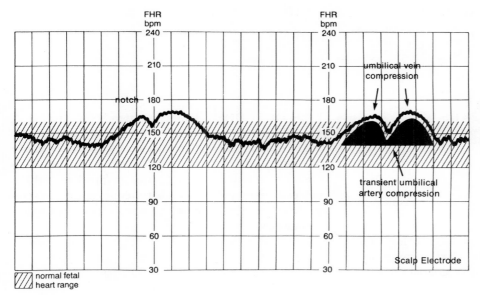

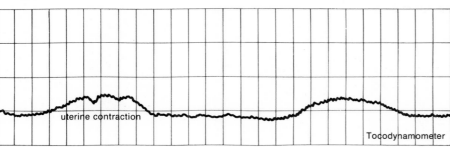

Pattern Characteristic:
Periodic Accelerations: Uniform, Double Form

Periodic Accelerations as Components of Variable Decelerations

*V*ariable decelerations typically contain an acceleration just preceding and following the deceleration. These are termed "primary" and "secondary" accelerations, respectively. The primary acceleration has also been termed "initial" acceleration, and the secondary acceleration is also called an "overshoot" (see Chap. 12 on Variable Decelerations). The accelerations have also been referred to as shoulders, compensatory accelerations, and pre- and postvariable deceleration accelerations.[15]

The proposed mechanism underlying the fetal heart rate pattern of variable decelerations is that of baroreceptor activity triggered by transition through partial and complete cord compression with recovery.

According to this theory, the primary acceleration occurs as the umbilical vein is compressed, resulting in egress of blood from the fetus without return from the placenta. The resulting hypotension results in a baroreceptor-induced increase in the heart rate. Upon complete umbilical cord compression, the deceleration is a consequence of the obstruction of the umbilical arteries through baroreceptor reflexes induced by the resulting hypertension. Hypoxemia further modifies the deceleration through chemoreceptor activity. The secondary acceleration occurs with reversal of the process. The presence of primary and secondary accelerations as part of the variable deceleration pattern is reassuring.[17,23]

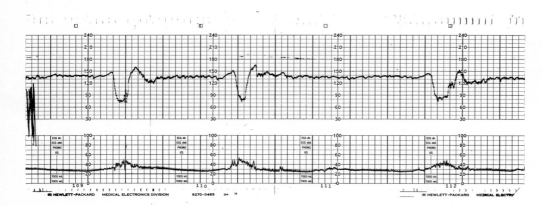

CASE INTERPRETATION: Class I

Baseline Information: normal rate and variability.

Periodic or Nonperiodic Changes: classical mild variable decelerations.

Uterine Activity: regular contractions as measured by a tocodynomometer.

Significance: a healthy fetus is predicted at this time. Decelerations may be triggered by cord compression. Therefore, maternal repositioning is appropriate. Observation of the pattern for development of atypia in the deceleration or hypoxic changes is appropriate.

CASE OUTCOME: Twenty-eight-year-old gravida 2, para 1001, at 40 weeks' gestation delivered vaginally, with local and pudendal anesthesia, a 7 pound, 10 ounce (3459 gram) male; Apgar score 7/9. The fetus was in a vertex presentation. The cord was wrapped around the neck one time; and the newborn required oxygen transiently at delivery. Thereafter, the infant followed a normal newborn course.

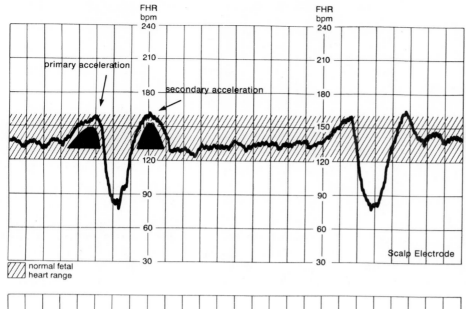

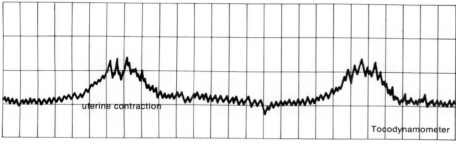

Pattern Characteristic:
Periodic Accelerations as
Components of Variable
Decelerations

Progression of Periodic Accelerations to Variable Decelerations

*O*bserving a continuum from periodic accelerations to variable decelerations may help our understanding of events associated with the individual patterns.

It is proposed that the uniform single form acceleration represents collapse of the thin-walled vein. The resulting hypotension, which occurs as the arteries continue to carry blood from the fetus without return from the placenta, produces a baroreceptor-stimulated heart rate increase.

As the artery becomes compressed, a baroreceptor response stimulates the heart rate decrease in response to the hypertension. This produces a notch. The notch progressively deepens through the double form configuration, until eventually an actual deceleration occurs as

progressive cord occlusion results from the effects of advancing labor. The accelerations produced by partial cord compression become the primary and secondary accelerations of the variable deceleration. Although conversion to variable decelerations with a smooth transition does not invariably occur in each patient, a search of the tracing containing one of the individual patterns often reveals one or more of the other patterns.

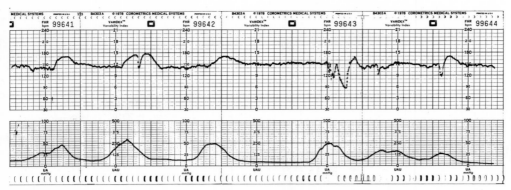

Recreation of original tracing

CASE INTERPRETATION: Class II

Baseline Information: normal rate, fair variability.

Periodic or Nonperiodic Changes: uniform single and double form periodic accelerations, mild W-shaped variable deceleration.

Uterine Activity: frequent uterine contractions.

Significance: this is a pattern probably reflecting progressive cord impingement with a healthy fetal response.

CASE OUTCOME: Seventeen-year-old primigravida delivered vaginally, with low elective forceps, at 39½ weeks' gestation a 6 pound, 9 ounce (2977 gram) female; Apgar score 8/9. A nuchal cord was noted at delivery. The infant followed an uncomplicated newborn course.

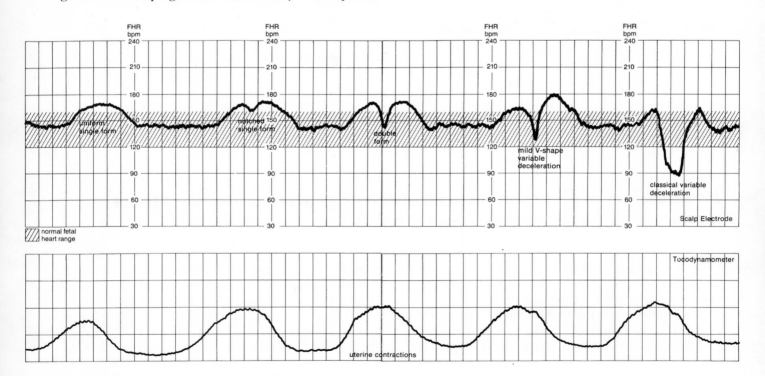

Pattern Characteristic:
Progression of Periodic Accelerations to Variable Decelerations

Periodic Variable Accelerations

*A*ccelerations may occur repeatedly or intermittently with uterine contractions. When these lack the smooth dome-shaped contour of uniform accelerations, they are termed "variable." The accelerations are a reassuring indicator of a responsive fetus. The configuration of the pattern is assumed to be a net result of increased sympathetic versus parasympathetic activity during acceler-ations. As with uniform periodic accelerations, a frequent association with variable decelerations has been noted.

Ultrasonography during uterine contractions has demonstrated a high correlation of this pattern with fetal activity.[46] The fetal activity may be a response to arousal, pain or hypoxemia or unknown causes.

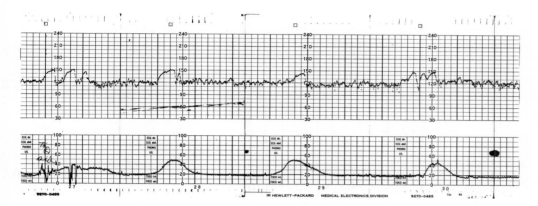

CASE INTERPRETATION: Class I

Baseline Information: normal rate and variability.

Periodic or Nonperiodic Changes: periodic accelerations, variable in appearance. On occasion there is a Lambda pattern.

Uterine Activity: regular contractions.

Significance: a healthy fetus is predicted.

CASE OUTCOME: Thirty-six-year-old gravida 3, para 2002, delivered at 40 weeks' gestation by primary cesarean section, under general anesthesia, performed for what was thought to be fetal distress developing in later labor, a 7 pound, 3 ounce (3260 gram) female; Apgar score 10/10. The fetus was in a vertex presentation. The infant followed a normal newborn course.

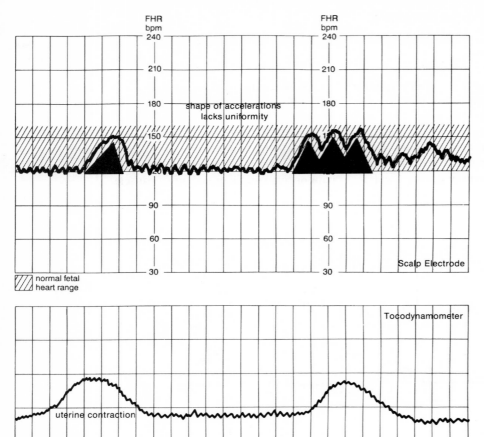

Pattern Characteristic:
Periodic Variable Accelerations

Accelerations Followed by Decelerations—Lambda Pattern

A Lambda pattern is a very common fetal monitoring finding, which is characterized by decelerations following accelerations.[12,48,52] This occurs in both the stressed and nonstressed fetus. It may be a periodic or a nonperiodic pattern. The postacceleration deceleration has also been termed an "undershoot."[12] It has been demonstrated to be dependent upon vagal activity, in contrast to the preceding acceleration, which is obliterated by sympathetic blockade and enhanced by parasympathetic withdrawal.[55] Other terms applied to the pattern have been "biphasic change"[55] and "combined accelerations" (with decelerations).

The frequency of Lambda patterns increases with fetal maturation.[30,51] The likelihood of a postacceleration deceleration increases with the duration of associated fetal activity, which may be spontaneous or induced by a

contraction. It is typically shallower in depth than the height of the associated acceleration.[52] When associated with contractions, a proposed mechanism is transient umbilical vein compression.[55] It is thus not surprising that clinical experience shows a frequent progression to variable deceleration when this pattern is present in the laboring patient.[55] However, progression to nonreassuring patterns is not expected.[2]

Although a fall in fetal tissue PO_2 has been identified with the pattern, it is important to note that a similar fall in PO_2 is commonly observed during contractions with other heart rate patterns of the normal fetus.[1,55] The reflex nature of the pattern, its spontaneous occurrence in the absence of contractions, and its association with benign outcomes warrants classification among heart rate patterns of the normal fetus.[2]

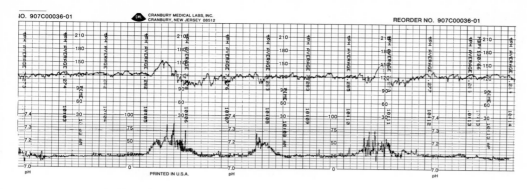

CASE INTERPRETATION: Class I

Baseline Information: low normal rate, normal variability.

Periodic or Nonperiodic Changes: periodic accelerations followed by brief decelerations.

Uterine Activity: regular contractions.

Significance: a healthy fetus is predicted.

CASE OUTCOME: Seventeen-year-old primigravida delivered vaginally, with pudendal anesthesia, at 43 weeks' gestation an 8½ pound (3674 gram) male; Apgar score 8/9. There was no meconium present and no abnormal cord position. The fetus was in a vertex presentation in a left occiput posterior position with spontaneous rotation to an occiput anterior position in late labor. The fetal scalp pHs were 7.3 to 7.4; tissue pHs were 7.18 to 7.26 (reflecting the usual 0.2 difference from scalp pHs); and umbilical cord pH was arterial 7.22, venous 7.31. The infant followed a normal newborn course.

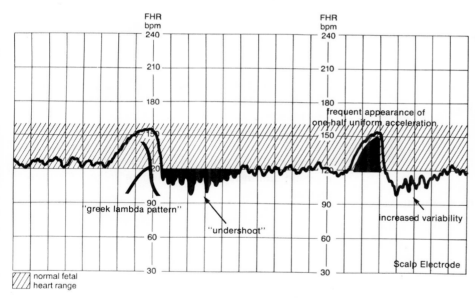

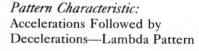

Pattern Characteristic:
Accelerations Followed by
Decelerations—Lambda Pattern

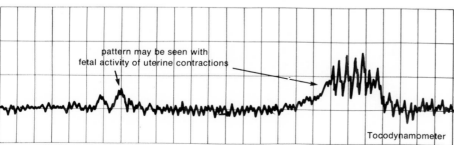

Periodic Late Accelerations

A rare fetal monitoring pattern that is characterized by the appearance of periodic, usually uniform accelerations, which are late in onset and recovery in relation to the uterine contraction, is termed "periodic late accelerations."

The pattern has been observed in association with an anencephalic fetus and after administration of atropine.[37] In both instances, it is proposed that sympathetic activity dominates in a setting defective in vagal influences.

Although generally reassuring, late accelerations may be recorded when a moribund fetus has a blunting of all the components of a variable deceleration except for the residual features of a prolonged secondary acceleration (see p. 144q).

A pattern of small accelerations late in occurrence, associated with a smooth baseline, has been described during initiation or recovery from some late deceleration patterns. Hypoxic cardiac depression, accompanied by vagal suppression and sympathetic activation, is implied by such a pattern.[26] The pattern should not be confused with a Lambda pattern (see page 188).

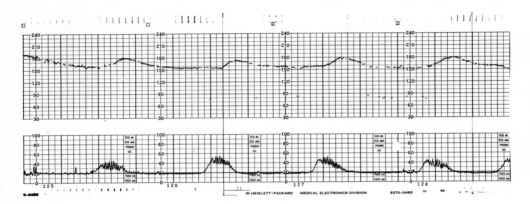

CASE INTERPRETATION: Class IV

Baseline Information: high normal rate, reduced beat-to-beat variability.

Periodic or Nonperiodic Changes: periodic, late uniform accelerations.

Uterine Activity: regular contractions with steep ascent, as is sometimes seen with oxytocin administration.

Significance: this is a rare fetal heart pattern that is reported to have an increased association with atropine administration and fetal anencephaly.

CASE OUTCOME: Nineteen-year-old primigravida at term delivered vaginally, from a vertex presentation with low forceps and epidural anesthesia, a 7 pound, 6½ ounce (3360 gram) male; Apgar score 9/10. The mother received meperidine and propiomazine during labor. Oxytocin augmentation was also given, but there was no atropine administration. The infant followed a normal newborn course.

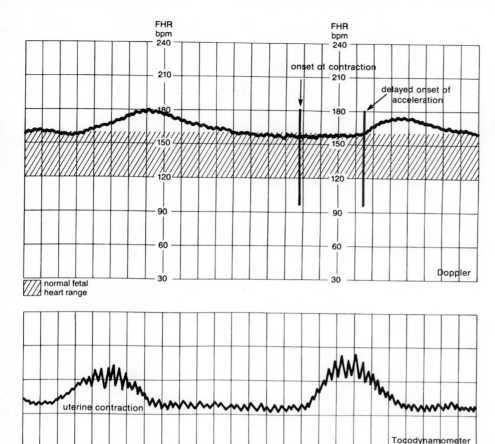

FHR
bpm

FHR
bpm

onset of contraction

delayed onset of acceleration

Pattern Characteristic:
Periodic Late Accelerations

normal fetal heart range

Doppler

uterine contraction

Tocodynamometer

Prolonged Accelerations

*A*t times the fetal heart may accelerate without a prompt return to baseline. The first step in interpreting such a pattern is to determine if this represents accelerations from a normal baseline with good beat-to-beat variability or an elevated smooth baseline from which decelerations with average variability are occurring. Studying several minutes of monitoring information usually clarifies the true baseline. Accelerations, like decelerations, usually have a rounded configuration, while the true baseline is relatively level.

Prolonged accelerations are often seen with marked fetal activity, especially when successive movements oc-cur within 30 seconds of each other.[52] There is typically loss of variability during the accelerations as sympathetic tone predominates. This is a normal physiologic phe-nomenon that does not represent the same mechanism or have the same significance as absent variability of the baseline fetal heart rate.

Although the stimulus for accelerations in some situ-ations may be mild hypoxemia, the increased heart rate is a compensatory response of a healthy fetus.

Accelerations increase in duration with advancing ges-tation. (See pages 133 and 166 for other examples of this pattern.)

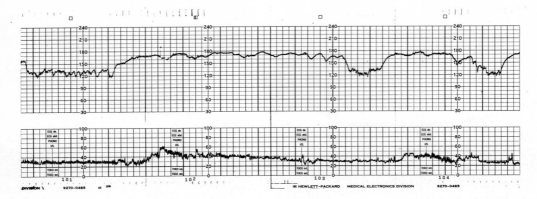

CASE INTERPRETATION: Class II

Baseline Information: normal heart rate of 120 to 130 bpm, normal variability.

Periodic or Nonperiodic Changes: prolonged accelerations.

Uterine Activity: there appear to be prolonged, skewed contractions.

Significance: a healthy fetal response that is possibly produced by mild hypoxia in this case.

CASE OUTCOME: Nineteen-year-old primigravida at 41 weeks' gestation, delivered by cesarean section performed for preeclampsia and dystocia unresponsive to oxytocin augmentation an 8 pound, 3 ounce (3714 gram) male; Apgar score 9/10. The mother received meperidine, propiomazine, and magnesium sulfate intrapartum. The infant followed a normal newborn course.

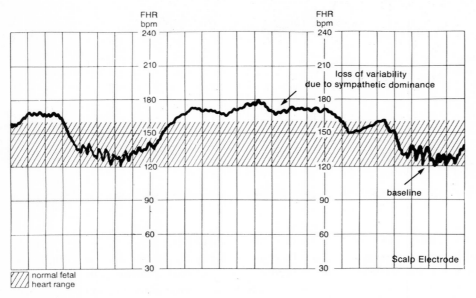

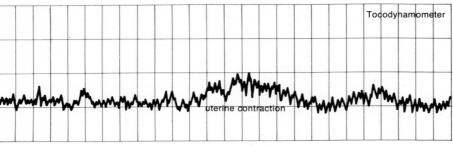

Pattern Characteristic:
Prolonged Accelerations

Marked Accelerations

*A*ccelerations increase in amplitude with advancing fetal gestational age and with decreasing basal heart rate.[9,30,39,47]

Marked accelerations are defined as fetal heart rate accelerations 30 bpm or greater above the baseline heart rate and lasting 30 seconds or more.[33] They are also called exaggerated accelerations.[36] The term "marked" is preferred because it is more consistent with other fetal monitoring terminology, reserving the term "exaggerated" to describe artifactual distortions.

This pattern has been reported to occur in approximately 12% of monitored labors. As with other accelerations, marked accelerations generally provide reassurance of a healthy fetus. However, when amplitude is in excess of 50 bpm, the acceleration may denote an unusual degree of baroreceptor response to hypotension, and may be accompanied by a fall in pH.[34,35]

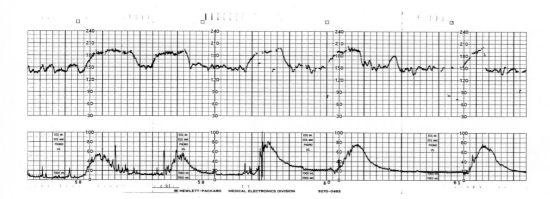

CASE INTERPRETATION: Class II

Baseline Information: upper limits of normal heart rate, normal variability.

Periodic or Nonperiodic Changes: uniform marked accelerations, many periodic.

Uterine Activity: normal except for skewing, the frequency is compatible with active labor.

Significance: a healthy fetus with probable partial cord impingement. Observation for a transition to variable decelerations is appropriate.

CASE OUTCOME: Twenty-year-old primigravida delivered vaginally, with pudendal anesthesia, at 40 weeks' gestation a 7 pound, 7 ounce (3374 gram) male; Apgar score 7/9. The fetus was in a vertex presentation. A nuchal cord was noted at delivery. The infant followed a normal newborn course.

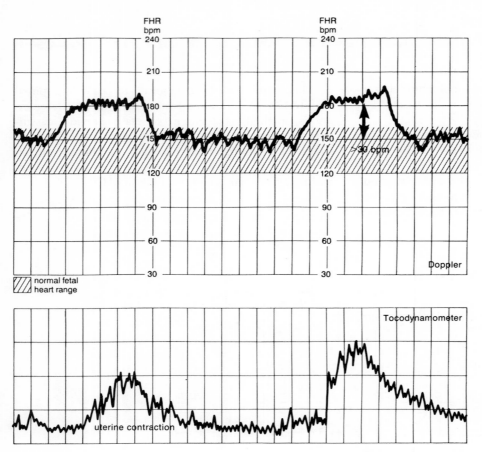

Pattern Characteristic:
Marked Accelerations

Atypical Accelerations Associated with Baseline Bradycardia

*A*n unusual type of acceleration may occur when baseline bradycardia is present in late labor. These fetal heart rate increases do not have the appearance of typical accelerations.

There is not the usual rounded shape of a classical acceleration. Instead, there are sharp ascending and descending limbs and flattened apices, the appearance of variable decelerations inverted.

There is also not consistent loss of variability, as occurs with a classical acceleration. Instead, varying degrees of long- and short-term variability may appear in the level apex.

A retrospective study of tracings with this pattern suggests that the fetal heart rate is returning intermittently to a former higher baseline. The degree of variability in

this "remembered" baseline may be observed as one indicator of fetal status. This pattern usually occurs in settings of normal or increased baseline variability in late labor.

The importance of distinguishing this pattern from classical accelerations is that it may denote a more stressed fetus. Full delineation of the significance awaits study. In formulating management decisions, one may consider the overall beat-to-beat variability, anticipated time of delivery, fetal and maternal risk factors, and the response to measures such as administering oxygen to the mother, decreasing maternal pushing, and diminishing uterine contractions. (See page 158 for another example of this pattern.)

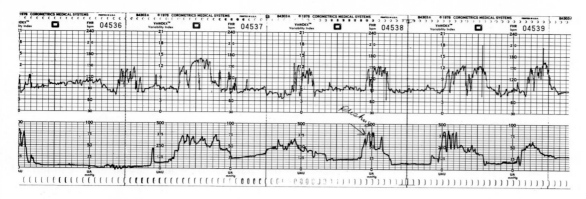

CASE INTERPRETATION: Class IV

Baseline Information: marked to moderate bradycardia, present but reduced variability in the baseline.

Periodic or Nonperiodic Changes: unusual "accelerations" with increased variability at the apex.

Uterine Contractions: regular, frequent contractions with maternal straining, some contractions are prolonged.

Significance: because of the sharp features of variability, this indicates stress of a healthy fetus in late labor. Management would be to diminish uterine activity if possible or deliver the fetus soon. Observation of the tracing for ominous changes such as the smoothing of either the oscillations or the baseline variability is appropriate.

CASE OUTCOME: Twenty-four-year-old gravida 3, para 2002, delivered vaginally, with a history of previous low transverse cesarean section and with pudendal anesthesia, a 7 pound, 15 ounce (3600 gram) female; Apgar score 8/9. There was no meconium. There was a nuchal cord. The mother received butorophanol tartrate during labor. The fetus was in a vertex presentation. The infant followed a normal newborn course.

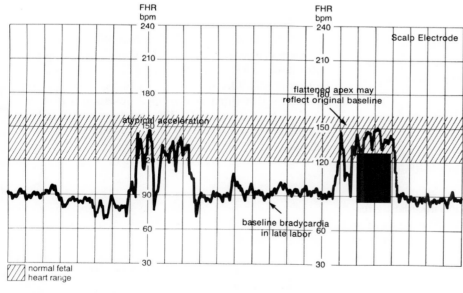

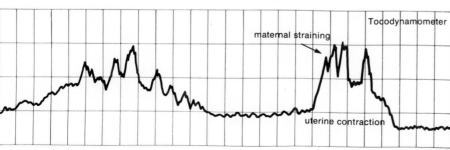

Pattern Characteristic:
Atypical Accelerations

Atypical Accelerations Produced by Partial Recovery from Late Decelerations

*R*ecurrent attempts of the fetal heart rate to return to baseline after recovery from late-occurring uniform or variable decelerations may give the appearance of accelerations. Such a pattern is typically seen in late labor with excessive uterine activity.

Without adequate time for recovery between contractions, the fetal heart rate between contractions progressively deepens. The return of the trace back to the general range of the original baseline coincides with the onset of the next contraction, thus producing the appearance of periodic accelerations. These do not share the same degree of reassuring significance as do classical accelerations, particularly when they are accompanied by a loss of short-term baseline variability and undulating long-term variability.

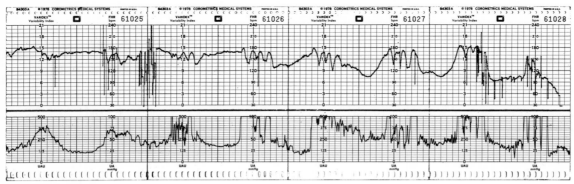

Recreation of original tracing

CASE INTERPRETATION: Class IV

Baseline Information: unstable baseline rate, progressively decreasing diminished short-term variability, undulating long-term variability.

Periodic or Nonperiodic Changes: the evolution of atypical accelerations with undulating long-term variability in the apex.

Uterine Activity: frequent contractions without a resting phase, maternal straining.

Significance: because of the smoothed undulating features, this is a nonreassuring pattern. Management is dictated by the clinical situation, including estimated time to delivery, gestation, and response to basic fetal supportive measures.

CASE OUTCOME: Eighteen-year-old primigravida at 37 weeks' gestation delivered vaginally, with pudendal anesthesia, a 5 pound, 15½ ounce (2710 gram) male; Apgar score 5/7. The fetus was in a frank breech presentation. It was a thirty-five weeks' gestation according to the newborn evaluation. The newborn exhibited mild respiratory distress, which did not require assisted ventilation.

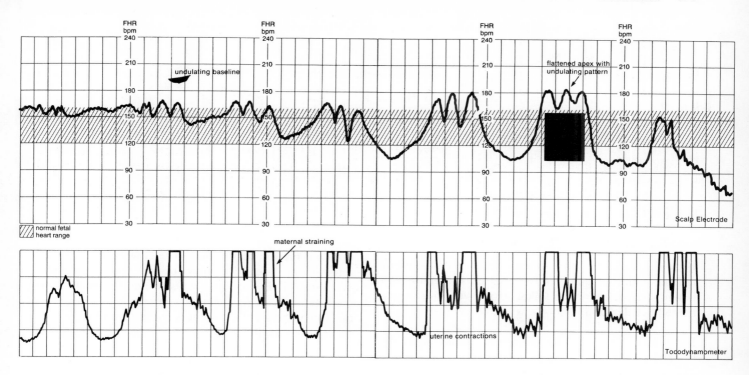

Pattern Characteristic:
Atypical Accelerations Produced by Partial Recovery from Late Decelerations

Accelerations Secondary to Double Counting: Artifact

Double counting, which simulates accelerations, is an artifact that is potentially detrimental to accurate fetal monitoring interpretation when it occurs as a result of decelerations and is unrecognized. Not only may it mask a pattern that could be indicative of fetal compromise, but it also may provide erroneously reassuring information, in that accelerations are usually interpreted as signs of good fetal condition. A distinguishing feature between true accelerations and the artifact produced by double counting is that doubling exaggerates variability while variability is diminished in true accelerations.

When the fetal heart being monitored by the Doppler transducer falls below 90 bpm, double counting can oc-cur with older as well as modern fetal monitors. The machines are programmed to reject rates outside the usual fetal heart range to minimize artifactual printing of sounds other than the fetal heart. The double counting may occur as a result of counting both systolic and diastolic movements at the slower rate.

One may identify double counting by halving the artifactual rate. The resulting numbers typically fall in a continuous pattern with the fetal heart trace, which precedes and follows the artifact.

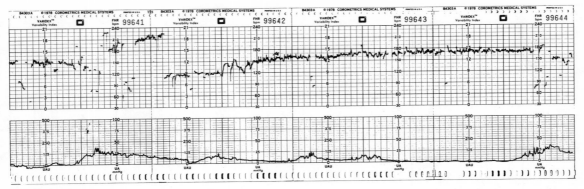

Recreation of original tracing

CASE INTERPRETATION: Class 0

Baseline Information: normal rate, variability is not reliable with a preautocorrelation external monitor. Rebound tachycardia occurs following recovery from a prolonged deceleration.

Periodic or Nonperiodic Changes: a prolonged deceleration is in response to an abnormal contraction. Doubling of the fetal heart rate during the deceleration tends to obscure the deceleration. No accelerations.

Uterine Activity: a prolonged, skewed contraction followed by regular contractions of a more normal appearance.

Significance: lack of reactivity with external monitor does not present reassurance of fetal well being. An internal scalp electrode may clarify this if feasible. Whether this is a healthy fetus responding to hypoxia produced by a single abnormal contraction or a sick fetus in a threatening environment is not resolved by this segment of the tracing.

CASE OUTCOME: Twenty-four-year-old primigravida delivered vaginally at 40½ weeks' gestation a 7 pound, 9½ ounce (3444 gram) male: Apgar score 6/9. Vertex presentation. Thick meconium managed by DeLee suctioning. Twenty percent placental abruption. Normal newborn course.

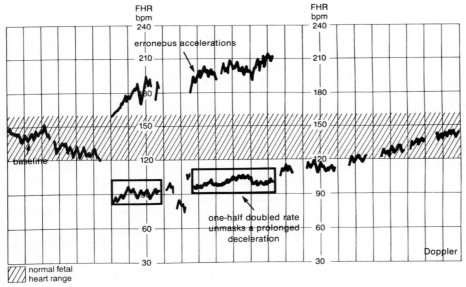

Pattern Characteristic:
Artifactual Accelerations: Double Counting

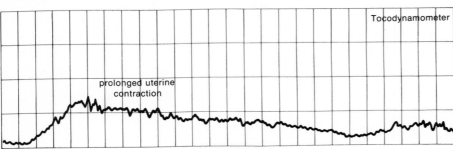

Accelerations Produced by Alternating Maternal and Fetal Heart Rate Recording: Artifact

*T*he external fetal monitor, whether or not it functions through autocorrelation or older technology, is prone to maternal heart rate monitoring artifact. The Doppler transducer is able to transmit the movement of maternal vessels, which may produce signals stronger than those of the fetus, especially when accompanied by wide pulse pressure produced during tachycardia, whether caused by illness or drug-derived. The artifact is enhanced when the fetal heart rate is outside the normal fetal heart range. Maternal heart rate artifact is also facilitated when the fetal and maternal heart rates are closely proximated.

The monitor recording may move so easily between the maternal and fetal signals that the trace is uninterrupted. This is termed "slipping," in keeping with the dictionary definition: "to move without attracting notice, to pass smoothly or easily, to slide accidentally, to overlook/miss."[54]

When the monitor predominately monitors the maternal heart rate, the brief, intermittent returns to the fetal heart rate, especially when slipping occurs, may be misinterpreted as accelerations.

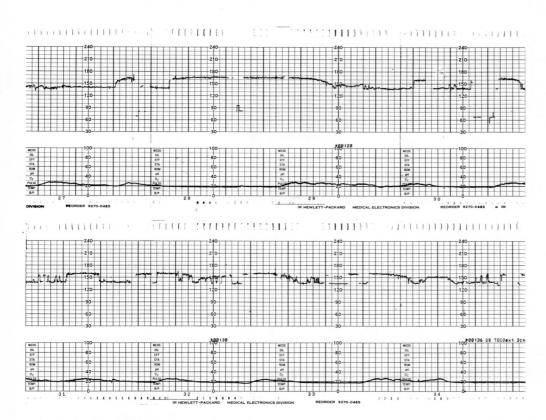

CASE INTERPRETATION: Class III

Baseline Information: two heart rates, both in normal fetal heart range, no variability is seen.

Periodic or Nonperiodic Changes: none seen. The pattern is hard to distinguish from decelerations and accelerations.

Uterine Activity: rapid vertical excursions that are superimposed on the contraction waveform, as seen with maternal tachypnea.

Significance: this is a probable maternal heart rate artifact because of the parallel flat double line appearance.

The appropriate management is to attempt a better fetal heart rate recording by altering the Doppler placement or employing scalp electrode monitoring. Dual monitoring of mother and fetus, if feasible, may help clarify when the monitor slips to the maternal heart rate.

CASE OUTCOME: Nineteen-year-old primigravida with sickle cell disease delivered vaginally at 26 weeks' gestation a 1 pound, 12½ ounce (806 gram) female; Apgar score 1/6. Local and pudendal anesthesia were administered. Study of the entire tracing and bedside observations confirmed that there was a maternal heart rate artifact. The newborn course was complicated by respiratory distress syndrome, hydrocephalus (ventriculoperitoneal shunt), and congenital cytomegalic viral hepatitis. The infant was dismissed at four months of age.

The etiology of the maternal tachypnea was acute chest syndrome. (See page 368 for a further tocodynamometry demonstration of maternal tachypnea.)

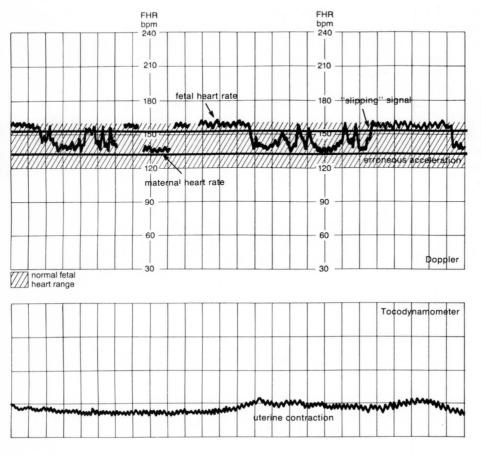

Pattern Characteristic:
Artifactual Accelerations:
Maternal Heart Rate
Interference

Accelerations or Decelerations?

A pattern is occasionally encountered in which it is difficult to determine which aspects of a fetal heart trace are baseline and which are periodic or nonperiodic changes.

The first step in interpreting such a pattern is to search the entire tracing for areas of clearly recorded stable baseline with normal appearing variability. If no area is found from which baseline identification can be established, known features of accelerations and decelerations, compared to the baseline, assist in making the distinction. Although it is possible to have a flat-line baseline with absent variability yet with variability appearing during decelerations, it is more common to have variability present in the baseline with disappearance of variability during accelerations. Accelerations and late and early decelerations usually have a rounded contour, while the baseline characteristically appears flat.[8] Variable decelerations, although sometimes flat at the base, usually have distinctive features. Prolonged accelerations that produce a flat line during the high rates create confusion. When followed by decelerations (Lambda pattern), the baseline may be further obscured. To help with the diagnosis, the tracing may be searched for accelerations of similar appearance but briefer duration.

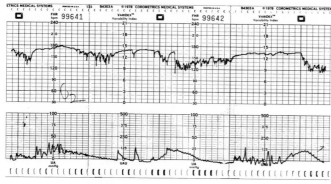

Recreation of original tracing

CASE INTERPRETATION: Class I

Baseline Information: good variability, normal baseline fetal heart rate of 130 to 140 bpm.

Periodic or Nonperiodic Changes: nonperiodic prolonged accelerations are possibly associated with fetal activity, with the loss of beat-to-beat variability in the accelerations.

Uterine Activity: skewed contractions.

Significance: Lambda pattern (decelerations after some prolonged accelerations) and normal variability are consistent with fetal well-being.

CASE OUTCOME: Nineteen-year-old at 39 weeks' gestation delivered by cesarean section for dystocia, with general anesthesia, a 6 pound, 5 ounce (2863 gram) female; Apgar score 7/9. The fetus was in a vertex presentation, in an occiput posterior position. Intermittent oxytocin augmentation was given to the mother during labor. The pattern appeared in early labor. Accelerations diminished as labor progressed, but a low normal baseline with normal variability persisted until delivery. Scalp pHs were 7.20 to 7.25, and the cord pH was 7.30. There were prolonged ruptured membranes (for 36 hours). The infant followed an uncomplicated newborn course.

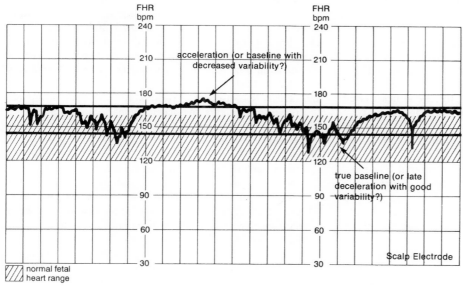

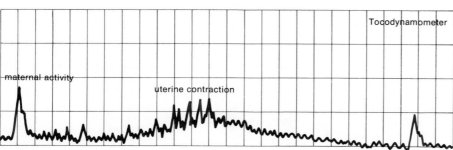

Pattern Characteristic:
Accelerations or Decelerations?

References

1. Aarnoudse JG, Huisjes HJ, Gordon H, et al: Fetal subcutaneous scalp PO_2 and abnormal heart rate during labor. *Am J Obstet Gynecol* 153:565, 1985.

2. Brubaker K, Garite TJ: The Lambda fetal heart rate pattern: An assessment of its significance in the intrapartum period. *Obstet Gynecol* 72:881, 1988.

3. Clark SL, Gimovsky ML, Miller FC: Fetal heart rate response to scalp blood sampling. *Am J Obstet Gynecol* 144:706, 1982.

4. Clark SL, Gimovsky ML, Miller FC: The scalp stimulation test: A clinical alternative to fetal scalp blood sampling. *Am J Obstet Gynecol* 148:274, 1984.

5. Devoe LD, Castillo R, Saad S, et al: Percent acceleration time: A new method of fetal assessment. *Obstet Gynecol* 67:191, 1986.

6. Devoe LD, McKenzie J, Searle N, et al: Nonstress test: Dimensions of normal reactivity. *Obstet Gynecol* 66:617, 1985.

7. Fox HE, Steinbrecher M, Ripton B: Antepartum fetal heart rate and uterine activity studies. I. Preliminary report of accelerations and the oxytocin challenge test. *Am J Obstet Gynecol* 126:61, 1976.

8. Freeman RK, Garite TJ: *Basic Pattern Recognition in Fetal Heart Rate Monitoring.* Baltimore, Williams & Wilkins, 1981, p. 79.

9. Gagnon R, Cambell K, Hunse C, et al: Patterns of human fetal heart rate accelerations from 26 weeks to term. *Am J Obstet Gynecol* 157:743, 1987.

10. Gagnon R, Hunse C, Carmichael L, et al: External vibratory acoustic stimulation near term: Fetal heart rate and heart rate variability responses. *Am J Obstet Gynecol* 156:323, 1987.

11. Gaziano EP, Freeman DW, Bendel RP: Fetal heart rate variability: Heart rate in second stage of labor. *Obstet Gynecol* 54:42, 1980.

12. Goodlin RC: Fetal Heart Rate Monitoring, in *Care of the Fetus.* Masson Publishing, 1979, p. 116.

13. Goodlin RC, Schmidt W: Human fetal arousal levels as indicated by heart rate recordings. *Am J Obstet Gynecol* 114:613, 1972.

14. Hon EH, Quilligan EJ: The classification of fetal heart rate. II. A revised working classification. *Connecticut Medicine*, November 1967, p. 779.

15. James LS, Yeh M, Morishima HO, et al: Umbilical vein occlusion and transient acceleration of the fetal heart rate. Experimental observations in subhuman primates. *Am J Obstet Gynecol* 126:267, 1976.

16. Kariniemi V, Ammala P: Interval index: A measure of fetal heart rate accelerations. *J Perinat Med* 9:248, 1981.

17. Krebs HB, Petres RE, Dunn LJ, et al: Intrapartum fetal heart rate monitoring. I. Classification and prognosis of fetal heart rate patterns. *Am J Obstet Gynecol* 133:762, 1979.

18. Krebs HB, Petres RE, Dunn LJ, et al: Intrapartum fetal heart rate monitoring. VI. Prognostic significance of accelerations. *Am J Obstet Gynecol* 142:297, 1982.

19. Kubli FW, Hon EH, Khazin AF, et al: Observations on heart rate and pH in the human fetus during labor. *Am J Obstet Gynecol* 104:1190, 1969.

20. Lee CY, DiLoreto PC, Logrand B: Fetal activity acceleration determination for the evaluation of fetal reserve. *Obstet Gynecol* 48:19, 1976.

21. Lee CY, DiLoreto PC, O'Lane JM: A study of fetal heart rate acceleration patterns. *Obstet Gynecol* 45:142, 1975.

22. Levenko KJ, Williams L, De Palmer RT, et al: Perinatal outcome in the absence of antepartum fetal heart rate acceleration. *Obstet Gynecol* 61:347, 1983.

23. Luerti M, Spagnolo D, Stefanoni S: Acclerations in "intrapartum" cardiotocographic recording. IV. Correlation with the presence of a funiculus pathology. *Clin Exp Obst Gyn* 8:31, 1981.

24. Luerti M, Stefanoni S, Busacca M: Accelerations in "intrapartum" cardiotocographic recording. I. Correlation with perinatal outcome. *Clin Exp Obst Gyn* 7:94, 1980.

25. Luerti M, Stefanoni S, Busacca M: Accelerations in "intrapartum" cardiotocographic recording. II. Present contemporaneously to prognostically unfavourable cardiotocographic aspects. *Clin Exp Obst Gyn* 7:101, 1980.

26. Martin CB: Regulation of the fetal heart rate and genesis of FHR patterns. *Seminars in Perinatology* 2:131, 1978.

27. Mendenhall HW, O'Leary JA, Phillips KD: The nonstress test: The value of a single acceleration in evaluating the fetus at risk. *Am J Obstet Gynecol* 136:87, 1980.

28. Milliez J, Legrand H, Goupil F, et al: Antepartum fetal heart rate monitoring. III. Fetal movements and accelerations in fetal heart rate. *Europ J Obstet Gynec Reprod Biol* 11:251, 1981.

29. Natale R, Nasello C, Turlenk R: The relationship between movements and accelerations in fetal heart rate at twenty-four to thirty-two weeks' gestation. *Am J Obstet Gynecol* 148:591, 1984.

30. Natale R, Nasello-Paterson C, Turlink R: Longitudinal measurements of fetal breathing, body movements, heart rate and heart rate accelerations and decelerations at 24 to 32 weeks of gestation. *Am J Obstet Gynecol* 151:256, 1985.

31. Navot D, Yaffe H, Sadovsky E: The ratio of fetal heart rate accelerations to fetal movements according to gestational age. *Am J Obstet Gynecol* 149:92, 1984.

32. Nyholm HC, Hansen T, Neldam S: Fetal activity acceleration during early labor. *Acta Obstet Gynecol Scand* 62:131, 1983.

33. Odendaal HJ, Sandenbergh HA: Acceleration patterns of the fetal heart rate before and during labor. *South African Med J* 52:473, 1977.

34. O'Gureck JE, Roux JF, Neuman MN: Neonatal depression and fetal heart rate patterns during labor. *Obstet Gynecol* 40:347, 1972.

35. O'Gureck JE, Roux JF, Neuman MN: A practical classification of fetal heart rate patterns. *Obstet Gynecol* 40:356, 1972.

36. Ott WJ: Significance of exaggerated fetal heart rate accelerations during active labor. *J Reprod Med* 29:661, 1984.

37. Parer JT: Late Accelerations, in: *Handbook of Fetal Monitoring*. Philadelphia. W.B. Saunders, 1983, p. 143.

38. Patrick J, Carmichael L, Chess L, et al: Accelerations of the human fetal heart rate at 38 to 40 weeks' gestational age. *Am J Obstet Gynecol* 148:35, 1984.

39. Patrick J, Carmichael L, Chess L, et al: The distribution of accelerations of the human fetal heart rate at 38 to 40 weeks' gestational age. *Am J Obstet Gynecol* 151:283, 1985.

40. Peleg D, Goldman JA: Fetal heart rate acceleration in response to light stimulation as a clinical measure of fetal well-being. A preliminary report. *J Perinat Med* 8:38, 1980.

41. Powell OH, Melville A, MacKenna J: Fetal heart rate acceleration in labor: Excellent prognostic indicator. *Am J Obstet Gynecol* 134:36, 1979.

42. Rabinowitz R, Persitz E, Sadovsky E: The relation between fetal heart rate accelerations and fetal movements. *Obstet Gynecol* 61:16, 1983.

43. Rice PE, Benedetti TJ: Fetal heart rate acceleration with fetal blood sampling. *Obstet Gynecol* 68:469, 1986.

44. Rochard F, Schifrin BS, Goupil F, et al: Nonstress fetal heart rate monitoring in the antepartum period. *Am J Obstet Gynecol* 126:699, 1976.

45. Sadovsky E, Navot D, Yaffe H: Antenatal evaluation of the FHR accelerations associated with fetal movements. *Int J Gynaecol Obstet* 19:441, 1981.

46. Sadovsky E, Rabinowitz R, Freeman A, et al: The relationship between fetal heart rate accelerations, fetal movements, and uterine contractions. *Am J Obstet Gynecol* 149:187, 1984.

47. Sato A, Chin E, Endo C, Dyosuka M, et al: The significance of nonstress test from 24 to 42 weeks' gestation. *Acta Obst Gynaec Jpn* 36:2634, 1984.

48. Schifrin BS: Interpretation hints in exercises in fetal monitoring. Los Angeles, bpm inc. 1985.

49. Smith CV, Phelan JP, Paul RH, et al: Fetal acoustic stimulation testing: A retrospective experience with the fetal acoustic stimulation test. *Am J Obstet Gynecol* 153:567, 1985.

50. Smith CV, Phelan JP, Paul RH: A prospective analysis of the influence of gestational age on the baseline fetal heart rate and reactivity in a low risk population. *Am J Obstet Gynecol* 153:780, 1985.

51. Sorotkin Y, Dierker LJ, Pillay SK, et al: The association between fetal heart rate patterns and fetal movements in pregnancies between 20 and 30 weeks' gestation. *Am J Obstet Gynecol* 143:243, 1982.

52. Timor-Tritsch IE, Dierker LJ, Zador I, et al: Fetal movements associated with fetal heart rate accelerations and decelerations. *Am J Obstet Gynecol* 131:276, 1978.

53. Vintzileos AM, Campbell WA, Nochimson D: Relation between fetal heart rate accelerations, fetal movements, and fetal breathing movements. *Am J Perinatology* 3:38, 1986.

54. *Webster's New World Dictionary of the American Language.* Second College Edition. New York, Simon and Schuster, 1980:1340.

55. Wood C, Walker A, Yardley R: Acceleration of the fetal heart rate. *Am J Obstet Gynecol* 134:523, 1979.

Uniform Decelerations: Early Decelerations

Early Decelerations

Although early decelerations are one of the best known basic fetal monitoring patterns, they are actually one of the rarest in pure form.

To qualify for this pattern decelerations must be uniform in appearance, that is, each must be similar to the next. A dictionary definition of uniform states: "not varying or changing in form, rate, degree or manner, having the same form and appearance as others in the same class, conforming to a given standard."[21] The configuration "standard" to which early decelerations conform is the shape of the uterine contraction, reversed—"mirror imaging." Since the uterine contraction is typically bell shaped, the uniform deceleration is typically bowl shaped, with gradual onset and gradual resolution.[10]

Further, criteria for early decelerations are that they be recurrent with each contraction (periodic) and confined to the time of the contraction (similar onset, peak/nadir, and resolution). Due to the use of the term "early," it is a common error to focus just on *timing*, overlooking the significance of *shape*.

Early decelerations usually occur within the normal fetal heart range, usually do not fall more than 20 to 30 bpm or below 100 bpm, usually last less than 90 seconds, and are usually proportional to the strength of the contraction.[12] Variability is unaffected by the deceleration.[6]

The mechanism of early decelerations is believed to be vagal discharge produced by head compression.[7] It is not surprising, therefore, that the pattern is associated with a vertex presentation, the active phase of labor, primigravid labor, a relatively large fetus for the pelvic size, and ruptured membranes.[3,13] Whether the pattern is baroreceptor or chemoreceptor mediated is a subject of controversy.[13]

The pattern of early decelerations is not associated with a low Apgar score, hypoxia, or fetal acidosis, therefore, no subclassification is necessary or meaningful.[15] Its simultaneous occurrence in relationship to uterine contractions distinguishes it from hypoxia-produced late decelerations, which are also uniform in configuration. Therefore, it is appropriate to analyze the pattern closely, confirming the *absence* of subtle degrees of a "shift to the right."

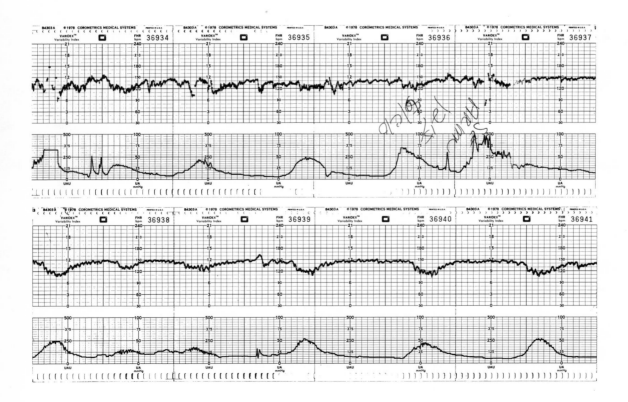

CASE INTERPRETATION: Class I

Baseline Information: normal rate and variability.

Periodic or Nonperiodic Changes: periodic early decelerations appear after rupture of the membranes.

Uterine Activity: normal frequency and configuration of contractions for active labor.

Significance: head compression, usually primigravida, a vertex presentation, or ruptured membranes. It is ap-

propriate to observe the pattern for a mixture with or transition to variable decelerations.

CASE OUTCOME: Twenty-seven-year-old gravida 4, para 3003, delivered vaginally at 41½ weeks' gestation, with local anesthesia, an 8 pound, 12 ounce (3969 gram) female; Apgar score 8/9. The infant followed a normal newborn course. The membranes were artificially ruptured just prior to the appearance of the early decelerations.

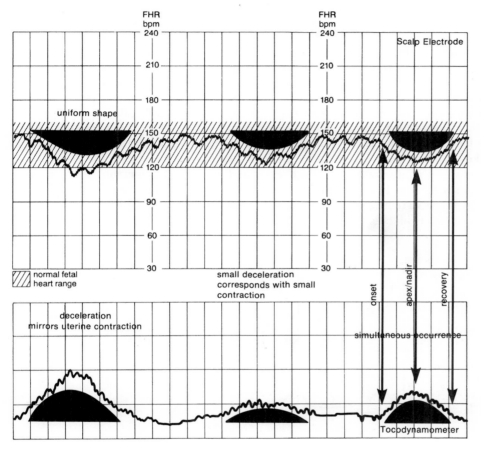

Pattern Characteristic:
Early Decelerations

Early and Variable Decelerations: Mixed Pattern

*W*hen early decelerations are diagnosed and the complete intrapartum tracing is reviewed, a mixed pattern with variable decelerations is often identified. Intrapartum occurrence rates of early decelerations vary from uncommon[8,17] to as frequent as 27%.[20] Such a wide discrepancy is perhaps influenced by whether a meticulous effort is made to distinguish early decelerations in

"pure" form from patterns mixed with variable decelerations,[11] assuming that there is a normal baseline pattern. The pure form is not associated with an unfavorable newborn outcome.[5] Interpretation with the mixed form varies with the appearance of the variable decelerations.

An increased frequency of both early and variable decelerations is associated with ruptured membranes,[2,3,9,19] so that the incidence of a mixed pattern varies according to the number of patients with ruptured membranes in any given series.

What appears to be a mixed pattern may simply reflect a difficulty in the diagnosis of the two types of deceleration. Some patterns that appear to be early decelerations may actually be atypical variable decelerations that are exhibiting the loss of primary and secondary accelerations. On the other hand, some patterns that appear to be variable decelerations may be early decelerations with an unusual presentation. For example, when contractions assume a peaked (inverted V) shape, mirror imaging produces a V-shaped deceleration resulting in mixed visual features of early and variable decelerations.

Mirror imaging is a feature of early decelerations. Intermittent slowing of the fetal heart rate is believed to be caused by a parasympathetic response to the cranial pressure produced by uterine contractions. The resulting decelerations mirror the bell-shaped uterine contraction waveform, resulting in a bowl shape. When uterine contractions have an atypical configuration such as rapid rise to maximum pressure, peaking, skewing, and polysystole, early decelerations may also assume a nonuniform configuration that may simulate features of variable decelerations. Mirror imaging is typically seen as a transient phenomenon at 4 to 6 centimeters cervical dilatation, when the cervical lip traverses the anterior fontanel of the fetus.[8] This association was suggested by the results of applying pressure to fetal or newborn heads using circular pessaries.[4]

Both early and variable decelerations may be altered by atropine administration.[12] Neither is expected to be affected by oxygen administration, with the exception of variable decelerations, which are frequent and prolonged.[12] A maternal position change is less likely to modify early decelerations than variable decelerations; the former are believed to be produced by the effects of head compression and the latter most commonly by the effects of cord compression but occasionally by the effects of head compression. The mechanisms of vagal stimulation through head compression are not fully understood. Present theories for the production of early decelerations include pressure deformations of the fetal head that produce flow-induced baroreceptor responses or local central nervous system hypoxia that stimulates chemoreceptors.[13,18] Theories for the production of variable decelerations include abrupt vagal discharge caused by fetal eye pressure (see page 00).

Both early and variable decelerations that are confined to the time of the uterine contraction were formerly called "type I dips."[3]

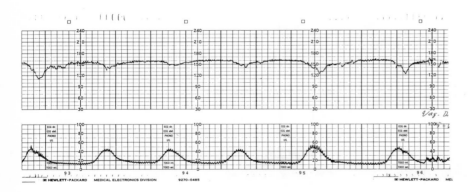

CASE INTERPRETATION: Class IV

Baseline Information: high to normal rate and decreased variability.

Periodic or Nonperiodic Changes: a mixed pattern of early decelerations and mild variable decelerations, with atypia characterized by absent primary and secondary accelerations, a delayed return to baseline, and diminished variability.

Uterine Activity: a normal configuration and frequency of contractions for active labor.

Significance: an absence of variability and atypia of variable decelerations predicts an increased risk of a low Apgar score and acidosis. Management is selected after an assessment of clinical factors, including the estimated time of vaginal delivery, gestation, response to the administration of oxygen and maternal position change, prior fetal status, and response to treatments used. The pattern needs to be differentiated from prolonged accelerations with a brief return to baseline by studying larger segments of the tracing.

CASE OUTCOME: Twenty-eight-year-old gravida 2, para 1001, delivered vaginally, with low forceps and ketamine anesthesia, a 6 pound, 12½ ounce (3076 gram) male; Apgar score 9/9. The fetus was in an occiput anterior position. The umbilical cord was not noted to be entrapped. Oxytocin augmentation was administered during labor. The infant followed an uncomplicated newborn course.

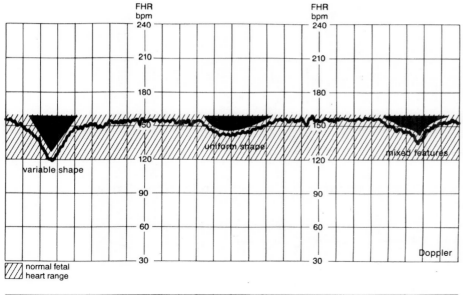

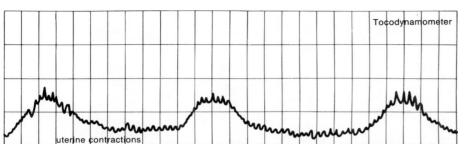

Pattern Characteristic:
Early Decelerations and Variable
Decelerations: Mixed Pattern

Progression from Early to Variable Decelerations

*E*arly decelerations are typically a transient pattern of a midactive phase of labor when the dilating cervix traverses the pressure-sensitive anterior fontanel. Variable decelerations, which are also usually pressure-induced, typically increase in occurrence as the active phase of labor progresses.[1] It is not surprising, therefore, to find a transition from early decelerations to variable decelerations in the same fetus as labor progresses, particularly in the presence of ruptured membranes.[2,3,19]

Early decelerations may be visually indistingishable from atypical shallow variable decelerations with loss of primary and secondary accelerations. Variable decelerations may be indistinguishable from V-shaped early de-

celerations that are produced not by cord compression but by mirror imaging a peaked uterine contraction.

The difference in pathogenesis of the patterns may help in distinguishing the two in a given set of clinical circumstances. A minimum intracranial pressure of 40 mm Hg and an intrauterine pressure of 40 to 50 mm Hg is required to produce early decelerations. Variable decelerations occur with only mild pressures that are sufficient to induce umbilical cord vessel occlusion, but cord vulnerability may not occur until late labor.[14,16] Some variable decelerations are not produced by cord compression but by other vagal effects (see Chap. 12).

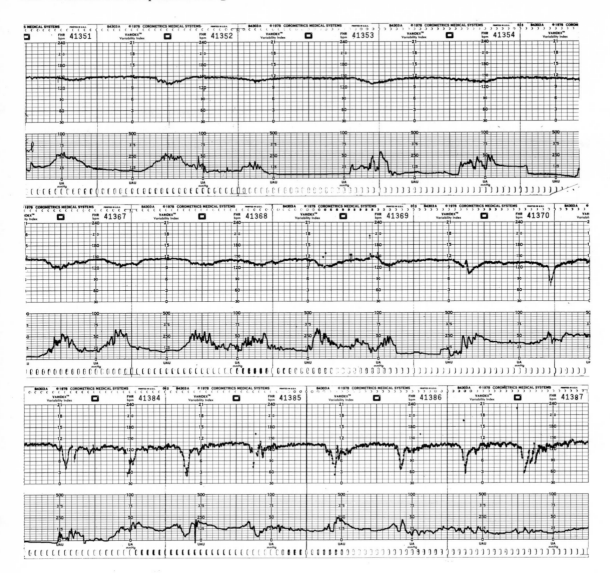

CASE INTERPRETATION: Class I

Baseline Information: normal rate and normal variability in some areas, decreased variability in others.

Periodic or Nonperiodic Changes: progression from early periodic decelerations to mild V-shaped variable decelerations.

Uterine Activity: not clearly recorded; frequent contractions, some of which are skewed.

Significance: diminished variability warrants close observation of the progress of the pattern, but the classic appearance of variable decelerations is reassuring.

CASE OUTCOME: Twenty-year-old primigravida at 40 weeks' gestation delivered vaginally, with pudendal and local anesthesia, a 7 pound, 7 ounce (3374 gram) male; Apgar score 7/9. Meconium was present. A nuchal cord was noted at delivery. The fetus was in a vertex presentation, in an occiput anterior position. The infant followed a normal newborn course.

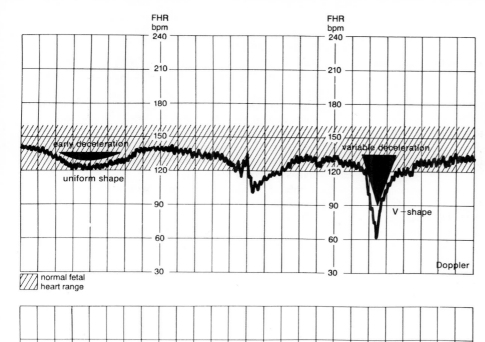

Pattern Characteristic:
Progression From Early to
Variable Decelerations

References

1. Beard RW, Filshie GM, Knight CA: The significance of the changes in the continuous fetal heart rate in the first stage of labor. *J Obstet Gynecol Br Commonw* 78:865, 1971.
2. Caldeyro-Barcia R, Schwarcz RL, Althabe O: Effects of rupture of membrane on fetal heart rate pattern. *Int J Gynaecol Obstet* 10:169, 1972.
3. Caldeyro-Barcia R, Schwartcz R, Belizan JM, et al: Adverse perinatal effects of early amniotomy during labor, in Gluck L (ed): *Modern Perinatal Medicine*. Chicago, Medical Publishers, 1974, p. 431ff.
4. Chung F, Hon EH: The electronic evaluation of the fetal heart rate. I. With pressure on the fetal skull. *Obstet Gynecol* 13:633, 1959.
5. Cibils LA: Clinical significance of fetal heart rate patterns during labor. VI. Early decelerations. *Am J Obstet Gynecol* 136:392, 1980.
6. Cibils LA: Early decelerations, in *Electronic Fetal-Maternal Monitoring: Antepartum, Intrapartum*. Boston, PSG Publishing, 1981, p. 294ff.
7. Freeman RK, Garite TJ: Basic pattern recognition, in *Fetal Heart Rate Monitoring*. Baltimore, Williams & Wilkins, 1981, p. 67.
8. Freeman RK, Garite TJ: The physiologic basis of fetal monitoring, in *Fetal Heart Rate Monitoring*. Baltimore, Williams & Wilkins, 1981, p. 12.
9. Gabert HA, Stenchever MA: Effect of ruptured membranes on fetal heart rate patterns. *Obstet Gynecol* 41:279, 1973.

10. Hon EH: *An Introduction to Fetal Heart Rate Monitoring.* Los Angeles, University of Southern California School of Medicine, 1973.

11. Hon EH: Severe variable decelerations in fetal heart rate. *CMA Journal* 115:491, 1976.

12. Hon EG, Quilligan EJ: Electronic evaluation of fetal heart rate. IX. Further observations on "pathologic" fetal bradycardia, in Quilligan EJ (ed): *Clinical Obstetrics and Gynecology.* New York, Harper and Row, 1968, p. 149ff.

13. Hutson JM, Mueller-Heubach E: Diagnosis and management of intrapartum reflex fetal heart rate changes. *Clinics in Perinatology* 9:325, 1982.

14. Kelly JV: Instrument delivery and the fetal heart rate. *Am J Obstet Gynecol* 87:529, 1963.

15. Kubli FW, Hon EH, Kazin AF, et al: Observations on heart rate and pH in the human fetus during labor. *Am J Obstet Gynecol* 104:1190, 1969.

16. Mann LI, Carmichael A, Duchin S: The effect of head compression on FHR, brain metabolism and function. *Obstet Gynecol* 39:721, 1972.

17. Parer J: Heart rate patterns, in: *Handbook of Fetal Heart Rate Monitoring.* Philadelphia: W.B. Saunders, 1983, p. 90.

18. Paul WM, Quilligan EJ, MacLachlan T: Cardiovascular phenomenon associated with fetal head compression. *Am J Obstet Gynecol* 90:824, 1964.

19. Schwarcz RL, Althabe O, Belitzky R, et al: Fetal heart rate patterns in labors with intact and with ruptured membranes. *J Perinat Med* 1:153, 1973.

20. Shenker L: Clinical experiences with heart rate monitoring of one thousand patients in labor. *Am J Obstet Gynecol* 115:1111, 1973.

21. *Webster's New World Dictionary, Second College Edition.* New York, Simon and Schuster, 1980:1551.

Uniform Decelerations: Late Decelerations

Chapter 11

Late Decelerations with Good Variability

*L*ate decelerations are characterized by a "uniform" configuration.[22] A dictionary definition of uniform is "having the same form and appearance as others in the same class, not varying or changing in form, rate, degree or manner, conforming to a given standard."[48] As with early decelerations, the standard for defining the shape of the late deceleration is the shape of the uterine contraction, reversed. Thus, a gradual onset and gradual resolution of each late deceleration is a prerequisite for diagnosis (assuming a typical uterine contraction waveform).

Unlike early decelerations, late decelerations have a delay in occurrence in relation to the uterine contraction. Each, and usually all, of the following events may be delayed: onset (latency period), nadir in relationship to contraction peak (lag time), and return to baseline (recovery time).[16] The late deceleration in a fetus who is not moribund reflects a varying intensity of uterine contractions with a varying depth of deceleration.[10,35]

There are two etiologies of late decelerations.[21,27,36] Those associated with preservation of beat-to-beat variability are believed produced by a vagal response to chemoreceptors triggered by hypoxia.[26,42] These represent a compensated stress pattern. The onset typically precedes the loss of accelerations.[40] The deceleration does not occur immediately with the onset of the uterine contraction because the fetus is initially able to continue to extract sufficient oxygen from the blood until levels fall to those that stimulate the receptors. It is therefore apparent that the sooner the onset of critical hypoxia, the closer to the uterine contraction the onset appears (shorter latency period).[41] However, recovery duration increases with the severity, reflecting the time restoration of uteroplacental flow and fetal oxygenation.[37]

Of greater significance in predicting a potentially compromised fetus are the late decelerations produced by myocardial depression.[28] These are typically associated with absent variability. The degree of acidosis correlates with the depth of the deceleration *except* in certain very moribund fetuses, in whom there is a tendency for the decelerations to become shallower as the fetal condition worsens. Late decelerations may manifest varying degrees of both mechanisms.[11]

The management of late decelerations with good variability is directed at improving fetal oxygenation. Fetal mechanisms for response to the hypoxemia include shunting the blood from nonvital to vital vascular beds and increasing the extraction of oxygen at the site of placental exchange as well as through changes in the heart rate.[10,13] It is not surprising, therefore, that producing maternal hyperoxia has been demonstrated to improve fetal PO_2 and to eradicate this type of late deceleration.[15,49,50] These effects may be temporary if the oxygen is not continued or the underlying disease process is not corrected. Improving maternal position, hydration, correction of maternal hypotension, and other measures to maximize uterine blood flow are also adjuncts in "unstressing" the fetus who is exhibiting this pattern, since reduced uterine blood flow is one mechanism of producing or enhancing fetal hypoxemia.[1,6,8,11] In the case of hypoxemia derived from maternal anemia, resolution has been demonstrated to accompany correction of the anemia by transfusion.[7]

Late decelerations with reduced variability are discussed in ensuing pages.

If late decelerations cannot be abolished, preparations for delivery are appropriate in many clinical situations, even in the presence of variability.[33]

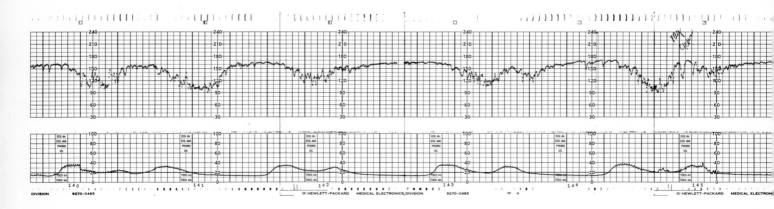

CASE INTERPRETATION: Class II

Baseline Information: high normal rate with rebound tachycardia upon recovery from some decelerations; normal variability, which is increased in decelerations.

Periodic or Nonperiodic Changes: late decelerations that maintain good variability in the decelerations.

Uterine Activity: coupled or polysystolic contractions, as measured by external monitoring.

Significance: the pattern denotes mild hypoxia which is usually responsive to administration of oxygen to the mother. Repositioning of the patient and hydration may also be beneficial. Obtaining a fetal pH level or performing a fetal stimulation test may be an adjunct if delivery is not imminent, the pattern does not improve, and the baseline variability declines. The timing of preparations for a potential cesarean section vary with the availability of resources.

CASE OUTCOME: Twenty-six-year-old primigravida at 41 weeks' gestation delivered vaginally, with epidural anesthesia and outlet forceps, a 5 pound, 15 ounce (2693 gram) male; one minute Apgar score of 6 was influenced by meconium suctioning. The five minute Apgar score was 6/8. The infant followed a normal newborn course.

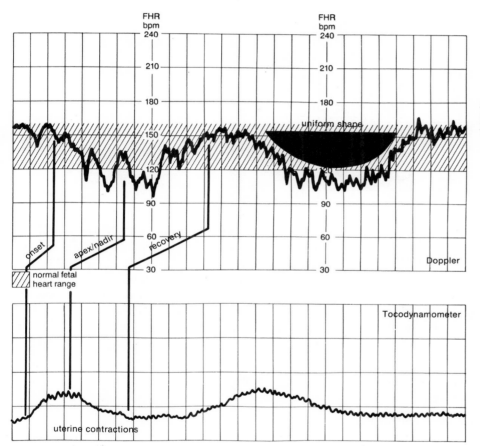

Pattern Characteristic:
Late Decelerations with Good Variability

Late Decelerations with No Variability—Low Apgar Score

*W*hen late decelerations are associated with the absence of beat-to-beat variability, an increased incidence of a low Apgar score and fetal acidosis is predicted. Late decelerations are produced by hypoxemia.[4] When fetal compensatory responses to the hypoxemia are insuffi-cient to meet metabolic needs, anaerobic glycolysis typically occurs, producing circulating acids and a fall in pH.[20] This is accompanied by diminished beat-to-beat variability. There are other less ominous potential causes of decreased variability in the presence of late decelerations. In situations of diminished variability, therefore, pH studies or fetal stimulation testing may assist delivery planning. In situations of late decelerations with no variability, delivery without delay is also appropriate.

Attempts to improve a mixed pattern of late decelerations and absent variability by maternal oxygen administration, hydration, maternal position change, and reduction of uterine activity may be unsuccessful. Therefore, although those are appropriate adjuncts to achieving an optimal fetal condition at delivery, simultaneous efforts toward facilitating delivery are often appropriate. However, if the pattern improves by such measures while preparing for delivery, a reassessment of the urgency of delivery may be made.

When the uterine waveform includes a steep rise in maximum intensity and skewing, some late decelerations assume a configuration simulating a check mark. This is exaggerated by a one or two centimeter paper speed.

Late decelerations in an asphyxiated fetus may become so continuous that the baseline is obscured—full recovery from one deceleration does not occur before the onset of the next late deceleration, resulting in a coarse, undulating pattern (nonsinusoidal premortem) (see page 136). This is often associated with uterine hyperactivity as a factor influencing the continuum from hypoxia to acidosis.

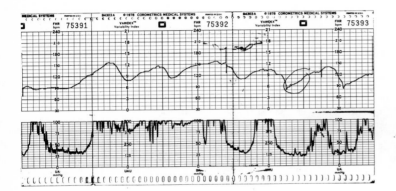

CASE INTERPRETATION: Class V

Baseline Information: decreased variability, obscured baseline.

Periodic or Nonperiodic Changes: periodic decelerations; late decelerations, most with uniform shape and some with a "check mark" shape so continuous that there is obliteration of the baseline and an undulating appearance.

Uterine Activity: increased uterine activity in frequency and duration; maternal straining efforts.

Significance: the pattern may have been ameliorated earlier by administering oxygen and decreasing uterine activity, but the fetus now may be at too high a risk of a low Apgar score and acidosis to justify a prolonged delay in delivery.

CASE OUTCOME: Twenty-year-old primigravida at 39 weeks' gestation delivered by emergency cesarean section, with inhalation anesthesia, for probable fetal distress a 6 pound (2722 gram) female; Apgar score 1/7. The newborn required transient oxygen by hood and was treated for hyponatremia. Thereafter, the infant followed an uncomplicated newborn course. No pH studies were done.

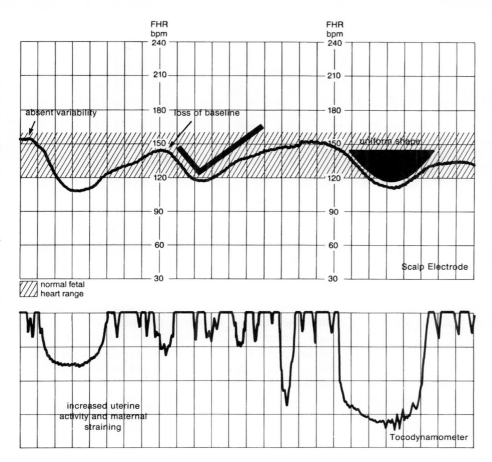

normal fetal
heart range

Late Decelerations with No Variability—Unfavorable Outcome

*T*he combination of late decelerations in a mixed pattern with absent beat-to-beat variability is associated with an increased incidence of acidosis and a low Apgar score. Failure to recover from one deceleration before the onset of the next further denotes an increased likelihood of significant fetal compromise.[24] Prompt delivery is often appropriate. If an immediate fetal pH is available, it may assist delivery planning and not delay appropriate intervention.

While preparing for delivery, if the measures taken to produce an optimal fetal status abolish the pattern, the need for emergency delivery may then be reassessed. Maternal oxygen administration and hydration, lateral positioning, and reduction of uterine hyperactivity are appropriate measures accompanying preparations for delivery.[23,39]

The fetal monitor pattern of late decelerations is increased in frequency in clinical situations of reduced placental exchange, for example, preeclampsia and other hypertensive disorders, placental abruption, diabetes mellitus, intrauterine growth retardation, and postdate pregnancy.[5,10,11,34] The effect of these problems is enhanced in the older patient.[10] The outcome in the presence of late decelerations is also poorer for preterm newborns.[11] Late decelerations are also increased in clinical situations of maternal hypoxemia (e.g., sickle cell disease), fetal hypoxemia (e.g., erythroblastosis fetalis), or reduced maternal blood pressure.[11,12,22]

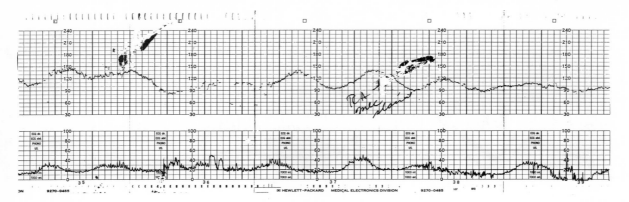

CASE INTERPRETATION: Class V

Baseline Information: baseline obscured by decelerations, absent variability.

Periodic or Nonperiodic Changes: recurrent late decelerations with absent variability of such frequency that each begins before recovery from the previous one.

Uterine Activity: not well recorded, frequent contractions without resting intervals.

Significance: high probability of a low Apgar score and acidosis. Delivery is appropriate in most clinical situations. While preparing for delivery, maternal oxygen administration, position change, and hydration may improve the fetal status at delivery.

CASE OUTCOME: Twenty-seven-year-old primigravida, at 38 weeks' gestation, delivered vaginally, with epidural anesthesia, a 6 pound, 12 ounce (3062 gram) female; Apgar score 2/2. The fetus was in an occiput anterior position. The newborn expired one hour after birth with meconium aspiration and intracerebral hemorrhage.

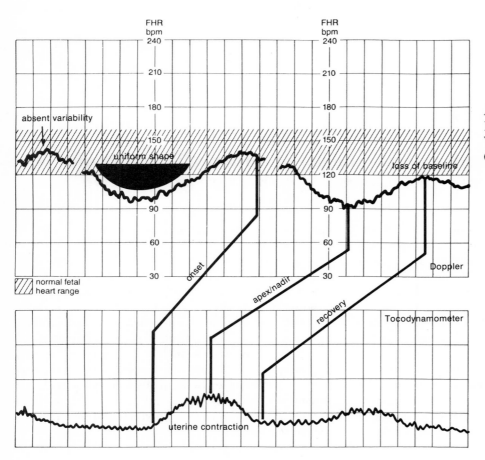

Pattern Characteristic:
Late Decelerations with No Variability—Unfavorable Outcome

Late Decelerations with No Variability—Favorable Outcome

*L*ate decelerations with the preservation of good variability represent a reflex vagal response to hypoxemia for which the healthy fetus is usually able to compensate. The pattern is produced when a fall in PO$_2$ induced by uterine contractions exceeds 5 mm Hg, particularly a fall below 15 to 20 mm Hg.[4,8,25,29,37] This corresponds to a hemoglobin saturation with oxygen of less than 25% to 30%.[2] The pattern of late decelerations with good variability appears before sufficient hypoxia has occurred to produce neurologic consequences.[2] This pattern has been demonstrated to be correctable by oxygen administration to the mother as well as improved uterine perfusion.[3]

Since variability can be obliterated by causes other than acidosis, for example, a drug effect, it is possible to have a fetal monitoring pattern of late decelerations with absent variability in the healthy stressed fetus without asphyxia.[39] The ability to predict a sick fetus by this pattern is as poor as 50%.[38,47] However, the incidence of a low Apgar score and fetal acidosis with such a pattern is sufficiently high to make it unwise to *assume* that the fetus is not in jeopardy.[14,33]

Preparations for delivery are usually in order when this pattern is encountered. In those situations in which the depth of decelerations are minimal or intermittent and previous excellent variability preceded drug administration, intermittent fetal pH studies may selectively be used for clarification.[46] Instantaneous pH capability would be an advantage for such a pattern.[51] Fetal stimulation studies or pH studies are useful with cases in which there is a pattern of diminishing variability and late decelerations and vaginal delivery is imminent.[43] Likewise, demonstrating eradication of the abnormal fetal monitoring pattern *while* proceeding with preparations for delivery supports a change to more conservative management.

If pH studies are not available or a reassuring response to fetal stimulation does not occur, delivery is usually appropriate in the presence of persistent late decelerations and reduced variability.

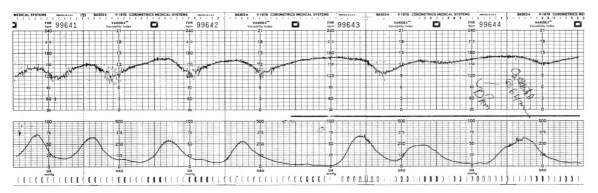

Recreation of original tracing

CASE INTERPRETATION: Class V

Baseline Information: the heart rate is obscured by decelerations; there is probably a high-normal heart rate or moderate tachycardia and absent variability, as measured by an external monitor without autocorrelation. Artifactual "jitter" is noted.

Periodic or Nonperiodic Changes: recurrent late decelerations with absent variability, occurring with such frequency that the next deceleration begins upon recovery of the previous one.

Uterine Activity: skewed and polysystolic contractions without a resting interval.

Significance: a high incidence of acidosis or a low Apgar score. Prompt delivery is usually appropriate. Maternal administration of oxygen, position change, and hydration may be effected while preparing for delivery.

Rarely, the pattern may be abolished and conservative management reinstituted.

CASE OUTCOME: Sixteen-year-old primigravida delivered by cesarean section for cephalopelvic disproportion, with general anesthesia, a 5 pound, 1/2 ounce (2282 gram) male; Apgar score 8 at one minute, five minute Apgar score was only stated to be "more than 7." The mother had severe preeclampsia; the labor was spontaneous. The mother received magnesium sulfate, meperidine, propiomazine, scopolamine, and levallorphan tartrate intrapartum.

The patient was lying on her back receiving buccal oxytocin at the time of the tracing segment. The pattern improved with a maternal position change, oxygen therapy, and discontinuation of the oxytocin. The fluid was clear. The newborn followed an uncomplicated newborn course.

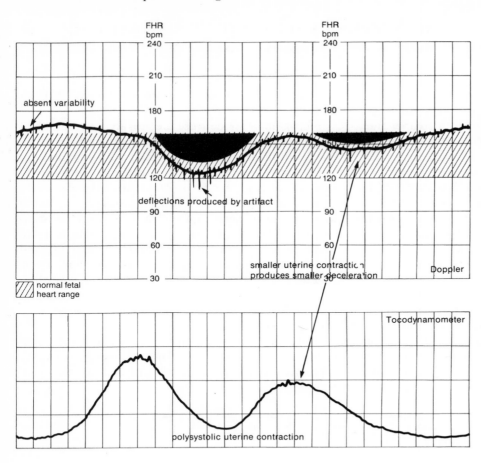

Pattern Characteristic:
Late Decelerations with No
Variability—Favorable Outcome

Shallow Late Decelerations

*E*arly in the continuum of hypoxia to acidosis, deepening late decelerations correlate with increasing hypoxemia, which is produced by an increasing chemoreceptor response. For this reason, late decelerations were once graded as mild, moderate, and severe by depth, but this classification is now considered less clinically useful than identification by the presence or absence of variability.[31,44] Late in the course of hypoxia changing to acidosis, late decelerations become progressively shallower as myocardial depression eradicates the ability of the fetus to respond any longer to stimuli by slowing the heart rate. The postdate fetus is particularly susceptible to this pattern.[18]

Decelerations may eventually become *imperceptible*, resulting in a flat-line pattern that is associated with decreased or absent short- and long-term variability.[9] Hence, it may benefit some fetuses to be delivered when exhibiting flat-line intrapartum patterns *unless* there are pH studies available for fetal surveillance or other information indicative of a good fetal condition exists.

Beat-to-beat electronic fetal heart rate monitoring is a valuable adjunct in elucidating this pattern because this subtle degree of late deceleration cannot be identified with auscultation alone.[45]

It may not be possible to reverse this pattern in a timely way in utero because fetal compromise may have progressed beyond the usual fetal-placental compensatory mechanisms for recovery.

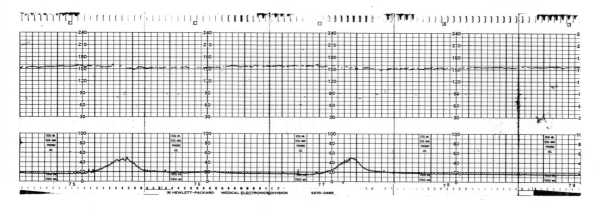

CASE INTERPRETATION: Class V

Baseline Information: high normal rate, absent variability.

Periodic and Nonperiodic Changes: shallow, late decelerations with absent variability.

Uterine Activity: infrequent contractions of normal configuration, as measured by external monitoring.

Significance: this may be a severely asphyxiated fetus with myocardial depression. Delivery is usually appropriate if the pattern is not promptly corrected by oxygen, maternal position changes, and hydration.

CASE OUTCOME: Twenty-eight-year-old gravida 3, para 1011, at 42 weeks' gestation delivered from a vertex presentation by cesarean section, with inhalation anesthesia, a growth retarded 3 pound, 9½ ounce (1630 gram) female; Apgar score 1/1. The newborn expired after 15 days of life; the infant's course was complicated by renal failure and hypoglycemia.

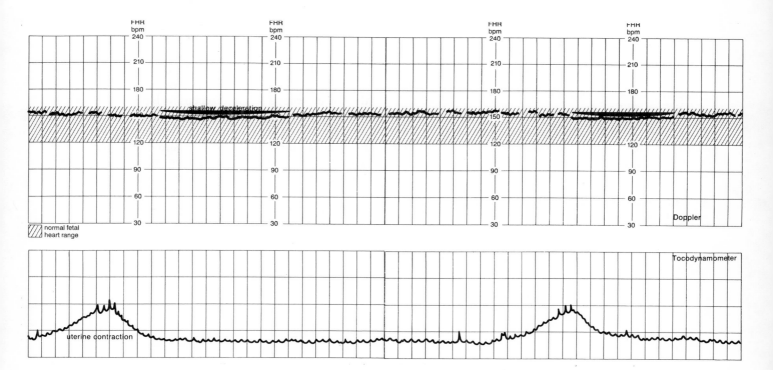

Pattern Characteristic:
Shallow Late Decelerations

Transient Late Decelerations, Recovery Phase of Prolonged Deceleration

*L*ate decelerations may appear during recovery from prolonged decelerations.[17] Usually, the prolonged deceleration was produced by uterine hyperactivity.[30] The late decelerations become progressively shallower with recovery in this instance.[11] Full recovery to the preceding baseline should be anticipated within 30 minutes if the fetus is able to appropriately use compensatory mechanisms for in utero resuscitation. The long-term, potentially subtle effects on the neonate of a prolonged recovery phase that exhibits transient hypoxemia are unknown. Administration of oxygen to the mother, optimum maternal positioning, hydration, and reduction of uterine hyperactivity are appropriate adjuncts in the resuscitation process.

Delivery need not be required in the healthy term fetus unless progressive recovery is not demonstrated or recurrent progressive hypoxic episodes occur despite therapy. The fetus with intrauterine growth retardation, postmaturity syndrome, immaturity, thick meconium, or who is in a pregnancy with preeclampsia is at greater risk than the normal term fetus when encountering this pattern.

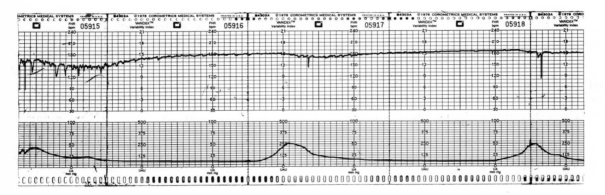

CASE INTERPRETATION: Class II

Baseline Information: moderate to severe tachycardia, rising baseline, decreased baseline variability.

Periodic or Nonperiodic Changes: average variability within the first of three late decelerations that become progressively shallower, small jagged V-shaped variable decelerations within each late deceleration.

Uterine Activity: infrequent but prolonged polysystolic, skewed contractions.

Significance: a pattern seen upon recovery from a prolonged deceleration that produced transient local tissue hypoxia.

CASE OUTCOME: Twenty-three-year-old primigravida at 40 weeks' gestation delivered, with local and pudendal anesthesia and midforceps for a persistent occiput posterior position, a 7 pound, 5 ounce (3317 gram) male; Apgar score 6/8. There was thick meconium. The infant followed an uncomplicated newborn course. Prolonged decelerations occurred during a maternal seizure. The tracing reverted to a normal pattern, and delivery occurred 1¼ hours later. (See page 393 for the pattern during the seizure in this case.)

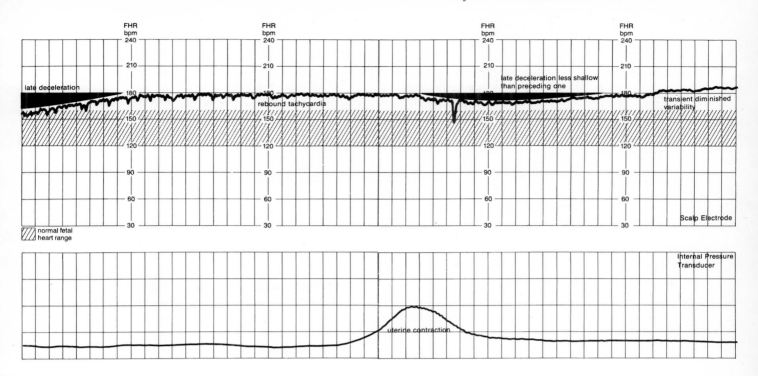

Pattern Characteristic:
Transient Late Decelerations, Recovery Phase of Prolonged Deceleration

Late Increased Variability

*B*oth late decelerations and increased variability are fetal heart rate responses to hypoxemia. When episodes of increased variability occur late, they may be managed clinically in a way similar to late decelerations with good variability and are, in fact, possibly variants of the same pattern. The presence of increased variability may obscure recognition of the presence of coexisting late decelerations.

When encountered in antepartum testing, late increased variability is not reassuring and management of the test results should be much like that for a suspicious or positive stress test.

When encountered intrapartum, the demonstration of good variability indicates that the fetus is in no immediate jeopardy but that responses to stress have been elicited. Administration of oxygen to the mother and steps to improve uterine blood flow are appropriate measures. (See page 79 for a similar pattern.)

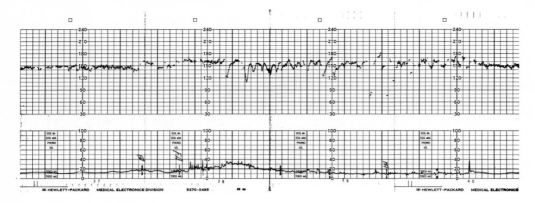

CASE INTERPRETATION: Class II

Baseline Information: normal rate, decreased variability except following uterine contractions when there is an episode of increased variability.

Periodic or Nonperiodic Changes: late decelerations that are obscured by the increased variability with which they are associated.

Uterine Activity: single contraction, appears skewed.

Significance: a pattern of mild hypoxia. Appropriate management is the same as with findings of late decelerations and average variability. When encountered in antepartum testing, this pattern does not give assurance that the fetal condition will remain good for one week.

CASE OUTCOME: Twenty-six-year-old gravida 5, para 3013 at 42½ weeks' gestation, upon arrival in the labor unit, spontaneously delivered vaginally, with local anesthesia, an 8 pound, 10 ounce (3912 gram), male; Apgar score 2/6. The fetus was in a vertex presentation. The newborn expired at 12 hours of life, with severe meconium aspiration. The maternal course was complicated by asthma. The delivery occurred one week after this tracing was obtained.

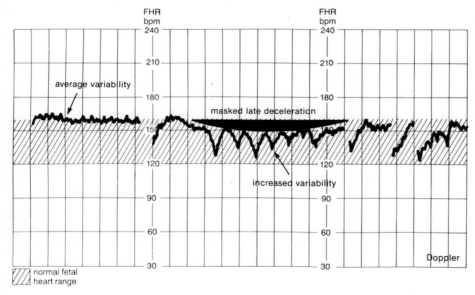

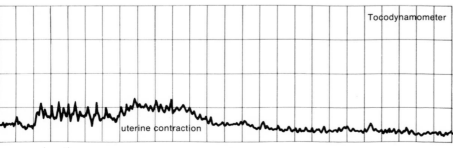

Pattern Characteristic:
Late Increased Variability

Late Decelerations with Variable Decelerations—Combined Pattern

*L*ate decelerations may denote hypoxia with potential myocardial ischemia if they are associated with loss of variability, especially with shallow depth. Certain configurations in atypical variable decelerations may also denote hypoxia. Prolonged secondary acceleration and slow recovery are two examples of this. In the latter context, umbilical cord impingement is suggested as a factor in producing hypoxia.

When both atypical variable decelerations and late decelerations occur together with a loss of baseline variability, the risks of an unfavorable outcome are compounded.[19,21] The pattern has a high association with increased uterine activity.[27] (See pages 254 and 291 for other examples and further discussion of this pattern.)

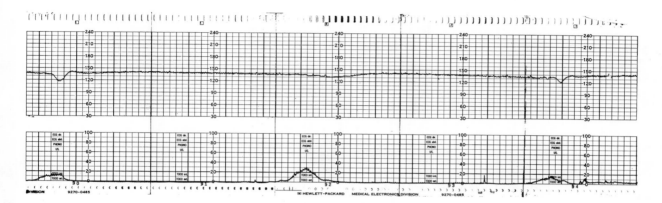

CASE INTERPRETATION: Class V

Baseline Information: normal heart rate, absent variability, gradual downward shift of baseline between contractions.

Periodic or Nonperiodic Changes: combined mild atypical variable decelerations and shallow late decelerations interspersed with shallow late decelerations.

Uterine Activity: infrequent contractions of a normal configuration.

Significance: an increased risk of a low Apgar score and fetal hypoxia with acidosis. Delivery planning is usually appropriate while performing measures to improve fetal oxygenation during preparation.

CASE OUTCOME: Fifteen-year-old primigravida delivered at 30 weeks' gestation by cesarean section with general anesthesia, performed for possible fetal distress and eclampsia a 3 pound, 7 ounce (1559 gram) female; Apgar score 1/5. The fetus was in a vertex presentation. The patient required an emergency postpartum tracheostomy for an upper airway obstruction (laryngeal edema). The mother received magnesium sulfate intrapartum as well as meperidine and promethazine. The newborn was transferred from a tertiary to a secondary hospital at 24 days of life.

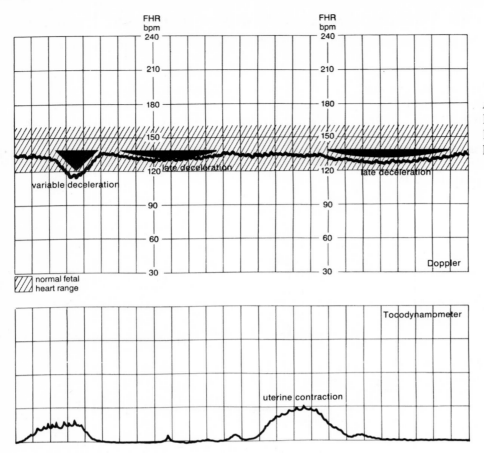

Pattern Characteristic:
Late Decelerations with Variable
Decelerations—Combined
Pattern

Late or Variable Decelerations?

*I*t is not always possible to conclusively distinguish between late decelerations and variable decelerations that are occurring late.

Variable decelerations may assume a uniform shape when atypia is present, as characterized by a loss of primary (initial) and secondary accelerations. Variable decelerations may occur late, either because of timing of a cord impingement, or an associated hypoxia.

Late decelerations may maintain the criteria for uniformity while reflecting an unusually peaked uterine contraction that produces a V-shaped deceleration.

The importance of distinguishing late from variable decelerations is somewhat academic if the pattern is associated with a loss of baseline variability, smoothness of the deceleration, and slow recovery. Although the etiology of the hypoxic mechanisms may vary in each case, clinical management is essentially the same for each. That is, preparations for delivery because of an increased risk of acidosis and a low Apgar score, unless the pattern is abolished by measures to improve fetal oxygenation while preparing for delivery or other information is available assuring good fetal condition.

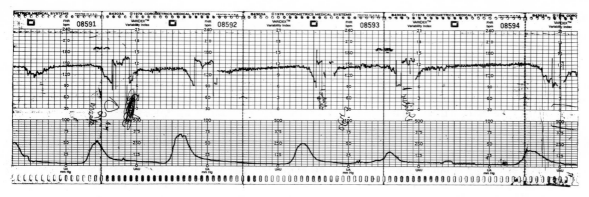

CASE INTERPRETATION: Class IV/V

Baseline Information: normal rate, absent variability.

Periodic or Nonperiodic Changes: late decelerations (with some features of atypical variable decelerations) partially obscured by the double counting phenomenon; a slow return to the baseline follows each deceleration.

Uterine Activity: peaked, skewed contractions.

Significance: regardless of whether the decelerations are late or are variable decelerations that are occurring late, the baseline loss of variability and slow drifting back to a 140 to 150 bpm heart rate after each deceleration is not reassuring. Doubling, which produces a rate of approximately 150 bpm, gives a visual illusion that the decelerations are not as profound as they actually are. Internal fetal heart rate monitoring would clarify the pattern, if this is feasible, and delivery may be indicated if the pattern is not promptly obliterated by oxygen, a maternal position change, and hydration. (See page 363 for a discussion of peaked contractions.)

CASE OUTCOME: Twenty-year-old primigravida at 30 weeks' gestation delivered by primary cesarean section for possible fetal distress, inhalation of anesthesia, and a vertex presentation a 2 pound, 3 ounce (990 gram) male; Apgar score 5/7. The pregnancy was complicated by severe preeclampsia, meconium passage, and placental abruption.

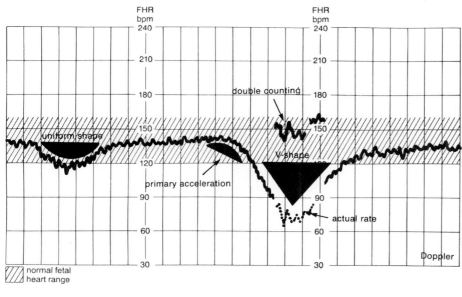

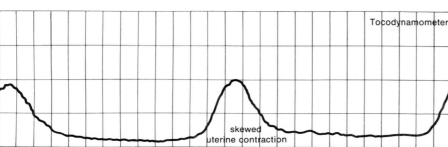

Pattern Characteristic:
Late or Variable Decelerations?

References

1. Abitbol MM: Supine position in labor and associated fetal heart rate changes. *Obstet Gynecol* 65:481, 1985.

2. Adamsons K, Myers RE: Late decelerations and brain tolerance of the fetal monkey to intrapartum asphyxia. *Am J Obstet Gynecol* 128:893, 1977.

3. Althabe O, Schwarcz RL, Pose EV, et al: Effects on fetal heart rate and fetal PO₂ of oxygen administration to the mother. *Am J Obstet Gynecol* 98:858, 1967.

4. Arnoudse JG, Huisjes HJ, Gordon H, et al: Fetal subcutaneous scalp PO₂ and abnormal heart rate during labor. *Am J Obstet Gynecol* 153:565, 1985.

5. Bekedam DJ, Visser GHA: Effects of hypoxemic events on breathing, body movements, and heart rate variation: A study in growth-retarded human fetuses. *Am J Obstet Gynecol* 155:52, 1985.

6. Bocking AD, Harding R, Wickham FJD: Effects of reduced uterine blood flow on accelerations and decelerations in heart rate of fetal sheep. *Am J Obstet Gynecol* 154:329, 1986.

7. Cabaniss ML: Clinical observations.

8. Caldeyro-Barcia R, Rose SV, Poseiro JJ, et al: Effects of several factors on fetal PO₂ recorded continuously in the fetal monkey, in: Gluck L (ed): *Intrauterine Asphyxia and the Developing Fetal Brain*. Chicago, Yearbook Medical Publishers, 1977, p. 237ff.

9. Cetrulo CL, Schifrin BS: Fetal heart rate patterns preceding death in utero. *Obstet Gynecol* 48:521, 1976.

10. Cibils LA: Clinical significance of fetal heart rate patterns during labor. II. Late decelerations. *Am J Obstet Gynecol* 123:473, 1975.

11. Cibils LA: *Late Decelerations in Electronic Fetal Monitoring*. Boston, PSG Publishing, 1981, p. 306.

12. Cruz AC, Spellacy WN, Jarrell M: Fetal heart rate tracing during sickle cell crisis: A cause for transient late decelerations. *Obstet Gynecol* 54:647, 1979.

13. Edelstone DI, Peticca BB, Goldblum LJ: Effects of maternal oxygen administration on fetal oxygenation during reductions in umbilical blood flow in fetal lambs. *Am J Obstet Gynecol* 152:351, 1985.

14. Emmon L, Huisjes HJ, Aaronoudse JG, et al: Antepartum diagnosis of the "terminal" fetal state by cardiotocography. *Br J Obstet Gynaecol* 82:353, 1975.

15. Fall O, Ek B, Nilsson BA, et al: Time factor in oxygen transfer from mother to fetus. *Gynecol Obstet Invest* 10:231, 1979.

16. Freeman RK, Garite TJL: *Basic Pattern Recognition in Fetal Heart Rate Monitoring*. Baltimore, Williams & Wilkins, 1981, pp. 68, 69.

17. Freeman RK, Garite TJL: *The Clinical Management of Fetal Distress in Fetal Heart Rate Monitoring*. Baltimore, Williams & Wilkins, 1981, p. 89.

18. Garite TJ, Freeman RK: Decelerations subtle when pregnancy is prolonged. *Contemp Obstet Gynecol* 20:35, 1982.

19. Gaziano EP: A study of variable decelerations in association with other heart rate patterns during monitored labor. *Am J Obstet Gynecol* 135:360, 1979.

20. Gimovsky ML, Caritis SN: Diagnosis and management of hypoxic fetal heart rate patterns. *Clinics in Perinatology* 9:313, 1982.

21. Harris JL, Krueger TR, Parer TJ: Mechanisms of late decelerations of the fetal heart rate during hypoxia. *Am J Obstet Gynecol* 144:491, 1982.

22. Hon EH: *An Introduction to Fetal Heart Rate Monitoring*. Los Angeles, University of Southern California School of Medicine, 1973.

23. Hon EH: The fetal heart rate patterns preceding death in utero. *Am J Obstet Gynecol* 78:47, 1959.

24. Hon EH, Lee ST: Electronic evaluation of the fetal heart rate. VIII. Patterns preceding fetal death, further observations. *Am J Obstet Gynecol* 87:814, 1963.

25. Huch A, Huch R, Schneider H, et al: Continuous transcutaneous monitoring of fetal oxygen tension during labour. *Br J Obstet Gynaecol* 84:4, 1971.

26. Hutson JM, Mueller-Heubach E: Diagnosis and management of intrapartum reflex fetal heart rate changes. *Clinics in Perinatology* 9:325, 1982.

27. Ingemarsson E, Ingemarsson I, Westgren M: Combined decelerations-clinical significance and relation to uterine activity. *Obstet Gynecol* 58:35, 1981.

28. Itskovitz J, Goetzman BW, Rudolph AM: The mechanism of late deceleration of the heart rate and its relationship to oxygenation in normoxemic and chronically hypoxemic fetal lambs. *Am J Obstet Gynecol* 142:66, 1982.

29. James LS, Morishima HO: Mechanism of late deceleration of the fetal heart rate. *Int J Gynaecol Obstet* 10:182, 1972.

30. Klaven M: Prolonged deceleration patterns, in: *Clinical Concepts of Fetal Heart Rate Monitoring*. Chester, PA, 1973, p. 51.

31. Kubli FW, Hon EH, Khazin AF, et al: Observations on heart rate and pH in the human fetus during labor. *Am J Obstet Gynecol* 104:1190, 1969.

32. Lin C, Schulman H, Saldana LR: Deceleration/contraction ratios as an index of fetal health during labor. *Obstet Gynecol* 51:666, 1978.

33. Low JA, Boston RW, Pancham SR: The role of fetal heart rate patterns in the recognition of fetal asphyxia with metabolic acidosis. *Am J Obstet Gynecol* 109:922, 1971.

34. Low JA, Pancham SR, Worthington D: Fetal heart deceleration patterns in relation to asphyxia and weight-gestational age percentile of the fetus. *Obstet Gynecol* 47:14, 1976.

35. Martin CB: Regulation of the fetal heart and genesis of FHR patterns. *Seminars in Perinatology* 2:131, 1978.

36. Martin CB, de Haan J, van der Wildt B, et al: Mechanisms of late decelerations in the fetal heart rate. A study

with autonomic blocking agents in fetal lambs. *Europ J Obstet Gynec Reprod Biol* 9:361, 1979.

37. Mendez-Bauer C, Arnt IC, Gulin L, et al: Relationship between blood pH and heart rate in the human fetus during labor. *Am J Obstet Gynecol* 97:530, 1967.

38. Miller FC: Prediction of acid-base values from intrapartum fetal heart rate date and their correlation with scalp and funic values. *Clinics in Perinatology* 9:353, 1982.

39. Morishima HO, Daniel SS, Richards RT, et al: The effect of increased maternal PO$_2$ upon the fetus during labor. *Am J Obstet Gynecol* 123:257, 1975.

40. Murata Y, Martin CB, Ikenoue T, et al: Fetal heart rate accelerations and late deceleration during the course of intrauterine death in chronically catheterized rhesus monkeys. *Am J Obstet Gynecol* 144:218, 1982.

41. Myers RE, Mueller-Heubach E, Adamsons K: Predictability of the state of fetal oxygenations from a quantitative analysis of the components of late deceleration. *Am J Obstet Gynecol* 115:1083, 1973.

42. Parer JT: Late decelerations, in: *Handbook of Fetal Monitoring*. Philadelphia, W.B. Saunders, 1983, p. 94.

43. Parer JT, Krueger TR, Harris JL: Fetal oxygen consumption and mechanisms of heart rate response during artificially produced late decelerations of fetal heart rate in sheep. *Am J Obstet Gynecol* 136:478, 1980.

44. Paul RH, Petrie RH: *Fetal Intensive Care*. Corometrics Medical Systems, Inc., Wallingford, CT, 1979. p. III 20.

45. Paul RH, Suidan AK, Yeh S, et al: Clinical fetal monitoring VII. The evaluation and significance of intrapartum baseline FHR variability. *Am J Obstet Gynecol* 123:206, 1975.

46. Tejani N, Mann LI, Bhakthavathsalam A, et al: Correlation of fetal heart rate—uterine contraction patterns with fetal scalp blood pH. *Obstet Gynecol* 46:392, 1975.

47. Thomas G: The aetiology characteristics and diagnostic relevance of late deceleration patterns in routine obstetric practice. *Br J Obstet Gynaecol* 82:121, 1975.

48. Webster's New World Dictionary. Second College Edition. New York, Simon and Schuster, 1980:1551.

49. Willcourt RJ, King JC, Indyk L, et al: The relationship of fetal heart patterns to the fetal transcutaneous PO$_2$. *Am J Obstet Gynecol* 140:760, 1981.

50. Willcourt RJ, King JC, Queenan JT: Maternal oxygenation administration and the fetal transcutaneous PO$_2$. *Am J Obstet Gynecol* 146:714, 1983.

51. Young BK, Katz M, Klein SA: The relationship of heart rate patterns and tissue pH in the human fetus. *Am J Obstet Gynecol* 134:685, 1979.

Variable Decelerations

Variable Decelerations with a Trigeminal Rhythm

Variable Decelerations with Cardiac Asystole: Transient

Variable Decelerations with Cardiac Asystole: Prolonged

Variable Decelerations with Overlap Phenomenon

Agonal Variable Decelerations

Variable Decelerations with Premature Gestation

Masked Variable Decelerations

Progression from Mild to Severe Variable Decelerations

Variable Deceleration at Fetal Expulsion

Severe Variable Decelerations with Atypia and Baseline Tachycardia: Mixed Pattern

Severe Variable Decelerations with Atypia and Decreased Baseline Variability: Mixed Pattern

Severe Variable Decelerations with Atypia and No Baseline Variability and Tachycardia: Mixed Pattern

Variable Deceleration and Late Deceleration: Combined Pattern

Variable Deceleration Produced by Hold Mode: Artifact

The "Variable," Variable Deceleration

*V*ariable decelerations are appropriately named. Each deceleration typically varies in configuration in comparison to those preceding and following it.[33,34,43] The decelerations also may vary in timing in relationship to the uterine contractions.[33,34,43] Although the classic appearance of a variable deceleration is an initial (primary) acceleration preceding a V-shaped decelerative component that is followed by a secondary acceleration, innumerable shapes are seen in labor. These are produced by a variation in the duration, degree, and nature of causative stimuli; a variety of cardiac responses to abrupt heart rate deceleration; superimposed effects of hypoxia; the basal fetal condition; and many other factors.

Although such a fetal monitoring pattern potentially provides a large quantity of information to be "read" for purposes of predicting the fetal condition, the wide variation in information makes it one of the most difficult patterns to interpret. Each case must be individually managed, correlating specific pattern information with specific clinical circumstances.

As with all fetal monitoring interpretation, the baseline variability is critical in assessment.[24]

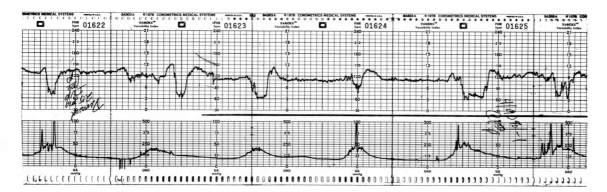

CASE INTERPRETATION: Class I-II

Baseline Information: moderate bradycardia, average variability.

Periodic or Nonperiodic Changes: variable decelerations, mild to moderate, generally exhibiting classical features, widely varying in configuration and displaying a variable relationship to contractions.

Uterine Activity: skewed contractions of moderate intensity, a high resting tone.

Significance: a healthy fetus is predicted, here demonstrating a normal response to stress, which is probably secondary to abnormal uterine activity and cord impingement. Maternal position change and other measures taken to improve umbilical perfusion may resolve or improve the pattern. The pattern is appropriately observed for the appearance of atypical features and baseline changes.

CASE OUTCOME: Thirty-year-old primigravida at 42 weeks' gestation delivered by primary cesarean section for fetal distress a 7 pound, 11 ounce (3487 gram) female; Apgar score 2/6. There was a "tight" nuchal cord. The newborn course was complicated by transient tachypnea, which was treated with oxygen delivered by mask. Thereafter, the infant followed a normal newborn course.

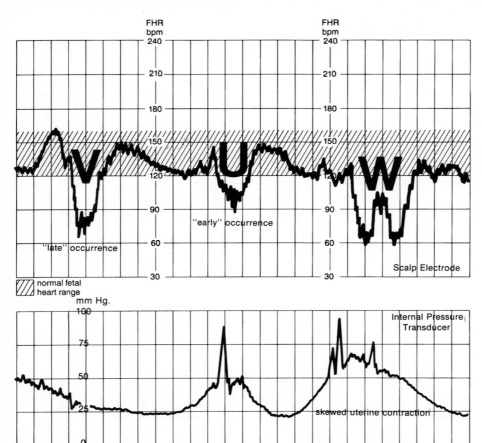

Classic Variable Decelerations, Mild

A mild variable deceleration is defined as a deceleration of less than 30 seconds in duration, irrespective of the level; or a deceleration to no less than 80 bpm, irrespective of the duration, or a deceleration to 70 to 80 bpm, with a duration of less than 60 seconds.[48] Classification of variable decelerations by depth and duration alone has been found to be insufficient in predicting fetal outcomes.[47] The other features of the configuration of the variable deceleration must also be taken into account.

Classic mild variable decelerations typically maintain a V-shaped configuration with jagged features and the presence of primary or secondary accelerations. Usually, the decelerative components are not precipitous enough or to a low enough level to produce sinus node suppres-

sion. The baseline remains stable after the deceleration. The pattern is usually caused by transient umbilical cord occlusion of such brief duration that if hypoxia occurs, it is not of sufficient duration in the basally healthy fetus to produce acidosis.[5,6,30,50,74] In the face of excellent variability, the pattern is of no greater concern than the classic normal tracing of average variability with accelerations present,[20] but the fetus may benefit from continued observation, at least intermittently, for an increase in the duration or depth of the variable decelerations and an onset of atypia with or without baseline changes.

This pattern has also been termed a "first degree" variable deceleration.[61]

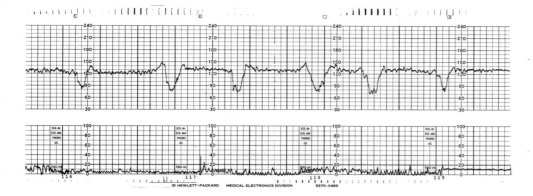

CASE INTERPRETATION: Class I

Baseline Information: normal rate and variability, stable.

Periodic or Nonperiodic Changes: mild variable decelerations ("classic" or "pure").

Uterine Activity: not recorded except for respiratory movements.

Significance: a reassuring pattern that is usually seen in late labor, often secondary to cord impingement. An appropriate intervention is a maternal position change in a term gestation in late labor. Amnioinfusion is an option in selected cases. The pattern is appropriately observed for transition to decelerations with atypia.

CASE OUTCOME: Twenty-two-year-old gravida 3, para 1011, at 39 weeks' gestation delivered by primary cesarean section, with epidural anesthesia, performed for what was believed to be possible fetal distress a 7 pound, 1½ ounce (3218 gram) male; Apgar score 9/10. The fetus was in a vertex presentation. The location of the umbilical cord was not noted at delivery. The infant followed a normal newborn course.

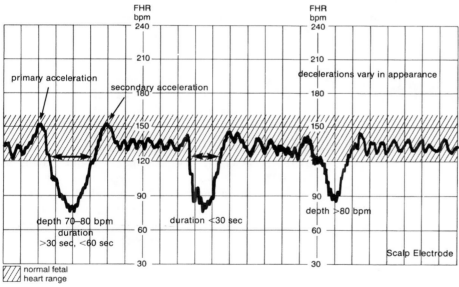

Pattern Characteristic:
Classic Variable Decelerations, Mild

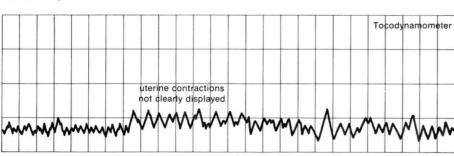

Classic Variable Decelerations, Moderate

A moderate variable deceleration is defined by a depth of less than 70 bpm at greater than 30 but less than 60 seconds duration or by a depth of 70 to 80 bpm with a duration of greater than 60 seconds.[48] In its classic form, the trace maintains a jagged stroke. There is a trend away from a V-shape toward an open-sided square, and primary and secondary accelerations are present.[10] Although the precise role of fetal baroreceptor responsiveness has been questioned, the most accepted basis for these accelerations is a baroreceptor response to the hypotension that is produced by a transient vein-only phase of umbilical cord compression.[11,82] The decelerative component of the variable deceleration pattern reflects a baroreceptor response to hypertension that is produced by total cord occlusion.[10,15,37,49] When decelerations extend beyond 15 seconds, hypoxia-induced chemoreceptor heart rate changes are also believed to be operative.[5,6,50,57]

Although usually produced by vagal effects of cord compression, which produces at least a 50% reduction in umbilical flow, an abnormal cord position may not be noted at delivery.[28,31,58,73] On the other hand, when an abnormal location of the umbilical cord is noted at delivery, almost 90% of intrapartum tracings demonstrate variable decelerations.[73] The pattern is also increased when the fetus is in an occiput posterior position, which is believed to be secondary to vagal reflex responses to pressure on the fetal face or head.[35] Variable decelerations with classic features have a higher correlation with abnormal cord position than those with a decelerative component only.[23]

In the presence of good variability and a stable baseline, the pattern may be managed expectantly in an uncomplicated term pregnancy, while attention is given to measures to improve umbilical cord perfusion that are appropriate to the clinical situation.

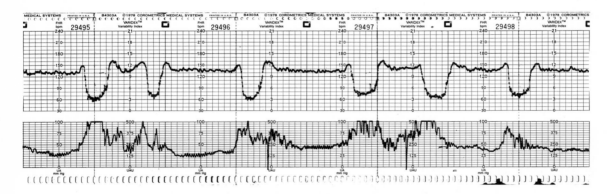

CASE INTERPRETATION: Class II

Baseline Information: normal rate and average variability.

Periodic or Nonperiodic Changes: moderate variable decelerations with classic features.

Uterine Activity: prolonged polysystolic or paired contractions with maternal straining, suggesting late labor.

Significance: a stress pattern. Measures taken to improve the umbilical flow such as maternal position change and amnioinfusion may improve the pattern.

CASE OUTCOME: Twenty-three-year-old gravida 3, para 2002, at 37 weeks' gestation precipitously delivered vaginally with no anesthesia, a 5 pound, 7 ounce (2466 gram) male; Apgar score 8/9. The fetus was in a vertex presentation. No abnormal cord position was detected. The infant followed an uncomplicated newborn course.

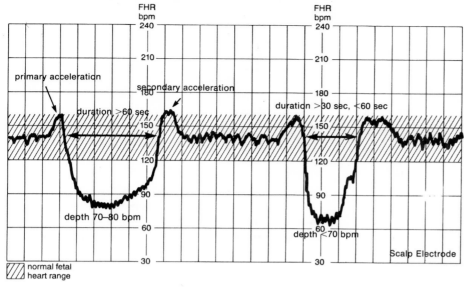

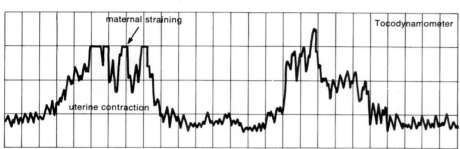

Pattern Characteristic:
Classic Variable Decelerations,
Moderate

Classic Variable Decelerations, Severe: Duration

*V*ariable decelerations are termed severe if they last longer than 60 seconds with a nadir of less than 70 bpm.[48] The classic severe variable deceleration still displays a primary and secondary acceleration and a jagged waveform. In the absence of atypia, the pattern in its classic form usually denotes umbilical cord impingement, and is of no greater concern than milder degrees of classic variable decelerations.[23,47] Hence, the term "severe" selected in this text because of its long-standing usage, is an unfortunate one in that it implies more jeopardy than

is appropriate in most cases. However, although in its classic form it does not denote a severely distressed fetus, it does represent a pattern in which the fetus is called upon to exercise compensatory measures for homeostasis and, therefore, warrants therapeutic measures to relieve stress as reducing uterine activity, changing the maternal position to achieve optimum uterine flow, and taking measures to improve fetal oxygenation. Amnioinfusion may relieve cord impingement in selected cases.[56]

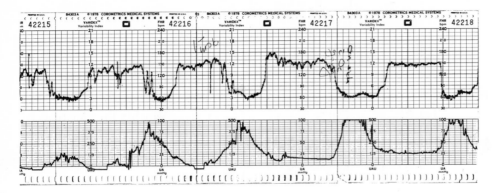

CASE INTERPRETATION: Class II

Baseline Information: normal rate with a loss of stability between some contractions, good variability.

Periodic or Nonperiodic Changes: severe variable decelerations with classic features, several lasting greater than one minute, a depth of 60 or greater.

Uterine Activity: peaked contractions (as sometimes seen in patients with preeclampsia). Maternal straining effects are superimposed.

Significance: a good baseline variability and sharp or jagged features of the variable decelerations are reassuring if delivery is imminent. Measures are taken in order to improve umbilical flow. This pattern is appropriately observed for further baseline instability and/or tachycardia and progressive atypical features, particularly a smoothing of the pattern.

CASE OUTCOME: Twenty-two-year-old gravida 4, para 3003, at 43 weeks' gestation delivered vaginally, with pudendal anesthesia, a 5 pound, 7 ounce (2466 gram) female; Apgar score 8/9. The fetus was in a vertex presentation, in an occiput anterior position. There was a double nuchal cord. The newborn course included ligation of an extra digit. The mother did not have preeclampsia.

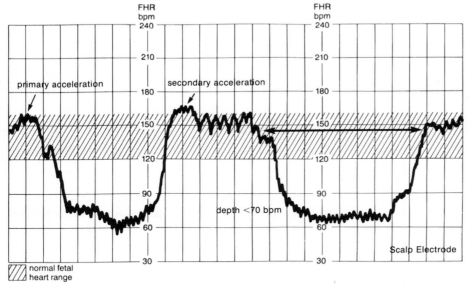

Pattern Characteristic:
Classic Variable Decelerations, Severe: Duration > 60 Seconds

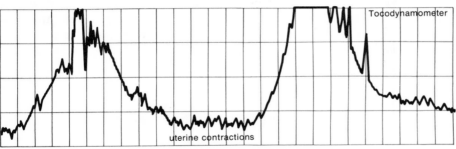

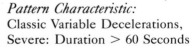

Classic Variable Decelerations, Severe: Depth

*V*ariable decelerations are classified as severe when the depth is less than 70 bpm, with a duration of greater than one minute. It is also popular to use a depth below 60 bpm according to Goodlin's "rule of 60s": (a duration of greater than 60 seconds, a depth of less than 60 bpm or falling more than 60 beats from the baseline level).[63]

The absolute depth to which a severe variable deceleration falls is important because with low nadirs cardiac arrhythmias are common, and perfusion may be reduced to critical levels. Severe variable decelerations that maintain classic features with a normal stable baseline rate with good variability are of less concern than those with atypical features or baseline changes.[20,47] In many cases, measures to improve umbilical cord perfusion such as maternal position change and amnioinfusion are appropriate considerations, as is reduction of uterine activity.[55]

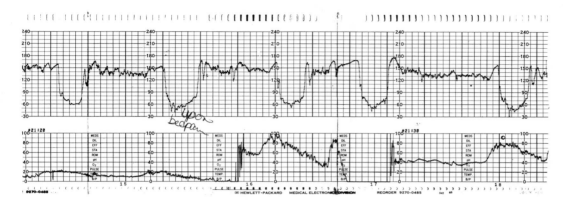

CASE INTERPRETATION: Class II

Baseline Information: normal rate, average variability. There is a slight downward shift in baseline.

Periodic or Nonperiodic Changes: moderate and severe variable decelerations with classic features.

Uterine Activity: skewed contractions without a resting phase, as measured by external monitoring; an area of no recording.

Significance: good variability and classic features of decelerations are reassuring, although, transient respiratory acidosis of the newborn may be noted. Intervention decisions are influenced by gestation, estimated duration until vaginal delivery, anticipated ease of delivery, and any subsequent change in the pattern. There is a high likelihood of cord impingement. Measures taken to improve umbilical flow are in order.

CASE OUTCOME: Twenty-three-year-old gravida 2, para 1001, at 35 weeks' gestation delivered vaginally, with pudendal anesthesia, a 5 pound, 4 ounce (2381 gram) male; Apgar score 9/9. The fetus was in a vertex presentation. The mother received oxytocin augmentation for premature ruptured membranes at term. A double nuchal cord was noted at delivery. The infant followed an uncomplicated newborn course.

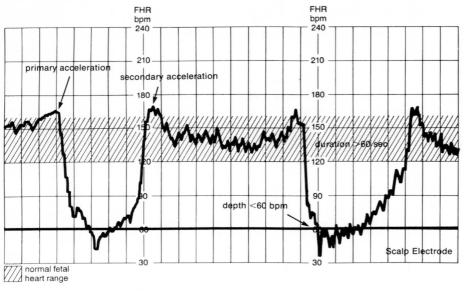

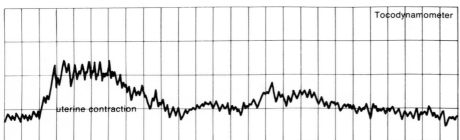

Pattern Characteristic:
Classic Variable Decelerations,
Severe: Depth < 60–70 BPM

Classic Variable Decelerations, Severe: Range

*T*he skilled interpreter of fetal monitoring tracings soon abandons specific numerical criteria for grading variable decelerations and turns his or her attention to the composite pattern made up of the basic shape, the presence or absence of atypical features, and the relationship to baseline findings.

Using the absolute depth at nadir of a variable deceleration to assess severity has some limitations because the baseline from which it falls may vary greatly, influencing the significance of the variable deceleration. For example, a variable deceleration at a depth of 50 bpm is of greater concern if it falls from a baseline of 180 bpm than from a baseline of 100 bpm. Therefore, the range of the deceleration has also been added to the distinguishing features of severe variable decelerations. A drop of greater than 60 bpm from the baseline is part of Goodlin's rule of 60s (a greater than 60 second duration, a depth of less than 60 bpm, or a drop of 60 bpm).[63] A deceleration of greater than one minute duration may not fall below 60 bpm but still qualifies as severe if there is a greater than 60 bpm drop from a high baseline.

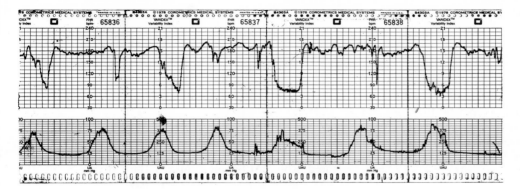

CASE INTERPRETATION: Class II

Baseline Information: moderate tachycardia, normal variability.

Periodic or Nonperiodic Changes: "variable," variable decelerations: varying in configuration and relationship to contractions, two are severe in range and duration but maintain classical features.

Uterine Activity: frequent contractions, most are normal configurations, some are skewed. Elevated resting tone, as measured by an internal pressure transducer.

Significance: classical features are reassuring, but the association of these severe variable decelerations with baseline tachycardia is less reassuring. There is probable cord impingement. Measures to improve umbilical perfusion and oxygenation are in order. A vigorous fetus is predicted if delivery is imminent. Subsequent management is influenced by the predicted ability of the fetus to tolerate stress and by its response to intervention measures.

CASE OUTCOME: Twenty-eight-year-old gravida 3, para 2002, at 40 weeks' gestation delivered vaginally, with pudendal anesthesia, a 6 pound, 5 ounce (2863 gram) male; Apgar score 8/9. The fetus was in a vertex presentation, with a nuchal cord. The infant followed a normal newborn course.

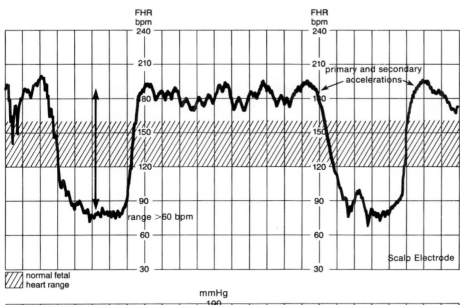

Pattern Characteristic:
Classic Variable Decelerations,
Severe: Range > 60 BPM

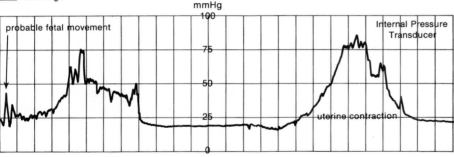

Atypical Variable Decelerations: Loss of Primary Acceleration

*W*hen variable decelerations retain the classic features that were presented on the preceding pages and are accompanied by normal and stable baseline findings, the fetus is demonstrating a successful ability to compensate for pressure changes with or without hypoxia, whether they are induced by cord impingement or other causes of abrupt vagal discharge.[2] The risk of fetal compromise is small.

Aberrations from the classic configuration of variable decelerations have been identified that are associated with an increased incidence of poor perinatal outcome.[14]

Seven features, producing "atypical variable" decelerations by Krebs and coworkers, have been associated with an increased risk of a low Apgar score and acidosis.[45,47] They may be present in mild, moderate, and severe variable decelerations. The seven typical features are:

1. loss of initial (primary) acceleration
2. slow return to the baseline fetal heart rate
3. loss of secondary acceleration
4. prolonged secondary acceleration
5. biphasic deceleration
6. loss of variability during deceleration
7. continuation of the baseline at a lower level

Loss of primary acceleration is the most frequently encountered atypical feature, occurring in over two-thirds of variable decelerations in the last 30 minutes of monitored labor. Although almost a third of the newborns with this fetal heart rate pattern have an Apgar score of less than 7 at one minute, less than 7% have an Apgar score of less than 7 at five minutes.[47]

Loss of the primary acceleration may reflect an abrupt total cord occlusion without a vein-only compression phase.[23,38] This pattern, especially when co-existing with the loss of a secondary acceleration, may cause a variable deceleration to be similar in appearance to an early deceleration, producing a diagnostic challenge (see page 207).

Loss of primary and secondary accelerations have been reported with the deep variable decelerations that are associated with an occiput posterior position. In such a case, the deceleration is believed to be caused by a vagal stimulus other than cord compression, for example, eyeball or tracheal pressure, so that there is no partial cord compression phase to elicit accelerations.

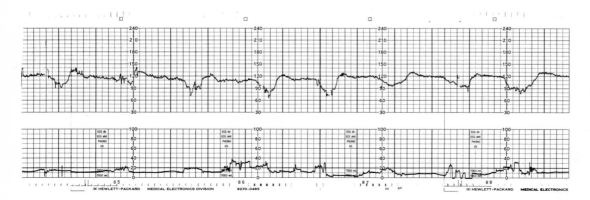

CASE INTERPRETATION: Class IV

Baseline Information: low normal heart rate to moderate bradycardia, fair variability.

Periodic or Nonperiodic Changes: mild variable decelerations with an atypical feature of the loss of primary acceleration, also occasional prolongation of secondary acceleration and the smoothing of the variability within the deceleration.

Uterine Activity: frequent, small contractions, poorly recorded. Maternal straining appears to be present.

Significance: there is a slightly increased risk of a low Apgar score and acidosis. Maternal repositioning may de-crease the cord impingement. Management is influenced by the duration to and anticipated ease of delivery. There is increased concern in the case of a premature gestation. If the fetus is not delivered, it is appropriate to observe the tracing for further baseline changes and atypical features. A fetal pH or fetal stimulation test may be of help in this case because of diminished baseline variability.

CASE OUTCOME: Thirty-eight-year-old gravida 3, para 2002, delivered vaginally, with local and pudendal anesthesia, a 5 pound, 10¾ ounce (2572 gram) male; Apgar score 6/9. Meconium was present. A nuchal cord was identified. The fetus was in a vertex presentation, in a left occiput anterior position. There was DeLee suction- ing at the perineum and visualization of the cord after delivery. The infant followed an uncomplicated newborn course.

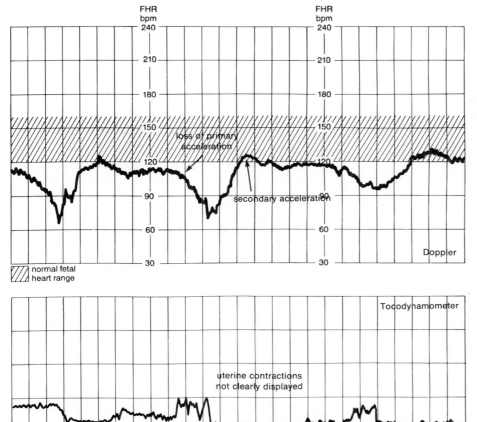

Pattern Characteristic:
Atypical Variable Decelerations:
Loss of Primary Acceleration

Atypical Variable Decelerations: Loss of Secondary Acceleration

*L*oss of secondary acceleration is one of the atypical features of variable decelerations, denoting an increased risk of a low Apgar score or fetal acidosis.[47] This is the third most common of the seven atypical changes. It is of slightly more concern than loss of primary acceleration, predicting a 39% risk of a low Apgar score at one minute and a 14% risk of a low Apgar score (less than 7) at five minutes.

The pattern may reflect an abrupt release of total cord compression, without a gradual vein-only compression phase. The slightly increased association with a depressed fetus may reflect an overlap of this pattern with a slow return to baseline, a pattern recognized as reflecting persistent fetal hypoxia beyond the duration of the contraction.

When decelerations are profound, loss of both primary and secondary accelerations have been associated with an occiput posterior position, the decelerative vagal stimulus believed to be other than cord-compression induced.[35]

When decelerations are shallow and both the primary and secondary acceleration are missing, the pattern may be easily confused with early decelerations (see page 207).

Intrapartum management in a situation in which a fetus exhibits a loss of secondary acceleration, as with other atypical variable decelerations, is influenced by the presence of co-existing atypical features or baseline changes, the individual clinical setting, and the response exhibited by the fetus to measures taken to improve the fetal umbilical cord perfusion and fetal oxygenation.

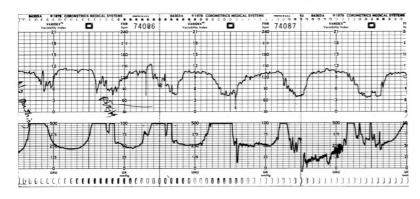

CASE INTERPRETATION: Class IV

Baseline Information: normal rate, reduced short-term variability.

Periodic or Nonperiodic Changes: some atypical variable decelerations with a loss of primary and secondary accelerations, distinguished from uniform decelerations by a flat base and a more classic appearance elsewhere on the segment.

Uterine Activity: brief contractions without a resting period and maternal straining are present, suggesting late labor.

Significance: there is an increased risk of a low Apgar score, but management is dictated by the clinical situation such as the estimated duration to delivery, gestation, and response to standard measures to improve the fetal environment.

CASE OUTCOME: Nineteen-year-old primigravida at 39 weeks' gestation delivered vaginally, with pudendal anesthesia, a 6 pound, 13 ounce (3090 gram) female; Apgar score 8/9. The fetus was in a vertex presentation, with a double nuchal cord. There was thin meconium present. The infant followed a normal newborn course.

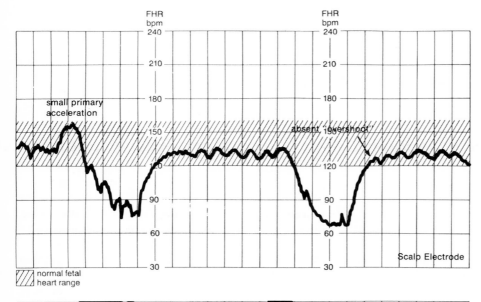

Pattern Characteristic:
Atypical Variable Decelerations:
Loss of Secondary Accelerations

Atypical Variable Decelerations: Prolonged Secondary Acceleration

A prolonged secondary acceleration, also termed "overshoot," frequently indicates an abnormal cord position and is thought to be produced by a fetal hypoxic insult that is rapidly relieved.[25] The secondary acceleration is a baroreceptor response to hypotension that transiently occurs upon release of the cord compression. In the presence of mild hypoxemia, it may become prolonged. The pattern is believed to be mediated by sympathetic stimulation, in that it is not obliterated by atropine in a research model. It may be more common in the immature organism.

Prolonged secondary acceleration, as an abnormal component of a variable deceleration, is one of the seven atypical variable decelerations associated with an increased risk of fetal hypoxia. It is the fourth most common of the seven atypical variable decelerations.[47] Thirty percent of the cases with a prolonged secondary acceleration have a one minute Apgar score less than 7, but only 10% have a five minute Apgar score less than 7.

This pattern usually reflects a mildly hypoxic fetal state for which the fetus usually readily compensates, but when it is combined with other atypical features and baseline changes such as tachycardia and decreased variability, it may indicate a fetus further along on the continuum between hypoxia and metabolic acidosis. The combined pattern of no baseline variability and variable decelerations with an overshoot has been retrospectively identified in fetal heart rate monitoring tracings of some infants with cerebral palsy, as have tracings with no aberrations whatsoever.[70]

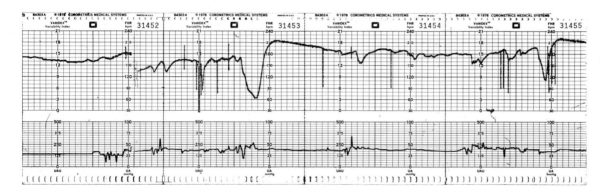

CASE INTERPRETATION: Class IV

Baseline Information: high normal heart rate to moderate tachycardia, decreased short-term variability, some instability, undulation of long-term variability.

Periodic or Nonperiodic Changes: severe variable decelerations, with sloping side limbs and the atypical features of prolonged secondary acceleration and loss of variability.

Uterine Activity: there appear to be regular uterine contractions with a minimal deflection of the tocodynamometer.

Significance: a nonreassuring pattern that is associated with an increased risk of fetal hypoxia and a low Apgar score.

CASE OUTCOME: Eighteen-year-old primigravida, at 30 weeks' gestation delivered vaginally, with pudendal anesthesia, a 1 pound, 10 ounce (737 gram) female; Apgar score 8/9. There was a premature rupture of the membranes for one week, chorioamnionitis, and a maternal fever of 100.3°F intrapartum. The cord location was not noted at the time of delivery. The newborn's problems included effects of intrauterine growth retardation and bronchopulmonary dysplasia. The newborn was dismissed at three months of life.

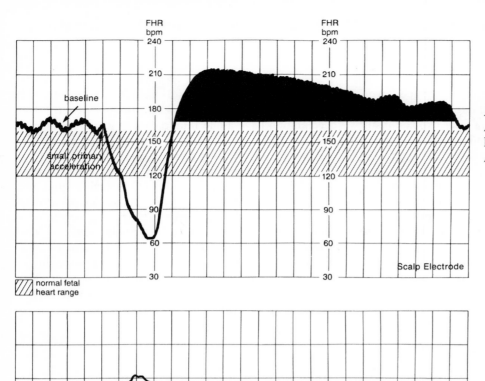

Pattern Characteristic:
Atypical Variable Decelerations:
Prolonged Secondary
Acceleration

Atypical Variable Decelerations: Slow Return

A delayed return to the baseline of the ascending (return) limb of a variable deceleration is the characteristic feature of one of the seven atypical variable decelerations, which may be used to predict a fetus with an increased risk of a low Apgar score or acidosis.[47] This pattern has also been termed variable decelerations with "hypoxic components."[9] This is to be distinguished from a combined deceleration (variable plus late deceleration), a pattern in which the late deceleration occurs after the variable deceleration has returned to baseline. In both situations, the compounding effects of cord compression and a diminished oxygen supply from the intervillous space are implied. In an earlier classification, this pattern was termed a third degree variable deceler-

ation when recovery extended 25 seconds beyond recovery of the contraction.[61] On some occasions, the delayed recovery mirrors a skewed uterine contraction. Even though in such a case, the deceleration does not extend beyond the duration of the contraction, there is still reason for concern because it may reflect a hypoxic environment for the fetus.

This pattern occurs in 60% of atypical variable decelerations and is thus second only to the loss of initial acceleration in frequency as an atypical feature.[47] It is associated with a one minute Apgar score of less than 7 in 47% of fetuses with variable decelerations in the last 30 minutes of monitored labor, but only 10% have a five minute Apgar score of less than 7.

This pattern is frequently seen in combination with atypical biphasic variable decelerations or combined late and variable decelerations.

Management may include maternal oxygen administration and efforts to relieve prolonged uterine activity as well as measures to improve umbilical perfusion. In addition to assessment of the fetal response to these measures, delivery decisions are influenced by the presence or absence of other atypical features or baseline changes and antepartum and intrapartum risk factors.

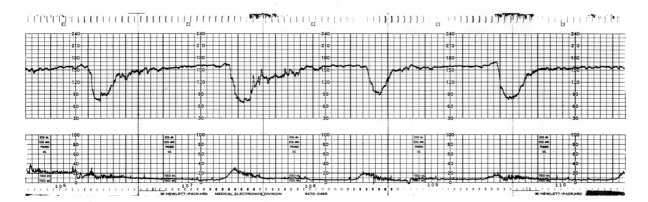

CASE INTERPRETATION: Class IV

Baseline Information: high normal rate. Fair variability when the baseline is re-established after decelerations.

Periodic or Nonperiodic Changes: moderate variable decelerations with atypical features of a slow return to baseline, accompanied by a loss of secondary acceleration. Variability in the variable decelerations, including the return limb, is normal.

Uterine Activity: regular contractions that appear to have a long skewed phase that corresponds somewhat to the prolonged recovery phase of the variable decelerations.

Significance: atypical variable decelerations with an increased risk of a low Apgar score. The preservation of variability allows clinical judgment to include conservative management if delivery is imminent. Measures to minimize cord compression are appropriate during the conservative management.

CASE OUTCOME: Twenty-nine-year-old gravida 3, para 1102, at 37½ weeks' gestation delivered vaginally, with epidural anesthesia and low elective forceps, a 6 pound, 1½ ounce (2764 gram) female; Apgar score 6/8. A two vessel cord was noted at delivery. The fetus was in a vertex presentation. Oxytocin augmentation was used as management for the premature rupture of membranes. The infant followed a normal newborn course.

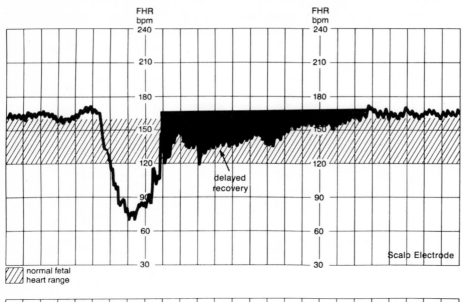

Pattern Characteristic:
Atypical Variable Decelerations:
Slow Return

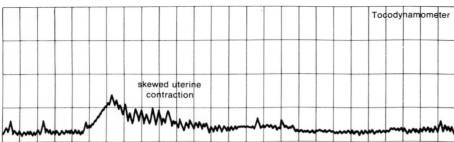

Atypical Variable Decelerations: Continuation of the Baseline at a Lower Level

*T*he least common atypical variable deceleration is characterized by the continuation of the baseline at a lower level after the deceleration recovery.[47] This pattern probably overlaps with the atypical feature of a slow return to the baseline. The next deceleration may occur before there is time for full recovery to the original baseline. When the pattern persists beyond 10 minutes, a new baseline is created that may progressively deepen if no improvement occurs spontaneously or with clinical intervention (see page 153).

This pattern occurs in only 7.5% of atypical variable decelerations in the last 30 minutes of monitored labor.[47]

Although 43% of the fetuses exhibiting this pattern are predicted to have a low Apgar score at one minute, only 7% have an Apgar score less than 7 at five minutes.

Clinical management is aimed at the treatment of fetal hypoxia in conjunction with measures taken to improve the umbilical blood flow.

Delivery planning is influenced by whether this is an isolated fetal monitoring pattern or whether it is seen in combination with other atypia and baseline changes as well as by the individual clinical circumstances.

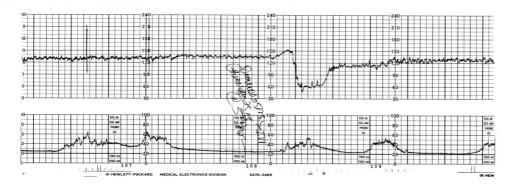

CASE INTERPRETATION: Class IV

Baseline Information: a normal baseline rate of 130 to 140 bpm followed by a baseline rate of 120 to 130 bpm following recovery from a variable deceleration. Average variability.

Periodic or Nonperiodic Changes: severe variable deceleration with atypia characterized by a delayed return to a lower baseline, accounting also for a loss of secondary acceleration.

Uterine Activity: polysystolic, skewed irregular contractions.

Significance: an increased risk of a low Apgar score at delivery. Normal variability and a lack of recurrence war-

rants initial conservative management, including changing maternal position and maternal oxygen administration. Whether or not, in this patient, there is an association of the pattern with bolus narcotic administration is unclear.

CASE OUTCOME: Twenty-six-year-old gravida 3, para 2002, at 40 weeks' gestation delivered vaginally, with local anesthesia, a 6 pound (2722 gram) male; Apgar score 9/9. The fetus was in a vertex presentation. Thin meconium was present. The infant followed an uncomplicated newborn course.

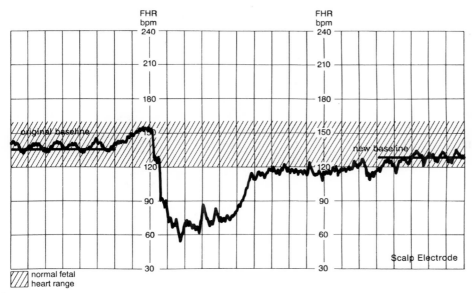

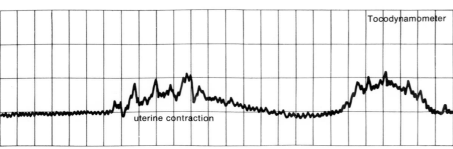

Pattern Characteristic:
Atypical Variable Decelerations:
Continuation of Baseline at
Lower Level

Atypical Variable Decelerations: Loss of Variability

*L*oss of variability in the variable deceleration is the most ominous of the seven atypical features predicting an increased risk of a low Apgar score or fetal acidosis.[47]

It is important to recognize that loss of variability in this case does not refer to baseline variability, which may or may not be preserved, but to variability within the deceleration itself. The presence of variability in both the baseline and deceleration is most reassuring. A diminished variability in the variable deceleration with preservation of good baseline variability is of intermediate concern, and loss of both the baseline and deceleration variability is most ominous. When a loss of variabil-

ity smooths the deceleration itself, 67% of fetuses are predicted to have a low one minute Apgar score and 22% still have a low Apgar score at five minutes.

Such a pattern has also been termed "second degree variable deceleration."[61]

Management is influenced by the particular clinical setting, including gestation, fetal growth, the presence or absence of meconium, anticipated duration to delivery, and the anticipated ease of delivery. Whether an expectant course or one of intervention is chosen, measures to improve fetal oxygenation and umbilical flow are appropriate.

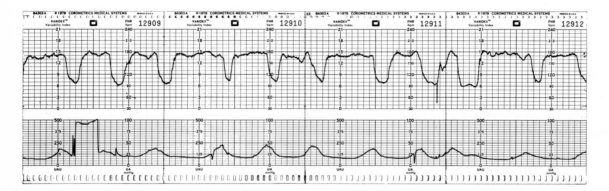

CASE INTERPRETATION: Class IV

Baseline Information: moderate tachycardia, fair variability.

Periodic or Nonperiodic Changes: mild and moderate variable decelerations with atypia characterized by loss of variability within the deceleration. Decelerations are late in occurrence and vary in configuration.

Uterine Activity: small, normally shaped frequent contractions, as measured by external monitoring.

Significance: the combination of a loss of variability within the variable deceleration, baseline tachycardia, and reduced variability predicts an increased risk of a low Apgar score. Cord impingement is a likely factor. A change in the maternal position is thus appropriate. Delivery timing is influenced by gestation, the estimated time to vaginal delivery, predicted ease of vaginal delivery, as well as other clinical features.

CASE OUTCOME: Seventeen-year-old primigravida at 34 weeks' gestation delivered vaginally, with no anesthesia, following the premature rupture of membranes for 30 hours, a 4 pound, 13 ounce (2183 gram) female; Apgar score 1/5. The maternal temperature was 101.8°F during labor, secondary to chorioamnionitis. There was a double nuchal cord. The newborn course was complicated by hyaline membrane disease and sepsis. The infant was dismissed at 14 days of life.

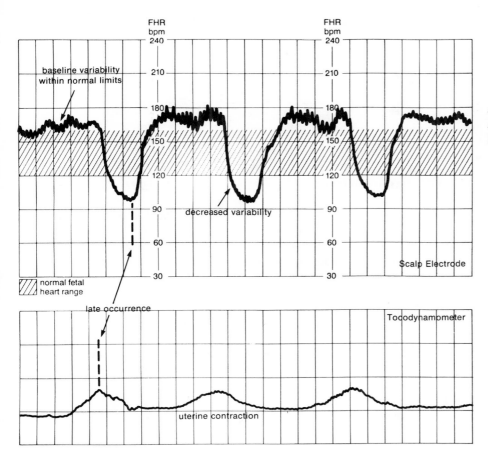

Pattern Characteristic:
Atypical Variable Decelerations:
Loss of Variability

Atypical Variable Decelerations: Biphasic

*B*iphasic variable decelerations have been the subject of much interest and controversy as clinical experience and research in fetal monitoring have evolved.

As one of the seven atypical variable decelerations presented by Krebs, et al, this pattern predicts an increased risk of a low Apgar score and fetal acidosis.[47] This is the fifth most frequently occurring atypical feature. It predicts a 48% incidence of a low one minute Apgar score and a 12% persistence of a low Apgar score at five minutes.

The pattern is identified when, after an initial deceleration, the fetal heart rate begins to return to the baseline but a second decelerative component occurs before the baseline is reached. The second portion of the deceleration represents a late (hypoxic) component, but the overall configuration remains that of a variable deceleration, as distinct from a combined variable and late pattern (see p 225 & 291) or a slow return to baseline without two separate components (see p 246).[44] The resulting pattern is depicted as a W-shape.[43]

There are multiple possible causes for two components of a variable deceleration, hence the confusion concerning the significance of the pattern. These causes include: (1) Impingement of the umbilical cord by brief successive fetal movements that produce short periodic spikes.[44] (2) Impingement of the umbilical cord at more than one location at different times during the uterine contraction. This is supported by an increased association with long umbilical cords.[75] (3) Impingement of the cord intermittently during the contraction during bursts of increased intrauterine pressure that is produced by maternal straining (see page 253).[44] (4) Impingement and release of the cord, followed by reimpingement that is produced by polysystolic uterine contractions. (5) Impingement of the cord that is associated with hypoxia, thus producing a variable deceleration followed by a late decelerative component before recovery to the baseline (see page 252).[44]

The latter cause is the etiology for which the category of atypical variable deceleration is reserved. It is distinguished by the late occurrence of the second component. Because of the increased risk of a low Apgar score and fetal acidosis when associated with no baseline variability, it has been flagged by the term "W-sign" (see pages 254 and 256).[75] In the past, such a pattern has also been termed a "fourth degree variable deceleration."[61]

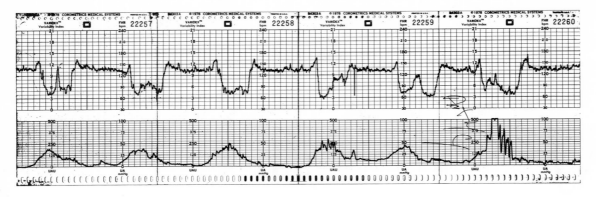

CASE INTERPRETATION: Class IV

Baseline Information: normal rate and variability.

Periodic or Nonperiodic Changes: moderate and severe variable decelerations with classical features, except for occasional biphasic atypia that produces a W-shape. On occasion, the second component of the W appears late in relation to the contraction.

Uterine Activity: normal, skewed and polysystolic contractions, as measured by external monitoring, frequently with a brief resting phase.

Significance: the maintenance of baseline variability and variability within the deceleration is reassuring de-

spite the biphasic pattern. There is probable umbilical cord impingement. It is appropriate to observe the pattern for baseline changes or further atypia. Measures taken to improve umbilical flow are also appropriate.

CASE OUTCOME: Twenty-three-year-old gravida 3, para 2002, at 39 weeks' gestation delivered vaginally, with no anesthesia, a 6 pound, 3 ounce (2807 gram) male; Apgar score 6/8. The fetus was in an occiput posterior position. There was a double nuchal cord. The infant followed a normal newborn course.

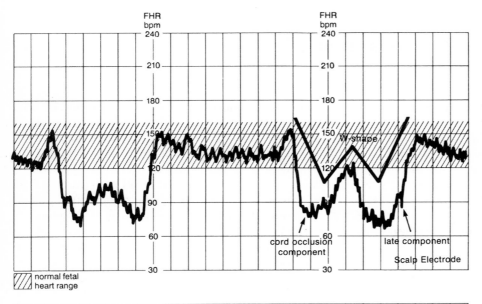

Pattern Characteristic:
Atypical Variable Decelerations:
Biphasic

Variable Decelerations: W-Shaped Associated with Maternal Straining

*N*ot all W-shaped or biphasic variable decelerations are atypical variable decelerations.

The multiple causes of two decelerative components range from the baroreceptor effects of transient episodes of successive impingement of the umbilical cord to hypoxia-induced fetal heart rate changes.[44,54] These are discussed on page 251.

One cause of multiple episodes of impingement occurs when there are intermittent bursts of maternal straining, as in the second stage of labor.[44] The contraction alone does not generate sufficient intrauterine pressure to occlude the umbilical cord but superimposed maternal straining does.

The abrupt cord occlusion produces a baroreceptor-mediated deceleration with a partial recovery between straining episodes. It is apparent that a first step in ameliorating this pattern may be directed at coaching the patient in modified pushing techniques such as with an open glottis.

The W-shaped pattern that is produced by brief increases and decreases in intrauterine pressure is distinguished from the biphasic atypical variable deceleration, because in the former case both decelerative components are within the confines of the uterine contraction. In the latter case there is clearly a late-*occurring* component.[44]

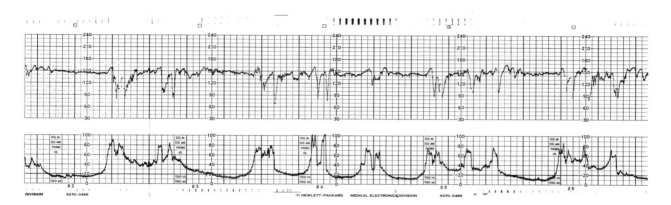

CASE INTERPRETATION: Class I

Baseline Information: normal rate and variability, a stable baseline.

Periodic or Nonperiodic Changes: brief, biphasic variable decelerations with a jagged waveform.

Uterine Activity: maternal straining efforts appear to be associated with the biphasic components of the variable decelerations.

Significance: a biphasic configuration, W-shaped variable decelerations but without atypia. The prognosis is excellent, similar to that for single V-shaped variable decelerations when they are associated with good baseline variability and no smoothing of features and no late component.

CASE OUTCOME: Twenty-five-year-old primigravida at 40 weeks' gestation delivered vaginally, with local anesthesia, a 7 pound, 6 ounce (3345 gram) female; Apgar score 9/9. The fetus was in a vertex presentation. The location of the cord was not noted at delivery. The infant followed an uncomplicated newborn course.

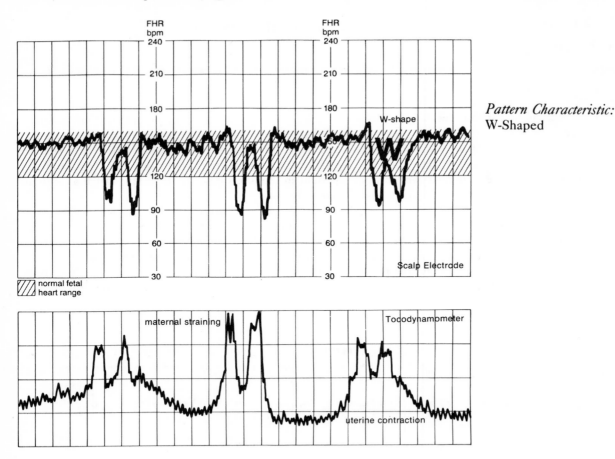

Pattern Characteristic:
W-Shaped

Variable Decelerations: W-Sign Evolution

The W-sign describes graphically the biphasic atypical variable deceleration when associated with no baseline variability. The deceleration is W-shaped, that is, there are two decelerative components, the second occurring before the recovery to the baseline of the first, with an overall configuration of a variable deceleration. The distinguishing feature of the W-sign from other W-shaped decelerations is that it is produced by a late hypoxic component following a cord impingement component.[44] The W-sign is distinguished from a combined variable and late deceleration in that, in the latter case, the baseline is recovered between decelerative components. It is also distinguished from a slow return to baseline, where the hypoxic delay in recovery appears as an extension of the return limb of the cord impingement deceleration rather than as a second decelerative component.

All three have a similar connotation: fetal hypoxia produced by a compromised umbilical cord perfusion co-existing with a form of placental insufficiency.[19] Various combinations of the three patterns may be seen in evolution of the W-sign.

Because of its most ominous connotation, the term "W-sign" in this text is reserved for the biphasic deceleration that is accompanied by a loss of baseline variability and a loss of variability in the deceleration.

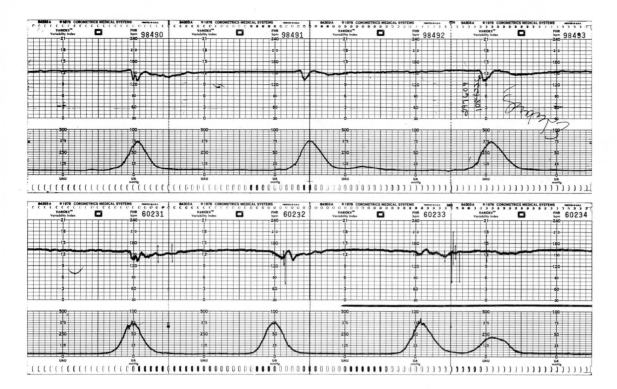

CASE INTERPRETATION: Class IV/V

Baseline Information: upper limits of normal rate, absent (flat-line) long- and short-term variability.

Periodic or Nonperiodic Changes: combined decelerations, mild atypical variable decelerations and late decelerations with prolonged recovery. Occasional W-sign.

Uterine Activity: contractions of normal configuration, occasional pairing.

Significance: an increased incidence of low Apgar scores and acidosis. In most clinical circumstances, delivery is appropriately expedited while improving the fetal milieu.

CASE OUTCOME: Thirty-six-year-old gravida 3, para 1011, who had little prenatal care delivered by cesarean section, with general anesthesia, performed for cephalopelvic disproportion a 9 pound, 12 ounce (4423 gram) female; Apgar score 2/8. The fetus was in a vertex presentation. The newborn course was complicated by a group B streptococcal infection, which responded to antibiotic therapy.

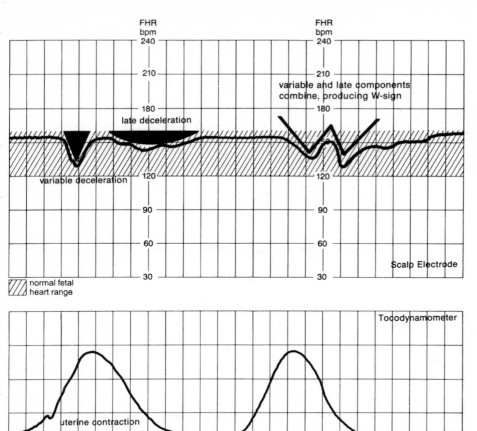

Pattern Characteristic:
Variable Decelerations:
Evolution of W-Sign

Variable Decelerations: W-Sign

*T*he unique biphasic atypical variable deceleration which is termed the "W-sign," predicts a potentially moribund fetus.[37,61] This is not the case for all W-shaped variable decelerations. The term W-sign is appropriately reserved for W-shaped decelerations that are composed of two distinct components: a primary cord-impingement deceleration followed by a secondary hypoxic late-occurring deceleration, without full recovery between them and with both baseline and deceleration variability diminished.

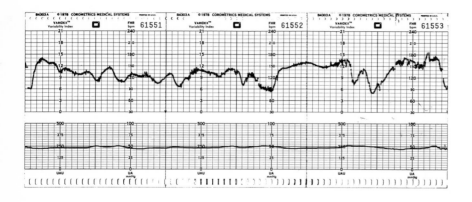

CASE INTERPRETATION: Class V

Baseline Information: an unstable baseline, ranging from low normal to high normal; decreased variability, even with external monitoring.

Periodic or Nonperiodic Changes: a biphasic deceleration of the W-shape, which is variable in appearance. W-sign.

Uterine Activity: contractions are poorly recorded, if at all. If the minimal deflections of the tocodynamometer represent contractions, they appear to be prolonged. Some suggest that this is due to pairing or polysystole.

Significance: the W-sign is associated with a significant increased risk of a decreased Apgar score and fetal acidosis.

CASE OUTCOME: Twenty-eight-year-old gravida 4, para 3003, at 25 weeks' gestation delivered vaginally a 1 pound, 9 ounce (737 gram) male stillborn. The fetus was in a breech presentation. The pregnancy was complicated by chorioamnionitis. The decision was made not to do a cesarean section in the case of possible fetal distress because of the very preterm gestation. Intrauterine fetal death occurred two hours after this segment was made.

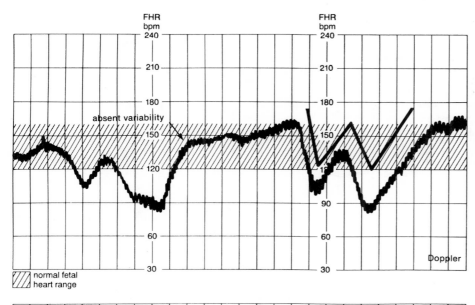

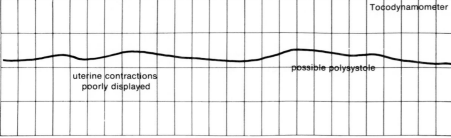

Pattern Characteristic:
Variable Decelerations: W-Sign

Variable Decelerations: Multiphasic

If variable decelerations with two decelerative components are termed "biphasic," then three decelerative components are appropriately called "triphasic," and more than three decelerative components may be termed "multiphasic."

A multiphasic deceleration may or may not maintain a jagged waveform.

It is frequently associated with maternal straining efforts, suggesting that one etiology is a sudden intermittent increase and decrease in intrauterine pressure.

At times, the pattern cannot be distinguished from increased variability that occurs as a mixed pattern with variable decelerations (see page 76). The distinction is probably not crucial, since both represent the stress of a responsive fetus when it is in the presence of good baseline variability.

When it is observed that the pattern is developing a smoothing of the waveform (a change from an oscillating to an undulating appearance), there should be an increased concern about the possibility of hypoxia or acidosis.

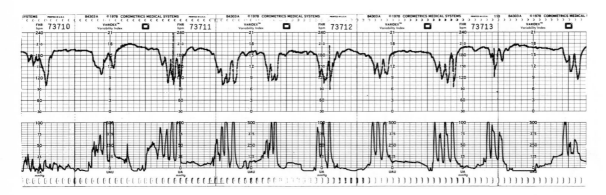

CASE INTERPRETATION: Class II

Baseline Information: tachycardia, fair beat-to-beat variability.

Periodic or Nonperiodic Changes: variable decelerations with jagged waveform, multiphasic.

Uterine Activity: multiple maternal straining efforts appear to be associated with the multiple decelerative components of the variable decelerations.

Significance: sharp waveforms are reassuring but the presence of baseline tachycardia and diminished variability raises concern that must be correlated with the clinical situation so as to design appropriate management. Factors to be considered include gestation, the estimated duration to delivery, the response to basic resuscitative measures, and antenatal risk factors.

CASE OUTCOME: Nineteen-year-old primigravida at 40 weeks' gestation delivered vaginally, with outlet forceps and pudendal anesthesia, a 9 pound, 2 ounce (4139 gram) female; Apgar score 8/9. The fetus was in an occiput anterior position. The delivery was complicated by shoulder dystocia. No abnormal cord position was noted at delivery. The infant followed an uncomplicated newborn course.

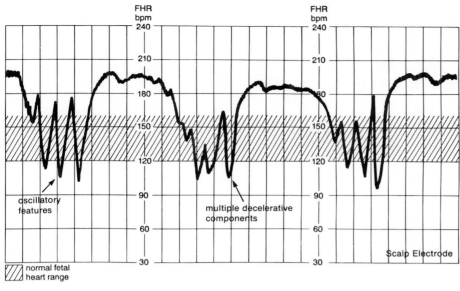

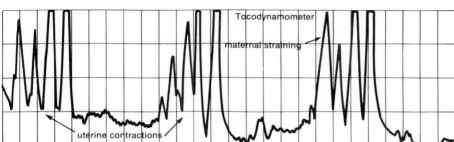

Pattern Characteristic:
Variable Decelerations:
Multiphasic

Variable Decelerations: V-Shaped

*E*arly classifications of variable decelerations have included describing the decelerations by using letters of the alphabet, for example, V, U, and W, to correspond with the configuration.[43] The V-shape implies maintenance of a jagged waveform, hence a good prognosis; the U implies some smoothing of the deceleration and a more prolonged and, therefore, potentially more ominous pattern; and W implies a possible late component, also potentially of increased concern. Although an adjunct in teaching, this classification system has not proven to be sufficient in understanding the varieties of variable decelerations and their significance.

V-shaped decelerations are abrupt brief decelerations, sharp in configuration. Such patterns, also termed "first degree variable decelerations," are defined as precipitous in onset and recovery, short in duration, and with a jagged waveform.[61] The etiology is usually a brief cord compression.

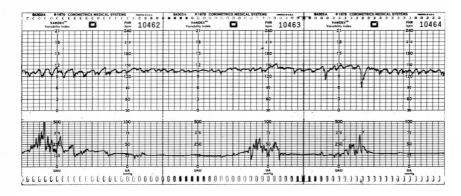

CASE INTERPRETATION: Class I

Baseline Information: normal rate and variability.

Periodic or Nonperiodic Changes: sporadic, small V-shaped variable decelerations. One appears to be associated with uterine contractions and the other with tocodynamometer deflection, suggesting fetal activity.

Uterine Activity: irregular contractions, as suggested by tocodynamometer and other deflections, possibly produced by fetal activity.

Significance: a reassuring pattern. Possible umbilical cord impingement.

CASE OUTCOME: Twenty-two-year-old gravida 2, para 1001, at 42 weeks' gestation delivered vaginally, with local anesthesia, a 7 pound, 3 ounce (3260 gram) male; Apgar score 9/9. A nuchal cord was noted. Variable decelerations progressed to moderate decelerations, retaining classic features. The infant followed a normal newborn course.

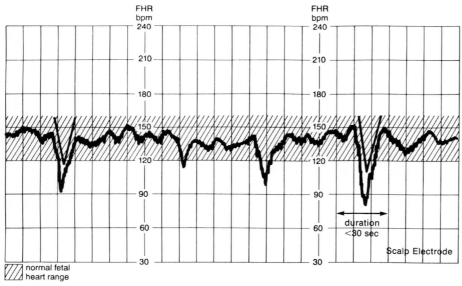

Pattern Characteristic:
Variable Decelerations:
V-Shaped

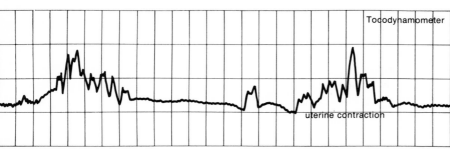

Variable Decelerations: V-Shaped, Associated with Fetal Movement

*T*he presence of brief variable decelerations during nonstress testing, occurring with episodes of fetal movement, has been associated with an increased incidence of variable decelerations with or without cord complications in labor.[39,62] When the decelerations are brief and retain classic and jagged features, the pattern is not associated with immediate fetal jeopardy.[53]

When the decelerations seen on antepartum fetal monitoring studies are brief and V-shaped with a jagged configuration, no response other than reassessment intrapartum is needed. When they are prolonged or appear with the presence of atypia, contraction stress testing or ultrasonography for the amount of amniotic fluid and cord position are of potential benefit.[67]

The fetal movement-triggered V-shaped deceleration is expected to appear with increased frequency in situations of cord vulnerability such as after ruptured membranes.[16] For further discussion of V-shaped variable decelerations as detected in antepartum monitoring, see page 298.

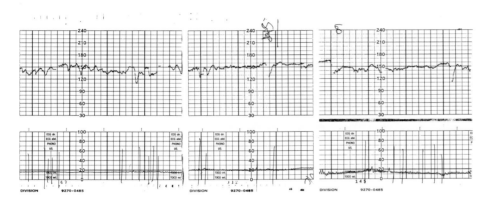

CASE INTERPRETATION: Class I

Baseline Information: three segments on different dates all with normal heart rate and variability, as measured by external monitoring.

Periodic or Nonperiodic Changes: one or more small, V-shaped decelerations on each segment. Small accelerations on two of the three segments.

Uterine Activity: none noted, fetal activity is noted by lines drawn by hand at the time of occurrence.

Significance: the fetus is not in immediate jeopardy, but there may be a vulnerable cord with an increased risk of cord compression patterns in labor.

CASE OUTCOME: Twenty-four-year-old gravida 2, para 1001, at 38½ weeks' gestation delivered vaginally, with pudendal anesthesia, a 6 pound, 7 ounce (2920 gram) female; Apgar score 8/9. Oxytocin augmentation was administered for secondary arrest of dilatation. The fetus was in a vertex presentation, in an occiput anterior position. The cord was around a shoulder at delivery. The newborn course was marked by detection of a cyst in the liver. The newborn was dismissed at 10 days of life.

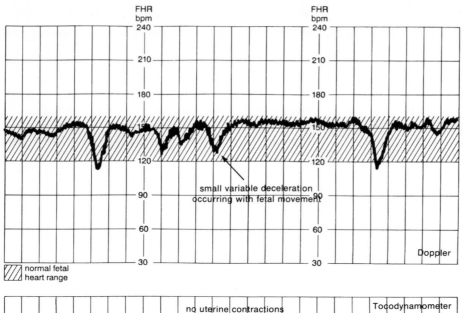

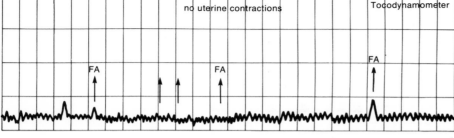

Pattern Characteristic:
Variable Decelerations:
V-Shaped, Associated with Fetal
Movement

Variable Decelerations: U-Shaped

*V*ariable decelerations have historically been identified with alphabet letters that correspond with certain configurations: V, U, and W.[43]

The U-shape is produced by a steep descending limb followed by a gradual drop to the nadir of the contraction, usually with minimal or no escape rhythm, followed by an initial gradual recovery from the nadir, then a steep return of the ascending limb. This is comparable to the atypical variable deceleration: loss of variability during

deceleration (see page 250).[47] Because the jagged waveform is lost to some extent, the U is less reassuring than the V, which implies a jagged waveform (good variability). When complete smoothing takes place, this pattern is comparable to the second degree variable decelerations of O'Gureck et al.[61] This pattern is easily distinguished from a uniform deceleration, which typically has a more gradual onset and recovery.

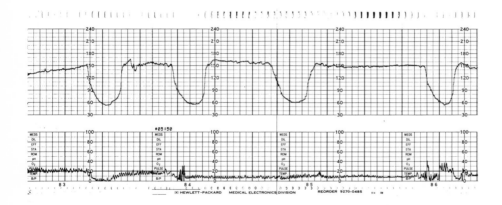

CASE INTERPRETATION: Class IV

Baseline Information: normal heart rate, decreased beat-to-beat variability.

Periodic or Nonperiodic Changes: severe variable decelerations with atypia, characterized by the loss or blunting of primary acceleration, the loss of variability in the deceleration, and some prolonged secondary accelerations.

Uterine Activity: poorly recorded, "reversed" uterine contractions that are associated with the decelerations.

Significance: multiple features of atypia in the variable decelerations plus the loss of baseline variability predicts an increased risk of a low Apgar score and acidosis. Management is influenced by the duration of the pattern, the anticipated time to vaginal delivery, the anticipated ease of delivery, and the response to measures taken to improve fetal oxygenation and umbilical flow.

CASE OUTCOME: Thirty-one-year-old gravida 2, para 1001, delivered at 38 weeks' gestation by cesarean section performed for probable fetal distress, with general anesthesia, a 5 pound, 6¾ ounce (2459 gram) male; Apgar score 3/6. The fetus was in a vertex presentation, in an occiput anterior position. The newborn was determined by neonatology evaluation to be at 34 weeks' gestational age. The newborn was diagnosed to have esophageal atresia. The scalp pHs were 7.00 and 7.08 minutes before delivery. The first newborn pH was 7.49. The maternal course was complicated by polyhydramnios, preeclampsia, and placental abruption.

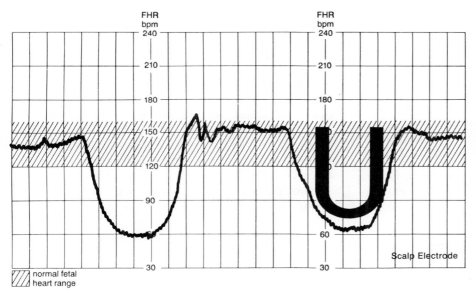

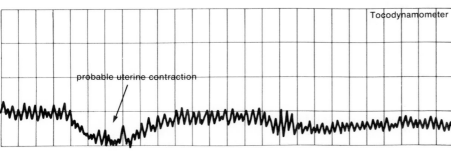

Pattern Characteristic:
Variable Decelerations:
U-Shaped

Variable Decelerations: Sloping Limbs

*T*he sloping limb of a variable deceleration, in contrast to vertical precipitous descending and return limbs, is occasionally seen as a variant of the atypical variable deceleration with loss of variability in the deceleration (see page 250).[14,27,47] It displays smoothing of the waveform or "loss of a jagged appearance," which is a prerequisite for the second degree variable deceleration of O'Gureck, et al, in whose classification such a deceleration represents mild cord involvement.[61]

The slope of the variable deceleration has been demonstrated to be a predictor of the fetal condition in sheep.[1]

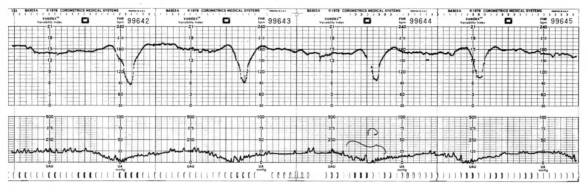

Recreation of original tracing

CASE INTERPRETATION: Class IV

Baseline Information: moderate tachycardia and an unstable baseline based on slow return to a normal baseline after recovery from the deceleration (prolonged secondary acceleration), decreased short-term variability.

Periodic or Nonperiodic Changes: moderate variable decelerations with atypia, characterized by absent variability and prolonged secondary accelerations. Sloping ascending and descending limbs.

Uterine Activity: contractions recorded as negative deflections in relationship to the baseline; they appear slightly skewed in configuration.

Significance: an increased risk of a decreased Apgar score. Management is influenced by the clinical situation, including the estimated duration until delivery, the fetal gestational age, and the response to standard measures taken to improve the fetal environment.

CASE OUTCOME: Nineteen-year-old gravida 2, para 0010, at 30 weeks' gestation delivered vaginally, with pudendal anesthesia, 85 minutes after this segment, a 2 pound, 14 ounce (1304 gram) male; Apgar score 7/7. The fetus was in a vertex presentation. The cord was wrapped around the right arm. The newborn course was complicated by a clubfoot and a large intraventricular hematoma that was diagnosed on the sixth day of life. The infant was dismissed on the 58th day of life.

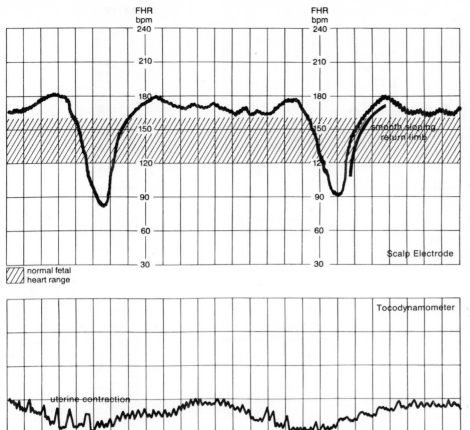

Pattern Characteristic:
Variable Decelerations: Sloping Limbs

Variable Decelerations: Slow Onset

*A*n unusual variant of the atypical variable deceleration with loss of variability in the deceleration is one in which the configuration is marked by a slow onset (gradual descent of the descending limb). This has been associated with a true knot in the umbilical cord.[17] However, the frequency of occurrence both in the presence and absence of a true knot has not been established. A slow rate of onset of the descending limb of the variable deceleration has a higher correlation with an acidemic than a nonacidemic fetus in sheep.[1] The slow onset, when accompanied by loss of variability in the deceleration, warrants similar interpretation as that of an atypical variable deceleration with a loss of variability.

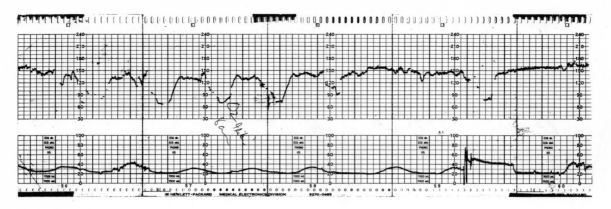

CASE INTERPRETATION: Class IV

Baseline Information: normal rate and variability, an episode of rebound tachycardia.

Periodic or Nonperiodic Changes: moderate atypical variable decelerations, late in occurrence with slow onset and loss of variability within decelerations.

Uterine Activity: small, frequent contractions as measured by external monitoring.

Significance: this pattern is seen at times with a true knot in the cord. Because of good baseline variability, despite atypia of decelerations, conservative management is appropriate if the fetus is of term gestation and vaginal delivery is imminent. It is appropriate to change the maternal position and to evaluate the tracing for further baseline changes or atypia.

CASE OUTCOME: Twenty-five-year-old gravida 2, para 1001, delivered at 40 weeks' gestation by cesarean section for possible "fetal distress" an 8 pound, 14 ounce (4026 gram) female; Apgar score 9/9. The mother was given oxytocin augmentation. There was a true knot in the cord. Thick meconium was present. The mother's postoperative recovery was uncomplicated, and the infant followed a normal newborn course.

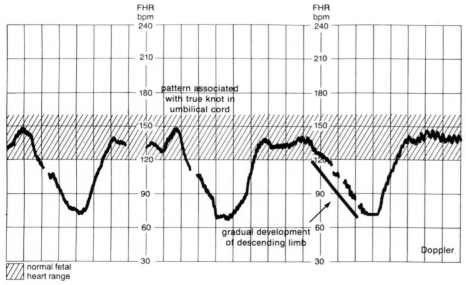

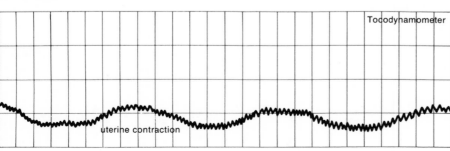

Pattern Characteristic:
Variable Decelerations: Slow Onset

Variable Decelerations: Nonperiodic

*V*ariable decelerations may have a varying relationship to the timing of the uterine contraction.[33,34] Because most variable decelerations are believed to be produced by cord impingement, most intrapartum variable decelerations occur simultaneously with uterine contractions (periodic). The pressure generated by the uterine contractions produces cord occlusion, which triggers the baroreceptor responses that result in the initial fetal heart rate change.

Cord occlusion can be produced by other mechanisms such as by fetal movement against a "vulnerable" cord segment. Variable decelerations may also be produced by other than cord impingement.[36] For these reasons, variable decelerations need not have a fixed relationship to contractions (nonperiodic).

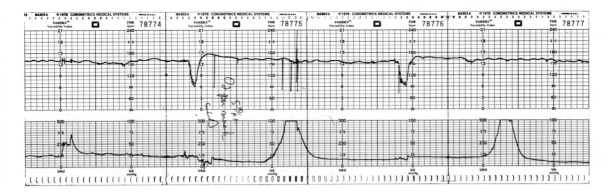

CASE INTERPRETATION: Class IV

Baseline Information: high normal heart rate to moderate tachycardia, decreased variability.

Periodic or Nonperiodic Changes: mild variable decelerations with atypia: loss of primary accelerations and a prolonged secondary acceleration. The occurrence is not related to uterine contractions.

Uterine Activity: infrequent contractions of greater than one minute duration, as measured by external monitoring.

Significance: an increased risk of a low Apgar score or acidosis is predicted by the baseline loss of variability (unless medication-induced) and the mild atypia of decelerations. Cord impingement is probable, therefore, changing the maternal position is appropriate. Delivery management is influenced by clinical factors, including the fetal gestational age, the anticipated time to vaginal delivery, the anticipated ease of vaginal delivery, as well as the response to measures taken to improve umbilical flow and fetal oxygenation.

CASE OUTCOME: Seventeen-year-old primigravida at 42 weeks' gestation delivered, with local anesthesia, a 7 pound, 6½ ounce (3360 gram) female; Apgar score 7/9. The fetus was in a vertex presentation. Thin meconium was present. No abnormal cord position was noted. Intrapartum fetal capillary pHs were 7.26 to 7.33. The patient had a clinical picture of mild preeclampsia. The infant followed a normal newborn course.

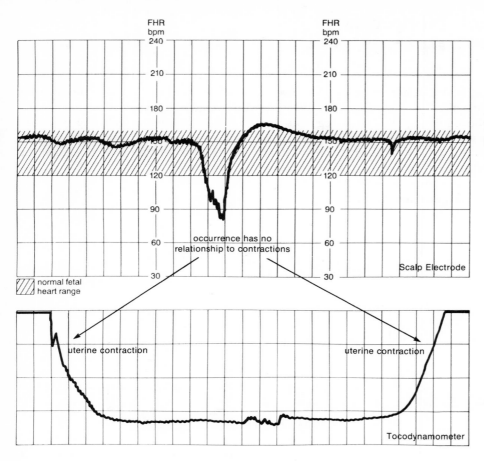

Pattern Characteristic:
Nonperiodic Variable
Decelerations

Variable Decelerations: Late Occurrence

Variable decelerations may be typically variable in timing in relationship to uterine contractions as well as variable in configuration. Therefore, the term "periodic" is usually omitted when describing variable decelerations.

Since most variable decelerations are caused by umbilical cord impingement and pressure generated by uterine contractions is the most common mechanism for cord impingement during labor, most intrapartum variable decelerations occur simultaneously with uterine contractions. A late-occurring variable deceleration is certainly less reassuring than a variable deceleration with onset and recovery confined to the timing of the uterine waveform.[81] However, late occurrence does not invariably imply a hypoxic etiology of the deceleration. Late occurrence may be produced by cord compression, occurring late in the timing of the uterine pressure curve. Late occurrence may also be produced by pressure on the cord that is not caused by the contraction but by fetal movement that tightens or compresses a vulnerable cord.

As with all variable decelerations, the key factor in interpretation is configuration.[18] A late-occurring variable deceleration with a smooth waveform and atypical features, especially with a loss of baseline variability or other baseline changes associated with fetal jeopardy, has an ominous connotation (see page 286). In contrast, a late-occurring variable deceleration with minimal or absent atypia, accompanied by a stable baseline with good variability is usually not cause for aggressive intervention.

This pattern is to be distinguished from a variable deceleration with slow recovery (see page 246), a variable deceleration with late component (atypical biphasic variable decelerations) (see page 251), late/variable decelerations (see Chap. 13), and combined variable and late decelerations (see pages 225,291).

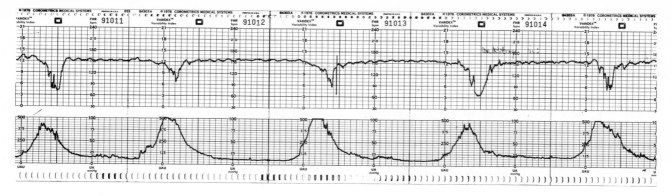

CASE INTERPRETATION: Class IV

Baseline Information: high normal rate, satisfactory variability.

Periodic or Nonperiodic Changes: mild and moderate variable decelerations with jagged features, late in occurrence in relationship to uterine contractions, some atypia: absent primary and secondary accelerations, and delayed return to baseline.

Uterine Activity: skewed contractions of a frequency compatible with active labor.

Significance: interpretation is based on features of the deceleration and not on timing alone. It is appropriate to observe the tracing for baseline changes or further atypia while performing measures to improve umbilical cord perfusion and fetal oxygenation.

CASE OUTCOME: Thirty-two-year-old gravida 2, para 0010, at 40 weeks' gestation spontaneously delivered vaginally, with local anesthesia, a 5 pound, 1 ounce (2296 gram) female; Apgar score 8/9. The fetus was in a vertex presentation, in a deflexed occiput posterior position. No abnormal cord position was detected. The infant followed an uncomplicated newborn course. Delivery occurred 5½ hours after this tracing segment was made. Variable decelerations increased in duration but never lost their jagged configuration.

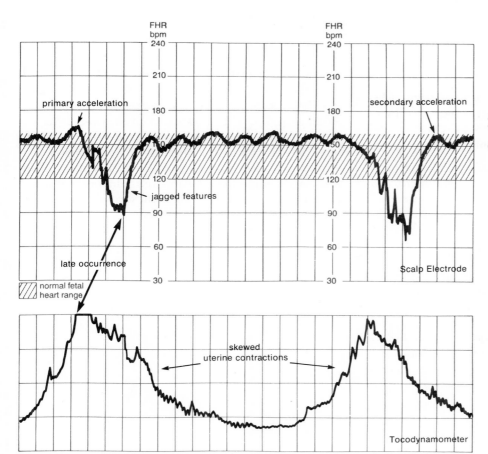

Pattern Characteristic:
Variable Decelerations: Late Occurrence

Variable Decelerations with Escape Rhythm

*T*he descending limb of a variable deceleration reflects a precipitous drop in heart rate that is produced by reflex stimulation of the vagus nerve (modifiable by atropine administration).[31] The abrupt slowing of the heart rate is believed to depict a parasympathetic suppression of the sinus node pacemaker. As a protective mechanism under such circumstances, lower pacemakers in the cardiac conduction system may generate impulses to prevent further slowing and fetal cardiac asystole.[79] Rates derived from junctional or ventricular pacemakers are typically slower, and because they are independent of autonomic nervous system regulation, produce no beat-to-beat vari-

ability. These escape rhythms account for the horizontal flat-line segments in the nadir of some variable decelerations. These usually occur at a rate of 60 or 70 bpm. The loss of variability by this mechanism has an entirely different significance from the loss of variability produced by fetal metabolic acidosis. It is usually the healthy fetus who demonstrates a well-demarcated escape entry and recovery.

When this pattern is encountered, typically the variable deceleration maintains jagged features and is usually moderate or severe.

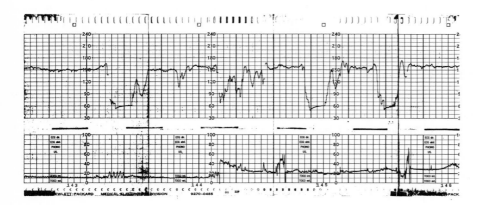

CASE INTERPRETATION: Class IV

Baseline Information: normal heart rate, diminished but present beat-to-beat variability, as measured by internal monitoring. A mixed pattern of increased variability with variable decelerations. Stable baseline.

Periodic or Nonperiodic Changes: moderate to severe variable decelerations with atypia, characterized by biphasic configuration and a slow return to baseline; a mixed pattern with increased variability. An escape rhythm in the base of decelerations.

Uterine Activity: not clearly displayed.

Significance: intermittent sinus node suppression with escape. The fetus is reacting to stressful stimuli, for example, cord compression. The outcome varies with the duration, gestation, and other clinical factors. It is appropriate to change the maternal position, evaluate for cord prolapse, and administer oxygen. Other decisions such as use of amnioinfusion, vary with the clinical circumstances.

CASE OUTCOME: Thirty-four-year-old gravida 4, para 2012, at 43 weeks' gestation delivered vaginally, with low forceps, a 6 pound, 15 ounce (3147 gram) male; Apgar score 7/9. The fetus was in a vertex presentation. Ketamine anesthesia was administered to the mother. The pregnancy was complicated by preeclampsia and anemia. Oxytocin augmentation for dysfunctional labor and magnesium sulfate therapy were administered intrapartum. The newborn had transient seventh nerve palsy.

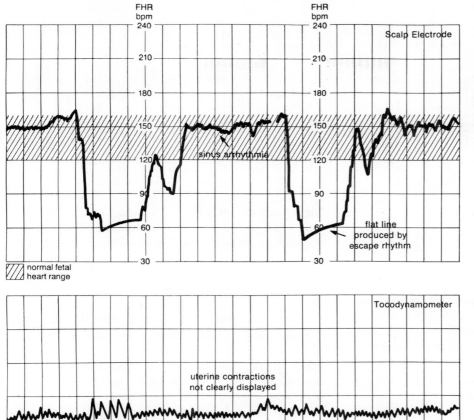

FHR bpm

240
210
180
150
120
90
60
30

normal fetal heart range

sinus arrhythmia

FHR bpm

240
210
180
150
120
90
60
30

Scalp Electrode

flat line produced by escape rhythm

Pattern Characteristic:
Variable Decelerations with Escape Rhythm

Tocodynamometer

uterine contractions not clearly displayed

Variable Decelerations with a Bigeminal Rhythm

A burst of parasympathetic activity, producing an abrupt slowing of the fetal heart, is the reflex-mediated mechanism that initiates a variable deceleration. The resulting suppression of the sinus node has been associated in the fetus with myocardial conduction defects that allow lower pacemakers to discharge.[79] When such pacemakers are in close proximity to the sinus node and the suppression is partial, a competitive interplay may occur between the two pacemakers, resulting in a bigeminal pattern. These produce characteristic double horizontal lines in the nadir of the variable deceleration. The pattern is usually seen as a higher heart rate (80–90 bpm) rather than as a pure escape rhythm (60–70 bpm).

The pattern is also seen as a baseline finding (see page 476) and during recovery from some prolonged decelerations (see page 325). The bigeminal pattern is not in itself an ominous finding in a setting of variable decelerations that retain good variability accompanied by normal baseline features.

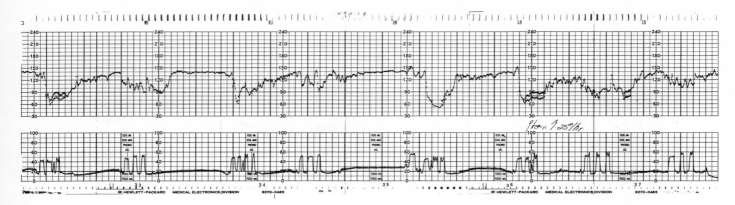

CASE INTERPRETATION: Class IV

Baseline Information: normal rate and variability, some fluctuation in the baseline level after decelerations (produced by a failure to return to original baseline *or* a slow return to the original baseline).

Periodic or Nonperiodic Changes: severe or moderate variable decelerations with minimal atypia characterized by a slow return to the baseline or return to a lower baseline. Many of the decelerations display a bigeminal rhythm in the nadir.

Uterine Activity: maternal contractions are indicated only by maternal straining deflections of the tocodynamometer.

Significance: because of reassuring baseline information, conservative management may be chosen despite the slow return to an unstable baseline, if delivery is imminent and the pattern does not display progressive atypia or baseline changes and the clinical circumstances indicate a fetus with good basal welfare.

CASE OUTCOME: Twenty-four-year-old primigravida delivered at 43½ weeks' gestation vaginally, with local and pudendal anesthesia, an 8 pound, 10 ounce (3912 gram) female; Apgar score 9/10. The fetus was in a vertex presentation. Oxytocin augmentation was given for premature rupture of the membranes. The infant followed a normal newborn course.

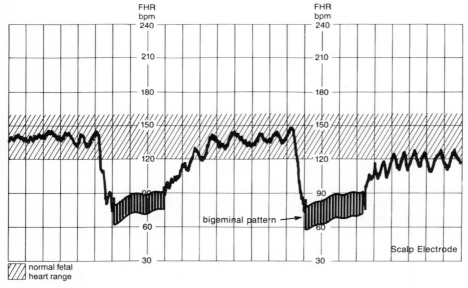

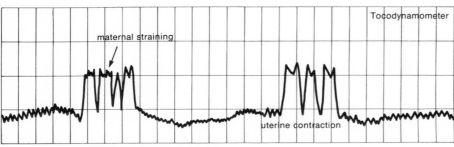

Pattern Characteristic:
Variable Decelerations with a Bigeminal Rhythm

Variable Decelerations with a Trigeminal Rhythm

*D*uring the sinus node suppression, which may occur at times of precipitous onset of variable deceleration, ectopic pacemakers may discharge impulses as part of the escape phenomenon of the cardiac conduction system.[79] This may produce a transient arrhythmia. Most often, a junctional escape rhythm occurs, producing a single horizontal flat-line at about 60 to 70 bpm (see page 111) in the nadir of the variable deceleration. It is not uncommon to see a bigeminal pattern when partial suppression occurs at slightly higher heart rates (see page 271). A

trigeminal pattern under such circumstances is a rare finding among fetal heart monitoring patterns. A similar pattern may occur during recovery from a prolonged deceleration as a transition to the resumption of sinus node control (see page 326). The pattern is in and of itself not ominous.

Management is based on the assessment of other features of the decelerations and baseline fetal heart rate findings.

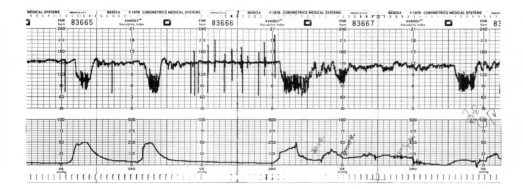

CASE INTERPRETATION: Class II

Baseline Information: normal rate, average variability.

Periodic or Nonperiodic Changes: moderate variable decelerations with transient arrhythmias occurring in the base of the deceleration, with features of bigeminy and trigeminy.

Uterine Activity: low intensity, skewed contractions with steep onset, as is often seen with oxytocin usage, as measured by an internal pressure transducer.

Significance: suppression of the sinus pacemaker during variable decelerations, accompanied by ectopic depolarizations. A healthy fetus is predicted by this pattern.

CASE OUTCOME: Thirty-four-year-old gravida 5, para 4004, at 37 weeks' gestation delivered vaginally, with low forceps and epidural anesthesia, an 8 pound, 14 ounce (4026 gram) male; Apgar score 4/8. The maternal course was complicated by diabetes mellitus. Oxytocin augmentation was given during labor. The delivery was complicated by shoulder dystocia. The newborn course was complicated by transient Erb's palsy.

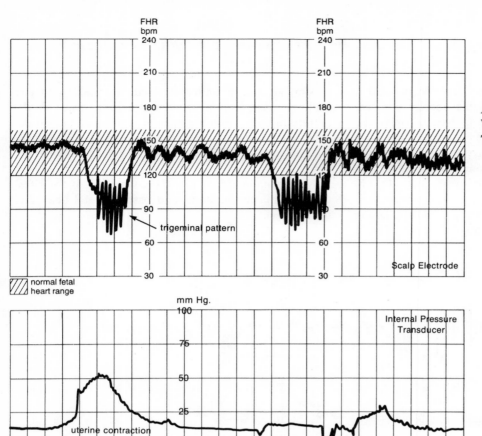

Pattern Characteristic:
Variable Decelerations with a
Trigeminal Rhythm

Variable Decelerations with Cardiac Asystole: Transient

*C*ardiac asystole has been arbitrarily defined as a pause in conducted impulses of greater than two seconds.[41] Such a phenomenon occurs occasionally during the phase of maximum heart rate slowing of a variable deceleration. The pattern often appears during an escape rhythm. In such circumstances, it represents a transient failure of the junctional pacemaker.[80] It is usually preceded by a fall of 40 beats or greater. The monitor displays a downward deflection of the fetal heart trace to the lowest limits of the heart rate portion of the graph. An upward deflection signifies recovery of impulses of greater than 30 bpm.

Although such a pattern has been reported prior to intrauterine death, the pattern is compatible with a healthy fetus who is displaying cardiac responses to excessive vagal tone.[21,40] Unless the episodes of cardiac asystole are prolonged, interpretation of the fetal condition is based on assessing other features of the variable decelerations and baseline findings.[41] In cases with prolonged asystole, potential cardiac arrest is a concern (see page 276). Although atropine may obliterate the pattern, it is debatable whether it is desirable to modify protective vagal responses in the fetus.[24,41,65,80]

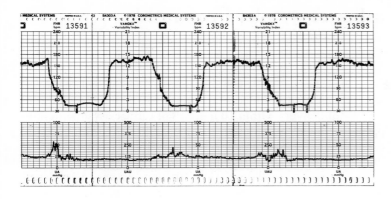

CASE INTERPRETATION: Class IV

Baseline Information: high normal rate, normal variability.

Periodic or Nonperiodic Changes: severe variable decelerations with atypia characterized by loss of variability in the decelerations and blunting of primary and secondary accelerations. Escape rhythm is present in the nadir of the deceleration, with episodes of probable cardiac asystole.

Uterine Activity: apparently regular contractions with minimal deflection of the tocodynamometer.

Significance: excessive vagal tone. Attempts to relieve cord compression are in order. Management is otherwise influenced by individual clinical circumstances. An electrocardiogram distinguishes transient asystole from artifact.

CASE OUTCOME: Nineteen-year-old gravida 3, para 2002, at 36 weeks' gestation delivered vaginally, with local anesthesia, a 5 pound, 12 ounce (2608 gram) female; Apgar score 8/9. The fetus was in a persistent occiput posterior position. A double nuchal cord was noted at delivery. The infant followed a normal newborn course.

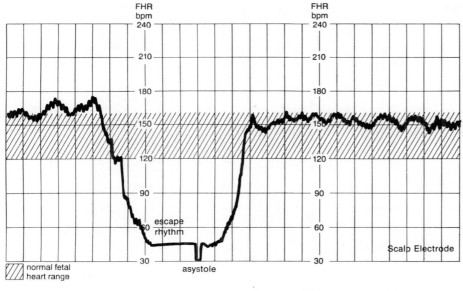

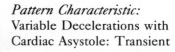

Pattern Characteristic:
Variable Decelerations with
Cardiac Asystole: Transient

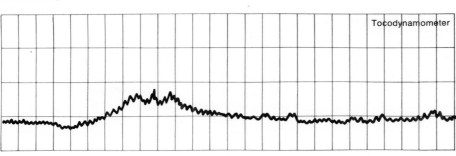

Variable Decelerations with Cardiac Asystole: Prolonged

*F*etal cardiac asystole, or a pause in fetal heart impulses for more than two seconds, is a phenomenon documented by electrocardiographic findings in the healthy fetus under conditions of excessive vagal tone. The pattern in and of itself is not an ominous finding. In situations in which cardiac asystole has been noted in the fetal heart rate tracings of the moribund fetus, such tracings demonstrated other features associated with an increased risk of fetal asphyxia.[40] Therefore, interpretation of the monitoring information about fetal status is focused on the baseline findings and other features of associated decelerations.[21]

However, when cardiac asystole is prolonged, concern increases regarding the risk of intrapartum death from cardiac arrest.[80] Such a phenomenon may explain the unexpected sudden intrapartum fetal death.[28] In the event of delivery within 10 minutes of cardiac asystole, umbilical acid base studies may not reflect the true fetal condition.[59] Prolonged cardiac asystole is a rare finding among fetal monitoring patterns and, therefore, a full range of possible clinical outcomes is yet to be developed. Atropine may modify the pattern, but the consequences of obliteration of (potentially protective) vagal responses is a subject of controversy.[24,65,80]

Fetuses with excessive vagal tone may continue to demonstrate delayed sympathetic system reactivity in the early neonatal course without asphyxia.[42]

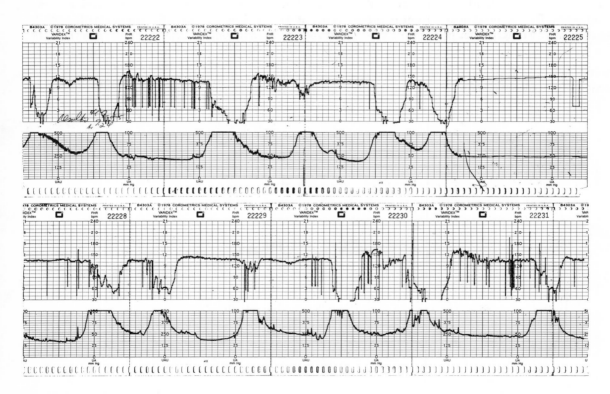

CASE INTERPRETATION: Class IV

Baseline Information: normal rate, some loss of baseline stability between contractions, normal variability.

Periodic or Nonperiodic Changes: severe variable decelerations with a precipitous fall to a depth of 30 bpm associated with episodes of probable prolonged asystole followed by precipitous recovery.

Uterine Activity: frequent, skewed contractions with little if any resting phase.

Significance: the fetus is at a possible risk for intrapartum death with prolonged periods of asystole, yet at the time of this segment the basal condition is healthy, as indicated by good variability. Management is influenced by the clinical situation such as the estimated time to vaginal delivery, the ability to reduce uterine activity, the presence of thick meconium, and the fetal gestational age. An electrocardiogram may clarify the precise cardiac impulse formation and conduction.

CASE OUTCOME: Thirty-six-year-old gravida 2, para 1001, at 40 weeks' gestation delivered by primary cesarean section for "fetal distress," with inhalation anesthesia, a 6 pound, 6½ ounce (2906 gram) male; a one minute Apgar score of 4 was influenced by management of

thick meconium (detected for the first time at delivery) through endotracheal suctioning; a five minute Apgar score was 8. The fetus was in an occiput posterior position. Intermittent loss of cardiac activity by auscultation as well as by monitoring. Intrapartum capillary pHs were 7.24 and 7.25; umbilical cord pHs were 7.19 arterial, 7.21 venous. The newborn course was complicated by persistent fetal circulation. The infant was dismissed at 18 days of life.

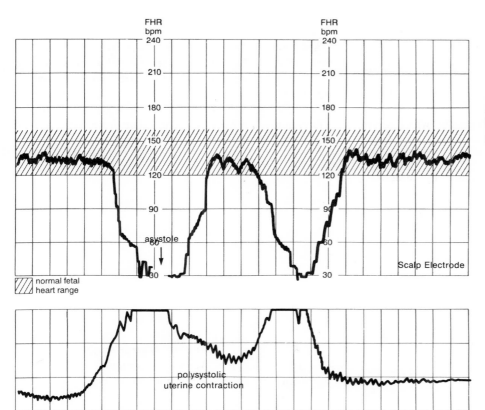

Pattern Characteristic:
Variable Decelerations with
Cardiac Asystole: Prolonged

Variable Decelerations with Overlap Phenomenon

A fetal heart rate phenomenon is termed "overlap" when decelerations occur in rapid succession with frequent uterine contractions.[5] Before recovery from one deceleration, the next is triggered, giving the impression that a new bradycardic baseline has developed.[46] When the decelerations are variable in configuration, the trace represents continuous "bases," which often are associated with a junctional rhythm that produces a smooth line, suggesting a loss of variability as well as bradycardia. Decreasing uterine activity is one method of relieving the stress of the fetus, who may be quite healthy. Without intervention, the fetus may eventually be jeopardized by diminished perfusion and resulting hypoxia.

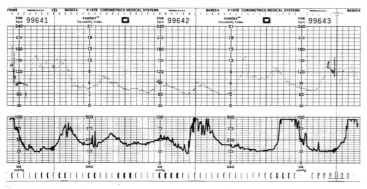

Recreation of original tracing

CASE INTERPRETATION: Class II

Baseline Information: normal rate of good variability.

Periodic or Nonperiodic Changes: a classical variable deceleration occurs with recovery followed by what appears to be a baseline shift to bradycardia, which is produced by incomplete recovery from subsequent decelerations before the next occurs.

Uterine Activity: increased frequency of contractions, no resting phase.

Significance: overlap phenomenon, reduction in uterine activity is appropriate.

CASE OUTCOME: Twenty-one-year-old gravida 3, para 2002, at 42½ weeks' gestation delivered vaginally, with epidural anesthesia from a vertex presentation, an 8 pound, 1 ounce (3657 gram) male; Apgar score 8/9. The delivery occurred soon after this segment was made. There was a nuchal cord. The infant followed a normal newborn course.

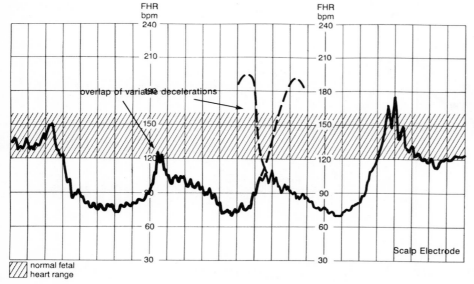

Pattern Characteristic:
Variable Decelerations: Overlap Phenomenon

Agonal Variable Decelerations

*T*he appearance of fetal heart rate patterns of a dying fetus vary with such factors as gestational age, etiology of the distress, and duration of the decompensation. The more immature the fetus the more periodic the changes in agonal patterns.[64]

When variable decelerations have been a feature of the monitoring tracing of a moribund fetus, progressive deterioration may be reflected by increasing atypia, particularly smoothing of the deceleration and appearance of late components; loss of baseline stability; decreased variability and tachycardia; and sinusoidal patterns.[32] Bradycardia may represent a failure of complete recovery of one deceleration before the onset of the next deceleration or an agonal baseline change.[29] A chaotic pattern ensues, and variability is lost.[7,69] As with late decelerations, features of variable decelerations that once denoted healthy reflex responses may become progressively blunted, until a smooth, barely wavering baseline replaces detectable decelerations.[64]

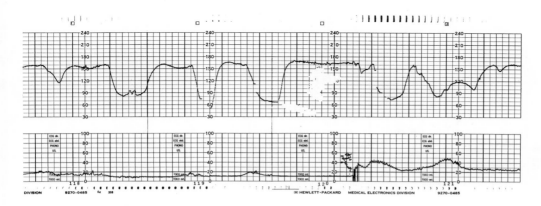

CASE INTERPRETATION: Class V

Baseline Information: moderate tachycardia, absent variability, loss of baseline stability.

Periodic or Nonperiodic Changes: severe variable decelerations with multiple atypical features, including loss of variability in the decelerations, prolonged secondary accelerations, and a W-sign.

Uterine Activity: regular uterine actions of normal configuration, as registered by a tocodynamometer.

Significance: this is a pattern often seen in association with a moribund fetus. Prompt delivery of a viable fetus is usually appropriate, but some patterns are produced by a deterioration of such duration that rapidity of delivery may offer no additional benefit.

CASE OUTCOME: Nineteen-year-old primigravida at 22 weeks' gestation delivered vaginally, with no anesthesia from a single footling breech presentation, a 1¼ ounce (461 gram) stillborn male. Intrauterine death occurred 50 minutes after this segment was made.

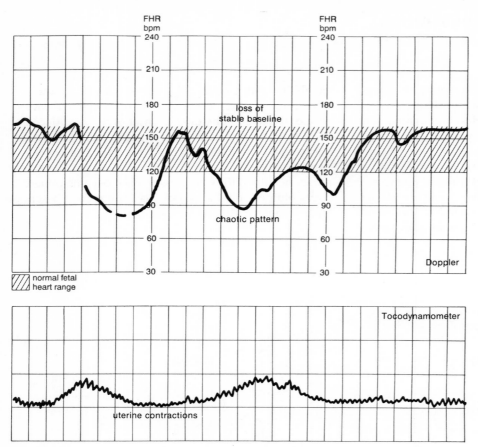

Pattern Characteristic:
Variable Decelerations: Agonal

Variable Decelerations with Premature Gestation

*T*he premature fetus presents a unique problem in assessing the significance of variable decelerations. Pattern interpretation is altered: Baseline variability may be diminished because of an incomplete parasympathetic system development, but a "silent" pattern may also reflect asphyxia.[40] Deceleration patterns may be less fully developed. Some small heart rate decelerations may be of more ominous significance than similar patterns in a term fetus.[77] Other decelerations may simply reflect inconsequential responses of an immature organism.[72] The umbilical cord is less developed and may be more vulnerable.[22] This is a particular problem in cases of premature ruptured membranes.[60] The fetus tolerates less hypoxia with an increased risk of intracranial hemorrhage and respiratory distress syndrome.[3,51] There may be a disproportionately poor neonatal outcome for the degree or duration of fetal monitoring pattern encountered.[77] This has been demonstrated, for example, by the finding of a

high association of low umbilical cord pH determinations and poor newborn performances in the presence of abnormal tracings such as those demonstrating decreased variability, the presence of severe variable decelerations, and late decelerations.[76,78,83]

For such reasons, it has been suggested that the premature fetus should have separate fetal monitoring interpretation criteria.[68] These interpretation problems are compounded by artifact: Contractions may be indistinctly registered by the small uterus, giving a false sense of security in assessing the fetal environment, and small decelerations may be masked even with modern monitors.[19]

Because premature newborns have multiple potential causes for low Apgar scores, umbilical cord pH studies have been demonstrated to be helpful in corroborating good fetal metabolic condition as predicted by a normal tracing.[3,4]

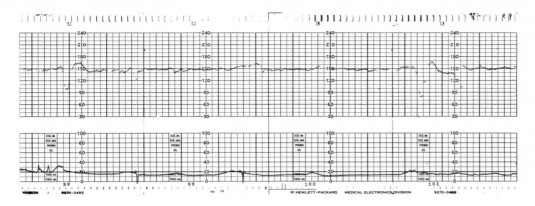

CASE INTERPRETATION: Class IV

Baseline Information: normal rate, decreased variability by external monitoring.

Periodic or Nonperiodic Changes: small, almost obscured atypical variable decelerations, late in relationship to the contractions, with a relatively prolonged secondary acceleration.

Uterine Activity: small, regular contractions, as indicated by a tocodynamometer.

Significance: increased risk of a low Apgar score and acidosis. Management varies with the clinical circumstances. When such a pattern is seen in a premature gestation, particularly in a situation of ruptured membranes, it is not reassuring but rather suggests that further fetal assessment may be needed to assure that there is a good fetal condition. Management may include relief of umbilical cord impingement through amnioinfusion in selected cases.

CASE OUTCOME: Twenty-one-year-old gravida 2, para 0010, at 29 weeks' gestation delivered by cesarean section, with general anesthesia, performed for possible fetal distress and breech presentation a 3 pound, 1 ounce (1389 gram) male; Apgar score 1/6. The pattern appeared in early labor. The placental culture was negative. The newborn survived, with dismissal at 24 days of life.

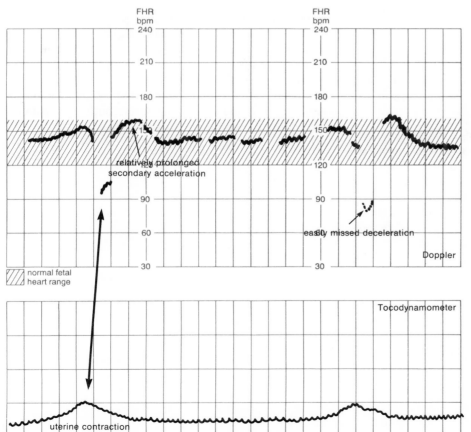

Pattern Characteristic:
Variable Decelerations with
Premature Gestation

Masked Variable Decelerations

Variable decelerations may be brief in duration while profound in range or depth. They may be so brief that with external monitoring the nadir of the deceleration is attributed to artifact and the primary and secondary accelerations are interpreted as usual fetal reactivity. This is particularly a problem with premature gestations.

It is a problem that can occur with fetal monitors that have autocorrelation as well as with other monitors.

Scalp electrode monitoring, if feasible, decreases the likelihood of a masked deceleration in a setting of concern about lost fetal heart rate signals. See page 405 for masked decelerations that were demonstrated with dual channel internal monitoring.

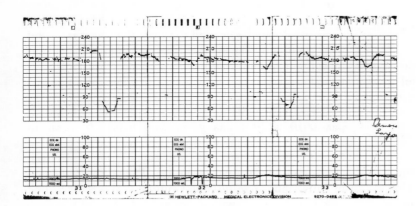

CASE INTERPRETATION: Class IV

Baseline Information: moderate to marked tachycardia, diminished variability with external monitoring, downward drifting of the baseline between contractions.

Periodic or Nonperiodic Changes: variable decelerations, moderate in duration but with a drop of 120 to 140 bpm. They are late in onset. Atypia: prolonged secondary acceleration.

Significance: an increased risk of a low Apgar score based on hypoxia, denoted by a prolonged secondary acceleration. Management is influenced by multiple factors, including the fetal gestational age, duration of the pattern, and the estimated time until delivery. It is appropriate to exclude umbilical cord prolapse and institute measures to improve umbilical flow as well as other management appropriate to the clinical situation.

CASE OUTCOME: Twenty-five-year-old gravida 4, para 1112, at 30 weeks' gestation delivered by cesarean section, with general anesthesia, performed for "fetal distress," a 2 pound, 13 ounce (1276 gram) female; Apgar score 1/3. The fetus was in a vertex presentation. The maternal antepartum course was complicated by intravenous drug use. The newborn expired at 80 days of life; the newborn course was complicated by group B streptococcal sepsis and necrotizing enterocolitis. The patient had ruptured membranes for 48 hours.

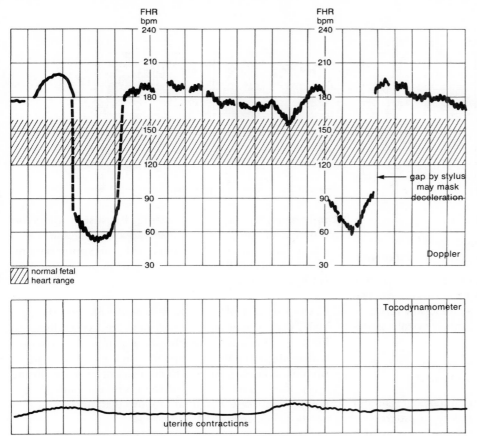

Pattern Characteristic:
Variable Decelerations: Masked

Progression from Mild to Severe Variable Decelerations

*V*ariable decelerations typically increase in frequency as labor progresses.[8] When a pattern changes from mild to severe variable decelerations rapidly, progressive umbilical cord impingement is a concern. Efforts are in order to improve umbilical cord perfusion. Should improvement in the pattern fail, cesarean section may be an appropriate intervention.[13] An end-stage deceleration may follow such a pattern (see page 322). The pattern has also been associated with an occiput posterior position.[71] The mechanism in the latter case is proposed to be fetal vagal stimulation other than cord compression, for example, eye pressure.[36] Variable decelerations produced by such a cause may not have primary and secondary accelerations because there is not a partial cord compression component in the mechanism of production of the pattern.

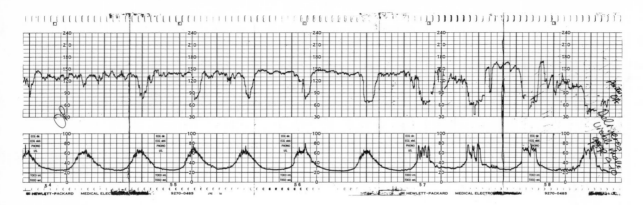

CASE INTERPRETATION: Class II

Baseline Information: normal rate, good variability, loss of stability after recovery from some decelerations.

Periodic or Nonperiodic Changes: progression from mild to severe variable decelerations with atypical features of loss of primary accelerations and a slow return to baseline; an episode of probable cardiac systole is denoted.

Uterine Activity: contractions are regular with little resting phase; maternal straining is indicated.

Significance: a healthy fetus with rapid progression of reflex decelerations, probably secondary to progressive umbilical cord compression, is indicated. Management is

influenced by the clinical setting. Because of the short duration of the pattern, conservative management in a viable fetus with delivery imminent is an appropriate response while instituting measures to improve umbilical cord perfusion and fetal oxygenation.

CASE OUTCOME: Twenty-two-year-old gravida, para 1001, at 43½ weeks' gestation delivered vaginally, with local and pudendal anesthesia, a 7 pound, 10 ounce male; Apgar score 9/10. Spontaneous rotation occurred from an occiput posterior to an anterior position during the pattern. The location of the umbilical cord was not noted at delivery. The infant followed an uncomplicated newborn course.

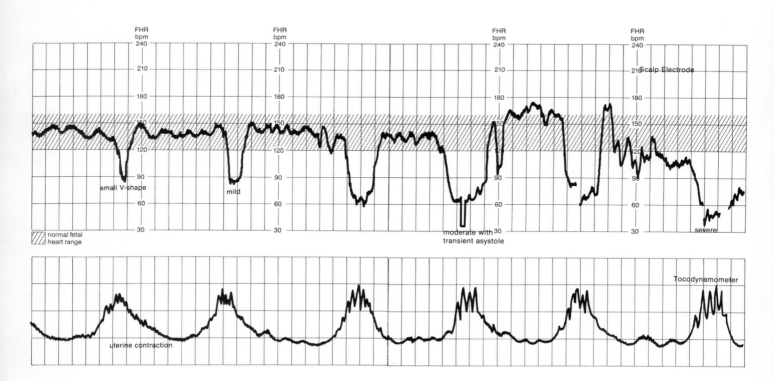

Pattern Characteristic:
Variable Decelerations, Progression from Mild to Severe

Variable Deceleration at Fetal Expulsion

A slowing of the fetal heart rate at expulsion during delivery from either a vertex or breech presentation has long been recognized.[84,85] The deceleration is best placed with variable decelerations, being nonuniform in configuration, unless its duration exceeds two and a half to three minutes, in which case it is termed a prolonged deceleration.

When such an "end-stage" deceleration (see page 322) lasts more than 10 minutes, it becomes a true bradycardia. Because of its occurrence just prior to delivery, it has in the past been called "terminal bradycardia." The same term is used for patterns of fetal heart rate that slow just prior to fetal death. It is preferable to reserve the word "terminal" for the latter situation (see page 322).

Expulsion bradycardia or deceleration is postulated to be produced by the vagal effects of marked head compression and not cord compression.[25,26] It is therefore no surprise that this finding is of increased frequency at deliveries of primigravidas.[52]

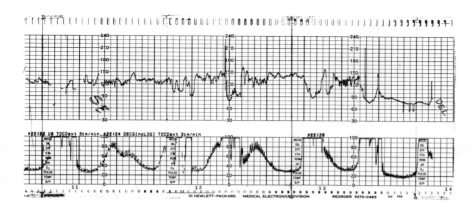

CASE INTERPRETATION: Class II

Baseline Information: normal rate, average variability.

Periodic or Nonperiodic Changes: mild variable decelerations precede a two minute deceleration with sinus node suppression and escape rhythm.

Uterine Activity: increased as recorded by external monitoring, with a pattern consistent with maternal straining.

Significance: The deceleration just prior to delivery is probably produced by fetal expulsion. Supporting this theory is a total lack of relationship to the maternal straining efforts, while prior to that deceleration, variable decelerations occurred only during straining.

CASE OUTCOME: Thirty-five-year-old gravida 4, para 0121, at 38 weeks' gestation delivered vaginally, with epidural anesthesia, from a vertex presentation a 7 pound, 5 ounce (3317 gram) male; Apgar score 9/9. The deceleration was observed during expulsion of the fetal head. Labor was induced for an indication of premature ruptured membranes. The infant followed an uncomplicated newborn course.

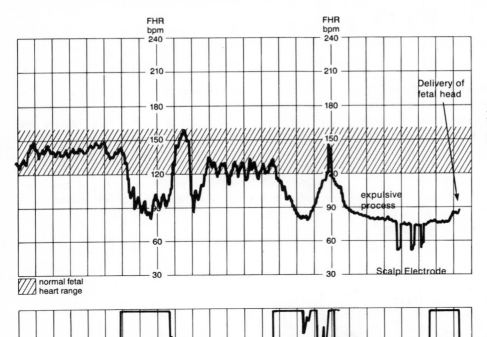

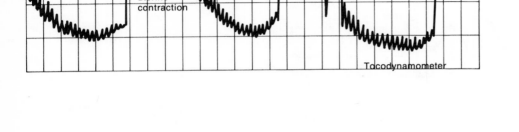

Pattern Characteristic:
Variable Deceleration at Fetal
Expulsion

Severe Variable Decelerations with Atypia and Baseline Tachycardia: Mixed Pattern

*T*he more atypical features identifiable with variable decelerations, the greater the risk of a low Apgar score and fetal acidosis.[47] When such features are seen in combination with baseline changes, particularly tachycardia and loss of variability, a compromised fetus is even more likely.[20] In fact, the presence of atypia and baseline changes are more important predictors of poor fetal condition than degree (mild, moderate, or severe) of the variable decelerations.[47]

In addition to rate and variability, changes in the baseline that may on occasion be associated with fetal stress or distress, a third feature is baseline stability. Loss of baseline stability (see Chap. 8) may occur with certain atypical variable decelerations when the fetal heart is still elevated in a prolonged secondary acceleration at the time of initiation of the next deceleration. The resulting trace has the appearance of a drifting baseline. It is possible for the heart rate to return to a lower than previous baseline, (see pages 144; 228), which also gives the appearance of instability.

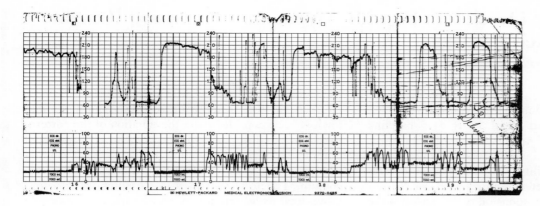

CASE INTERPRETATION: Class IV

Baseline Information: tachycardia, satisfactory variability, loss of baseline stability.

Periodic or Nonperiodic Changes: severe variable decelerations with atypia: prolonged secondary accelerations, loss of variability in the decelerations and biphasic configuration. An overlap phenomenon is also present.

Uterine Activity: indicated by maternal straining movements on a tocodynamometer, suggesting late labor.

Significance: an increased risk of a low Apgar score and acidosis. Management is based on the clinical situation such as duration of the pattern and the estimated time to delivery, fetal gestational age, and other clinical risk factors.

CASE OUTCOME: Twenty-year-old primigravida delivered at 41 weeks' gestation vaginally, with low forceps and local and pudendal anesthesia and ketamine anesthesia, a 6 pound, 15¼ ounce (3154 gram) male; Apgar score 4/6. The fetus was delivered from an occiput posterior position. A double nuchal cord was noted at delivery. A healthy newborn was dismissed at two days of life.

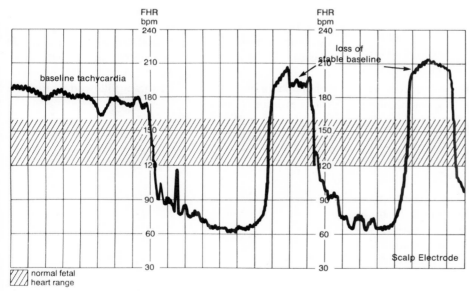

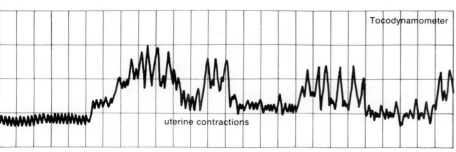

Pattern Characteristic:
Severe Atypical Decelerations
with Tachycardia: Mixed Pattern

Severe Variable Decelerations with Atypia and Decreased Baseline Variability: Mixed Pattern

*W*hen variable decelerations with atypical features are seen in combination with fetal heart rate baseline changes, the risk of a low Apgar score and fetal acidosis increases.[47] The most ominous baseline change in this regard is decreased variability. Multiple atypical features in the deceleration also denote an increased risk.[47]

The clinician has the responsibility of assessing the combination of multiple changes in decelerations and fe-tal heart baseline in the context of the clinical setting. Factors to be considered are the duration of the pattern, the anticipated duration to delivery, the gestation, and other underlying compounding risk factors such as intra-uterine growth retardation, or the presence of thick me-conium. The fetal responses to measures taken to improve fetal oxygenation may also be used for making a decision regarding delivery.

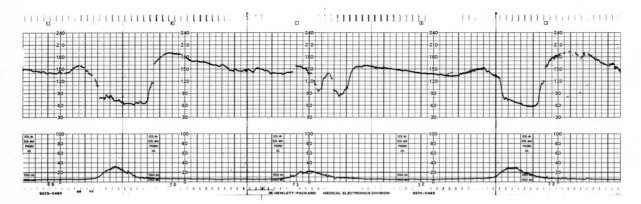

CASE INTERPRETATION: Class IV

Baseline Information: unstable because of a failure to return to normal baseline after contractions, decreased variability.

Periodic or Nonperiodic Changes: prolonged severe variable decelerations with multiple atypical features, prolonged secondary acceleration, loss of variability (sloping side limbs), biphasic.

Uterine Activity: regular contractions of a normal con-figuration.

Significance: an increased risk of a low Apgar score or acidosis. Management is influenced by clinical situations such as fetal gestational age and risk factors, fetal re-sponse to measures taken to improve oxygenation and umbilical perfusion, and anticipated delivery events.

CASE OUTCOME: Twenty-two-year-old gravida 3, para 1102, at 34 weeks' gestation delivered by primary cesarean section for possible fetal distress, with general anesthesia, a 4 pound, 3 ounce (1899 gram) female; Ap-gar score 6/7. The fetus was in a vertex presentation. There was a nuchal cord. The infant followed a satisfac-tory newborn course.

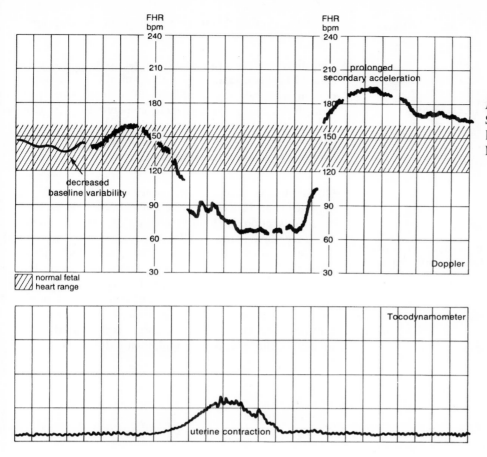

Pattern Characteristic:
Severe Atypical Decelerations,
Decreased Baseline Variability:
Mixed Pattern

Severe Variable Decelerations with Atypia and No Baseline Variability and Tachycardia: Mixed Pattern

An increased number of atypical features in variable decelerations increases the likelihood of a low Apgar score and acidosis.[47] Baseline changes such as increased tachycardia and decreased variability further increase the likelihood of acidosis and a depressed newborn.[2,20] When encountering a pattern with these mixed features, making preparations for a prompt delivery is usually appropriate while simultaneously instituting measures to improve fetal oxygenation and umbilical flow. Brief variable decelerations produced by umbilical cord impingement are not associated with an altered pH. As umbilical cord compression continues, initially a respiratory acidosis is produced, followed eventually, if unrelieved, by a metabolic acidosis.[34] Intermittent fetal pH values may vary during periods of umbilical cord impingement and release and, therefore, may be difficult to interpret. Clinical decisions may thus be appropriately based on assessment of the appearance of classic or atypical features of the decelerations and accompanying baseline changes.

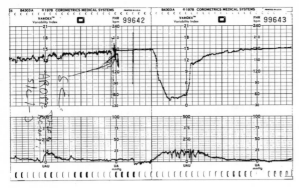

Recreation of original tracing

CASE INTERPRETATION: Class V

Baseline Information: moderate tachycardia absent variability, as measured by internal monitoring (misleading variability by external monitoring).

Periodic or Nonperiodic Changes: severe U-shaped variable decelerations with multiple features of atypia, prolonged return to baseline. Loss of variability in the deceleration, diminished primary acceleration.

Uterine Activity: prolonged contraction associated with the deceleration.

Significance: the combination of tachycardia and a decreased baseline variability with atypical variable deceleration increases the likelihood of a decreased Apgar score and acidosis. Management is dictated by the clinical situation. Prompt delivery with a viable fetus is usually appropriate, particularly in the presence of thick meconium, as was annotated on this tracing.

CASE OUTCOME: Thirty-nine-year-old gravida 6, para 4014, at 42 weeks' gestation delivered by primary cesarean section, with inhalation anesthesia, a 4 pound, 10 ounce (2098 gram) female; Apgar score 0/7. The fetus was in a vertex presentation. There was thick meconium. No meconium was present below the cords. The maternal course was complicated by hypertension, drug abuse, and asthma. The newborn course was complicated by respiratory distress, pneumothorax, and persistent fetal circulation. The newborn was dismissed at two months of life with bronchopulmonary dysplasia.

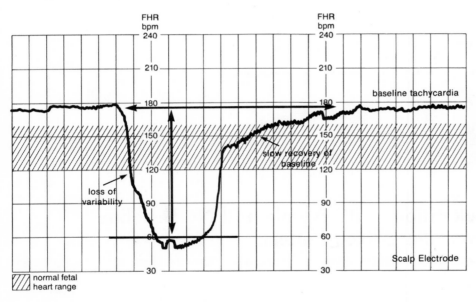

Pattern Characteristic:
Severe Atypical Decelerations, Tachycardia and No Baseline Variability: Mixed Pattern

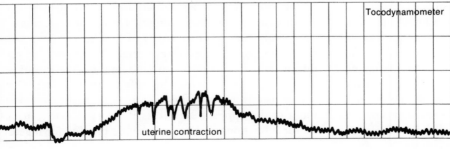

Variable Deceleration and Late Deceleration: Combined Pattern

Any combined pattern of periodic or nonperiodic components is characterized by the presence of two patterns in close proximation but with recovery occurring between them. The resulting pattern may depict the effects of two unrelated fetal stimuli. An example of a combined pattern is variable plus late decelerations. This should be distinguished from late occurring variable decelerations (see page 268), variable decelerations with a slow return to baseline (see page 246), late/variable decelerations (see Chap. 13), and variable decelerations with a late biphasic component (see page 251).

The interpretation of a combined pattern of variable and late decelerations may be approached by first assessing baseline variability and stability and then by interpreting each deceleration separately. Risk may then be assigned based on features of the more ominous of the two components in the context of the baseline indicators of the underlying fetal condition.

If variable decelerations retain classic features and the late decelerations are associated with good variability, a stress pattern is denoted. On the other hand, it is important to note that when hypoxic changes are seen in the variable deceleration and the late decelerations are associated with decreased variability, fetal jeopardy may be compounded[45] because there are most likely two contributing causes to the hypoxia: cord compression and placental insufficiency.[19]

The pattern has an increased association with an occiput posterior position and abnormal uterine activity.[36] Another similar combined pattern is late/variable deceleration and late deceleration (see page 304).

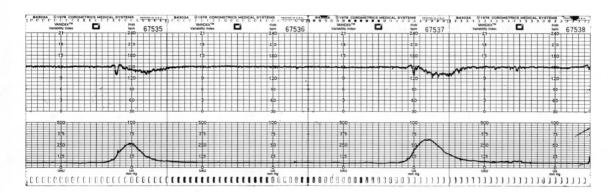

CASE INTERPRETATION: Class II

Baseline Information: the heart rate is normal and stable, decreased short-term variability.

Periodic or Nonperiodic Changes: combined small, mild variable decelerations and late decelerations both demonstrate normal variability in the decelerations. The variable decelerations have classic features.

Uterine Activity: infrequent, skewed contractions that generate greater than 50 mm Hg but Montevide units less than 200, as recorded by an internal pressure transducer.

Significance: this pattern indicates mild hypoxia and possible cord impingement. Management may include oxygen administration and a maternal position change.

Delivery plans are influenced by the response to the usual attempts taken to improve fetal oxygenation, the anticipated duration to delivery, and the anticipated ease of delivery.

CASE OUTCOME: Twenty-eight-year-old primigravida at 40 weeks' gestation delivered by cesarean section for cephalopelvic disproportion and possible macrosomia a 7 pound, 10½ ounce (3473 gram) female; Apgar score 8/9. The fetus was in a vertex presentation, in an occiput anterior position. "Moderate meconium" was stated to be present. The newborn course was complicated by hyperbilirubinemia, which was treated with phototherapy.

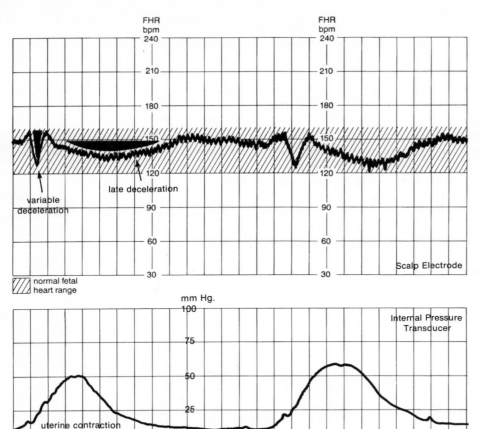

FHR bpm

Pattern Characteristic:
Variable Deceleration(s) and
Late Deceleration(s): Combined
Pattern

normal fetal heart range

Scalp Electrode

mm Hg.

Internal Pressure Transducer

uterine contraction

Variable Deceleration Produced by Hold Mode: Artifact

All fetal monitors are designed to reject artifact through electronic logic. This is activated when an unexpected signal or pause occurs. In some older monitors, the logic circuit first sampled each interval, and if it varied considerably from the previous interval, it was not accepted and the monitor entered a "hold mode" in which the monitor was instructed to keep the rate set at the same rate as the previously accepted interval. With such an artifact suppression system, after an arbitrary time or number of beats, the pen-lift was activated so that no printing resulted at all until a return to the accepted interval occurred.[66] This system is in operation on monitors with early external Doppler systems to avoid recording extraneous noise or movement that would obscure the fetal heart signal. However, with excessive degrees of hold mode the monitor loses true fetal heart data.

A second reason for loss of information in early Doppler systems was "averaging" intervals of at least three beats instead of beat-to-beat intervals. Without averaging the early monitor might print apparent increased variability since the sensing device cannot count the Doppler signal at exactly the same place on each cardiac cycle. With too much averaging there is a loss of important beat-to-beat information. With a three second averaging circuit, at a fetal heart rate of 140 bpm as many as seven beats may be averaged, destined to "smooth" the fetal heart rate. Resulting artifactual information may affect the accuracy of a clinical interpretation.

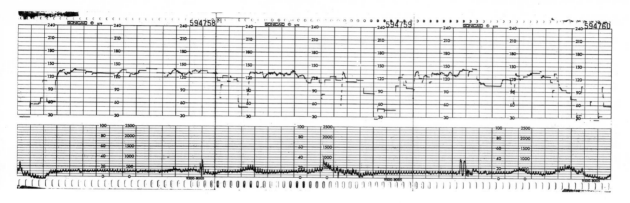

CASE INTERPRETATION: Class 0

Baseline Information: normal rate, areas with normal variability, others where pen holds up to 1½ cm.

Periodic or Nonperiodic changes: appearance of variable decelerations but features are unclear secondary to the hold artifact.

Uterine Activity: small deflections of the tocodynamometer, suggesting mild, infrequent contractions.

Significance: unsatisfactory for interpretation.

CASE OUTCOME: Thirty-year-old gravida 3, para 2002, delivered vaginally, with outlet forceps and pudendal anesthesia, a 9 pound, 2 ounce (4139 gram) male; Apgar score 9/9. The fetus was in a vertex presentation. The delivery was complicated by mild shoulder dystocia. The infant followed a normal newborn course.

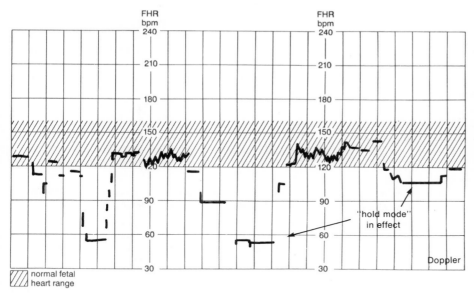

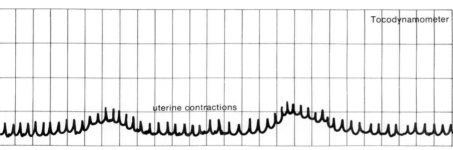

Pattern Characteristic:
Artifactual Variable
Decelerations: Produced by
Hold Mode

References

1. Akagi K, Okamura K, Endo C, et al: The slope of fetal heart rate deceleration is predictive of fetal condition during repeated umbilical cord compression in sheep. *Am J Obstet Gynecol* 159:516, 1988.

2. Beard RW, Filshie GM, Knight CA, et al: The significance of the changes in continuous fetal heart rate recordings. *J Obstet Gynaecol Br Commonw* 78:865, 1971.

3. Bowes WA, Gabbe CC, Dowes C: Fetal heart rate monitoring in premature infants weighing 1,500 grams or less. *Am J Obstet Gynecol* 137:791, 1980.

4. Braithwaite HDJ, Milligan JE, Shennan AT: Fetal heart rate monitoring and neonatal mortality in the very preterm infant. *Am J Obstet Gynecol* 154:250, 1986.

5. Caldeyro-Barcia R, Mendez-Bauer C, Poseiro JJ, et al: Control of human fetal heart rate during labor, in Cassels DE (ed): *The Heart and Circulation of the Newborn Infant*. New York, Grune and Stratton, 1966, p. 7ff.

6. Caldeyro-Barcia R, Schwarcz R, Belizan JM, et al: Adverse perinatal effects of early amniotomy during labor, in Gluck L (ed): *Modern Perinatal Medicine*. Chicago, Yearbook Medical Publishers, 1974, p. 431ff.

7. Cetrulo CK, Schifrin DS: Fetal heart rate patterns preceding death in utero. *Obstet Gynecol* 40:521, 1976.

8. Charonis NC, Wingate MD: Cord involvement bradycardia. *Int J Gynaecol Obstet* 11:5, 1973.

9. Cibils LA: Clinical significance of fetal heart rate patterns during labor. V. Variable decelerations. *Am J Obstet Gynecol* 132:791, 1970.

10. Cibils LA: Variable decelerations, in *Electronic Fetal-Maternal Monitoring: Antepartum, Intrapartum*. Boston, PSG Publishing, 1981, p. 341.

11. Dawes CC, Johnston DM, Walker DW: Relationship of arterial pressure and heart rate in fetal, newborn and adult sheep. *J Physiol* 307:405, 1980.

12. Douvas CC, Meeks CR, Graves C, et al: Intrapartum fetal heart rate monitoring as a predictor of fetal distress and immediate neonatal condition in low birth weight (less than or equal to 1,000 grams) infants. *Am J Obstet Gynecol* 140:300, 1984.

13. Feinstein CJ, Lodeiro JC, Vintzileos AM, et al: Intrapartum ultrasound diagnosis of nuchal cord as a decisive factor in management. *Am J Obstet Gynecol* 153:308, 1985.

14. Fischer WM: Grundlagen und klinishe Wertigkeit der Kardiotokographia, in Fischer WM (ed): *Kardiotodographia, Lehrbuch and Atlas*. Stuttgart, Goerg Thieme Verlag KC, 1976, p. 142ff.

15. Freeman RK, Garite TJ: Instrumentation, artifact detection, and fetal arrhythmias, in *Fetal Heart Rate Monitoring*. Baltimore, William & Wilkins, 1981, p. 12.

16. Gabbe CC, Ottinger DD, Freeman RK, et al: Umbilical cord compression associated with amniotomy: Laboratory observations. *Am J Obstet Gynecol* 126:353, 1976.

17. Garite TJ, Freeman RK: EFM today, case 2: Cord knot may cause atypical pattern. *Contemp Obstet Gynecol* Apr:27, 1983.

18. Garite TJ, Freeman RK: Were the decelerations variable, or late, or both? *Contemp Obstet Gynecol* 12:23, 1982.

19. Garite TJ, Ray DA: Mixed decelerations accompany PROM. *Contemp Obstet Gynecol*, Jan:30, 1987.

20. Gaziano EP: A study of variable decelerations in association with other heart rate patterns during monitored labor. *Am J Obstet Gynecol* 135:360, 1979.

21. Gaziano EP, Freeman DW: Analysis of heart rate patterns preceding fetal death. *Obstet Gynecol* 5:578, 1977.

22. Gimovsky ML, Bruce SL: Aspects of FHR tracings as warning signals. *Clin Obstet Gynecol* 29:51, 1986.

23. Goldkrand JW, Speichinger JP: "Mixed cord compression," fetal heart rate pattern and its relation to abnormal cord position. *Am J Obstet Gynecol* 122:144, 1985.

24. Goodlin RC: Inappropriate fetal bradycardia. *Obstet Gynecol* 40:117, 1976.

25. Goodlin RC, Lowe EW: A functional umbilical cord occlusion heart rate pattern. The significance of overshoot. *Obstet Gynecol* 43:22, 1974.

26. Goodlin RC, Haesslein HC: Fetal reacting bradycardia. *Am J Obstet Gynecol* 29:845, 1977.

27. Goodlin RC: Reacting Fetal Bradycardia, in *Care of the Fetus*. Masson Publishing, 1979:140.

28. Hayashi RH, Fox ME: Unforeseen sudden intrapartum fetal death in a monitored labor. *Am J Obstet Gynecol* 122:786, 1975.

29. Hon EH: The fetal heart rate patterns preceding death in utero. *Am J Obstet Gynecol* 78:47, 1959.

30. Hon EH: *An Introduction to Fetal Heart Rate Monitoring*. Los Angeles, Post-graduate Division, University of Southern California School of Medicine, 1973.

31. Hon EH, Bradfield AH, Hess OW: The electronic evaluation of the fetal heart rate. V. The vagal factor in fetal bradycardia. *Am J Obstet Gynecol* 9:291, 1961.

32. Hon EH, Lee CT: Electronic evaluation of the fetal heart rate. VIII. Patterns preceding fetal death, further observations. *Am J Obstet Gynecol* 87:014, 1963.

33. Hon EH, Quilligan EJ: Electronic evaluation of fetal heart rate. IX. Further observations in "pathologic" fetal bradycardia. *Clin Obstet Gynecol* 11:151, 1968.

34. Hutson JM, Mueller-Heubach E: Diagnosis and management of intrapartum reflex fetal heart rate changes. *Clinics in Perinatology* 9:325, 1982.

35. Ingemarsson E, Ingemarsson I, Solum T, et al: Influence of occipital posterior position on the fetal heart rate pattern. *Obstet Gynecol* 35:301, 1980.

36. Ingemarsson E, Ingemarsson I, Westgren M: Combined decelerations—clinical significance and relation to uterine activity. *Obstet Gynecol* 50:35, 1981.

37. Itkovitz J, LaGamma EF, Rudolph AM: Heart rate and blood pressure responses to umbilical cord compression in

fetal lambs with special reference to the mechanism of variable deceleration. *Am J Obstet Gynecol* 147:451, 1983.

38. James LS, Yeh M, Morishimer HO, et al: Umbilical vein occlusion and transient acceleration of the fetal heart rate. Experimental observations in subhuman primates. *Am J Obstet Gynecol* 126:267, 1976.

39. Judge NE, Mann LI, Lupe P, et al: Clinical associations of variable decelerations during reactive nonstress tests. *Obstet Gynecol* 74:351, 1989.

40. Kariniemi V, Jarvenpaa AL, Teramo K: Fetal heart rate patterns and perinatal outcomes of very low birthweight infants. *Br J Obstet Gynaecol* 91:18, 1984.

41. Kates RD, Schifrin BS: Fetal cardiac asystole during labor. *Obstet Gynecol* 67:549, 1986.

42. Katz M, Dokal MM, Lilling M, et al: Neonatal heart rate reactivity following variable decelerations during labor. *Am J Obstet Gynecol* 136:309, 1980.

43. Klaven M, Laver AT, Boscola MA: Periodic fetal heart rate (periodic patterns), in *Clinical Concepts of Fetal Heart Rate Monitoring*. Chester, PA, 1973, p. 50.

44. Krebs H-B: Fetal heart rate W-sign (letter to the editor). *Obstet Gynecol* 65:448, 1985.

45. Krebs H-B, Petres RE, Dunn LJ, et al: Intrapartum fetal heart rate monitoring. I. Classification and prognosis of fetal heart rate patterns. *Am J Obstet Gynecol* 133:762, 1979.

46. Krebs H-B, Petres RE, Dunn LJ: Intrapartum fetal heart rate monitoring. V. Fetal heart rate patterns in the second stage of labor. *Am J Obstet Gynecol* 140:435, 1981.

47. Krebs H-B, Petres RE, Dunn LJ: Intrapartum fetal heart rate monitoring. VIII. Atypical variable decelerations. *Am J Obstet Gynecol* 145:297, 1983.

48. Kubli FW, Hon EH, Khazin AF, et al: Observations on heart rate and pH in the human fetus during labor. *Am J Obstet Gynecol* 104:1190, 1969.

49. Kunzel W, Mann LI, Bhakthavathsalan A, et al: Metabolic fetal brain function and cardiovascular observations following total cord occlusion, in *Fetal and Newborn Cardiovascular Physiology*, Longo and Reneau (eds). Garland Publishing 1978, p. 301.

50. Martin CD: Regulation of the fetal heart rate and genesis of FHR patterns. *Seminars in Perinatology* 2:131, 1978.

51. Martin CD, Siassi D, Hon EH: Fetal heart rate patterns and neonatal death in low birthweight infants. *Obstet Gynecol* 44:503, 1974.

52. Mega M, Ceruth R, Miccoli P, et al: Usefulness of cardiotocography in expulsion period. *Clin Exp Obst Gyn* 8:111, 1981.

53. Meis PJ, Ureda JR, Swain M, et al: Variable decelerations during nonstress tests are not a sign of fetal compromise. *Am J Obstet Gynecol* 154:586, 1986.

54. Mendez-Bauer C, Canseco AR, Ruiz MA, et al: Early decelerations of the fetal heart rate from occlusion of the umbilical cord. *J Perinat Med* 6:67, 1970.

55. Miyasaki FS: Relieving variable decelerations. *Contemporary OB/GYN* Feb.:23, 1987.

56. Miyazaki FS, Nevarez F: Saline amnioinfusion for relief of repetitive variable decelerations: A prospective randomized study. *Am J Obstet Gynecol* 153:301, 1985.

57. Mueller-Heubach E, Battelli AF: Variable heart rate decelerations and transcutaneous PO₂ during umbilical cord occlusion in fetal monkeys. *Am J Obstet Gynecol* 144:796, 1982.

58. Murakami M, Kanzaki T, Utsu M, et al: Changes in the umbilical venous blood flow of human fetus in labor. *Acta Obst Gynaec Jpn* 37:776, 1985.

59. Nakamura KT, Smith BA, Erenberg A, et al: Changes in arterial blood gases following cardiac asystole during fetal life. *Obstet Gynecol* 70:16, 1987.

60. Nageotte MP, Freeman RK, Garite TJ, et al: Prophylactic intrapartum amnioinfusion in patients with preterm premature rupture of membranes. *J Obstet Gynecol* 153:557, 1985.

61. O'Gureck JC, Roux JF, Neuman MR: A practical classification of fetal heart rate patterns. *Obstet Gynecol* 40:356, 1972.

62. O'Leary JA, Andrinopoulos GC, Giordano PC: Variable decelerations and the nonstress test: An indication of cord compromise. *Am J Obstet Gynecol* 137:704, 1980.

63. Parer J: Basic patterns, their classification and in utero treatment, in *Handbook of Fetal Heart Rate Monitoring*. Philadelphia, W.B. Saunders, 1983, p. 99.

64. Parer J: Fetal heart rate patterns preceding death in utero, in *Handbook of Fetal Heart Rate Monitoring*. Philadelphia, W.B. Saunders, 1983, p. 147.

65. Paul RH, Petrie R: *Fetal Intensive Care*, Corometrics Medical Systems, Inc., 1979, p. III-4, vol 3, Wallingford, CT.

66. Penlift circuit, artifact suppression circuit, 3 second averaging circuit, in *Sonicaid Service Manual*. Fredericksburg, VA. Modular Fetal Monitor FM3 R, 1981, p. 17.

67. Phelan JP, Lewis PE: Fetal heart rate decelerations during a nonstress test. *Obstet Gynecol* 57:220, 1981.

68. Schifrin BS: Personal communication.

69. Serafini PC, Amisial PA, Murgalo JA, et al: Unusual fetal heart rate pattern associated with severe neonatal asphyxia and death. *Am J Obstet Gynecol* 140:715, 1981.

70. Shields JR, Schifrin BS: Perinatal antecedents of cerebral palsy. *Obstet Gynecol* 71:899, 1988.

71. Sokol RJ, Roux JF, McCarthy S: Computer diagnosis of labor progression. VI. Fetal stress and labor in the occipitoposterior position. *Am J Ob Gynecol* 122:253, 1975.

72. Sorokin Y, Bottoms SF, Dierker LJ, et al: The clustering of fetal heart rate changes and fetal movements in pregnancies between 20 and 30 weeks of gestation. *Am J Obstet Gynecol* 143:952, 1982.

73. Tejani NA, Mann LI, Sanghave M, et al: The association of umbilical cord complications and variable decelerations with acid-base findings. *Obstet Gynecol* 47:157, 1977.

74. Towell ME, Lysak I: Mild umbilical cord compression and arterial blood gases in the fetal lamb, in Longo and Kenean (eds).: *Fetal and Newborn Cardiovascular Physiology*, Garland Publishing, 1978, p. 290.

75. Welt GI: The fetal heart rate W-sign. *Obstet Gynecol* 63:405, 1984.

76. Westgrand M, Holmquist P, Ingemarsson I, et al: Intrapartum fetal acidosis in preterm infants: Fetal monitoring and long-term morbidity. *Obstet Gynecol* 63:355, 1984.

77. Westgrand M, Holmquist P, Svenningsen NW, et al: Intrapartum fetal monitoring in preterm deliveries: Prospective study. *Obstet Gynecol* 60:77, 1982.

78. Wood C, Yu V: Obstetric care of the very premature fetus. *Aust NZ J Obstet Gynaec* 20:28, 1980.

79. Yeh M-N, Morishima HO, Niemann WH, et al: Myocardial conduction defects in association with compression of the umbilical cord. Experimental observations on fetal baboons. *Am J Obstet Gynecol* 121:951, 1975.

80. Yeh S-Y, Zanini B, Petrie RH, et al: Intrapartum fetal cardiac arrest. A preliminary observation. *Obstet Gynecol* 50:571, 1977.

81. Young BK, Katz M, Wilson SJ: Fetal blood and tissue pH with variable deceleration patterns. *Obstet Gynecol* 56:170, 1980.

82. Young M, Cottom D: An investigation of baroreceptor responses in the newborn infant, in Cassells DE, ed. *The Heart and Circulation of the Newborn Infant*. New York, Grune and Stratton, 1966, p. 111.

83. Zanini B, Paul RH, Huey JR: Intrapartum fetal heart rate: Correlation with scalp pH in the preterm fetus. *Am J Obstet Gynecol* 136:43, 1980.

84. Zilianti M, Segura CL, Cabello F, et al: Studies on fetal bradycardia during birth process I. *Obstet Gynecol* 42:831, 1973.

85. Zilianti M, Segura CL, Cabello F, et al: Studies on fetal bradycardia during birth process II. *Obstet Gynecol* 42:840, 1973.

Late/Variable Decelerations

Chapter 13

Late/Variable Decelerations: S-Sign

A distinct fetal monitoring heart rate pattern has been identified in association with chronic oligohydramnios.[3,8,9] The pattern is characterized by late-occurring atypical variable decelerations with a loss of baseline *and* deceleration variability. Prolonged secondary accelerations combined with the smooth contour of the nadir of the deceleration and a sloping ascending limb produce a smoothly curved pattern with an S configuration.[18] Therefore, here it is given the term "S-sign." Study of the proposed etiology of the pattern leads to a better understanding of these characteristic features. The pattern has been associated with oligohydramnios of a chronic nature, which was first reported as a finding during oxytocin challenge tests that were performed in cases with growth-retarded fetuses.[3,8,9] The particular configuration is believed to be caused by umbilical cord impingement of a chronic nature (such as that caused by vulnerability secondary to oligohydramnios) and superimposed acute hypoxia (such as that caused by further cord impingement with uterine contractions). It is very likely that chronic uteroplacental insufficiency and its attendant fetal hypoxemia, or other causes underlying the intrauterine growth retardation, also contribute to the pattern.[3,4,9,20,26,29] Because subsequent outcomes in early reported cases indicated significant intrauterine growth retardation and poor newborn performance, prompt delivery has been recommended as an appropriate response when encountering this type of pattern with a viable fetus.[5,6,7,8]

A similar pattern may develop in the presence of oligohydramnios caused by other etiologies (see the following pages). This pattern has also been documented as a transient finding during a maternal systemic allergic reaction.[16] Occasionally, an S-shape appears in the ascending limb of an atypical variable deceleration that otherwise retains a jagged wave-form and has normal baseline features. Although the pattern atypia indicates concern, the implication is not as ominous as the fully developed S-sign.

Not all variable decelerations encountered during antepartum testing require such immediate intervention. Small, V-shaped decelerations with a jagged waveform are often encountered when monitoring the healthy fetus and are perhaps secondary to transient umbilical cord impingement produced by fetal movement (see page 261).[21] It is not surprising that various configurations of variable decelerations encountered during antepartum monitoring have been associated with an increased incidence of "vulnerable cord" locations, as noted by intrapartum heart rate patterns and at delivery.[1,2,27,28] The response to variable decelerations encountered in antepartum monitoring is individualized according to the appearance of the deceleration and the original indication for monitoring.[13,24,27,32] In some cases, management may include ultrasonography and contraction stress testing.[31]

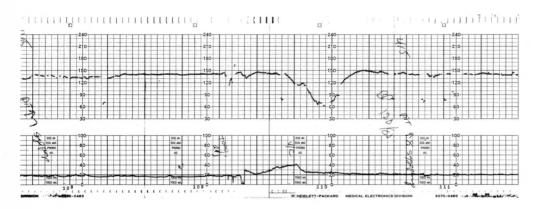

CASE INTERPRETATION: Class V

Baseline Information: normal rate, absent variability.

Periodic or Nonperiodic Changes: late/variable decelerations with an S configuration on an ascending limb that is produced by absent variability in the deceleration and prolonged secondary acceleration. S sign.

Uterine Activity: a single, small contraction that is slightly skewed, as measured by an external monitor.

Significance: a pattern seen with chronic oligohydramnios, as with intrauterine growth retardation or fetal oliguria. Prompt delivery is usually indicated if the fetus is viable.

CASE OUTCOME: Sixteen-year-old primigravida delivered at 33 weeks' gestation a 2 pound, 1¾ ounce (957 gram) stillborn female. This tracing was obtained seven days before the intrauterine fetal death. Intervention was not performed because an ultrasonographic study predicted a fetal weight below viability at that time (less than 500 grams) and severe oligohydramnios. The fetus had no detected anomalies. The patient became pregnant on two more occasions, both resulting in growth retarded infants who survived.

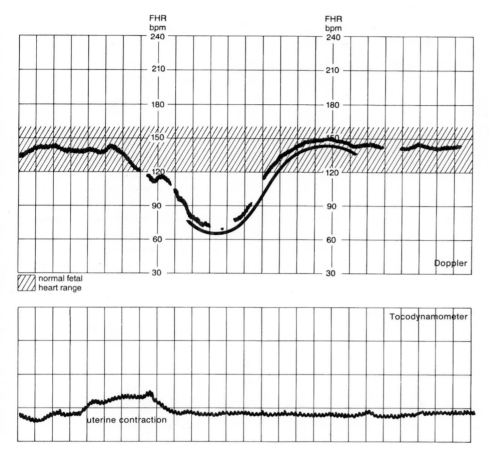

Pattern Characteristic:
Late/Variable Decelerations:
S-Sign Oligohydramnios
Intrauterine Growth Retardation

Late/Variable Decelerations: S-Shape

*L*ate/variable deceleration patterns may display an S-shape without the more ominous loss of deceleration and baseline variability features reserved for the S-sign (see page 298). The pattern has subsequently been identified with other causes of chronic oligohydramnios other than intrauterine growth retardation, including prolonged pregnancy and severe maternal hemoglobinopathy and major fetal congenital abnormalities.[14,22,25] Also included in this text are cases in which there is a lack of fetal urine contribution to the amniotic fluid secondary to urinary tract obstruction or a lack of urine production altogether.

The fetus with anuria on the basis of renal maldevelopment or obstruction has a milieu for chronic cord impingement. S-shaped late/variable decelerations have been detected in such circumstances.[30] However, this pattern is not pathognomonic of fetal anuria, nor does it appear in all situations of renal agenesis (see page 5a). The preservation of baseline variability in such patients suggests that chronic placental insufficiency must play an additional role in the development of the S-sign, as seen with oligohydramnios on the basis of intrauterine growth retardation.[3,9,20]

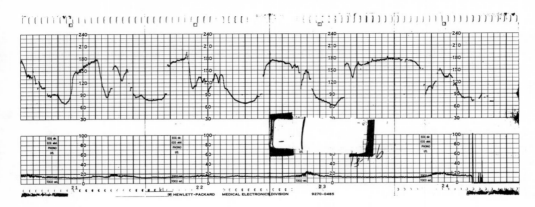

CASE INTERPRETATION: Class V

Baseline Information: moderate tachycardia, unstable diminished variability.

Periodic or Nonperiodic Changes: late/variable decelerations with an S configuration on an ascending limb, which is produced by the absence of variability in the deceleration and a prolonged secondary acceleration.

Uterine Activity: poorly displayed, denoted by change in maternal respiration intermittently.

Significance: the pattern retains some jagged features, although these may be exaggerated by external monitor-

ing. It is seen with chronic oligohydramnios, as is present with intrauterine growth retardation or absent fetal urinary output. Prompt delivery is usually indicated if the fetus is viable.

CASE OUTCOME: Twenty-seven-year-old gravida 2, para 1001, at 31 weeks' gestation delivered by repeat cesarean section, with inhalation anesthesia, a 3 pound, 6½ ounce (1545 gram) male; Apgar score 3/5. The labor was premature. The fetus was in a breech presentation. The newborn expired at 17 hours of age with renal agenesis and pulmonary hypoplasia.

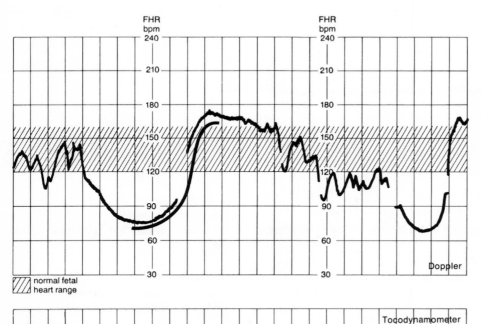

Pattern Characteristic:
Late/Variable Decelerations:
S-Shaped Oligohydramnios,
Renal Agenesis

Agonal Late/Variable Decelerations

*L*ate/variable decelerations are identified by an S configuration of the ascending limb of a smooth atypical variable deceleration that occurs late in relationship to uterine contractions. These are considered to have an "ominous" connotation when associated with loss of variability and loss of stability of the baseline heart rate, with the etiology believed to be hypoxia that is produced by the chronic and acute effects of umbilical cord impingement.

If labor progresses without intervention (as may be allowed to occur with a nonviable fetus because of immature gestation or anomalies that are believed to be lethal), the features that once were recognizable as those of variable decelerations may become so blunted as to simulate the smoother characteristics of late decelerations.[3,9]

When the smooth prolonged secondary acceleration is followed immediately by the next smooth deceleration, the overall pattern assumes an undulating appearance (nonsinusoidal premortem [see page 136]), which has been further associated with poor fetal outcome, and even fetal or newborn death.

Although on occasion such a pattern may be produced by causes of an acute nature, which are potentially reversible, it is more likely, despite prompt delivery upon encountering this pattern, to find an already compromised newborn, which emphasizes the chronic nature of the adverse fetal effects often underlying this pattern.[3,9,12,17,34]

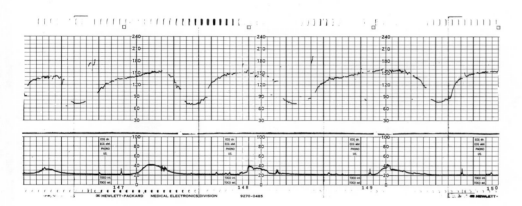

CASE INTERPRETATION: Class V

Baseline Information: almost obscured by decelerations, high normal rate, absent variability.

Periodic or Nonperiodic Changes: late/variable decelerations with an S configuration of an ascending limb, which is produced by absent variability and prolonged secondary acceleration. Onset of each deceleration occurs before the preceding deceleration recovers.

Uterine Activity: small, skewed contractions, as measured by external monitoring.

Significance: a pattern seen with chronic oligohydramnios, as in intrauterine growth retardation. Prompt delivery is indicated if the fetus is viable.

CASE OUTCOME: Thirty-three-year-old gravida 2, para 1001, at term delivered vaginally, with pudendal anesthesia, a 3 pound, 7 ounce (1559 gram) male stillborn. The fetus was in a vertex presentation. The cord was wrapped around the neck three times. There was severe oligohydramnios and intrauterine growth retardation, as detected by ultrasonography. The massive cystic dilatation of abdominal structures led to the decision not to do a cesarean section for fetal distress. The fetal death occurred intrapartum. An autopsy showed only intrauterine growth retardation, with no gastrointestinal anomalies.

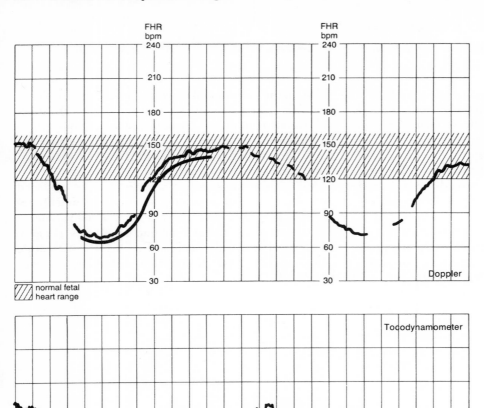

Pattern Characteristic:
Agonal Late/Variable
Decelerations: S-Sign
Oligohydramnios

Late/Variable Decelerations with Slow Return

*W*hen hypoxia produced by the effects of cord compression is seen in the same clinical situation as hypoxia produced by other causes such as placental insufficiency, mixed features may be seen in the resulting fetal heart rate pattern.

Cord impingement, per se, is reflected by variable decelerations of a classic configuration, with varying degrees of depth and duration. Atypical features, when present, suggest varying degrees of superimposed hypoxia and/or acidosis that result from the impingement. When atypical variable decelerations occur late, with a smoothing of the contour, both acute and chronic hypoxia secondary to the cord impingement is suggested,

as is seen with certain clinical situations involving prolonged oligohydramnios. Deficient transplacental oxygen exchange, whether it is secondary to placental surface or vascular limitations or to relative maternal hypoxia, is typically reflected by late decelerations. When the hypoxia changes appear simultaneously with variable decelerations, the net result is either a slow return to baseline for the variable decelerations, as illustrated here, or a combination pattern (see page 304).

An example of a clinical setting which has been associated with the production of such a pattern is diabetes mellitus coexisting with intrauterine growth retardation.[29]

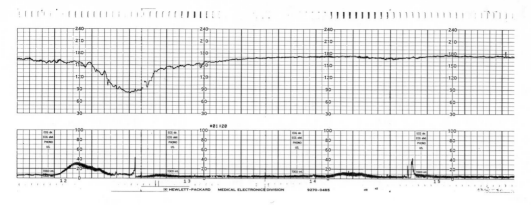

CASE INTERPRETATION: Class V

Baseline Information: a normal baseline rate and diminished beat-to-beat variability, loss of variability and rebound tachycardia during the recovery phase of deceleration.

Periodic or Nonperiodic Changes: a late/variable deceleration with an S-shape of the ascending limb that is partially obliterated by a slow return to baseline, possibly secondary to a polysystolic contraction or a late deceleration component.

Uterine Activity: skewed and polysystolic uterine contractions that are accentuated by maternal respiratory activity.

Significance: a pattern compatible with both hypoxia, as seen with chronic cord impingement produced by chronic oligohydramnios, and placental insufficiency.

CASE OUTCOME: Twenty-five-year-old gravida 3, para 1001, at 33 weeks' gestation delivered by repeat cesarean section a 6 pound, 5½ ounce (2877 gram) female; Apgar score 2/8. The fetus was in a vertex presentation. The maternal course was complicated by poorly controlled insulin-dependent diabetes (class C). The initial attempts to arrest premature labor with tocolytic therapy were abandoned. The newborn was dismissed with the mother at six days of life. No late third trimester ultrasonography was done.

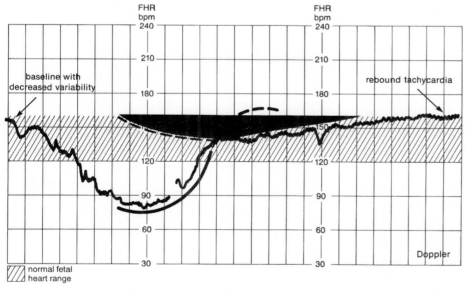

Pattern Characteristic:
Late/Variable Decelerations:
S-Sign Slow Recovery

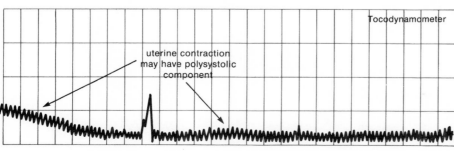

Late/Variable Decelerations with Late Decelerations: Combined Pattern

A single fetus may simultaneously demonstrate features of hypoxia secondary to the effects of cord impingement and the effects of insufficient transplacental oxygen exchange. Fetal monitoring patterns, when these occur independently of each other, are typically variable decelerations and late decelerations. When occurring simultaneously, they may either be seen as a mixed pattern (variable decelerations with slow recovery (see page 246) or as a combination pattern (variable decelerations followed by late decelerations), or as demonstrated here, late/variable decelerations followed by late decelerations.[15]

The fact that by such a pattern the fetus is demonstrating dual sources of hypoxia increases concern.[11,33] Interpretation is focused on individual features of the respective decelerations as well as on baseline changes. Management is directed at improving both transplacental oxygen exchange and umbilical flow, when feasible.

However, when the variable decelerations are identified as late/variable by their smooth configuration, prompt delivery is also an appropriate intervention for the fetus at a gestation compatible with viability since a chronic (less reversible) disease process is suggested as well as an acute process.

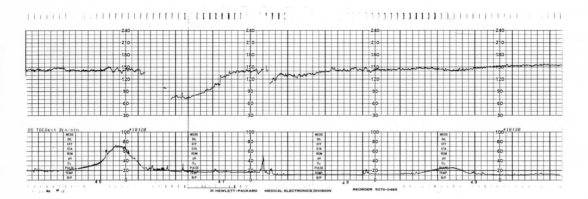

CASE INTERPRETATION: Class V

Baseline Information: normal rate, average to decreased variability.

Periodic or Nonperiodic Changes: late/variable decelerations with an S-shaped configuration of the ascending limb followed by late decelerations (combined pattern).

Uterine Activity: infrequent contractions of a normal configuration. Rapid maternal breathing is depicted.

Significance: this is a pattern seen with cord-impingement hypoxia of a chronic nature, which is associated with oligohydramnios such as is produced by intrauterine growth retardation or fetal anuria plus superimposed acute hypoxia in combination with placental insufficiency.

CASE OUTCOME: Thirty-one-year-old primigravida at 41 weeks' gestation delivered by cesarean section, with general anesthesia, for probable fetal distress, a 6 pound, 15 ounce (3147 gram) male; Apgar score 8/9. The fetus was in a vertex presentation. There was an intrapartum ultrasonic diagnosis of oligohydramnios and a fetal cystic abdominal mass that was believed to represent a urinary tract obstruction. The newborn was diagnosed as having a hydronephrotic left kidney and a multicystic dysplastic right kidney. The newborn underwent pyeloplasty of the left proximal ureter.

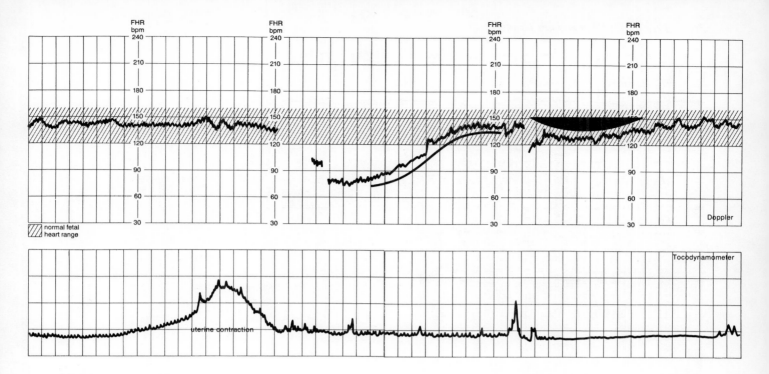

Pattern Characteristic:
Late/Variable Decelerations with Late Decelerations: Oligohydramnios,
Urinary Tract Obstruction—Combined Pattern

Late, or Late/Variable Decelerations?

*I*t may be difficult to distinguish late decelerations from late/variable decelerations, especially when the late variable decelerations exhibit a slow return to baseline.[10]

Hypoxia and acidosis may cause progressive smoothing of a late/variable deceleration sufficient enough to give a uniform appearance, especially when there is a loss of primary and secondary accelerations.

On the other hand, late decelerations may lose their uniform appearance and assume more of a "V"-shape when reflecting contractions that are peaked in configuration.

A delayed return to baseline may be present with both patterns. It may be produced by "late" components superimposed on late/variable decelerations or, in the case of late decelerations, by reflecting skewed contractions.

Except for helping to clarify the underlying pathophysiology of the fetal stimuli, the distinction is academic because both late and late/variable decelerations with poor variability in both the baseline and the decelerations suggest a compromised fetus with a high enough possibility of acidosis to usually warrant intervention by delivery.

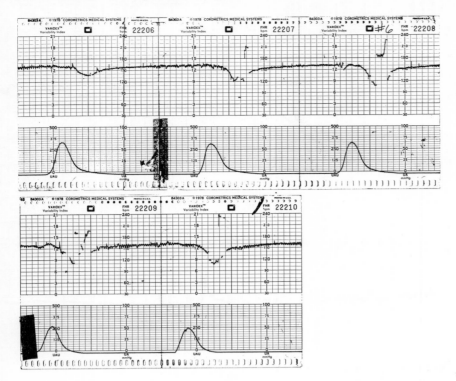

CASE INTERPRETATION: Class V

Baseline Information: high normal rate, absent variability.

Periodic or Nonperiodic Changes: late/variable decelerations with a slow return to baseline (combined pattern), a configuration reflecting skewed contractions or late decelerations.

Uterine Activity: peaked, minimally skewed contractions, as measured by external monitoring with the baseline set low on the paper, which potentially could result in loss of information.

Significance: suggests a chronically compromised fetus with both cord and placental contributions to hypoxia. Prompt delivery is in order if the fetus is viable in most clinical circumstances.

CASE OUTCOME: Twenty-one-year-old primigravida delivered at 27 weeks' gestation by cesarean section performed for probable fetal distress, with general anesthesia, a 2 pound, 8 ounce (1134 gram) female; Apgar score 1/6. The maternal course was complicated by eclampsia. The newborn survived without significant complications.

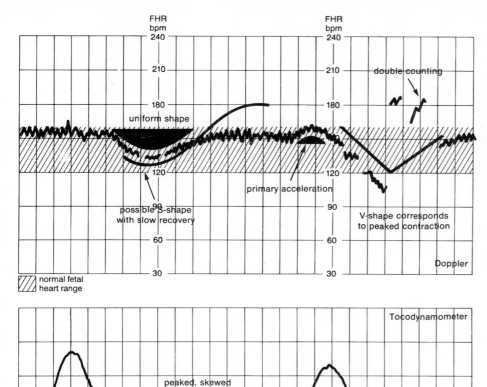

FHR
bpm

normal fetal
heart range

Pattern Characteristic:
Late, or Late/Variable
Decelerations? Mixed Features

Late-Occurring Variable Decelerations with S-Shape

*O*ccasionally, an S-shape appears in the ascending limb of an atypical variable deceleration in which there is both loss of variability in the deceleration and a prolonged secondary acceleration, but with otherwise normal variability in the baseline, in the other components of the variable deceleration, and in the accompanying decelerations. Such a deceleration meets the criteria for an atypical variable deceleration and, therefore, has an increased risk of a low Apgar score and/or fetal acidosis and hypoxia. The pattern, at least in part, may be expected to be produced by cord compression. However, the pres-

ervation of beat-to-beat variability in portions of the trace does not suggest the chronic hypoxic process associated with patterns that are reserved for the "S-sign." It may be that such a pattern is able to develop in labor, with cord impingement occurring during the course of oligohydramnios of a relatively short duration such as is encountered with postdate pregnancy and with premature rupture of membranes, a transient urinary tract obstruction, or even in a normal fetus with a normal milieu.[19,23,35]

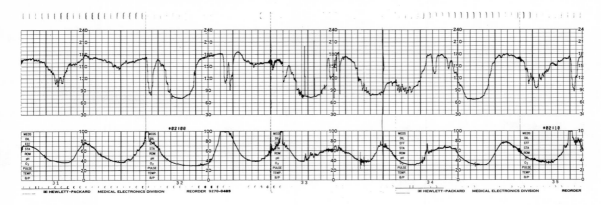

CASE INTERPRETATION: Class IV

Baseline Information: generally unstable and often obscured by frequent decelerations and secondary accelerations. Baseline variability appears to be average in some areas and diminished in others.

Periodic or Nonperiodic Changes: mild, moderate, and severe variable decelerations. Some retain classic features, others display various forms of atypica, including the loss of primary accelerations, the loss of variability, and prolonged secondary acceleration.

Uterine Activity: frequent skewed contractions with varying intensity, an absent resting phase, and an elevated uterine tone.

Significance: some decelerations occur during peak uterine activity and others are late in occurrence. This finding, plus multiple decelerative components in some of the decelerations (W-shape), suggest cord impingement in varying locations and to varying degrees.

CASE OUTCOME: Twenty-three-year-old primigravida delivered at 40 weeks' gestation by primary cesarean section for dystocia coupled with possible fetal distress a 7 pound, 4 ounce (3289 gram) female; Apgar score 3/8. Duplicate scalp pHs were 7.25; cord pHs were 7.13 arterial and 7.2 venous. An attempt was made to relieve cord impingement by amniofusion. Thick meconium was present. The newborn course was uneventful, and the infant was dismissed on the fifth day of life.

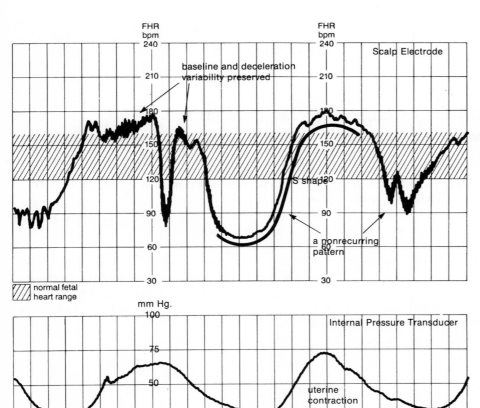

Pattern Characteristic:
Late-Occurring Variable
Decelerations with S Shape

References

1. Anyaegbunam A, Bruetman L, Divan M, et al: The significance of antepartum variable decelerations. *Am J Obstet Gynecol* 155:707, 1986.

2. Barrett JM, Salyer SL, Boehm FH: Variable decelerations on nonstress test of monoamniotic twins. *Am J Obstet Gynecol* 141:503, 1981.

3. Baskett TF, Sandy EA: The oxytocin challenge test: An ominous pattern associated with severe fetal growth retardation. *Obstet Gynecol* 54:365, 1979.

4. Bekedam DJ, Visser GHA, Mueder EJH, et al: Heart rate variation and movement incidence in growth-retarded fetuses: The significance of antenatal late heart rate decelerations. *Am J Obstet Gynecol* 157:126, 1987.

5. Bourgeois FJ, Thiagariah S, Harbert GM: The significance of fetal heart rate decelerations during nonstress testing. *Am J Obstet Gynecol* 153:213, 1984.

6. Caldeyro-Barcia R, Mendez-Bauer C, Poseiro JJ, et al: Control of human fetal heart rate during labor, in Cassels DE (ed): *The Heart and Circulation of the Newborn and Infant.* New York, Grune and Stratton, 1966, pp. 7–36.

7. Dashow EE, Read JA: Significant fetal bradycardia during antepartum heart rate testing. *Am J Obstet Gynecol* 148:187, 1984.

8. Fairbrother PF, Van Coeverden De Groot HA, Coetzee EJ, et al: The significance of prelabour type II deceleration of fetal heart rate in relation to Braxton-Hicks contractions. *S.A. Medical Journal* November 30, p. 2391, 1974.

9. Freeman RK, James J: Clinical experience with the oxytocin challenge test. *Obstet Gynecol* 46:255, 1975.

10. Garite TJ, Freeman RK: Equal time—were the decelerations variable, or late, or both? *Contemporary OB/GYN* 19:23, 1982.

11. Garite TJ, Ray DA: Mixed decelerations accompanying PROM. *Contemp Obstet Gynecol* Jan:30, 1987.

12. Gaziano EP: A study of variable deceleration in association with other heart rate patterns during monitored labor. *Am J Obstet Gynecol* 135:360, 1979.

13. Hagay ZJ, Mazor M, Lieberman JR, et al: The significance of single sporadic deceleration during a nonstress test. *Europ J Obstet Gynec Reprod Biol* 15:165, 1983.

14. Hughes RS, Gonik B, Rivera-Alsina ME, et al: Continuous fetal monitoring during partial exchange transfusion in a patient with sickle cell disease crisis. *Am J Obstet Gynecol* 149:819, 1984.

15. Ingemarsson E, Ingemarsson I, Westgren M: Combined decelerations: Clinical significance and relation to uterine activity. *Obstet Gynecol* 58:35, 1984.

16. Klein VR, Harris AP, Abraham RA, et al: Fetal distress during a maternal systemic allergic reaction. *Obstet Gynecol* 64:158, 1984.

17. Langer O, Sonnendecker EWW, Jacobson MJ: Categorization of terminal fetal heart-rate patterns in antepartum cardiotocography. *Brit J Obstet Gynaecol* 89:179, 1982.

18. Lee CY, Drukker B: The nonstress test for the antepartum assessment of fetal reserve. *Am J Obstet Gynecol* 134:460, 1979.

19. Leveno KJ, Quirk JG, Cunningham FG, et al: Prolonged pregnancy. I. Observations concerning the cause of fetal distress. *Am J Obstet Gynecol* 150:465, 1984.

20. Lin C-C, Devoe LD, River P, et al: Oxytocin challenge test and intrauterine growth retardation. *Am J Obstet Gynecol* 140:282, 1981.

21. Meis PJ, Ureda JR, Swain M, et al: Variable decelerations during nonstress tests are not a sign of fetal compromise. *Am J Obstet Gynecol* 154:586, 1986.

22. Moberg LJ, Garite TH, Freeman RK: Fetal heart rate patterns and fetal distress in patients with preterm premature rupture of membranes. *Obstet Gynecol* 64:60, 1984.

23. Molloy C, Bernstine R: Fetal heart rate deceleration patterns during antepartum nonstress testing. *Journal of ADA* 85:637, 1985.

24. Myazaki FS, Myazaki BA: False reactive nonstress test in postterm pregnancies. *Am J Obstet Gynecol* 140:269, 1981.

25. Navot D, Mor-Yosef S, Granat M, et al: Antepartum fetal heart rate pattern associated with major congenital malformations. *Obstet Gynecol* 63:414, 1984.

26. Odendall H: Fetal heart rate patterns in patients with intrauterine growth retardation. *Obstet Gynecol* 48:187, 1976.

27. Odendaal HJ: Variable decelerations of the fetal heart rate during antenatal monitoring. *S Afr Med J* 59:979, 1981.

28. O'Leary JA, Andrinopoulos GC, Giordano PC: Variable decelerations and the nonstress test: An indication of cord compromise. *Am J Obstet Gynecol* 137:704, 1980.

29. Pazos R, Vuolo K, Aladiem S, et al: Association of spontaneous fetal heart rate decelerations during antepartum nonstress testing and intrauterine growth retardation. *Am J Obstet Gynecol* 144:574, 1982.

30. Peleg D, Dicker D, Samuel N, et al: FHR patterns in Potter's syndrome. *J Perinat Med* 11:179, 1983.

31. Phelan JP, Lewes PE: Fetal heart rate decelerations during a nonstress test. *Obstet Gynecol* 57:228, 1981.

32. Trimbos JB, Keires MJNC: Nonspecific decelerations in fetal heart rate during high-risk pregnancy. *Brit J Obstet Gynec* 84:732, 1977.

33. Tushuizen PGT, Stoot JEGM, Ubachs JMH: Fetal heart rate monitoring of the dying fetus. *Am J Obstet Gynecol* 120:922, 1974.

34. Visser GHA, Redman CWG, Huisies HJ, et al: Nonstressed antepartum heart rate monitoring: Implications of decelerations after spontaneous contractions. *Am J Obstet Gynecol* 138:429, 1980.

35. Vintzileos AM, Campbell WA, Nochimson DJ, et al: Degree of oligohydramnios and pregnancy outcome in patients with premature rupture of membranes. *Obstet Gynecol* 66:162, 1985.

Prolonged Decelerations

Chapter 14

Prolonged Deceleration Associated with Maternal Hypotension

*P*rolonged decelerations are defined as decelerations lasting more than two to three minutes.[18] The term "bradycardia" is reserved for decreases in fetal heart rate that exceed 10 minutes in duration.[20] It is not necessary to use terms such as "late" or "variable" or "periodic" or "nonperiodic" in describing prolonged decelerations. Most begin with sinus node suppression that is induced by a burst of vagal activity. The etiology may vary from a relatively benign reflex response such as to scalp electrode placement to significant fetal hypoxic effects of increased uterine activity or maternal hypotension. Less frequent causes are umbilical cord impingement or prolapse, placental abruption, uterine rupture, maternal seizure, status asthmaticus, local decreased perfusion secondary to paracervical block or maternal cardiorespiratory collapse.[4,38,41] Also described are prolonged decelerations that are believed to be produced by fetal sucking or grunting.[25]

Prolonged decelerations produced by maternal hypotension are most commonly associated with a supine position. This may be aggravated by the sympatholytic effects of regional anesthesia or any other cause of decreased uterine blood flow.[1,8,9,26,40] The supine position allows progressive compression of the vena cava and aorta.[2,44] Maternal brachial blood pressure may not reflect the true hypoperfusion in the uterus because uterine circulation is distal to the aortic compression.[5] Maternal hypotension is minimized by hydration and a lateral position in labor.[32,58]

A prolonged deceleration resulting from a hypoxic fetal insult often demonstrates increased variability at onset followed by sinus node suppression with an escape rhythm and, again, a demonstration of increased variability upon recovery. If the hypoxic episodes stimulated the protective compensatory mechanism of shunting blood from less critical structures to vital organs, the recovery phase typically exhibits rebound tachycardia that is believed to be secondary to circulating catecholamines and a transient loss of variability that is caused by the mobilization of acids produced by anaerobic metabolism during the transient hypoxia. Occasionally, a prolonged recovery, including transitory late decelerations and a sinusoidal pattern, is seen.[12] The long-term effects on the newborn of prolonged decelerations with prolonged recovery episodes are unknown.[59]

Although normal fetuses have been delivered after prolonged decelerations (acute bradycardia) lasting more than 15 minutes, steps to effect delivery are usually appropriate with the failure of initiation of recovery after five minutes of attempted in utero resuscitation or after progressive recurrence without an identifiable correctable cause.[19,34,37] Such delivery is ideally accomplished by 10 to 15 minutes after the initial deceleration, longer duration to delivery times may be acceptable when continued fetal perfusion is satisfactory for oxygenation. See p. 320 for a discussion of the problem of failure of recovery from prolonged decelerations in postdate pregnancy.

The previously uncompromised fetus is unlikely to suffer a sufficient enough insult to produce permanent neurologic sequelae if the recovery phase exhibits a prompt progression toward a resumption of predeceleration status with only brief periods of increased variability, rebound tachycardia, and decreased variability.[12,51] These reflect normal compensatory mechanisms of the healthy fetus.

Management is directed toward correcting the inciting mechanism. Such measures may include a position change and hydration (if supine aortocaval compression is an etiologic factor), discontinuing drug treatment (if drug-induced uterine tetany produced the deceleration), tocolytic therapy (if spontaneous uterine hyperactivity has occurred), examination and relief of pressure on a prolapsed cord, or treatment of a maternal seizure.[23] Saline amnioinfusion has been effective in the relief of repetitive prolonged decelerations in some instances.[46]

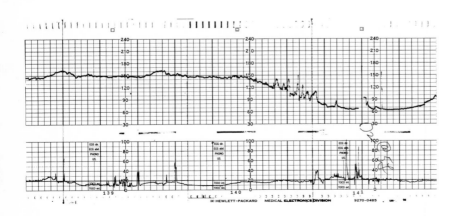

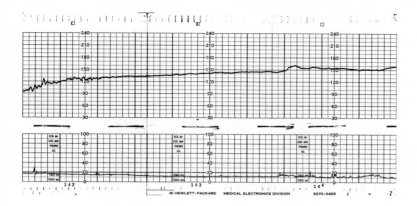

CASE INTERPRETATION: Class II

Baseline Information: normal rate and variability.

Periodic or Nonperiodic Changes: a prolonged deceleration that is eight minutes in total duration.

Uterine Activity: none recorded.

Significance: rapid recovery suggests a transient acute insult, for example, supine hypotension or uterine hyperactivity. This pattern indicates a basically healthy fetus, who is probably not significantly postdate.

CASE OUTCOME: Twenty-three-year-old primigravida at 40 weeks' gestation delivered vaginally, with outlet forceps and epidural anesthesia, an 8 pound, 9 ounce (3884 gram) male; Apgar score 9/9. The fetus was in a vertex presentation, and the mother was supine and undergoing catheterization of the urinary bladder at the time of the deceleration. The mother was immediately turned to the right and left side. She delivered 20 minutes later. The infant followed a normal newborn course.

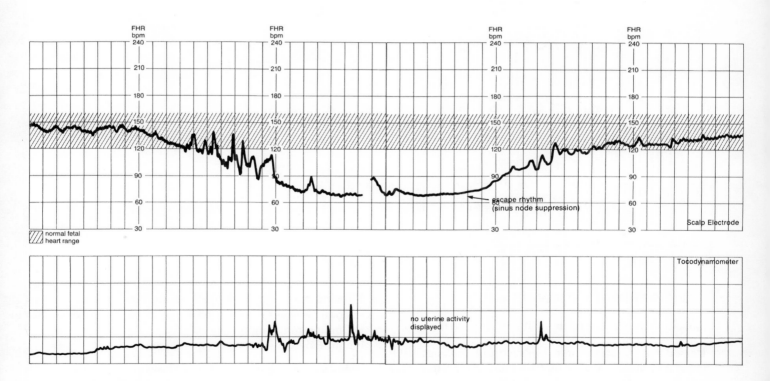

Pattern Characteristic:
Prolonged Decelerations, Maternal Hypotension

Prolonged Deceleration Associated with Increased Uterine Activity

*U*terine hyperactivity is one of the major causes of prolonged decelerations. Such hyperactivity may be spontaneous or induced such as by nipple stimulation or by intravenous bolus administration of pharmacologic agents.[13,17,30,54,63] One theory about the mechanisms of prolonged decelerations produced by paracervical administration of a local anesthetic is that uterine hypertonicity is stimulated by a decreased uterine vascular flow.[17] Antepartum management involves evaluating the fetal response to normal uterine activity if hyperactivity was induced, versus determining the frequency of prolonged uterine contractions in the context of the clinical situation if hyperactivity was spontaneous.

Initial intrapartum management is the discontinuation of drug therapy (e.g., oxytocin) that stimulates uterine activity. Uterine relaxants such as betamimetic agents or magnesium sulfate may be used in treating acute uterine hyperactivity.[33]

Because of an increased risk of fetal acidosis, prompt delivery is necessitated if there is a failure to correct uterine hyperactivity, when associated with recurring and progressive spontaneous episodes of decelerations that are unresponsive to treatment.[14,51]

Further supportive measures are maternal oxygen therapy, hydration, and the assumption of a lateral maternal position to maximize uterine blood flow.

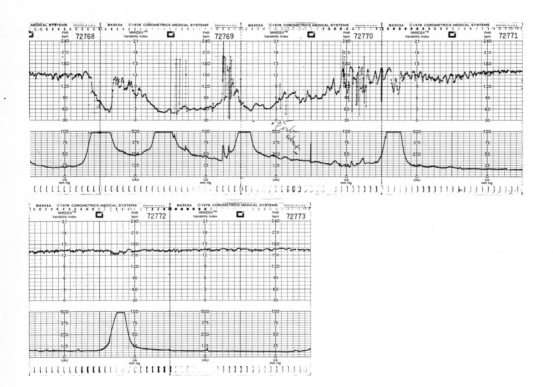

CASE INTERPRETATION: Class II

Baseline Information: normal rate and variability.

Periodic or Nonperiodic Changes: a prolonged deceleration lasting a total of 10 minutes, preceded by a variable deceleration and followed by rebound tachycardia. Increased variability is noted in the recovery phase and decreased variability is noted during rebound tachycardia.

Uterine Activity: prolonged, skewed polysystolic contractions without a resting phase, as measured by external monitoring. Improvement may be secondary to terbutaline therapy or may be spontaneous.

Significance: a healthy fetus showing a normal response to acute stress. It is appropriate to take measures to remove the possible inciting causes and to precede with an early delivery in some circumstances if there is a progressive reoccurrence.

CASE OUTCOME: Twenty-four-year-old gravida 2, para 1001, at 40 weeks' gestation delivered by cesarean section, with general anesthesia, for possible fetal distress a 5 pound, 12 ounce (2608 gram) male; Apgar score 2/9. Thick meconium was present. The cord pH was 7.31. Subcutaneous terbutaline was administered during a prolonged deceleration, which appeared to be caused by spontaneous increased uterine activity. The newborn was dismissed with the mother at five days of life.

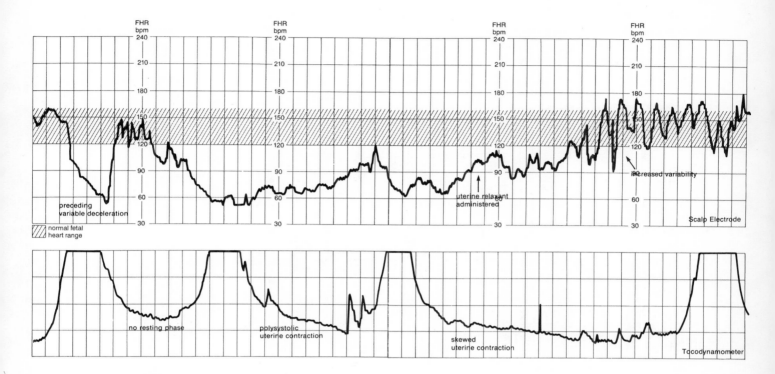

Pattern Characteristic:
Prolonged Deceleration(s), Increased Uterine Activity

Prolonged Decelerations Associated with a Prolapsed Cord

A prolonged deceleration produced by a prolapsed cord often displays profound sinus node suppression with very slow escape rhythms. Varying degrees of recovery occur with individual clinical circumstances.[21,31]

Management is directed at minimizing cord impingement by various methods of displacement of the pre-senting part of the fetus while preparing for emergency delivery.

Amnioinfusion has been useful in improving pro-longed decelerations induced by cord impingement in some situations of occult cord prolapse.[46]

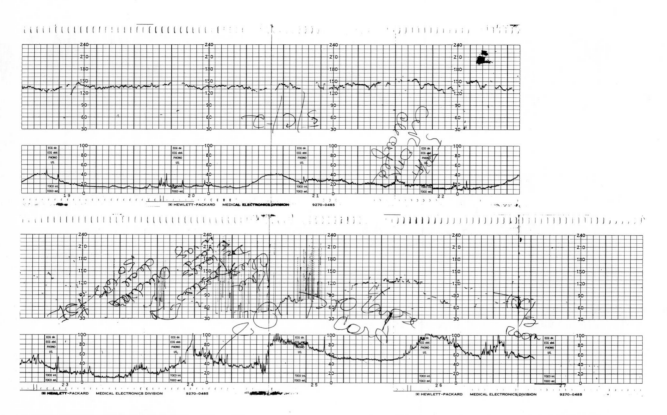

CASE INTERPRETATION: Class V

Baseline Information: normal rate and variability.

Periodic or Nonperiodic Changes: prolonged decel-eration of seven minutes duration with partial recovery and recurrence for three minutes without recovery at the end of the segment. An escape rhythm of less than 50 bpm is present at the base of the deceleration.

Uterine Activity: an increased frequency of contrac-tions, with a minimal resting phase, as recorded by an external monitor.

Significance: a differential diagnosis includes maternal supine hypotension, uterine hyperactivity, placental abruption, and a prolapsed cord. Clinical responses in-clude a maternal position change and evaluation for evi-dence of placental abruption, cord prolapse, and exces-sive uterine activity.

CASE OUTCOME: Twenty-five-year-old gravida 4, para 3003, at 40 weeks' gestation delivered by emer-gency cesarean section, with general anesthesia, for a prolapsed cord that occurred upon artificial rupture of the membranes a 10 pound, 11 ounce (4848 gram) male; Ap-gar score 7/8. The fetus was in a vertex presentation. The infant followed an uncomplicated newborn course.

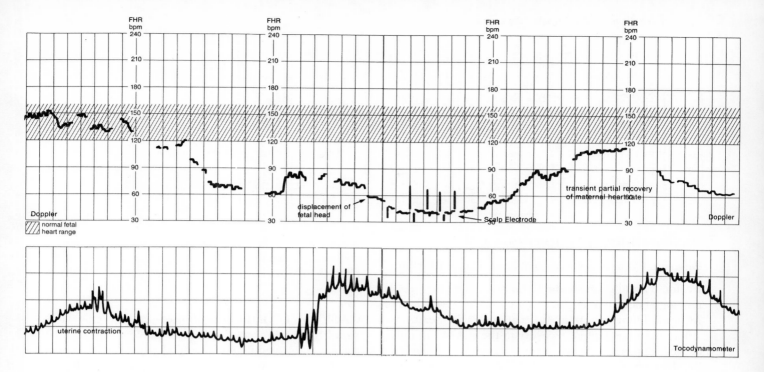

Pattern Characteristic:
Prolonged Deceleration(s), Prolapsed Cord

Prolonged Decelerations Associated with Placental Abruption

Prolonged decelerations associated with placental abruption may display sinus node suppression with an escape rhythm. However, it is more typical to see a decrease in heart rate to 70 to 120 bpm, often with maintenance of a sinus arrhythmia (beat-to-beat variability), although erratic.[51] If such a pattern persists for more than 10 minutes, it is appropriately termed a bradycardia. To review bradycardia associated with placental abruption see page 38.

This pattern suggests a different etiology from the more common vagally mediated prolonged decelerations presented earlier in this chapter. Areas of unabrupted placental surface may allow the fetus to continue to extract oxygen during placental passage of fetal blood even in the presence of a critically impaired supply of maternal oxygenated blood to the intervillous space.[64]

Despite the preservation of variability in a bradycardic range, prompt delivery is usually indicated when the etiology of the prolonged deceleration is a significant placental abruption.

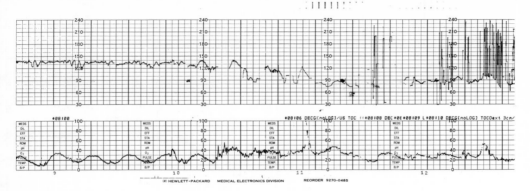

CASE INTERPRETATION: Class V

Baseline Information: normal rate, average variability.

Periodic and Nonperiodic Changes: eight minutes of prolonged deceleration are recorded to the lowest rate of 74 bpm. There are erratic fluctuations in the heart rate. There is an incomplete recovery in the last two minutes of what appears to be an average variability throughout the deceleration.

Uterine Activity: frequent contractions of less than one minute duration, with no resting phase, produce an undulating trace by external monitoring.

Significance: the uterine activity displays a pattern that is seen with placental abruption. The prolonged deceleration may be produced by hypoxia from the increased uterine activity or from loss of placental surface for exchange. Management is usually prompt delivery, if the clinical information is consistent with placental abruption.

CASE OUTCOME: Twenty-five-year-old gravida 2, para 0101, at 34 weeks' gestation delivered by cesarean section performed for possible fetal distress, with general anesthesia, a 4 pound, 8 ounce (2041 gram) female; Apgar score 2/4. The fetus was in a vertex presentation. A 25% to 30% placental abruption was noted at delivery. The umbilical cord pH was 6.9 (venous and arterial). The newborn required intubation at delivery and transient respiratory assistance. The newborn was dismissed at eight days of life.

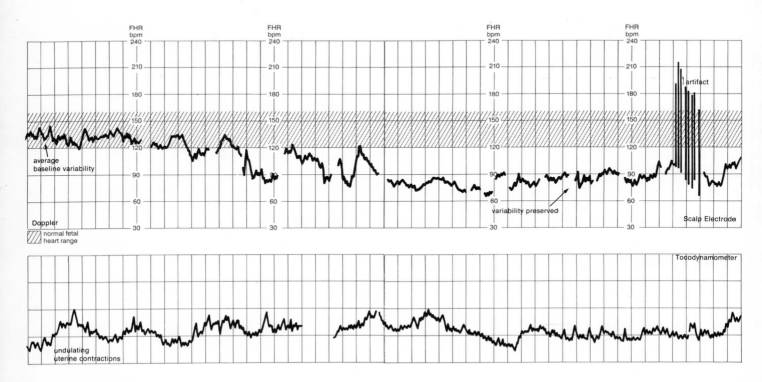

Pattern Characteristic:
Prolonged Deceleration(s), Placental Abruption

Prolonged Deceleration Associated with Maternal Seizure

*T*he etiology of a prolonged deceleration secondary to a seizure is usually secondary to prolonged uterine hypertonus, which commonly occurs simultaneously with seizures, the onset of the seizures usually coinciding with the onset of a contraction. Less commonly, maternal hypoxia from apnea during the seizure may contribute to acute fetal distress.[60] With external monitoring, it is not unusual to lose the fetal heart trace with the activity of the seizure. With internal monitoring, artifacts caused by maternal activity may help document the timing of the onset of the seizure. Prolonged decelerations may accompany seizures regardless of whether the etiology is preeclampsia or epilepsy.[7]

Management is protection of the mother from hypoxia, aspiration, and injury as well as treatment of the seizure and associated uterine tetany. Intervention for the latter may be accomplished with tocolytic therapy.[3] If fetal heart rate recovery does not begin within five minutes, preparations for emergency delivery to rescue a fetus of viable gestation may be indicated if maternal condition permits. Recovery may subsequently begin during the next few minutes, during preparation for delivery. If such is the case, emergency delivery efforts may be abandoned.

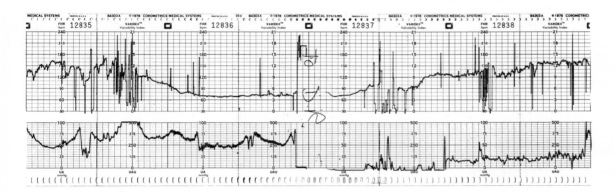

CASE INTERPRETATION: Class V, II

Baseline Information: normal rate and variability.

Periodic or Nonperiodic Changes: there was a prolonged deceleration that lasted five minutes before the mother was transferred to the delivery room; recovery began about one minute after she was remonitored, with eventual full recovery.

Uterine Activity: increased uterine activity appears to be present, onset of a seizure is accompanied by a uterine contraction, both of which persist (by external monitoring) during the five minutes prior to transfer to the delivery room.

Significance: acute fetal distress occurs during the increased uterine activity associated with a seizure. After ensuring maternal safety, measures to relax the uterus or deliver the fetus may become necessary.

CASE OUTCOME: Seventeen-year-old primigravida at 42 weeks' gestation delivered vaginally, from an occiput posterior position by outlet forceps with pudendal anesthesia, a 6 pound, 4 ounce (2835 gram) male; Apgar score 6/8. After full recovery from an eclamptic seizure, the patient pushed for several minutes in the delivery room prior to the forceps delivery. The infant followed a normal newborn course.

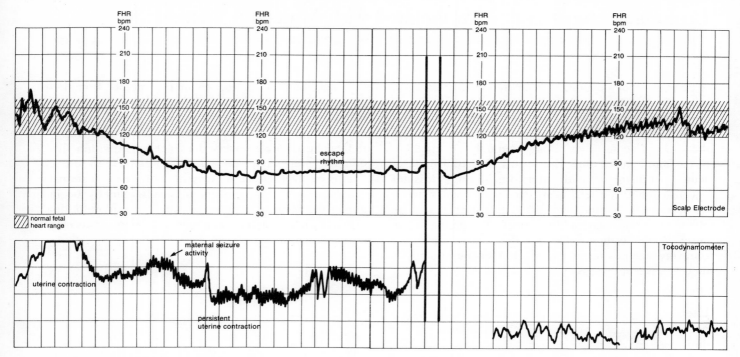

Pattern Characteristic:
Prolonged Deceleration(s), Maternal Seizure

Prolonged Deceleration without Recovery Associated with Postdate Pregnancy

*T*he significantly postdate pregnancy is unique in that when sinus node suppression occurs due to whatever cause, the capability for normal recovery may not be present. This may be the case even when the etiology of the sinus node suppression is as unthreatening as the vagal effects of the application of a scalp electrode. Decelerations on occasion may be so profound that maternal QRS signals are amplified and recorded with internal monitoring even in the presence of a live fetus.

Sudden intrapartum death has been recognized in the postdate pregnancy for decades.[47] Its circumstances are now documented by electronic fetal heart rate monitoring, but the mechanisms are far from elucidated.[15,48,49,50,51] Oligohydramnios and the associated umbilical cord compression are believed to play a major role in the fetal heart rate patterns of a postdate fetus.[19,39,45,52,56] It is important to note, however, that dysfunctional labor, the deterioration of the placenta's ability to produce the metabolic and respiratory functions necessary for resuscitation in utero, and limitations in the fetal compensatory mechanisms to respond to lack of adequate oxygen supply are also significant factors in certain cases.[57,64] The postdate pregnancy tracing may have falsely reassuring baseline variability since the parasympathetic nervous system develops with advancing gestational age. But risk of asphyxia also increases with postterm advancing gestational age.[28] Late decelerations heralding significant fetal distress are often absent, but variable decelerations, tachycardia, or a saltatory pattern may precede severe prolonged decelerations.[36,45,57] Besides prolonged decelerations without recovery, terminal patterns in postdate pregnancies include a sinusoidal pattern.[11,39,53]

Liberal usage of intrapartum pH studies or fetal scalp stimulation in postdate pregnancy, particularly in the presence of thick meconium, is an adjunct to electronic fetal monitoring.[43,51,55,64,65]

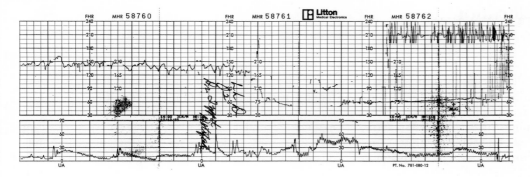

CASE INTERPRETATION: Class V

Baseline Information: normal rate and variability.

Periodic or Nonperiodic Changes: unheralded prolonged deceleration lasting eight minutes prior to discontinuation of monitoring. The scalp electrode is applied after the onset of deceleration.

Uterine Activity: initially, frequent skewed contractions are suggested. Uterine activity is not interpretable during the deceleration, but increased uterine activity is suggested.

Significance: immediate delivery is indicated because of the failure to recover from a prolonged deceleration.

This pattern is seen with postdate pregnancy and total cord prolapse. The heart rate pattern is less typical of total placental abruption, although it could be an etiologic factor.

CASE OUTCOME: Thirty-year-old primigravida at 41 weeks' gestation delivered by emergency cesarean section, with general anesthesia, an 8 pound, 1 ounce (3657 gram) male; Apgar score 3/8. No placental abruption or abnormal cord location was noted at delivery. The infant followed an uncomplicated newborn course. Deceleration occurred at less than two centimeters dilatation (therefore, it was not an end-stage deceleration).

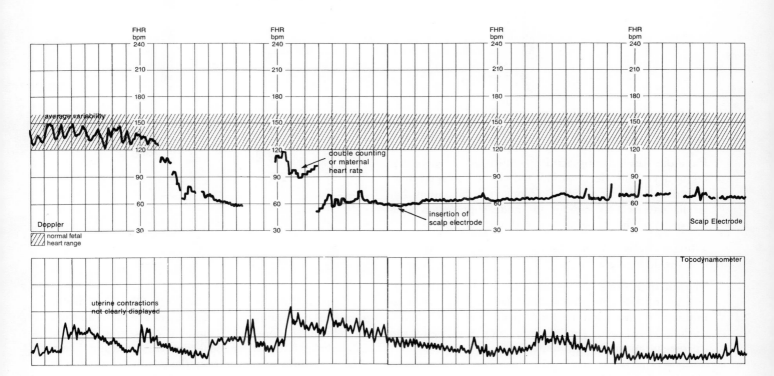

Pattern Characteristic:
Prolonged Deceleration(s), Recovery Postdate Pregnancy

End-Stage Deceleration

A very specific prolonged deceleration that occurs with the descent of the presenting fetal part in the second stage of labor is the end-stage deceleration.

This profound deceleration which, in its classic form, is characterized by failure of the fetal heart rate to recover, often occurs in the presence of a previously normal tracing, creating a true obstetrical emergency.

The deceleration is believed to be produced by umbilical cord impingement such as is created by a short cord or tight nuchal cord.[6] Management necessitates delivery by the quickest but also easiest route, a clinical judgment that must be individualized for each case. Persistence of the pattern beyond 15 minutes does not predict with certainty, ultimate neurologic consquences for the neonate.[16]

"End-stage deceleration" is a more appropriate term for this pattern than "terminal bradycardia." The term "bradycardia" may be assigned when the deceleration extends beyond 10 minutes without recovery, but "terminal" is best reserved for patterns preceding fetal death.[17] This pattern may certainly precede fetal death, the "terminal" events being consequences of acute severe asphyxia if delivery cannot be achieved.

However, the pattern more appropriately titled terminal bradycardia is one accompanying chronic in utero asphyxia in which bradycardia is a terminal event preceded by other monitoring patterns, including tachycardia; agonal periodic changes; and, always, loss of baseline variability.[10]

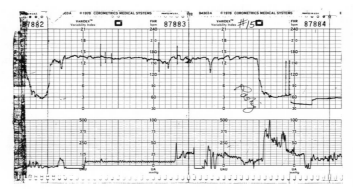
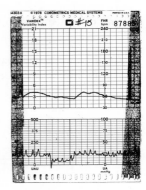

CASE INTERPRETATION: Class V

Baseline Information: normal rate and variability.

Periodic and Nonperiodic Changes: a moderate atypical variable deceleration and small V-shaped variable deceleration precede a prolonged deceleration that is characterized by rapid sinus node suppression with transition to an escape pattern without recovery.

Uterine Activity: the onset of maternal pushing coincides with deceleration.

Significance: this is a typical pattern of end-stage deceleration. Since the deceleration lasted longer than 10 minutes, it meets criteria for a baseline change (bradycardia). Management is the emergency delivery by the easiest and most efficient route.

CASE OUTCOME: Twenty-nine-year-old primigravida at 40 weeks' gestation, delivered from a vertex presentation with emergency forceps, a 6 pound, 9 ounce

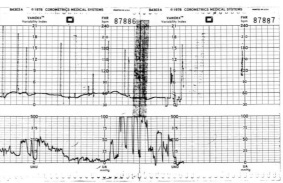

(2977 gram) female; Apgar score 1/5. The patient had received an epidural anesthesia earlier in labor and was in a birthing room fully equipped to accommodate an emergency delivery. A nuchal cord was noted at delivery. The newborn was carried from the hospital against medical advice on the fourth day of life, while feeding poorly. A review of the entire tracing shows a single variable deceleration preceding the end-stage deceleration.

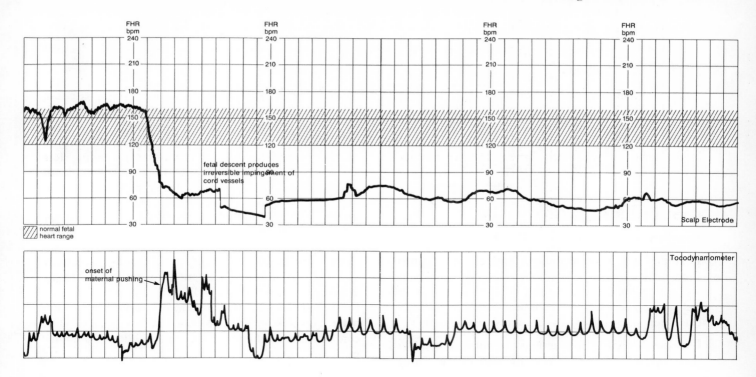

Pattern Characteristic:
End-Stage Deceleration

Progression from Mild Variable Deceleration to End-Stage Deceleration

*B*ecause end-stage deceleration is believed to be a precipitous and relentless sinus node suppression produced by impingement on the umbilical cord in the second stage of labor, it is not surprising that the fetal heart rate pattern will often *but not always* be preceded by evidence of cord vulnerability. Variable decelerations may be mild and sporadic, if present at all, or may show a progressive increase in severity and atypia as labor progresses. In the latter case, advance preparation for emergency delivery may facilitate responses should an end-stage deceleration emergency occur. Compromised umbilical cord perfusion usually is the underlying cause.

Neonatal outcome has a better prognosis when end-stage deceleration occurs in the presence of a previously normal tracing than when it occurs superimposed on a previously stressed fetus.[29,34] Neonatal acidosis is, of course, decreased in incidence if baseline variability is normal.[22] In fact, an exception to management by immediate delivery may be made when excellent to increased variability is present in the deceleration (in the absence of a significant placental abruption).

The pattern is a prolonged deceleration when duration exceeds two to three minutes.[18] Prolonged decelerations are frequently encountered during the spontaneous expulsion process of both vertex and breech deliveries[24,35,42,61,62,66,67] and during instrumental delivery (see page 285). Such a pattern after 10 minutes in duration is appropriately termed a baseline shift to bradycardia. Although often called terminal bradycardia, the word "terminal" is best reserved for use with a dying fetus.[27]

The initial configuration of an end-stage deceleration is usually that of a variable deceleration.

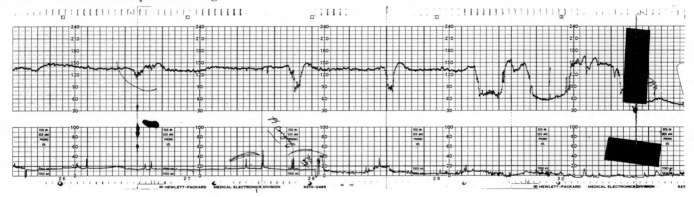

CASE INTERPRETATION: Class II

Baseline Information: normal rate and variability.

Periodic and Nonperiodic Changes: a progression from small variable decelerations through mild, moderate, and severe classical variable decelerations to an atypical variable deceleration (technically not a prolonged deceleration because only two minutes were recorded).

Uterine Activity: contractions are not well displayed, they appear to precede or coincide with decelerations.

Significance: this pattern suggests progressive cord impingement. If this is the second stage, and no recovery occurs, management is emergency delivery by the quickest and easiest route.

CASE OUTCOME: Twenty-two-year-old gravida 3, para 1011, at 38 weeks' gestation was transferred to the delivery room, where she delivered, with epidural anesthesia and low forceps, a 5 pound, 7 ounce (2466 gram) male; Apgar score 9/10. Meconium was present. The cord was around the neck. The infant followed a normal newborn course.

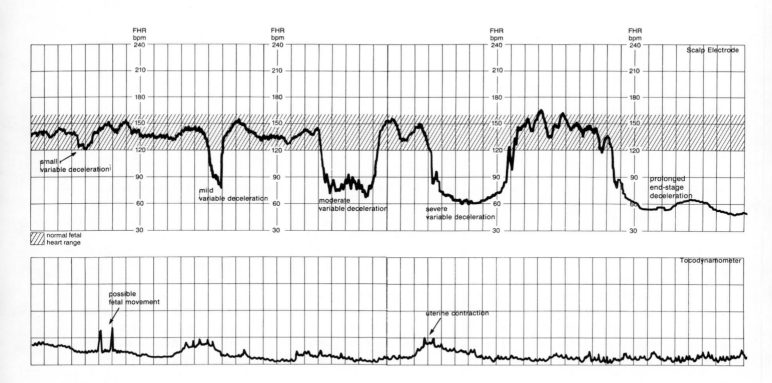

Pattern Characteristic:
Progression from Mild Variable Deceleration to End-Stage Deceleration

Bigeminal Rhythm in Prolonged Deceleration

*W*hen a bigeminal pattern appears in a previously normal fetal heart rate tracing it is often associated with a decrease in heart rate (deceleration) below the usual normal range (120–160 bpm) but above 70 to 80 bpm. This suggests a partial degree of sinus node suppression. Pacemakers near the sinus node may intermittently produce conducted signals.

A bigeminal pattern is therefore seen at times in shallow, prolonged decelerations and in some variable decelerations as well as during subtle downward baseline shifts (see page 476).

Although the fetuses displaying these patterns are usually healthy, exhibiting cardiac compensatory responses to a slowing of the heart rate, the pattern has also been reported in the dying fetus.[10] Therefore, it is not the presence or absence of the bigeminal pattern that predicts the fetal condition but the associated baseline variability and reactivity. Further reassurance is obtained by restoration of a normal pattern, evidencing full recovery from the prolonged deceleration.

Bigeminal patterns are recognized by two parallel horizontal lines connected by vertical parallel spikes. The alternating rates may vary from a few beats per minute to greater than 110 bpm.

Electrocardiography or echocardiography may aid in identification of the pattern and the level in the conduction system of the ectopic focus.

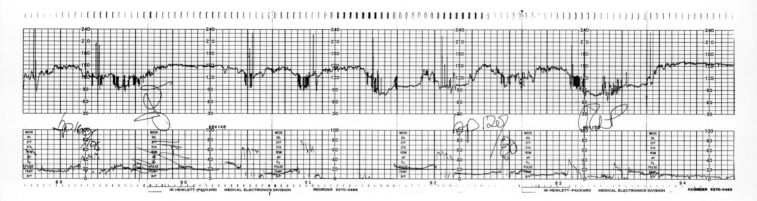

CASE INTERPRETATION: Class IV

Baseline Information: a normal stable rate and average variability.

Periodic or Nonperiodic Changes: variable decelerations, which are mild to moderate, with atypia characterized by the loss of primary and secondary accelerations and shallow prolonged decelerations of two to three minutes that exhibit a bigeminal pattern intermittently.

Uterine Activity: poorly recorded contractions every two to three minutes, with the appearance of maternal straining.

Significance: although atypia increases the risk of a low Apgar score, the average baseline variability predicts a normal outcome if delivery is imminent and the pattern does not worsen.

CASE OUTCOME: Twenty-year-old primigravida at 42 weeks' gestation, delivered with epidural anesthesia and elective low forceps, a 7 pound, 4 ounce (3289 gram) female; Apgar score 8/9. The fetus was in a vertex presentation, in an occiput anterior position. The infant followed an uncomplicated newborn course.

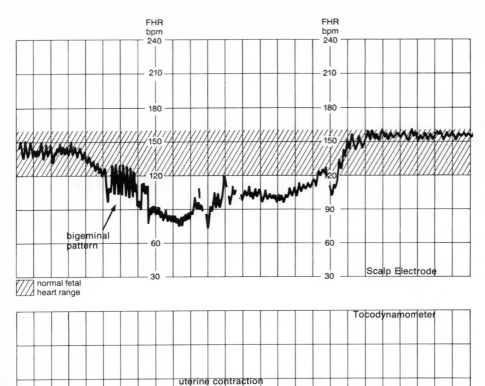

FHR
bpm

FHR
bpm

bigeminal
pattern

normal fetal
heart range

Scalp Electrode

Tocodynamometer

uterine contraction
not clearly displayed

Pattern Characteristic:
Bigeminal Rhythm in Prolonged
Deceleration

Trigeminal Rhythm in Prolonged Deceleration

*U*nder usual circumstances, the fetal heart, like the adult heart, is paced by automatic signals arising in the sinus node. With suppression of the sinus node such as by a vagally mediated slowing of the heart rate, signals may be able to be conducted from slower ectopic foci.

The most common fetal heart response to sinus node suppression is a flat-line produced by an escape rhythm from atrial, junctional, or ventricular foci at 50 to 70 bpm. This is seen in variable decelerations and prolonged decelerations such as those produced by abrupt vagal effects, for example, cord compression or scalp electrode application.

When heart rate deceleration is less precipitous and in the range of 70 to 120 bpm, bigeminal and trigeminal patterns are sometimes seen, bigeminal being the most common. The pattern suggests only a partial degree of sinus node suppression.

The trigeminal pattern is recognized as three parallel lines, the middle one reflecting the usual cardiac cycle. The lines are connected by vertical parallel spikes when machine logic is disengaged.

An ectopic focus other than the sinus node is conducting signals every third beat. The upper line on the fetal monitoring heart rate trace reflects this premature beat and the lower reflects the compensatory pause.

Fetal welfare is determined by the baseline variability and reactivity and the quality of recovery from the prolonged deceleration.

Electrocardiography and echocardiography may assist in identification of the pattern, including the level in the conduction system of the ectopic focus.

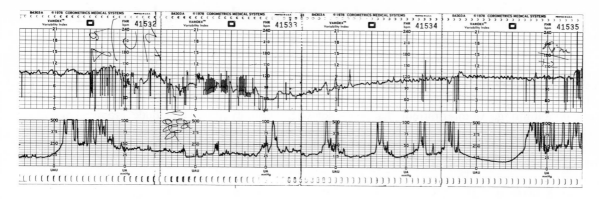

CASE INTERPRETATION: Class II

Baseline Information: normal heart rate and variability.

Periodic or Nonperiodic Changes: prolonged deceleration lasting nine minutes, with complete recovery. A trigeminal pattern in the onset limb of the deceleration.

Uterine Activity: small, frequently skewed contractions with maternal straining, no resting phase.

Significance: a normal fetus demonstrating an appropriate response to stress. It is appropriate to continue conservative management unless the pattern recurs in a progressive fashion. The increased uterine activity may be a contributing factor to the prolonged deceleration. Diminishing the amount of oxytocin, if in use, may improve the pattern.

CASE OUTCOME: Seventeen-year-old primigravida at 41 weeks' gestation delivered vaginally, with pudendal anesthesia from a vertex presentation, a 7 pound, 1 ounce (3203 gram) female; Apgar score 8/9. The infant followed an uncomplicated newborn course.

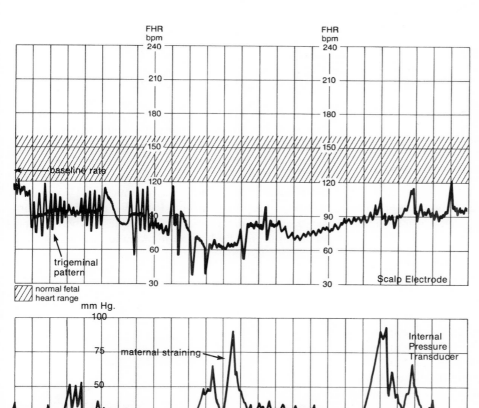

Pattern Characteristic:
Trigeminal Rhythm in
Prolonged Deceleration

Prolonged Deceleration Produced by Maternal Heart Rate: Artifact

A maternal heart rate recording should be considered as a cause when there appears to be a prolonged deceleration during external monitoring. An intermittent change of the Doppler incoming signal from the fetal heart to the maternal vessel source occurs most often when fetal and maternal rates are increased or closely proximated or with fetal movement away from the Doppler transducer.

The differentiation of fetal versus maternal signal often requires careful patient assessment for clarification. The maternal pulse is palpated for synchrony with the Doppler signal and a fetal scalp electrode may be applied if feasible. Dual maternal and fetal monitoring is an ideal way of clarifying this artifact. Characteristics of the monitor trace often provide distinguishing features. Usually, a true fetal heart prolonged deceleration falling to rates below 120 bpm causes a sinus node suppression and resulting smooth escape rhythm that is produced by lower cardiac pacemakers. In contrast, a maternal signal usually displays some degree of variability (sinus arrhythmia). Tracings exhibiting frequent maternal heart rate artifact produce a characteristic appearance of parallel double lines with abrupt interchanges. However, a smooth transition ("slipping") may occur between fetal and maternal heart rates because of machine characteristics designed to produce a clear signal (see page 199 and page 416).

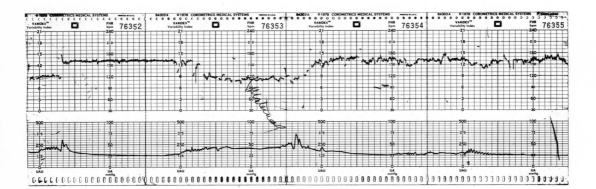

CASE INTERPRETATION: Class 0

Baseline Information: high normal fetal heart rate, variability appears normal in some areas and diminished in others (external monitor without autocorrelation limits interpretation).

Periodic or Nonperiodic Changes: appears to be three to four minutes deceleration, flat, without sinus node suppression.

Uterine Activity: increased level of trace suggests a five-minute contraction.

Significance: a maternal heart rate artifact (the tracing is labeled "maternal" in this case). The artifact is especially common when both the fetus and the mother have tachycardia. Although there appears to be a continuity between the two rates, the pattern does not have the usual characteristics of a fetal heart rate deceleration, although there *appears* to be continuity between the two rates ("slipping").

CASE OUTCOME: Twenty-four-year-old gravida 2, para 0010, at 30 weeks' gestation delivered vaginally, with pudendal anesthesia, a 3 pound, 6 ounce (1531 gram) female; Apgar score 4/7. The patient was receiving ritodrine. The pregnancy was complicated by placental abruption and possible chorioamnionitis. A 15% to 20% placental abruption was noted at delivery. The newborn was hospitalized for three weeks. The newborn course was complicated by hyaline membrane disease, making ventilatory assistance necessary.

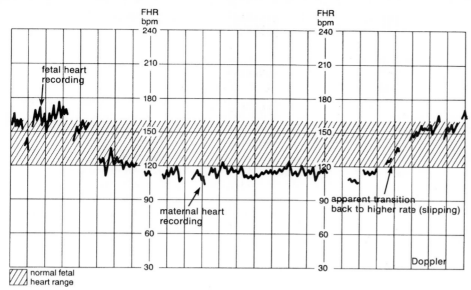

Pattern Characteristic:
Artifactual Prolonged
Deceleration Produced by
Maternal Heart Rate Artifact

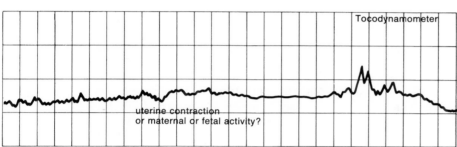

References

1. Abboud TK, Khoo SS, Miller F, et al: Maternal, fetal, and neonatal responses after epidural anesthesia with bupivacaine, 2-chloroprocaine, or lidocaine. *Anesth Analg* 61:638, 1982.

2. Abitbol MM: Supine position in labor and associated fetal heart rate changes. *Obstet Gynecol* 65:481, 1985.

3. Barrett JM: Fetal resuscitation with terbutaline during eclampsia-induced uterine hypertonus. *Am J Obstet Gynecol* 150:895, 1984.

4. Barrows JJ: A documented case of amniotic fluid embolism presenting as acute fetal distress. *Am J Obstet Gynecol* 143:599, 1984.

5. Bieniarz J, Branda LA, Maqueda E, et al: Aortocaval compression by the uterus in late pregnancy. III. Unreliability of the sphygmomanometric method in estimating uterine artery pressure. *Am J Obstet Gynecol* 102:1106, 1968.

6. Boehm FH: Prolonged end state fetal heart rate deceleration. *Obstet Gynecol* 45:579, 1975.

7. Boehm FH, Growdon JH: The effect of eclamptic convulsions on the fetal heart rate. *Am J Obstet Gynecol* 120:851, 1974.

8. Booking AD, Harding R, Wickham PJD: Effects of reduced uterine blood flow on accelerations and decelerations in heart rate of fetal sheep. *Am J Obstet Gynecol* 154:329, 1986.

9. Brotanek V: Fetal distress after artificial rupture of membranes. *Am J Obstet Gynecol* 101:542, 1968.

10. Cetrulo CL, Schifrin BS: Fetal heart rate patterns preceding death in utero. *Obstet Gynecol* 48:521, 1976.

11. Cibils LA: Agonal patterns, in: *Electronic Fetal-Maternal Monitoring: Antepartum, Intrapartum.* Boston, PSG Publishing, 1981, pp. 369ff.

12. Cibils LA: Bradycardia, in: *Electronic Fetal-Maternal Mon-*

itoring: Antepartum, Intrapatum. Boston, PSG Publishing, 1981, p. 284.

13. Dashow EE, Read JA: Significant fetal bradycardia during antepartum heart rate testing. *Am J Obstet Gynecol* 148:187, 1984.

14. Druzin ML, Cratacos J, Keegan KA, et al: Antepartum fetal heart rate testing. VII. The significance of fetal bradycardia. *Am J Obstet Gynecol* 139:194, 1981.

15. Dyson DC, Miller PD, Armstrong MA: Management of prolonged pregnancies: Induction of labor versus antepartum fetal testing. *Am J Obstet Gynecol* 156:928, 1987.

16. Farine D, Warrem W, Sutton J, et al: *Prolonged Fetal Bradycardia with Good Fetal Outcome.* Society of Perinatal Obstetricians Eighth Annual Meeting, Las Vegas, February 3–6, 1988.

17. Freeman RK, Garite TJ: *Basic Pattern Recognition in Fetal Heart Rate Monitoring.* Baltimore, William & Wilkins, 1981, p. 96.

18. Freeman RK, Garite TJ: *Management of Fetal Distress in Fetal Heart Rate Monitoring.* Baltimore, William & Wilkins, 1981, p. 96.

19. Freeman RK, Garite TJ, Modanlou H, et al: Postdate pregnancy: Utilization of contraction stress testing for primary fetal surveillance. *Am J Obstet Gynecol* 140:128, 1981.

20. Garite TJ, Freeman RK: Prolonged decelerations that don't respond to repositioning. *Contemp Obstet Gynecol* 19:29, 1982.

21. Garite TJ, Freeman RK: Case 1: Pelvic exam needed to rule out cord prolapse. *Contemp Obstet Gynecol* Apr:27, 1983.

22. Gilstrap LC, Hauth JC, Toussaint S: Second state fetal heart rate abnormalities and neonatal acidosis. *Obstet Gynecol* 62:209, 1984.

23. Gimosvsky ML, Caritis SN: Diagnosis and management of hypoxic fetal heart rate patterns. *Clinics in Perinatology* 9:313, 1982.

24. Goodlin RC: Reacting fetal bradycardia in care of the fetus, in *Care of the Fetus.* New York, Masson Publishing, 1979:127.

25. Goodlin RC: Importance of the lateral position during labor. *Obstet Gynecol* 37:698, 1971.

26. Goodlin RC, Haesslein HC: Fetal reacting bradycardia. *Am J Obstet Gynecol* 129:845, 1977.

27. Goodlin RC, Haesslein HC: When is it fetal distress? *Am J Obstet Gynecol* 128:440, 1977.

28. Grausz JP, Heimlev R: Asphyxia and gestational age. *Obstet Gynecol* 62:175, 1983.

29. Herbert CM, Boehm FH: Prolonged end-state fetal heart rate deceleration: A reanalysis. *Obstet Gynecol* 57:589, 1981.

30. Hill LM: Fetal distress secondary to vancomycin-induced maternal hypotension. *Am J Obstet Gynecol* 153:74, 1985.

31. Hon EH: The fetal heart rate patterns preceding death in utero. *Am J Obstet Gynecol* 78:47, 1959.

32. Hon EH, Reid BL, Hehre FW: The electronic evaluation of fetal heart rate. II. Changes with maternal hypotension. *Am J Obstet Gynecol* 79:209, 1960.

33. Ingemarsson I, Arulkumaran S, Ratnam SS: Single injection of terbutaline in term labor. I. Effect on fetal pH in cases with prolonged bradycardia. *Am J Obstet Gynecol* 153:859, 1985.

34. Katz M, Shani N, Meizner I, et al: Is end-state deceleration of the fetal heart ominous? *Br J Obstet Gynaecol* 89:186, 1982.

35. Kelly JV: Instrument delivery and the fetal heart rate. *Am J Obstet Gynecol* 87:529, 1963.

36. Klapholz H, Friedman EA: The incidence of intrapartum fetal distress with advancing gestational age. *Am J Obstet Gynecol* 127:405, 1977.

37. Krebs HB, Petres RE, Dunn LJ: Intrapartum fetal heart rate monitoring. V. Fetal heart rate patterns in the second stage of labor. *Am J Obstet Gynecol* 140:435, 1981.

38. LeFevre ML: Fetal heart rate pattern and postparacervical fetal bradycardia. *Obstet Gynecol* 64:343, 1984.

39. Leveno KJ, Quirk G, Cunningham G, et al: Prolonged pregnancy. I. Observations concerning the causes of fetal distress. *Am J Obstet Gynecol* 150:465, 1984.

40. Maltau JM: The frequency of fetal bradycardia during selective epidural anaesthesia. *Acta Obstet Gynaecol Scandinav* 54:478, 1975.

41. Maymon R, Shulman A, Pomeranz M, et al: Uterine rupture at term pregnancy with the use of intracervical prostaglandin E_2 gel for induction of labor. *Am J Obstet Gynecol* 165:368, 1991.

42. Mega M, Cerutti R, Miccoli P, Giorgino FL: Usefulness of cardiotocography in expulsion period. *Clin Exp Obst Gyn* 8:111, 1981.

43. Miller FC, Read JA: Intrapartum assessment of the postdate fetus. *Am J Obstet Gynecol* 141:516, 1981.

44. Milsom I, Forssman L: Factors influencing aortocaval compression in late pregnancy. *Am J Obstet Gynecol* 148:764, 1984.

45. Miyazaki FS, Miyazaki BA: False reactive nonstress tests in postterm pregnancies. *Am J Obstet Gynecol* 140:269, 1981.

46. Miyazaki FS, Taylor NA: Saline amnioinfusion for relief of variable or prolonged decelerations. A preliminary report. *Am J Obstet Gynecol* 146:670, 1983.

47. Nesbitt REL: Postmature pregnancy. A clinical and pathologic appraisal. *Obstet Gynecol* 8:157, 1956.

48. Parer J: Fetal heart rate patterns, in: *Handbook of Fetal Heart Rate Monitoring.* Philadelphia: W.B. Saunders, 1983, p. 108.

49. Paul RH, Petrie R: *Fetal Intensive Care.* Wallingford, CT, Corometric Medical Systems, Inc., 1979, pp. II, 4, 21, 23, 40.

50. Perkins RP: Sudden fetal death in labor. The significance of antecedent monitoring characteristics and clinical circumstances. *J Reprod Med* 25:309, 1980.

51. Quilligan EJ, Katigbak E, Hofschild J: Correlation of fetal heart rate patterns and blood gas values. II. Bradycardia. *Am J Obstet Gynecol* 91:1123, 1965.

52. Rayburn WF, Motley ME, Stempel LE, et al: Antepartum prediction of the postmature infant. *Obstet Gynecol* 60:148, 1982.

53. Ron M, Adoni A, Hochner-Celnikier D, et al: The significance of baseline tachycardia in the postterm fetus. *Int J Gynaecol Obstet* 18:76, 1980.

54. Ron M, Menashe M, Scherer D, et al: Fetal heart rate decelerations following the administration of meperidine-promethazine during labor. *Int J Gynaecol Obstet* 20:301, 1982.

55. Shaw K, Clark SL: Reliability of intrapartum fetal heart rate monitoring in the postterm fetus with meconium passage. *Obstet Gynecol* 72:886, 1988.

56. Silver RK, Dooley SL, Tamura RK, et al: Umbilical cord size and amniotic fluid volume in prolonged pregnancy. *Am J Obstet Gynecol* 157:716, 1987.

57. Silver RK, Dooley SL, MacGregor SN, et al: Fetal acidosis in prolonged pregnancy cannot be attributed to cord compression alone. *Am J Obstet Gynecol* 159:666, 1988.

58. Spinnato JA, Sibai BM, Anderson GD: Fetal distress after hydralazine therapy for severe pregnancy-induced hypertension. *South Med J* 79:559, 1986.

59. Tejani N, Mann LI, Bhakthavathsalan A, et al: Prolonged fetal bradycardia with recovery—its significance and outcome. *Am J Obstet Gynecol* 122:975, 1975.

60. Teramo K, Hiilesmaa V, Bardy A, et al: Fetal heart rate during a maternal grand mal epileptic seizure. *J Perinat Med* 7:3, 1979.

61. Teteris NJ, Botschner AW, Ullery JC, et al: Fetal heart rate during breech delivery. *Am J Obstet Gynecol* 107:762, 1970.

62. Ullery JC, Teteris NJ, Botschner AW, et al: Traction and compression forces exerted by obstetric forceps and their effect on fetal heart rate. *Am J Obstet Gynecol* 85:1066, 1963.

63. Viegas DAC, Arulkumaran S, Gibb DMF, et al: Nipple stimulation in late pregnancy causing uterine hyperstimulation and profound fetal bradycardia. *Brit J Obstet Gynaecol* 91:364, 1984.

64. Vorherr H: Placental insufficiency in relation to postterm pregnancy and fetal postmaturity. Evaluation of fetoplacental function; management of the postterm gravida. *Am J Obstet Gynecol* 123:67, 1975.

65. Yeh S, Bruce SL, Thornton YS: Intrapartum monitoring and management of the postdate fetus. *Clinics in Perinatology* 9:381, 1982.

66. Zilianti M, Segura CL, Cabello F, et al: Studies on fetal bradycardia during birth process: I. *Obstet Gynecol* 42:831, 1973.

67. Zilianti M, Segura CL, Cabello F, et al: Studies in fetal bradycardia during birth process: II. *Obstet Gynecol* 42:840, 1973.

UTERINE/MATERNAL/
FETAL ACTIVITY

The uterine contraction trace is an essential part of the fetal monitoring record. Even though it does not provide direct information about the fetal condition, information regarding the intrauterine environment of the fetus and the labor pattern may influence decisions that affect the fetus. Even more important, relating the timing of the fetal heart trace information to uterine activity may provide significantly more information than can be learned by viewing the fetal heart pattern alone.

Whether uterine activity is inefficient or excessive cannot be fully determined without coupling that information with the labor progress and fetal response. Contractions that are mild by usual criteria may be excessive for a particular fetus and quite effective as judged by the labor's progress. On the other hand, contraction traces that meet the usual criteria for increased uterine activity may be present in a clinical setting in which this amount of activity is needed for progress, while at the same time this uterine activity is well tolerated by a fetus who is neither chronically compromised nor acutely stressed.

In addition to uterine contraction waveforms and intrauterine pressure information (when the internal pressure transducer is employed), the uterine trace also presents information about maternal activity and, occasionally, fetal activity. Such information allows the correlation of some maternal or fetal events with the fetal heart rate status or changes in status. This is of particular interest in the presence of maternal seizures or pathologic maternal respiratory activity.

Uterine Activity

Increased Uterine Activity Associated with Total
Placental Abruption

Exaggerated Contraction Frequency Secondary
to Paper Speed: Artifact

Exaggerated Peaking of Contractions Secondary
to Paper Speed: Artifact

Normal Uterine Activity—External Monitor

The tocodynamometer produces a uterine contraction trace from data derived from the varying pressure of the contracting uterus against a pressure-sensitive instrument that converts the signal electronically. The external monitor provides a permanent documentation of contraction frequency and approximate duration but is not able to measure resting tone or intensity. The external monitor also provides a record of the contraction regularity or rhythmicity and displays the uterine contraction waveform.

The frequency of contractions typically increases as delivery approaches, averaging 3.5 per 10 minutes.[33] The contraction duration shows no significant change with advancing labor, although the duration may increase or decrease in individual cases. The regularity of the contraction pattern usually improves as labor progresses. The "normal" uterine contraction is bell-shaped, with the descending (relaxation) limb returning to the same basal level (resting tone) as preceded the ascending (contraction) limb.[31]

Manual palpation may detect onset, duration, and frequency and may offer a crude estimation of the intensity. Manual palpation detects a uterine contraction at about 10 mm Hg. The patient senses a uterine contraction at about 15 mm Hg. Tocodynamometry may detect the onset of a uterine contraction before intrauterine intensity actually rises if it is very sensitive, or it may only record the "tip" of a contraction, depending upon transducer placement, baseline placement, patient position, obesity, gestation, and other factors.[19]

Transducer placement is affected not only by the pressure of the uterus against the transducer at the site selected but also by the timing of the muscular contraction in different parts of the myometrium (usually fundal dominance and downward propagation during normal labor).[6]

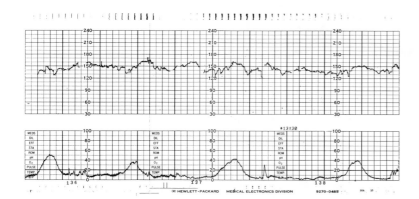

CASE INTERPRETATION: Class I

Baseline Information: normal rate and variability.

Periodic or Nonperiodic Changes: nonperiodic uniform accelerations.

Uterine Activity: normal uterine contraction frequency and configuration.

Significance: a pattern with a high reliability in predicting a healthy fetus.

CASE OUTCOME: Twenty-three-year-old gravida 2, para 1001, at 39 weeks' gestation delivered vaginally, with pudendal anesthesia, a 7 pound, 11 ounce (3487 gram) male; Apgar score 9/9. The fetus was spontaneously rotated from an occiput posterior to an occiput anterior position. The infant followed an uncomplicated newborn course.

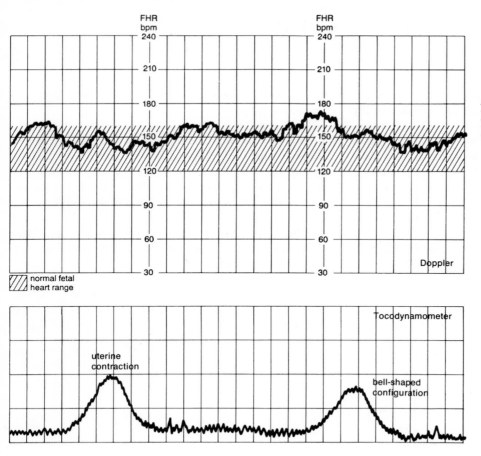

Pattern Characteristic:
Normal Uterine Activity—
External Monitor

Normal Uterine Activity—Internal Monitor

The internal monitor provides a uterine trace from data derived from the varying pressure generated within the uterus at rest and during contractions. Earliest internal pressure monitoring involved transmission of pressure through a column of fluid in a catheter continuous with the amniotic fluid. The pressure transmitted by the fluid within the "closed" system thus formed is sensed by a transducer that converts it to an electronic signal. Newer systems use a pressure transducer inserted directly into the amniotic cavity.

The internal monitor not only demonstrates the frequency, duration, configuration, and rhythmicity of contractions (all of which are provided by external monitoring) but it also documents the resting tone and the intensity occurring at any point in time during a contraction.

Both contraction intensity and tone typically increase with advancing labor.[33] Uterine activity increases as cervical dilatation progresses but also becomes more efficient in achieving cervical dilatation.[27,41]

Less uterine work is encountered in multiparous than in primigravid labors.[27,48,67]

Uterine activity in labor is quantitated by varying methods.[41,64] The one most widely used clinically is

Montevideo Units (MU): the amplitude of the contraction (peak intensity minus resting tone) times the frequency per 10 minutes.

Uterine activity is usually 80 to 120 MU at the onset of labor. In an unobstructed labor, 200 MU are generally sufficient for progress in cervical dilatation. In unstimulated labor, 250 MU are the maximum that are usually seen.[7]

Levels of up to 300 MU are not unusual with oxytocin-stimulated labor.[24] The calculation of MU is compatible with on-line systems for the quantitation of uterine activity.[60]

Another widely used method that measures, via computer, the area under the uterine pressure curve is *Uterine Activity Units* (UAU): the number of TORR/min (1 mm Hg occurring every minute) over a period of 10 minutes.

This method has the advantage of being less influenced by maternal straining in evaluating uterine activity.[26,72] It is obtained by an on-line voltage-controlled oscillator system or by off-line computer techniques.[25,39,59]

Approximately 210 to 375 UAU are compatible with an effective contraction intensity.[41] There is generally a progressive rise of UAU with progress in labor. This method is advantageous in comparison to MU in the presence of maternal straining. Also, when the contraction height is low in comparison to the duration, uterine activity is less likely to be underrated. This method is compatible with on-line systems for quantitation (print-out) of uterine activity.[42]

Other methods of evaluating uterine activity are: (1) *Alexandria Units* (similar to MU, but contraction duration is included in the calculations);[4,16] (2) *Active Planimeter Units* (measures the entire area under the uterine pressure curve over 10 minutes, excluding the baseline tone). This has been reported in KPas (kilopascal seconds)/10 minutes.[13] One MU is approximately equal to 6 KPas Units.[7] (3) *Total Planimeter Units* (same as Active Planimeter Units plus baseline tone and average rate of rise).

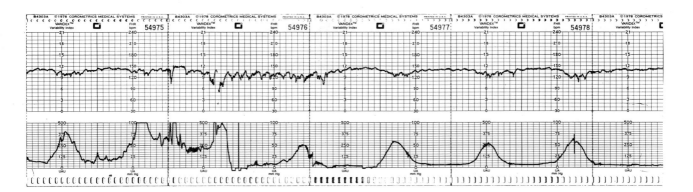

CASE INTERPRETATION: Class I

Baseline Information: normal rate and variability.

Periodic or Nonperiodic Changes: confluent accelerations of low amplitude simulate a pattern of early decelerations.

Uterine Activity: the pressure gauge demonstrates contractions of normal configuration and adequate intensity.

Significance: progressive cervical dilatation is predicted if there is normal term gestation and adequate pelvic size for the fetus, with a normal presentation. A good fetal outcome is predicted.

CASE OUTCOME: Twenty-two-year-old primigravida at 40 weeks' gestation delivered by cesarean section for cephalopelvic disproportion an 8 pound, 14½ ounce (4040 gram) male; Apgar score 8/9. The fetus was in a vertex presentation. The infant followed an uncomplicated newborn course.

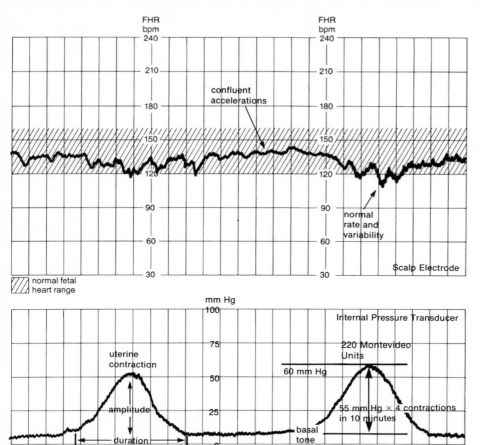

Pattern Characteristic:
Normal Uterine Activity—
Internal Monitor

Comparison of Presentation of Uterine Activity by Internal and External Monitoring

*T*he tocodynamometer offers the advantage of using a noninvasive system for producing a permanent record of uterine contractions for labor assessment and correlation with fetal heart rate data. It may thus be used in patients with contraindications for internal monitoring such as all antepartum patients and intrapartum patients with intact membranes or an undilated cervix. The contraction frequency is reliably recorded. The contraction waveform may be partially obscured by trace deflections that are produced by maternal activity. The recording of the contractions' duration is not consistently reliable.

The external monitor may have a delay in the display of an upswing at the onset of the uterine contraction and a return to "baseline" before true completion of the contraction, resulting in a waveform of artifactually short duration because of low pressure against the transducer that is influenced by such factors as transducer placement, belt tightness, maternal position, and obesity. On the other hand, the tocodynamometer trace may indicate an earlier contraction onset and delayed return in comparison to the internal monitor when it is very sensitive to pressure.[19] The internal pressure gauge will not indicate a change from the baseline until the intrauterine pressure generated by the myometrial contraction results in a change in the intrauterine pressure above the baseline tone, in contrast to a sensitive tocodynamometer that may detect movement produced by an early myometrial contraction before increased pressure is generated.

Although external monitor information is not useful regarding contraction intensity, and no information is acquired regarding uterine tone during relaxation, there is sufficient information obtained to safely monitor uterine activity in most clinical situations.[34]

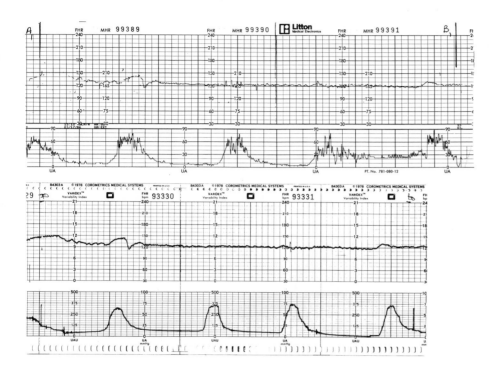

CASE INTERPRETATION: Class I

Baseline Information: low normal heart rate, decreased beat-to-beat variability.

Periodic or Nonperiodic Changes: nonperiodic accelerations present with a variable configuration.

Uterine Activity: skewed contractions every 2½ minutes, which are longer in duration as measured by external monitor then by internal monitor, achieving an intensity greater than 50 mm Hg and MUs greater than 200 and a resting tone less than 20 mm Hg.

Significance: accelerations are reassuring despite decreased beat-to-beat variability, especially if normal variability is preceded by drug administration. The contraction pattern is adequate for labor progress.

CASE OUTCOME: Sixteen-year-old primigravida at 34 weeks' gestation delivered vaginally, from a vertex presentation with pudendal and local anesthesia, a 4 pound, 6 ounce (1984 gram) male; Apgar score 8/9. The maternal course was complicated by preeclampsia. The mother received magnesium sulfate intravenously intrapartum. The infant followed an uncomplicated newborn course for his weight and gestation.

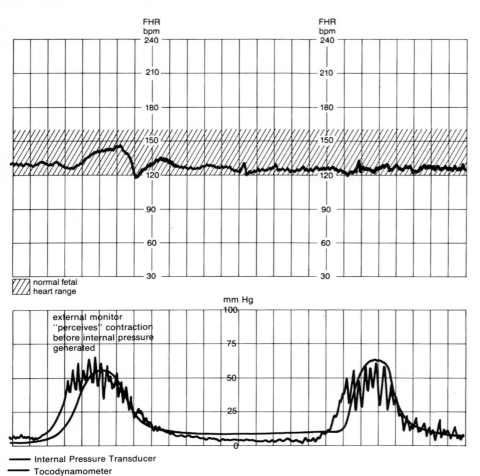

Pattern Characteristic:
Uterine Activity Comparison of
Internal and External Monitor

Decreased Uterine Activity: Hypocontractility and Hypotonia
Internal Pressure Transducer Clarification

When contractions are less than 25 to 30 mm Hg at their peak or recur less than every five minutes in the active phase of labor and last less than 45 seconds, hypocontractility is present, even if it is accompanied by progress in labor.[5,10,31] The mechanisms are probably a combination of multiple factors that may include decreased glucose supply, myometrial exhaustion, the effect of analgesic medication, anesthesia, and the scarring or overstretching of muscle.[5,19,48,57]

Manual uterine palpation, pain perception by the patient, and tocodynamometry are less precise than internal pressure monitoring in assessing uterine hypocontractility.

The waveform displayed by the internal monitor with hypocontractile labor typically shows a slow rate of rise to a low amplitude and a slow rate of fall, albeit not as slow as is encountered with contractions of similar height associated with otherwise "normal" labor.[61]

Whether contractions are mild, infrequent, or short in duration, progress in labor may still occur, depending on such factors as parity and cervical resistance. When uterine hypocontractility associated with the failure of progress in labor is diagnosed, oxytocin infusion may be selected as therapy if no contraindications exist. The lowest dosage necessary for progress in cervical change is appropriate.

A decreased resting tone (less than 8–10 mm Hg) may be encountered early in a progressive spontaneous labor.[23] Hypotonia may occur with epidural anesthesia and is of course, a goal of tocolytic therapy. It also may accompany secondary arrest of dilatation.[31]

Artifactual hypotonia may be produced by placing the internal pressure strain gauge above the pubic symphysis, by technical problems with calibration, by "zeroing" to atmospheric pressure, or by unsatisfactory placement of the catheter tip.[17,31,43]

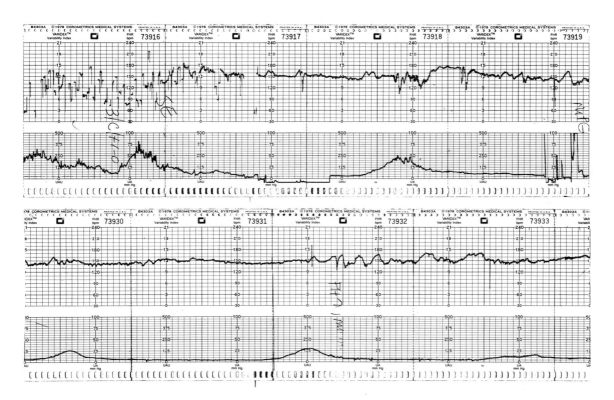

CASE INTERPRETATION: Class I

Baseline Information: normal rate and variability.

Periodic or Nonperiodic Changes: small variable accelerations and V-shaped variable decelerations are present.

Uterine Activity: internal pressure transducer shows uterine pressure that may be insufficient to produce labor progress.

Significance: a healthy fetus predicted. Oxytocin augmentation is appropriate if there are no contraindications to usage and no progress in labor.

CASE OUTCOME: Twenty-four-year-old primigravida at 42 weeks' gestation delivered by cesarean section for cephalopelvic disproportion after oxytocin augmentation, subsequent to this segment, an 8 pound, 2 ounce (3685 gram) female; Apgar score 8/9. The infant followed an uncomplicated newborn course.

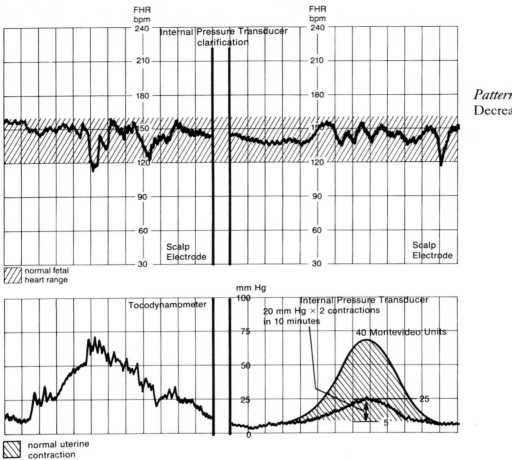

Pattern Characteristic:
Decreased Uterine Activity

Decreased Uterine Activity Produced by Air in the Internal Monitoring System: Artifact

*I*nternal pressure monitoring systems, which depend on transmission of the pressure signal through a column of water, require a closed system in order for the intrauterine pressure to be transmitted accurately to the pressure transducer. Although the uterus is "open" by the fact that the amniotic membranes are ruptured, the intrauterine environment still appears to function as a closed system unless marked leakage of amniotic fluid is occurring, probably because of the "seal" produced by the fetal presenting part.[43]

Within such a closed system, the presence of air dampens the transmission of the pressure-derived sig-

nal.[40] Air is compressible and therefore "cushions" the effect of the pressure, resulting in a uterine waveform displaying less amplitude.[14] This is partially corrected by flushing air from the line and transducer.[49]

The quality of readings may also be influenced by the technique of zeroing to atmosphere, the position of the transducer level in relationship to the level of the uterus, and any obstruction or leaking within the system. Newer transducers place the pressure sensor directly in the uterine cavity and thus do not produce such an artifact.

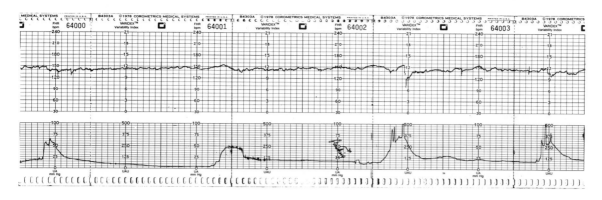

CASE INTERPRETATION: Class I

Baseline Information: normal rate and variability.

Periodic or Nonperiodic Changes: accelerations of low amplitude and mild variable decelerations.

Uterine Activity: a more accurate uterine pressure wave is portrayed after flushing air from the internal pressure gauge line. Polysystolic contractions are unmasked.

Significance: a healthy fetus is predicted. Abnormal uterine activity may contribute to an abnormal labor progress.

CASE OUTCOME: Sixteen-year-old primigravida at 35 weeks' gestation delivered vaginally a 5 pound, 9 ounce (2523 gram) male; Apgar score 7/9. Labor was induced for premature rupture of the membranes. The fetus was in a vertex presentation, in an occiput anterior position. The newborn course was complicated by necrotizing enterocolitis. The newborn survived and was dismissed at 24 days of life.

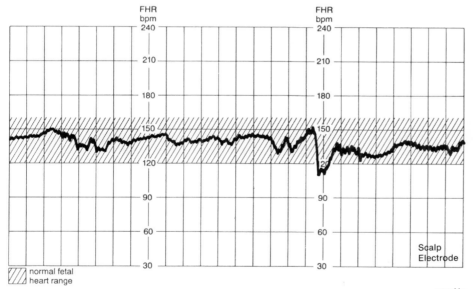

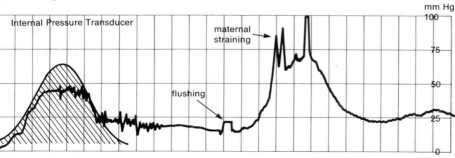

Pattern Characteristic:
Decreased Uterine Activity—
Artifact: Air in System

Decreased Uterine Activity Produced by Tocodynamometer Placement: Artifact

*T*o produce a record characterized by a rise and fall with uterine contractions, the tocodynamometer depends upon a rising and falling pressure against a pressure-sensitive button or membrane. This is usually best achieved by placement of the tocodynamometer at the point of maximum protrusion of the dome of the uterus against the abdominal wall. The myometrial contraction usually causes the fundus of the uterus to rise against the pressure sensor.

It is possible, however, for the uterus to contract away from the transducer, creating a negative deflection, especially at a premature gestation.

The uterine wave may be affected by belt tension, obesity, and also maternal position. Contractions that only produce a pressure signal at their peak also appear to be short in duration.[19]

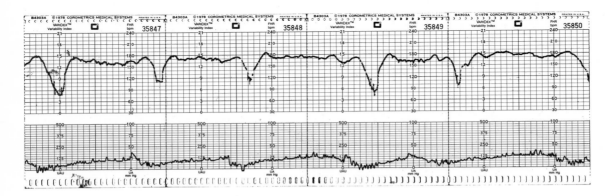

CASE INTERPRETATION: Class IV

Baseline Information: high normal rate to moderate tachycardia, decreased variability.

Periodic or Nonperiodic Changes: moderate variable decelerations with atypia: decreased variability within the decelerations and prolonged secondary accelerations. Also, sloping descending and ascending limbs.

Uterine Activity: a relatively small negative deflection is produced by contractions that appear slightly skewed if the trace is reversed.

Significance: there is a need to replace the tocodynamometer so that the uterus rises against instead of contracts from the tocodynamometer. See page 264 for a discussion of fetal heart pattern.

CASE OUTCOME: Nineteen-year-old gravida 2, para 0010, at 30 weeks' gestation delivered vaginally, with pudendal anesthesia, a 2 pound, 14 ounce (1304 gram) male; Apgar score 7/7. The newborn had equinovarus. The infant had a protracted hospitalization (50 days) because of a large intraventricular hematoma.

The nurses' annotations on other areas of the tracing verified that contractions were occurring simultaneously with "negative" trace deflections.

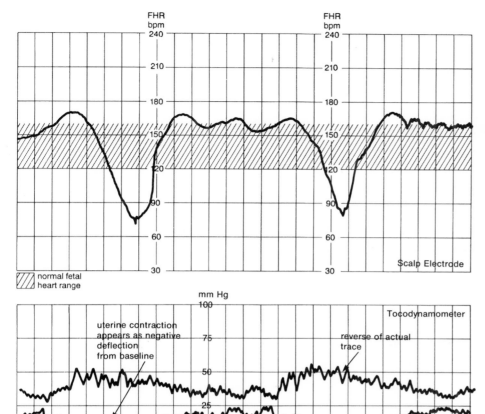

FHR
bpm
240
210
180
150
120
90
60
30

FHR
bpm
240
210
180
150
120
90
60
30

/// normal fetal
/// heart range

Scalp Electrode

mm Hg
100
75
50
25
0

uterine contraction
appears as negative
deflection
from baseline

reverse of actual
trace

Tocodynamometer

Pattern Characteristic:
Decreased Uterine Activity—
Artifact: Tocodynamometer
Placement Effect

Decreased Uterine Activity Produced by Baseline Adjustment: Artifact

*T*he tocodynamometer records the uterine contraction waveform, frequency, and, to some degree of accuracy, duration. It does not reflect the actual quantity of baseline tone or contraction amplitude. The baseline is arbitrarily adjusted by regulators on the fetal monitor and/or transducer. For optimum results, the baseline is arbitrarily set a distance above the zero line on the graph, for example, at "20" (although not truly indicating a 20 mm Hg intrauterine pressure). By placing the baseline purposefully above zero, if movement of the transducer or a patient position change causes the trace to drift to a lower level, it is less likely to fall all the way below the zero line. The instrument cannot record below zero, so any further reduction of pressure is simply displayed as

a flat-line at the bottom of the graph. This may result in the presentation of only the "tips" of contractions, giving the appearance of a lower "relative" amplitude and shorter duration than is actually the case. Furthermore, features of the contraction shape may be lost such as skewing and polysystole, and relatively small contractions may not appear at all. This artifact may influence decisions in the regulation of oxytocin dosage. The artifact is recognized by the smoothness of the "baseline" external monitor trace, positioned at the "zero" level. The maternal patient almost always produces sufficient movement through respirations or other activity to cause some fluctuations of the tocodynamometer-derived uterine trace if it is not set below zero.

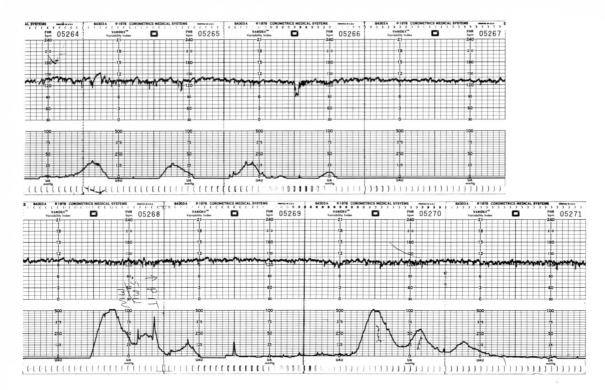

CASE INTERPRETATION: Class I

Baseline Information: a normal stable rate with average variability.

Periodic or Nonperiodic Changes: single small acceleration, single mild variable deceleration.

Uterine Activity: with the baseline uterine activity measured by a tocodynamometer set below zero, uterine contractions appear only every two to two and a half minutes, and oxytocin is increased; after placement of the baseline above zero, polysystolic contractions (in uterine "trigeminy") appear, which may have been previously masked.

Significance: a healthy fetus is predicted, despite the dysfunctional uterine activity. Baseline adjustment improves the assessment of uterine activity for oxytocin regulation.

CASE OUTCOME: Nineteen-year-old primigravida at 40 weeks' gestation delivered vaginally, with local anesthesia, a 9 pound, 9 ounce (4337 gram) male; Apgar score 9/9. The fetus was in a vertex position. A nuchal cord was present. The infant followed an uncomplicated newborn course.

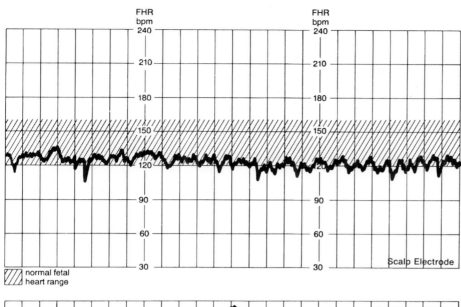

Pattern Characteristic:
Decreased Uterine Activity—
Artifact: Baseline Adjustment
Effect

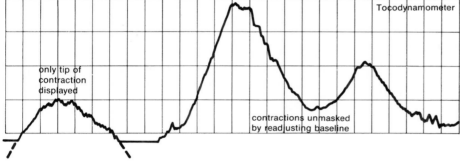

Discoordinate Uterine Activity

The constancy of the intervals between uterine contractions determines the degree of coordination or rhythm of uterine activity. When a marked interval variation occurs from contraction to contraction, the resultant pattern is termed "discoordinate labor." It has also been called "incoordinate labor," "dystonic labor," and "uterine arrhythmia" or "dysrhythmia."[10,15,31] This is less common than coordinate labor. It is associated with poorer progress than coordinate labor,[30] but it is not incompatible with progress in cervical dilatation and vaginal delivery. Discoordinate uterine activity in early labor may become rhythmic as labor advances.[30] There appears to be no association with parity, maternal age, gestational age, or fetal size.[15]

Intramyometrial pressure recordings and multichannel tocodynamometers have helped to clarify this labor abnormality.[5,6,52,68] The cause is believed to be localized myometrial contractions occurring asynchronously at sites that then become refractory during the propagation of the next contraction wave, resulting in variations in contraction frequency and configuration.[10,14] Because contractions may be generated from alternate uterine cornua as well as from other sites, frequent low-intensity contractions are a typical finding. Uterine hypertonus may result from the constantly contracting state of some area in the myometrium.[6,10] Extreme degrees of this phenomenon have been named "uterine fibrillation."[1,35]

With excessive oxytocin dosages, this, as well as any form of uterine hyperactivity, may be encountered.[5] However, oxytocin in physiologic dosages may actually improve such a pattern by causing all areas of the myometrium to contract and relax in a synchronous fashion.[50,57] Agents that diminish myometrial contractility may also therapeutically modify the abnormal patterns.

This pattern may be aggravated by the supine position.[17]

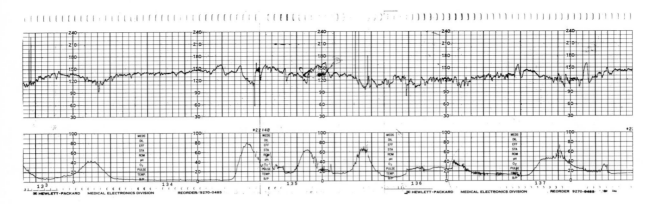

CASE INTERPRETATION: Class I–II

Baseline Information: normal rate to moderate bradycardia, average short- and long-term variability, slight instability.

Periodic or Nonperiodic Changes: nonperiodic accelerations, possible late decelerations (not seen with every uterine contraction).

Uterine Activity: discoordinate pattern characterized by an absent to prolonged resting phase, intermittent tachysystole, and variations in contraction contour. Also suggested (not diagnosed with tocodynamometry) are variations in the intensity and resting tone.

Significance: discoordinate uterine activity. Failure of progress may be managed by a change in maternal positioning and the selective use of myometrial stimulatory and/or relaxing agents.

CASE OUTCOME: Twenty-one-year-old primigravida at 40 weeks' gestation delivered by cesarean section for cephalopelvic disproportion, with spinal anesthesia, a 7 pound, 4 ounce (3289 gram) male; Apgar score 9/10. The discoordinate pattern improved with oxytocin, but an arrest in cervical change occurred at 6 cm dilatation. The infant followed a normal newborn course.

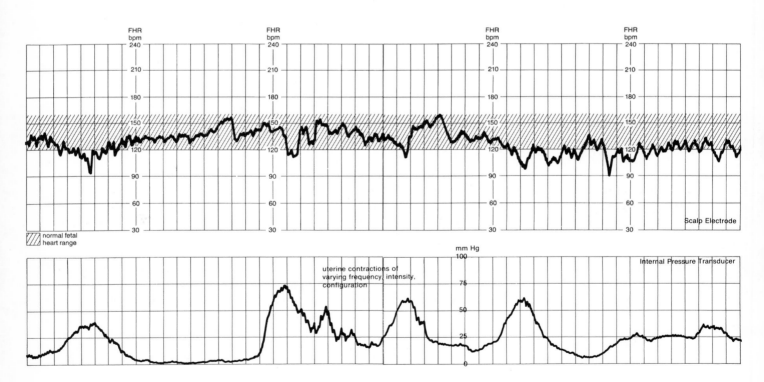

Pattern Characteristic:
Discoordinate Labor

Increased Uterine Activity: Skewed Contractions

A skewed contraction is characterized by a prolongation of the descending limb (relaxation phase) of the uterine contraction[65] and is often seen in a mixed pattern with polysystole.

It is a common pattern and is often associated with a nonprogressive spontaneous labor. This pattern has been described with oxytocin administration, but there is no evidence that physiologic doses of oxytocin increase the occurrence.[8]

This type of uterine contraction, because of the prolongation of decreased oxygen exchange at the inter-villous space, may be associated with "hypoxic" fetal monitoring patterns (e.g., increased variability or late decelerations), even in a basally healthy fetus. The same fetus may demonstrate no stress response to a contraction of normal configuration. Despite this, it is not appropriate to assume that the fetal response is inconsequential since both healthy and sick fetuses may demonstrate fetal heart rate changes only in response to prolonged contractions. Furthermore, the healthy fetus may eventually deplete compensatory mechanisms in response to the hypoxia induced by the contractions.

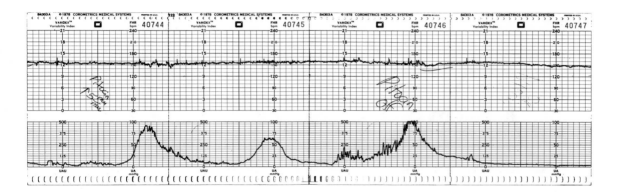

CASE INTERPRETATION: Class III

Baseline Information: high normal rate, decreased short- and long-term variability, short-term variability appears in association with the contractions.

Periodic or Nonperiodic Changes: a shallow drift in the baseline after the onset of contractions suggests late decelerations.

Uterine Activity: skewing of contractions.

Significance: abnormal uterine activity may contribute to abnormal labor progress. The fetal condition needs further assessment unless good variability recently preceded this segment.

CASE OUTCOME: Thirty-one-year-old gravida 2, para 0010, at 40 weeks' gestation delivered by cesarean section for cephalopelvic disproportion, with general anesthesia, a 6 pound, 15½ ounce (3161 gram) male; Apgar score 3/7. Moderate meconium was present. The newborn followed an uncomplicated newborn course.

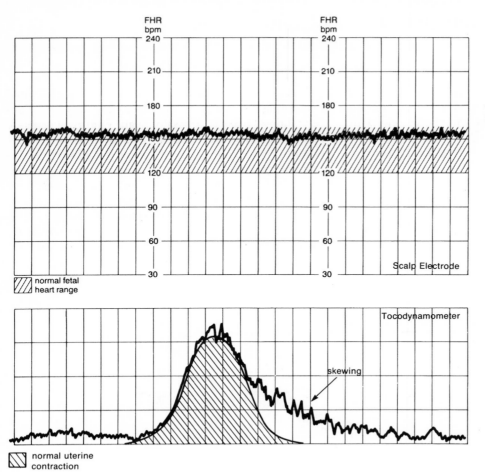

Pattern Characteristic:
Skewed Contractions

//// normal fetal
//// heart range

Scalp Electrode

Tocodynamometer

skewing

▨ normal uterine
contraction

Increased Uterine Activity: Polysystole

*P*olysystole is a common abnormal uterine waveform that is characterized by a single contraction with two or more peaks.[65] It is also described as two or more contractions in juxtaposition without full return to the baseline between each.[21]

When the two peaks occur, it is also called "coupling" or "uterine bigeminy." Usually the second peak is of lower amplitude than the first.

The theoretic pathophysiologic basis for this occurrence is the separate foci of autorhythmicity in the right and left cornual areas of the uterus. It is not unusual for this pattern to be associated with poor progress in labor.

The pattern occurs commonly in spontaneous labor.[21] Studies are conflicting regarding the increased or decreased occurrence with oxytocin use.[26,57] This is perhaps because, although all types of increased uterine activity have been described with excessive oxytocin use, oxytocin may also improve a pattern with polysystole by effecting a more coordinated contraction phase and refractory (resting) interval.[19,50]

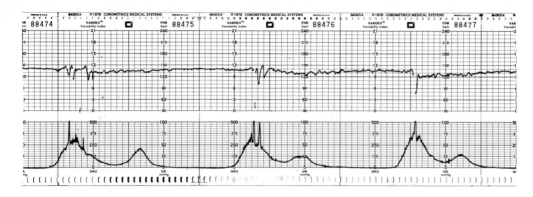

CASE INTERPRETATION: Class II

Baseline Information: normal rate, fair variability.

Periodic or Nonperiodic Changes: small V-shaped variable decelerations with jagged features; a shallow drift in the baseline after onset of the contractions suggests late decelerations.

Uterine Activity: polysystolic contractions of normal intensity.

Significance: abnormal uterine activity may contribute to abnormal labor progress. No intervention for fetal wel-

fare is indicated at this time but observation of the pattern for further development of late decelerations or further diminished variability is appropriate.

CASE OUTCOME: Twenty-one-year-old gravida 2, para 1001 delivered at 42 weeks' gestation by primary cesarean section for cephalopelvic disproportion and possible fetal distress a 7 pound, 15 ounce (3600 gram) female; Apgar score 8/8. No oxytocin was administered. The infant followed an uncomplicated newborn course.

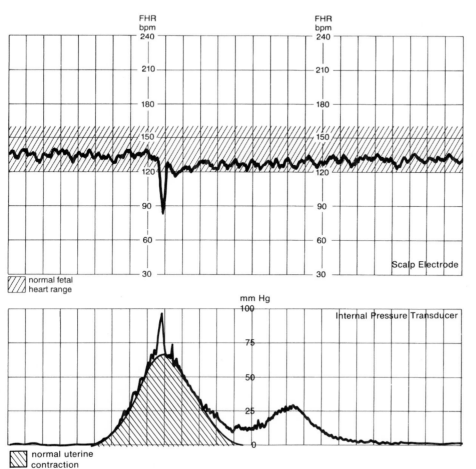

Pattern Characteristic:
Polysystole

Increased Uterine Activity: Paired Contractions

*P*aired contractions are a form of increased uterine contraction frequently characterized by one uterine contraction in close temporal relationship to a second uterine contraction, with the waveform returning to baseline between the two contractions.[65] It is often seen in a mixed pattern with polysystole (see page 352). Usually, the second contraction is smaller in amplitude. The smaller contraction may be a product of uterine activity propagated from the nondominant uterine cornual area. This uterine contraction pattern may be spontaneous or associated with oxytocin-induced or augmented labor. It is often associated with poor progress in labor. It is often a feature of discoordinate labor. As such, the pattern may improve with oxytocin administration.[50]

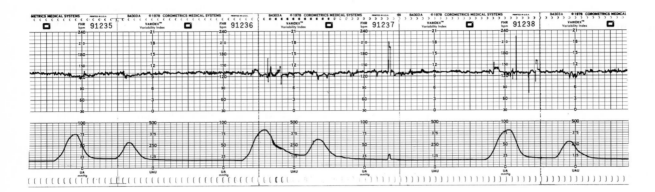

CASE INTERPRETATION: Class I

Baseline Information: low normal rate, average variability.

Periodic or Nonperiodic Changes: shallow periodic early decelerations.

Uterine Activity: paired uterine contractions, polysystolic contractions on other areas of the segment.

Significance: abnormal uterine activity that may contribute to abnormal labor progress.

CASE OUTCOME: Eighteen-year-old primigravida at 40 weeks' gestation delivered vaginally, with epidural anesthesia, a 7 pound, 15 ounce (3600 gram) female; Apgar score 8/9. The fetus was in a vertex presentation, in an occiput anterior position. The infant followed an uncomplicated newborn course.

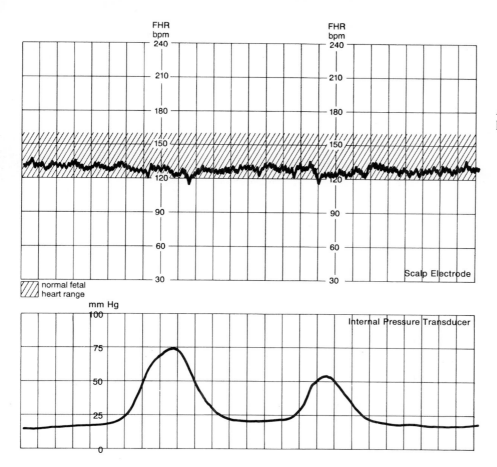

Chart labels:
- FHR bpm 240, 210, 180, 150, 120, 90, 60, 30 (left and right panels)
- normal fetal heart range
- Scalp Electrode
- mm Hg 100, 75, 50, 25, 0
- Internal Pressure Transducer

Pattern Characteristic:
Paired Contractions

Increased Uterine Activity: Tachysystole

Uterine contractions typically increase in frequency from three to five per 10 minutes to five per 10 minutes in late labor.[5] Tachysystole is defined as increased uterine contraction frequency, (e.g., greater than every two minutes).[65] Because of the inevitable accompanying diminished or absent resting interval, decreased fetal oxygenation has been associated more often with this form of uterine hyperactivity than with increased intensity or duration of the uterine contraction. However, increased uterine activity of any type does not infer fetal stress or distress.[51] Increased uterine activity may be well tolerated by some fetuses, whereas others may demonstrate stress even with uterine activity of a low intensity.

Tachysystole may be associated with preeclampsia or placental abruption.[22,45] When tachysystole occurs in the former condition, the contractions are frequently of high intensity.[18] In the latter condition, contractions are often of low intensity. Low-amplitude, frequent contractions may be observed in the antepartum patient with no apparent clinical abnormality or consequence. Low amplitude contractions of increased frequency also are noted with a supine antepartum or intrapartum position.[5] As with any form of uterine hyperactivity, this pattern may appear with oxytocin administration.[8,38]

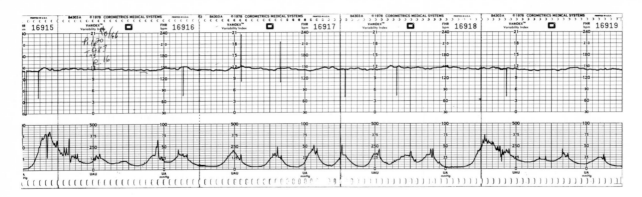

CASE INTERPRETATION: Class III

Baseline Information: normal rate, decreased short-term variability, wavering baseline.

Periodic or Nonperiodic Changes: none seen; possible shallow accelerations.

Uterine Activity: small contractions of normal configuration but excessive frequency as measured by external monitor; a minimal relaxation phase.

Significance: tachysystole. The fetal heart pattern is nonreassuring. Further assessment is indicated, unless study of the entire tracing provides information in support of a good fetal condition.

CASE OUTCOME: Twenty-year-old gravida 3, para 0020, at 39 weeks' gestation delivered vaginally, with pudendal anesthesia, a 6 pound, 2 ounce (2778 gram) male; Apgar score 8/9. The fetus was in a vertex presentation. The infant followed a normal newborn course.

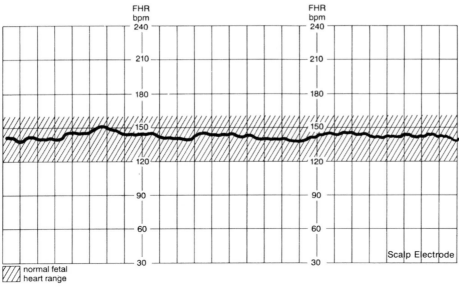

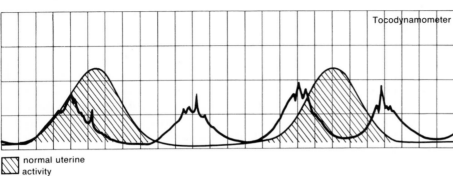

Pattern Characteristic:
Tachysystole

Increased Uterine Activity:
Tachysystole with Progressive Hypertonia

*P*rogressive hypertonia, usually associated with tachysystole, is a form of uterine dysfunction.[66] It represents incomplete relaxation between frequently occurring contractions.[8] It may also be seen after a bolus intravenous administration of drugs (see page 372). Almost any drug can produce a transient episode of increased uterine activity if it is administered rapidly.[47]

The pattern is also associated with oxytocin use and placental abruption.[8] The hyperactivity may exceed fetal tolerance even when the basal condition is healthy.

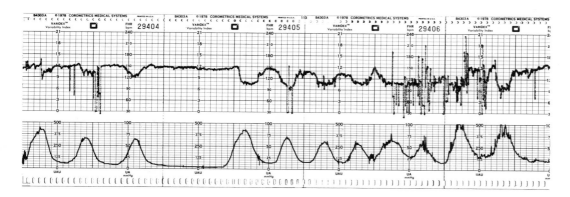

CASE INTERPRETATION: Class II

Baseline Information: normal heart rate, areas of average beat-to-beat variability.

Periodic or Nonperiodic Changes: mild to moderate variable decelerations become progressively closer and merge, producing a prolonged deceleration secondary to an overlap phenomenon, which is followed by recovery.

Uterine Activity: a rise in uterine tone from 4 mm Hg to greater than 25 mm Hg, as measured by an internal monitor.

Significance: the fetal heart rate changes reflect the changes in the uterine trace, with recovery occurring upon the resolution of increased uterine activity.

CASE OUTCOME: Seventeen-year-old primigravida at 41 weeks' gestation delivered vaginally, with epidural anesthesia, a 6 pound, 3 ounce (2807 gram) female; Apgar score 8/9. Thin meconium was present. The fetus was in a vertex presentation, in an occiput anterior position. The infant followed an uncomplicated newborn course.

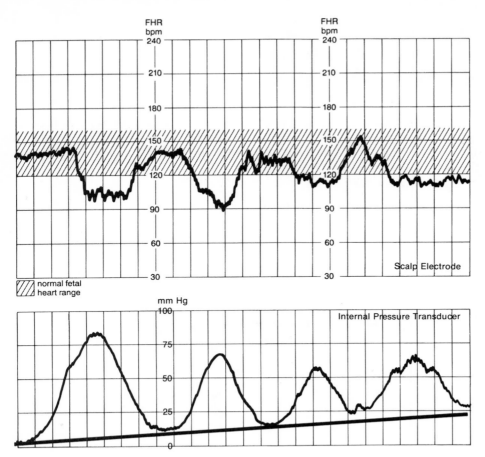

Pattern Characteristic:
Tachysystole with Progressive
Hypertonia

Increased Uterine Activity: Tachysystole with Progression to Tetany

*P*rogressive uterine hypertonus, characterized as a rising baseline tone, is often accompanied by tachysystole.[65]

During the relaxation phase, the uterine tone does not completely return to the prior resting phase level before the next contraction begins. This may progress to tetany.[65] Such a pattern of uterine hyperactivity may be accompanied by a fetal heart rate response in the form of a stress pattern, even in cases in which the underlying fetal condition is a healthy one, because of progressive diminishing to an absent oxygen exchange at the intervillous space.

Internal monitoring is needed to document the rising baseline intrauterine pressure, but the abdominal palpation characteristics of the uterine contraction waveform and observation of the fetal response may assist in making a diagnosis during external monitoring. The pattern may occur spontaneously, may be a response to bolus intravenous drug administration, may be encountered in oxytocin-induced or augmented labors, or may be associated with a pathologic condition such as placental abruption.[53]

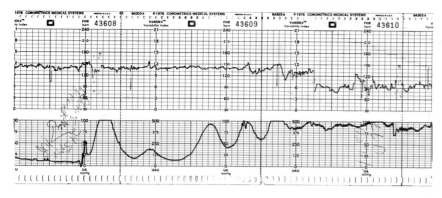

CASE INTERPRETATION: Class II

Baseline Information: normal heart rate and fair variability, as recorded with an external monitor.

Periodic or Nonperiodic Changes: small, variable decelerations that are replaced by a prolonged deceleration without sinus node suppression, which is associated with the increased uterine activity.

Uterine Activity: return of each contraction to a progressively higher level until continuous tetanic contraction. This pattern may be produced by tocodynamometer displacement, but the appearance and fetal response support a true abnormal uterine activity.

Significance: the appropriate management is to diminish uterine activity if feasible. Exclusion of the maternal

heart rate artifact as a cause of the fetal heart rate change is also indicated.

CASE OUTCOME: Thirty-four-year-old gravida 4, para 3003 at 40 weeks' gestation delivered vaginally a 6 pound, 14½ ounce (3132 gram) male; Apgar score 9/9. The fetus was in a vertex presentation. Thin meconium was present. Abnormal uterine activity occurred after the intravenous injection of meperidine and promethazine hydrochloride. The excessive uterine activity was managed by immediate administration of terbutaline 0.25 mg subcutaneously. The scalp pHs taken upon recovery from the acute episode averaged 7.31. The infant followed an uncomplicated newborn course.

Pattern Characteristic:
Tachysystole with Progression to Tetany

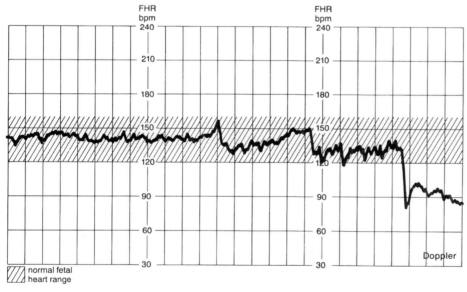

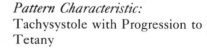

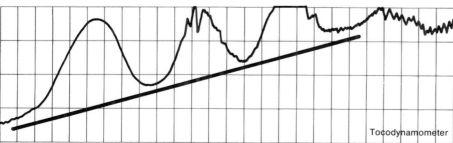

Increased Uterine Activity: Hypertonia

*U*terine tone is the lowest pressure between contractions. In a pregnancy that is near term, 8 to 12 mm Hg is a normal basal tone.

Uterine hypertonia, also termed "hypertonus," is classified as weak (12–20 mm Hg), medium (20–30 mm Hg), and strong (greater than 30 mm Hg).[5]

Tone typically increases as labor progresses. A baseline tone of 15 to 20 mm Hg is not unusual for late labor.[19] Therefore, hypertonia of greater than 20 mm Hg is that which is usually defined as pathologic.[7] Hypertonus as great as 80 mm Hg has been documented.[5] Uterine hypertonia has been associated with placental abruption, the administration of oxytocin or prostaglandin, an occiput posterior position, and cephalopelvic disproportion.[3,23,28,57] Hypertonus typically accompanies hydramnios of greater than five liters because of the overstretched myometrium.[5] Iatrogenic hydramnios has also been associated with hypertonia.[65]

In addition, any intravenous bolus drug administration may cause transient increased uterine activity, including hypertonus.[47] Uterine hypertonia is not typically seen with preeclampsia.[2] A sitting position has been determined to increase the resting uterine tone, which is potentially beneficial to labor duration.[9]

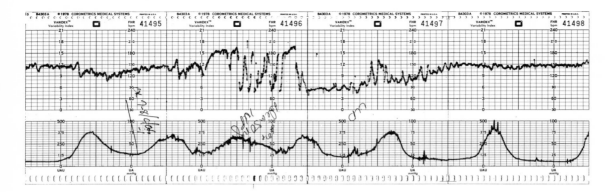

CASE INTERPRETATION: Class II

Baseline Information: normal variability and rate; a dramatic marked degree of increased variability occurs prior to deceleration and again during recovery.

Periodic or Nonperiodic Changes: a prolonged deceleration lasting four minutes, with full recovery; minimal sinus node suppression.

Uterine Activity: elevated resting tone as measured by an internal pressure transducer.

Significance: this is a healthy fetus responding appropriately to a diminished placental exchange. Intravenous narcotics may have aggravated an already increased uterine activity. Reduction of uterine activity, if feasible, is an appropriate response.

CASE OUTCOME: Nineteen-year-old gravida 2, para 1001, at 40 weeks' gestation delivered vaginally, with pudendal and local anesthesia, a 7 pound, 6½ ounce (3359 gram) male; Apgar score 8/9. The fetus was in a vertex presentation, in an occiput anterior position. The infant followed an uncomplicated newborn course.

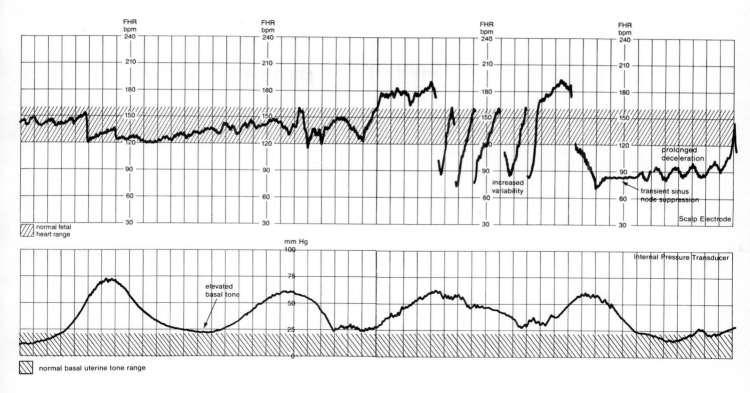

Pattern Characteristic:

Hypertonia

Increased Uterine Activity: Absent Resting Interval

*D*uring the resting phase between uterine contractions the fetus "recovers" from the hypoxic effects of the preceding contraction. The lack of a resting phase is believed to result in a critical decrease in uterine blood flow and fetal oxygenation, as is often evidenced by fetal heart rate responses, especially if the fetus is already compromised.[32] This pattern may be spontaneous and has also been associated with oxytocin use.

Both internal and external uterine contraction monitoring as well as manual palpation and patient perception are methods of assessing this abnormality.

If decelerations occur in response to the uterine contractions, an overlap phenomenon may occur (see page 277) with this pattern, with the next deceleration occurring before recovery from the previous.

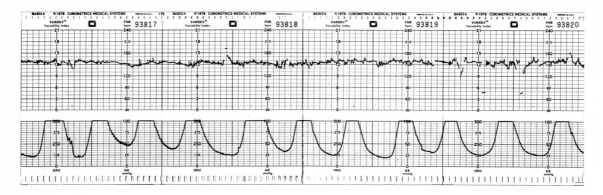

CASE INTERPRETATION: Class III

Baseline Information: normal rate, average variability (but external monitoring without autocorrelation may erroneously amplify variability).

Periodic or Nonperiodic Changes: possible small sporadic accelerations.

Uterine Activity: contractions of excessive frequency, with each contraction beginning before the resolution of the previous one, resulting in no resting phase.

Significance: a reduction of the uterine activity is appropriate if it is feasible. A healthy fetus is suggested because of no periodic changes despite the excessive uterine activity, but the external monitoring pattern is nondiagnostic.

CASE OUTCOME: Thirty-two-year-old gravida 6, para 5005 at 40½ weeks' gestation delivered vaginally, with local anesthesia, a 9 pound (4082 gram) male; Apgar score 8/9. Thick meconium was managed with DeLee suctioning. The infant followed an uncomplicated newborn course. There was no evidence of placental abruption.

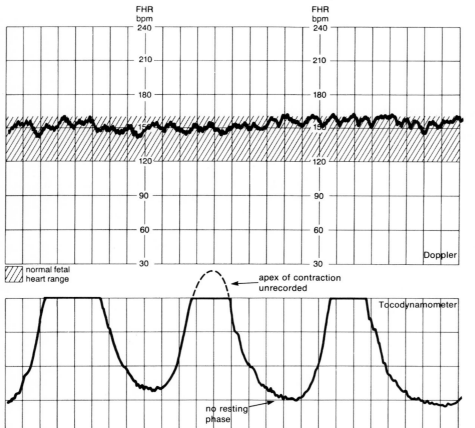

Pattern Characteristic:
Absent Resting Interval

Increased Uterine Activity: Peaked Contractions

A contraction pattern of high intensity and frequency, with a peaked contour, has been associated with preeclampsia and eclampsia.[18] The unusual configuration has been described as an inverted V.[31] The resting tone is typically not elevated.[2] This pattern is not limited to patients with preeclampsia, nor does it occur in every case of preeclampsia.

Oxytocin use in the presence of high intensity contractions of preeclampsia is not contraindicated in selected circumstances, but it may be additive, resulting in the production of uterine activity beyond the tolerance of fetal homeostatic mechanisms, which is eventually demonstrated by heart rate monitoring patterns of hypoxia such as late decelerations.[71] Such hypoxic patterns may occur in cases of preeclampsia without oxytocin use and without achieving intrauterine pressures as high as 50 mm Hg in situations in which the underlying disease process and its associated placental insufficiency, and not uterine activity per se, are predominant factors in the fetal stress.

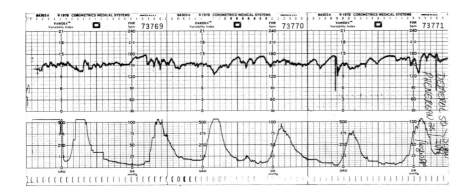

CASE INTERPRETATION: Class I

Baseline Information: normal rate, average variability.

Periodic or Nonperiodic Changes: variable nonperiodic accelerations, a single V-shaped variable deceleration.

Uterine Activity: tall, peaked contractions, as measured by a tocodynamometer.

Significance: this is a pattern seen with, but not limited to, preeclampsia.

CASE OUTCOME: Twenty-year-old primigravida at 29 weeks' gestation delivered vaginally, with spinal anesthesia, a 6 pound, 11 ounce (3033 gram) female; Apgar score 9/9. The maternal course was complicated by preeclampsia. The mother received magnesium sulfate, but no oxytocin, intrapartum. The infant followed an uncomplicated newborn course.

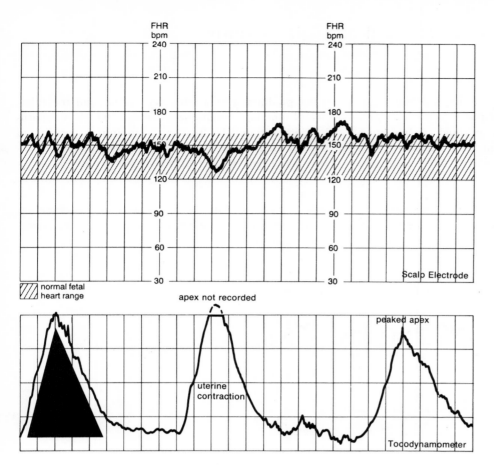

Pattern Characteristic:
Peaked Contractions

Increased Uterine Activity: Hypersystole

The amplitude of intensity is the mm Hg difference between the peak of the uterine contraction and the uterine tone preceding the contraction. Intensity increases on the average with the progressive cervical dilatation. During normal labor, strength varies from 30 mm Hg (early) to 50 mm Hg in the late first stage to 20 to 30 mm Hg in the second stage.[5,19]

Hyperstole is defined as greater than 60 mm Hg maximum pressure.[4]

Contractions of greater than 60 mm Hg are seen with pharmacologically overstimulated or spontaneous abnormal labor.[8] The intensity is usually greater in primigravidas than in multiparas.[67]

Hyperstole may occur in the presence of preeclampsia, placental abruption, and infection. It may be accompanied by fetal heart decelerations, which disappear at lower contraction intensity.[7]

Increased contraction intensity in comparison with normal labor has been reported with oxytocin usage.[58] However, in some nonprogressive labors with low amplitude but long duration of contractions, production of hypersystole by oxytocin augmentation may be therapeutic. Improved contractility may improve the myometrial contraction rhythm and produce a more complete resting phase.

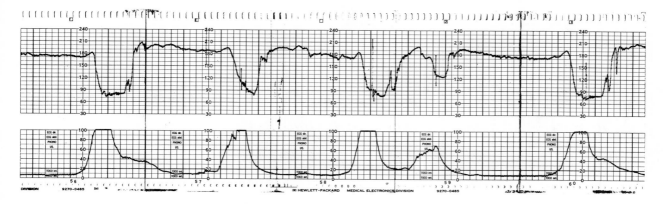

CASE INTERPRETATION: Class IV-V

Baseline Information: moderate to marked tachycardia with average to decreased beat-to-beat variability and some loss of stability.

Periodic or Nonperiodic Changes: severe variable decelerations with atypia, characterized by a loss of variability in the decelerations, some delayed return to baseline, and some prolongation of secondary accelerations.

Uterine Activity: documented contractions of at least 100 mm Hg, skewed and polysystolic, as measured by an internal pressure transducer, and a normal resting tone.

Significance: an increased risk of a low Apgar score and acidosis because of a combination of severe variable decelerations with atypia and baseline changes.

CASE OUTCOME: Twenty-one-year-old gravida 2, para 1001 at 34½ weeks' gestation delivered by cesarean section for secondary arrest of cervical dilatation at 9 centimeters and possible fetal distress a 5 pound, 14½ ounce (2679 gram) male; Apgar score 1/4. The fetus was in a vertex presentation, in an occiput posterior position. No intrapartum pH studies were done. No abnormal cord location was noted at delivery, but the subcutaneous tissues of the baby's head were blue and edematous, suggesting an unusual degree of neck compression by the excessively contracting uterine corpus musculature. The newborn course was complicated by transient tachypnea of the newborn and hyperbilirubinemia.

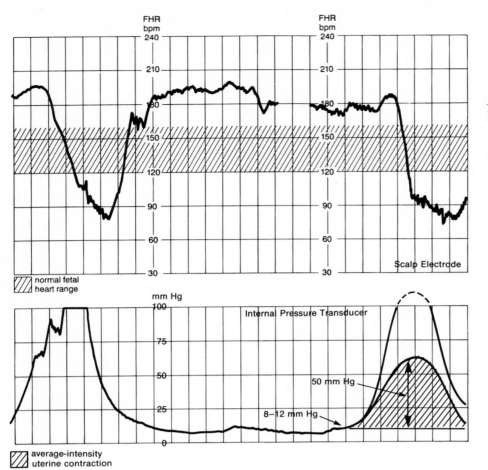

FHR
bpm

normal fetal
heart range

mm Hg

Internal Pressure Transducer

Scalp Electrode

50 mm Hg

8–12 mm Hg

average-intensity
uterine contraction

Pattern Characteristic:
Hypersystole

Increased Uterine Activity: Rate of Rise to Maximum Pressure

*O*xytocin, when used in an appropriate fashion for the induction or augmentation of labor, may be accompanied by a safety record that approaches that of normal labor.[70] Its use may even offer therapeutic advantages in settings with certain types of spontaneous hyperstimulated labor by improving the timing and coordination of uterine contractions.[50] Contraction patterns produced by oxytocin may be similar to those of spontaneous labor. On the other hand, oxytocin-induced uterine activity may also include contraction waveform characteristics that are associated with uterine hypercontractility of a different nature than is usually seen with either spontaneous or even prostaglandin-induced labor.[63] Such a waveform characteristic is a high rate of rise to a maximum pressure.[61,62] This is calculated by dividing active pressure (peak contraction pressure minus uterine resting pressure) by the time of the pressure rise.[14]

When seen in spontaneous labor, it is usually produced by the effects of maternal straining. Other findings associated with the exogenous oxytocin effect are combinations of skewing, polysystole, hypersystole, and tachysystole. With internal monitoring, an elevated baseline tone may also, on occasion, be documented with oxytocin use.

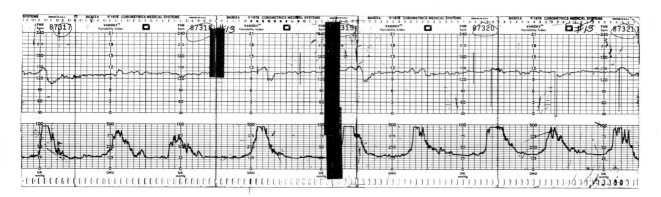

CASE INTERPRETATION: Class IV

Baseline Information: normal rate, decreased beat-to-beat variability with the preservation of long-term variability; an unstable baseline.

Periodic or Nonperiodic Changes: small accelerations are present, mild variable decelerations with atypia, characterized by loss of secondary accelerations and a slow return to baseline (contributing to the appearance of an unstable baseline).

Uterine Activity: contractions every one and a half to two and a half minutes, as measured by an external monitor, with a rapid ascent to peak amplitude followed by a skewed relaxation phase.

Significance: a contraction pattern seen with, but not limited to, oxytocin's effect in a patient who is not straining. The particular atypical variable decelerations present a small risk of increased acidosis or a low Apgar score. Management is influenced by the duration anticipated to delivery, improvement in the pattern with a position change, oxygen administration, and the decreasing of oxytocin if it is being infused, as well as information regarding overall beat-to-beat variability and the general fetal condition prior to medication use.

CASE OUTCOME: Twenty-four-year-old gravida 2, para 1001 at 40 weeks' gestation delivered vaginally, with local anesthesia, a 7 pound, 8 ounce (3402 gram) male; Apgar score 8/9. The fetus was in a vertex presentation. Oxytocin augmentation was performed for management of the premature rupture of membranes at term gestation. A nuchal cord was noted at delivery. The patient had a marginal placental abruption, which was noted at delivery as a possible factor in the increased uterine activity in addition to the use of oxytocin. The infant followed an uncomplicated newborn outcome, except for the finding of a nonpalpable right testicle.

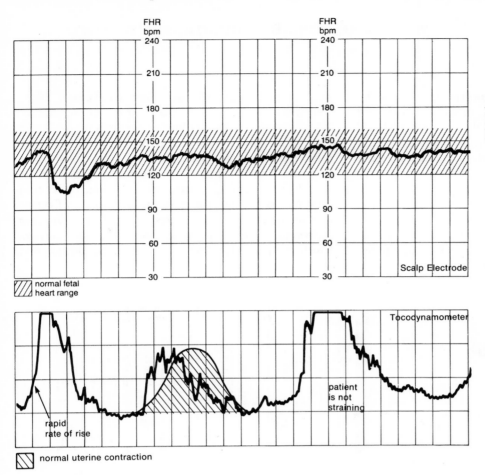

Pattern Characteristic:
Rapid Rate of Rise to Maximum Pressure

Increased Uterine Activity: Spontaneous Hyperstimulation

*H*yperstimulation may occur with nipple stimulation or with the use of uterotonic agents, such as oxytocin.[44,56,69] When a reactive fetus does not respond to uterine hyperstimulation with a fetal heart rate change, the situation suggests that excellent compensatory mechanisms for dealing with hypoxia are operative. However, the reserves of even a healthy fetus may be sufficiently taxed by some prolonged contractions, usually evidenced by an associated prolonged deceleration. Under such circumstances, discontinuing the source of stimulation and demonstrating a subsequent normal (negative) response to contractions of average duration is reassuring. Long-

term harmful effects of the transient stress do not usually occur.[44] The compromised fetus is distinguished from the healthy fetus by demonstrating abnormal responses to other fetal welfare indicators.

Prolonged uterine contractions may occur in the absence of uterotonic agents or nipple stimulation. Such spontaneous hyperactivity may be sporadic or recurrent. It may occur in the presence of a healthy fetus with no maternal risk factors or as a consequence of a pathologic condition. Factors reported to contribute to spontaneous uterine hyperstimulation are postdate pregnancy, maternal anxiety, maternal hyperbilirubinemia, preeclampsia, hydramnios, and placental abruption. A healthy fetus may display a deceleration in response to a prolonged contraction yet may produce no decelerations in response to contractions of normal duration and configuration. Nevertheless, recurrent episodes of prolonged contractions may gradually deplete fetal compensatory mechanisms for withstanding hypoxia. Therefore, the presence of prolonged contractions indicates a potential hostile environment for the fetus. If there is evidence of a good basal fetal condition (e.g., a reactive tracing), an appropriate management is the determination, through prolonged monitoring, that the prolonged contractions are occurring infrequently. In the absence of fetal reactivity, a decelerative response to a prolonged contraction may indicate that fetal compromise in the abnormal setting is already occurring and prompt steps to further evaluate the fetus are in order (such as by biophysical assessment with ultrasonography).

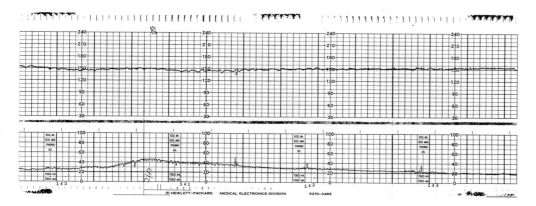

CASE INTERPRETATION: Class V

Baseline Information: normal heart rate, diminished short-term and long-term variability.

Periodic or Nonperiodic Changes: a shallow prolonged deceleration of seven to eight minutes, late onset, nadir and recovery in association with a uterine contraction.

Uterine Activity: a seven to eight minute skewed uterine contraction.

Significance: although a healthy fetus will potentially respond to a prolonged uterine contraction with a prolonged deceleration, there is no reassuring information (i.e., a reactive baseline) of a good basal fetal condition. Therefore, more information is necessary about the fetal welfare, as individualized by the clinical setting such as a biophysical profile, formal stress test, or prolonged monitoring.

CASE OUTCOME: Twenty-eight-year-old gravida 2, para 1001, at 38 weeks' gestation delivered by primary cesarean section for possible fetal distress a 6 pound, 11½ ounce (3040 gram) female; Apgar score 4/5. The first newborn pH was 7.04. There was thick meconium. A nuchal cord was present. The newborn was transferred from a Level II to a Level III center. The infant's course was complicated by persistent fetal circulation and seizures. The newborn was dismissed at nine days of life.

Spontaneous deceleration occurred at antepartum monitoring for possible intrauterine growth retardation. Antepartum monitoring one day after this segment showed late/variable decelerations.

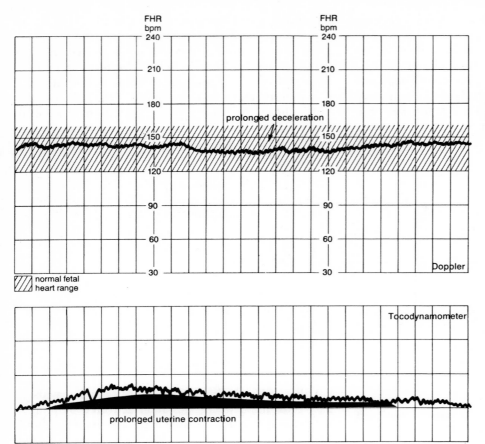

Pattern Characteristic:
Spontaneous Hyperstimulation

Increased Uterine Activity: Severe Hypercontractility

Severe hypercontractility refers to excessive uterine hyperactivity repeatedly occurring with each contraction, with or without progress in cervical dilatation. The phenomenon may be encountered in spontaneous labor without apparent cause: essential hypercontractility.[10] It may also accompany induced or augmented labor whether employing oxytocin, prostaglandin, or other uterotonic agents.[8] Spontaneous hypercontractility has been associated clinically with placental abruption, preeclampsia, maternal bilirubinemia, hydramnios, and in-

fection, or with no detectable cause (idiopathic).[10,22,54,66] Fetal and, occasionally, maternal jeopardy may require intervention. In the present case illustration, a fresh surgical scar in the uterine cornu may have played a role in the unusual labor pattern. Uterine contractions typically arise from the right fundus and propagate toward the cervix. Just as in the heart, foci of activity other than in the dominant pacemaker may occur, producing various patterns of abnormal muscular activity.

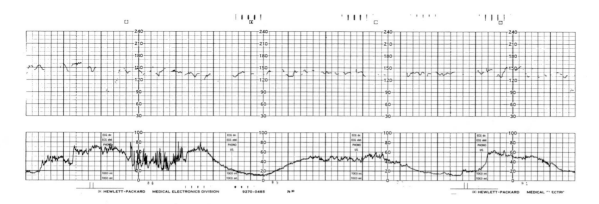

CASE INTERPRETATION: Class 0

Baseline Information: normal heart rate, average variability.

Periodic or Nonperiodic Changes: the signal fades and is lost in areas; there appear to be accelerations present. No decelerations are seen in this segment.

Uterine Activity: recurrent prolonged contractions lasting two to five minutes, as measured by external monitoring, a minimal resting phase.

Significance: excessive uterine activity. Discontinuation of oxytocin, if infusing, evaluation for underlying causes, and administration of a tocolytic agent, if feasible, are appropriate responses. Good fetal condition is suggested by the absence of a stress pattern in the presence of increased uterine activity.

CASE OUTCOME: Thirty-six-year-old gravida 7, para 6006, at 40 weeks' gestation delivered spontaneously from a vertex presentation a 7 pound, 12 ounce (3515 gram) female; Apgar score 6/7. Meconium was present. The infant followed a normal newborn course except for a heart murmur. A ruptured uterus in the left cornual region was diagnosed immediately after delivery and the patient underwent an emergency hysterectomy. The patient had a cornual resection of an ectopic pregnancy during the present pregnancy six and a half months earlier. Morphine sulfate was administered during labor in an attempt to reduce uterine activity. (This case management occurred prior to the use of beta sympathomimetic agents in labor.)

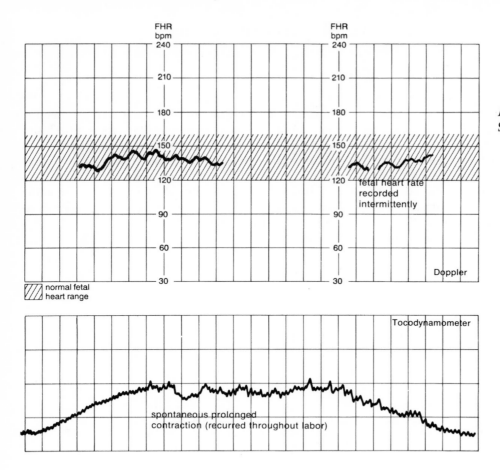

Pattern Characteristic:
Severe Hypercontractility

Increased Uterine Activity: Severe Tetany

A tetanic contraction is defined as a contraction that plateaus and does not return to normal baseline for two normal contraction cycles or five minutes. It has also been defined as a uterine contraction lasting longer than 180 seconds.[21]

Tetany may occur spontaneously, in a setting of nipple stimulation, with the use of uterotonic pharmacologic agents, or in the presence of placental abruption or infection.[20,21,56,57] It may be preceded by tachysystole.[65] Tetany occurring in oxytocin use may be a result of unusual patient sensitivity to the agent, or because of a cumulative effect of increasing the dosage, or even in a situation without dosage increase as the patient's contractions become more efficient with advancing labor, especially after ruptured membranes.[10] Uterine tetany may also accompany the bolus intravenous administration of drugs that are not usually considered uterotonic.[20]

Pharmacologic agents that produce uterine relaxation have been used to treat uterine tetany for many years. Use of various anesthetic drugs and morphine have been superceded by the bolus administration of B sympathomimetic agents and magnesium sulfate.[29,36,37,47]

A healthy fetus has compensatory mechanisms to endure the acute hypoxia and sinus mode suppression that typically occurs during tetany, but without spontaneous resolution of the contraction, these mechanisms may be depleted. Decompensation eventually results if intervention does not occur by either reduction of the uterine activity or delivery.

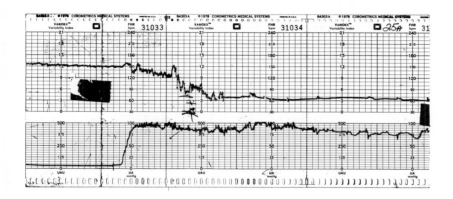

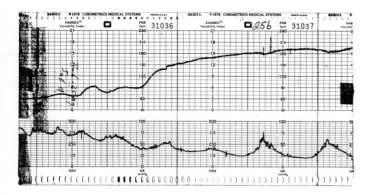

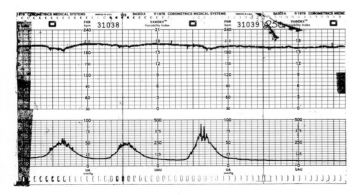

CASE INTERPRETATION: Class V

Baseline Information: normal rate and variability until deceleration (transient baseline changes); rebound tachycardia with decreased variability upon recovery.

Periodic or Nonperiodic Changes: a 12-minute prolonged deceleration; sinus node suppression with an escape; periodic, shallow late decelerations during the recovery phase.

Uterine Activity: tetany, as documented by an internal pressure monitor; tachysystole after resolution of the tetany.

Significance: acute, severe transient fetal heart response to uterine tetany, responding to uterine relaxation with terbutaline (0.25 mg subcutaneously) and discontinuation of oxytocin infusion.

CASE OUTCOME: Twenty-year-old primigravida at 40 weeks' gestation, after having ruptured membranes for 33 hours, delivered by cesarean section for cephalopelvic disproportion a 5 pound, 14 ounce (2665 gram) female; Apgar score 3/7. Labor was induced with oxytocin. The mother followed a febrile intrapartum course. Chorioamnionitis was diagnosed; placental cultures were positive for group B streptococcus. Oxytocin infusion at the time of tetany was 2.5 mU/min. The fetal heart recovery following the episode of severe tetany was protracted and included transient late decelerations, rebound tachycardia, and loss of beat-to-beat variability. The newborn followed an uncomplicated course and was dismissed with the mother at 5 days of life.

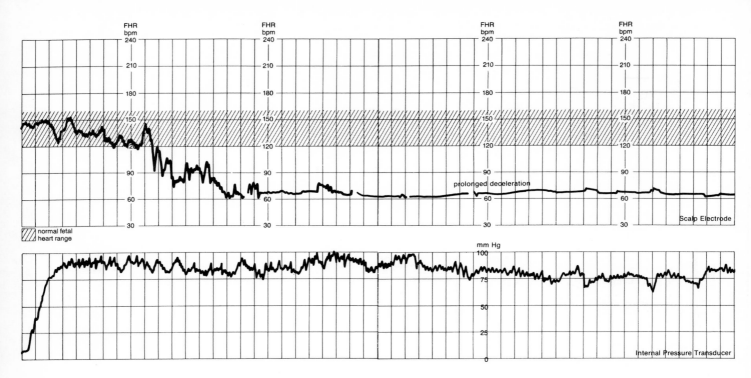

Pattern Characteristic:
Severe Tetany

Increased Uterine Activity Associated with Total Placental Abruption

*P*lacental abruption severe enough to cause intrauterine fetal death is typically associated with an increased frequency of uterine contractions averaging 8.4 per 10 minute period.[45] An increased uterine baseline tone is also characteristic of increased uterine activity with placental abruption. The mechanism for the increased uterine activity is believed to be the hollow organ's response to bleeding into its muscular wall.[10]

Several different uterine contraction patterns have been described with placental abruption.[12] Those without significant hypertonus (baseline tone less than 30 mm Hg) display normal activity, rhythmic low activity, or discoordinated low activity. Those with strong hypertonus show rhythmic contractions of increased frequency or discoordinated hyperactivity. Patterns with hypertonus are most likely to demonstrate fetal heart rate abnormalities.[28] Patterns with hypertonus are less likely to demonstrate change with the administration of oxytocin.[12]

The degree of hypertonus may or may not correlate with clinical features such as the degree of shock or the amount of retroplacental clot.[10] If the fetus is alive, fetal monitoring usually shows other than a normal pattern.[10]

Early detection of uterine hyperactivity in a patient suspected to have a placental abruption may lead to timely intervention prior to death of the fetus.[10,45,55] See pages 38 and 317 for fetal heart rate patterns associated with placental abruption.

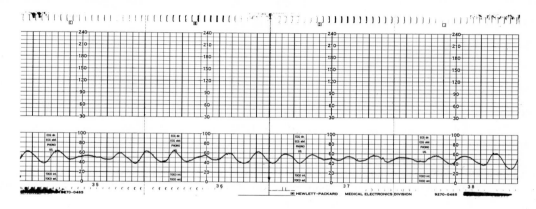

CASE INTERPRETATION: Class 0

Baseline Information: no heart rate trace recorded.

Periodic or Nonperiodic Changes: none recorded.

Uterine Activity: baseline tone elevation at 40 mm Hg with tachysystole, producing a pattern of undulating uterine contractions.

Significance: a pattern seen with severe placental abruption and usually accompanied by intrauterine fetal death.

CASE OUTCOME: Fourteen-year-old primigravida at 36 weeks' gestation delivered vaginally, with local and pudendal anesthesia, a 4 pound, 11 ounce (2126 gram) stillborn male from a vertex presentation. The patient was admitted with a clinical picture of intrauterine fetal death, preeclampsia, and placental abruption with disseminated intravascular coagulation. She received magnesium sulfate and blood products intrapartum. The membranes were ruptured artificially and internal pressure monitoring was performed.

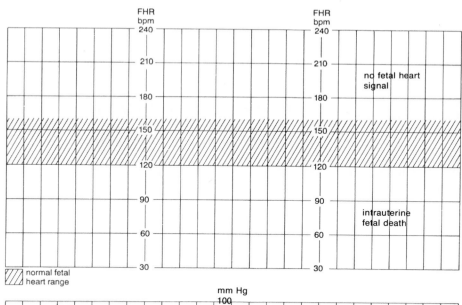

Pattern Characteristic:
Total Placental Abruption

Exaggerated Contraction Frequency Secondary to Paper Speed: Artifact

*I*n the United States, 3 cm/min is usually used as the basis for fetal monitoring interpretation. For prolonged monitoring of a single patient, one centimeter paper speed requires less paper, but the change in appearance makes interpretation depend on appropriate visual training for the altered speed. Modern US fetal monitors have deleted the paper speed options because 3 cm/min has evolved for most common use.[73]

Besides exaggerating apparent heart rate variability, periodic decelerations are altered in character so that subtle features may be masked.[11] Uterine contractions appear to be peaked, with an increased frequency and decreased resting phase.[46] Unless the slower speed is used regularly, failure to note the difference in speed could alter management.

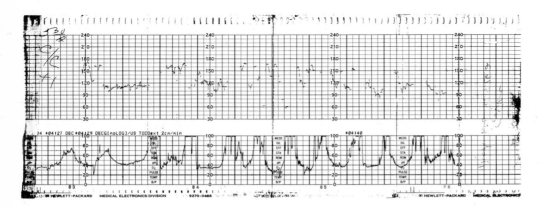

CASE INTERPRETATION: Class 0

Baseline Information: there appear to be two heart rates, one in the normal range and one in the moderate bradycardia range. Variability is good with the lower rate, normal to high with the upper rate.

Periodic or Nonperiodic Changes: none seen, although the pattern must be differentiated from intermittent prolonged decelerations.

Uterine Activity: contractions lasting one minute or less occur every minute without a resting phase. Straining is present.

Significance: the above interpretation, which is based on the usual paper speed, would signify excessive uterine activity as well as probable intermittent monitoring of the maternal heart rate, based on the flatness of the two rates. However, the observant interpreter would not miss that this pattern has the appearance of a pattern with a slower than 3 cm/min paper speed (especially in that the modern data entry system has printed 2 cm/min on the strip). Appropriate management is to correct the paper speed (unless the reader is visually trained in interpretation at this speed) and make a reevaluation as well as to reposition the Doppler transducer.

CASE OUTCOME:

Seventeen-year-old primigravida at 36½ weeks' gestation delivered vaginally, with local and pudendal anesthesia, a 7 pound (3175 gram) male; Apgar score 8/9. The infant followed an uncomplicated newborn course. This monitor had just arrived from Europe and was still set at the 2 cm/min speed.

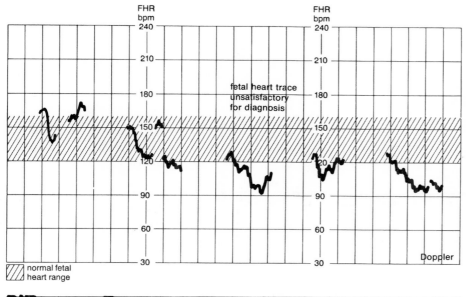

Pattern Characteristic:
Frequency Artifact: Paper Speed
Effect

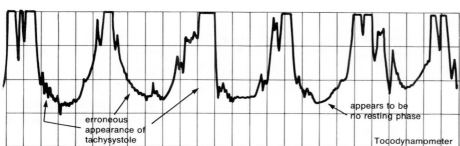

Exaggerated Peaking of Contractions Secondary to Paper Speed: Artifact

*J*ust as a slow paper speed (1 or 2 cm/min in contrast to 3 cm/min) alters the visual presentation of fetal heart information,[11] it also alters uterine activity information. Contraction frequency appears increased, there appears to be a more rapid rise to maximum amplitude, and the configuration is typically peaked. Contractions, of course, also appear to be shorter in duration. The overall effect may simulate the contraction pattern of a placental abruption. See pages 80, 376 for other examples of distortion produced by a variation in paper speed.

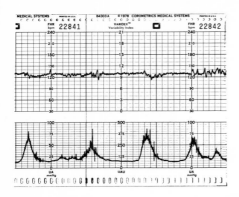

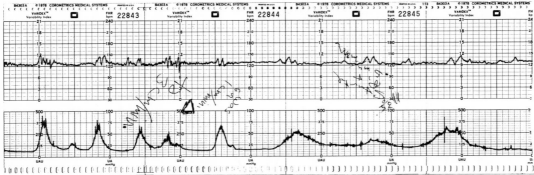

CASE INTERPRETATION: Class I

Baseline Information: normal rate, normal to increased variability changes to average variability with the paper speed change.

Periodic or Nonperiodic Changes: areas of apparent increased variability change to small variable accelerations with the paper speed change.

Uterine Activity: peaked contractions giving the appearance of tachysystole approximately every one to one and a half minutes change to contractions with a normal configuration approximately every two to four minutes.

Significance: visual distortion is produced by the 1 cm/min paper speed. The 3 cm/min portion predicts a normal fetal outcome.

CASE OUTCOME: Twenty-two-year-old primigravida at 40 weeks' gestation delivered by cesarean section for cephalopelvic disproportion with spinal anesthesia a 7 pound, 6 ounce (3345 gram) female; Apgar score 8/9. The fetus was in a vertex presentation. The infant followed an uncomplicated newborn course. The paper speed was changed from 1 cm/min to 3 cm/min during intrapartum monitoring.

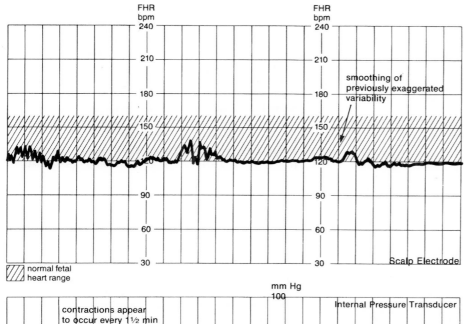

Pattern Characteristic:
Peaking Artifact: Paper Speed
Effect

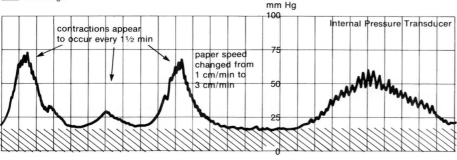

References

1. Alvarez H, Caldeyro-Barcia R: Fisiopatologia de la contraccion uterina y sus aplicaciones en clinica obstetrica. *II Cong Lat-Am Obstet Gynecol (Brasil)* 1:1, 1954.

2. Alvarez H, Pose SV, Caldeyro-Barcia R: La contractilidad uterina en la toxemia gravidica. *Proc First Peruv Cons Obstet Gynecol* 2:281, 1959.

3. Anderson GG, Hobbins JG, Speroff L: Intravenous prostaglandins E and F for the induction of term labor. *Am J Obstet Gynecol* 112:382, 1972.

4. Caldeyro-Barcia R, Poseiro JJ, Negreiros de Paiva C, et al: Effects of abnormal uterine contractions on a human fetus. *Mod Probl Pediat* 8:267, 1963.

5. Caldeyro-Barcia R, Poseiro JJ: Physiology of the uterine contraction. *Clin Obstet Gynecol* 3:386, 1960.

6. Caldeyro-Barcia R, Alvarez H, Reynolds SRM: A better understanding of uterine contractility through simultaneous recording with an internal and a seven channel external method. *Surg Gynecol and Obstet* 91:641, 1950.

7. Caldeyro-Barcia R, Poseiro JJ, Pantle G, et al: Effects of uterine contractions on the heart rate of the human fetus. *Digest of the 1961 International Conference on Medical Electronics*, New York, p. 1.

8. Cerevka J, Scheffs JS, Vasicka A: Shape of uterine contractions (intra-amniotic pressure) and corresponding fetal

heart rate. I. Spontaneous and oxytocin induced labors. *Obstet Gynecol* 35:695, 1970.

9. Chen S-Z, Aisaka K, Mori H, et al: Effects of sitting position on uterine activity during labor. *Obstet Gynecol* 69:67, 1987.

10. Cibils L: *Abnormal Uterine Contractility in Electronic Fetal-Maternal Monitoring: Antepartum, Intrapartum.* Boston, PSG Publishing, 1981, p. 111.

11. Cibils L: *Early Decelerations in Electronic Fetal-Maternal Monitoring.* Boston, PSG Publishing, 1981.

12. Cobo E, Quintero CA, Strada G, et al: Uterine behavior in abruptio placentae. 1. Contraction patterns and their reactivity to oxytocin. *Am J Obstet Gynecol* 92:1151, 1965.

13. Cowan DB, Van Middelkoop A, Philpott RH: Intrauterine-pressure studies in African nulliparae: Delay, delivery and disproportion. *Br J Obstet Gynaecol* 89:370, 1982.

14. Csapo A: The diagnostic significance of the intrauterine pressure part I: General considerations and techniques. *Obstet Gynecol Survey* 24:403, 1969.

15. Effer SB, Bertola RP, Urettos A, et al: Quantitative study of the regularity of uterine contractile rhythm in labor. *Am J Obstet Gynecol* 105:909, 1969.

16. El-Sahwi S, Gaafar AA, Toppozada HK: A new unit for evaluation of uterine activity. *Am J Obstet Gynecol* 98:998, 1967.

17. Freeman RK: Management of acute intrapartum fetal distress, in: *A Clinical Approach to Fetal Monitoring.* Berkeley, CA, Berkeley Bio-Engineering, Inc., 1974.

18. Freeman RK, Barden TP: Interpreting fetal heart tracings, in: *Management of High Risk Pregnancy,* Oradell, NJ, Queenan Medical Economics Co., 1980, pp. 175–182.

19. Freeman RK, Garite TJ: Uterine contraction monitoring, in: *Fetal Heart Rate Monitoring,* Baltimore, Williams & Wilkins, 1981, p. 55.

20. Friedman EA: Uterine tetany, in: *Obstetrical Decision Making,* Trenton, NJ, BC Decker, St. Louis, CV Mosby, 1982, p. 180.

21. Friedman EA, Sachtleben MR: Effect of oxytocin and oral prostaglandin E2 on uterine contractility and fetal heart rate patterns. *Am J Obstet Gynecol* 130:403, 1978.

22. Garite TJ, Freeman RK: Immediate cesarean for abruptio placentae. *Contemp Obstet Gynecol* 20:40, 1982.

23. Gross TL, Sokol RJ, Rosen MG: Clinical use of the intrapartum monitoring record. *Clin Obstet Gynecol* 22:633, 1979.

24. Hauth JC, Hankens GDV, Gilstrap LC, et al: Uterine contraction pressures with oxytocin induction/augmentation. *Obstet Gynecol* 68:305, 1986.

25. Hon EH, Paul RH: Quantitation of uterine activity. *Obstet Gynecol* 42:368, 1973.

26. Huey JR, Miller FC: The evaluation of uterine activity: A comparative analysis. *Am J Obstet Gynecol* 135:252, 1979.

27. Huey JR, Al-Hadjiev A, Paul RH: Uterine activity in the multiparous patient. *Am J Obstet Gynecol* 126:682, 1976.

28. Hurd WW, Miodovorik M, Hertzberg V, et al: Selective management of abruptio placentae: A prospective study. *Obstet Gynecol* 61:467, 1983.

29. Ingemarsson I, Arulkummaran S, Ratnam SS: Single in-

jection of terbutaline in term labor II. Effect on uterine activity. *Am J Obstet Gynecol* 153:865, 1985.

30. Karlson S: On the motility of the uterus during labour and the influence of the motility pattern on the duration of labour. *Acta Obstet Gynaecol Scand* 46:794, 1949.

31. Klaven M, Boscola MA: *A Guide to Fetal Monitoring.* Waltham, MA, Hewlett-Packard, 1973.

32. Klink F, Grosspietzsch R, Klitzing LV, et al: Uterine contraction intervals and transcutaneous levels of fetal oxygen pressure. *Obstet Gynecol* 57:437, 1981.

33. Krapohl AJ, Myers GG, Caldeyro-Barcia R: Uterine contractions in spontaneous labor. *Am J Obstet Gynecol* 106:378, 1970.

34. LaCroix GE: Monitoring labor by an external tocodynamometer. *Am J Obstet Gynecol* 101:111, 1968.

35. Lindgren L: The causes of foetal head moulding in labor. *Acta Obstet Gynecol Scand* 39:40, 1960.

36. Lipshitz J, Klose CW: Use of tocolytic drugs to reverse oxytocin-induced uterine hypertonus and fetal distress. *Obstet Gynecol* 66:165, 1985.

37. Lipshitz J: Use of a beta 2-sympathomemetic drug as a temporizing measure in the treatment of acute fetal distress. *Am J Obstet Gynecol* 129:31, 1977.

38. Liston WA, Campbell AJ: Dangers of oxytocin-induced labour to fetuses. *Brit Med J* 3:606, 1974.

39. Miller FC: Monitoring uterine activity. *Contemp OB/GYN* 13:35, 1979.

40. Miller FC, Paul RH: Intrapartum fetal heart rate monitoring. *Clin Obstet Gynecol* 21:561, 1978.

41. Miller FC, Yeh S-Y, Schifrin BS, et al: Quantitation of uterine activity in 100 primiparous patients. *Am J Obstet Gynecol* 124:398, 1976.

42. Miller FC, Mueller E, Veleck K: Quantitation of uterine activity: Clinical evaluation of a new method of data presentation. *Obstet Gynecol* 55:388, 1980.

43. Neuman MR: The biophysical and bioengineering bases of perinatal monitoring. Part II: Uterine contractions. *Perinatology/Neonatology* Sept-Oct 1978, p. 14.

44. Odendaal HJ: Hyperstimulation of the uterus during the oxytocin stress test. *Obstet Gynecol* 51:380, 1978.

45. Odendaal HJ: Uterine contraction patterns in patients with severe abruptio placentae. *S Afr Med J* 57:908, 1980.

46. Paul RH, Petrie R: *Fetal Intensive Care.* Wallingford, CT, Corometrics Medical Systems, Inc., 1979.

47. Petrie RH: How intrapartum drugs affect FHR. *Contemp Obstet Gynecol* 16:61, 1980.

48. Petrie RH, Wu R, Miller FC, et al: The effect of drugs on uterine activity. *Obstet Gynecol* 48:431, 1976.

49. Pillars SK, Chik L, Sokol RJ, et al: Fetal monitoring: A guide to understanding the equipment. *Clin Obstet Gynecol* 22:471, 1979.

50. Poseiro JJ, Noreiga-Guerra L: *Dose Response Relationships in Uterine Effect of Oxytocin Infusion.* London, Pergammon Press, 1960.

51. Reece EA, Antoine C, Montgomery J: The fetus as the final arbiter of intrauterine stress/distress. *Clin Obstet Gynecol* 29:23, 1986.

52. Reynolds SRM, Heard OO, Bruns P: Recording uterine

contraction patterns in pregnant women: Appreciation of a strain gage in multichannel tocodynamometer. *Science* 106:427, 1947.

53. Ron M, Menashe M, Scherer D, et al: Fetal heart rate decelerations following the administration of meperidine-promethazine during labor. *Int J Gynaecol Obstet* 20:301, 1982.

54. Roszkowski I, Pisarek-Miedzinska D: Jaundice in pregnancy II. Clinical course of pregnancy and delivery and condition of neonate. *Am J Obstet Gynecol* 101:500, 1968.

55. Saunderson PR, Steer PJ: The value of cardiotocography in abruptio placentae. *Br J Obstet Gynaecol* 85:796, 1978.

56. Schellpfeffer MA, Hoyle D, Johnson JWC: Antepartal uterine hypercontractility secondary to nipple stimulation. *Obstet Gynecol* 65:588, 1985.

57. Schifrin BS: Fetal heart rate patterns following epidural anaesthesia and oxytocin infusion during labour. *J Obstet Gynaecol Br Commonwealth* 79:332, 1972.

58. Schwarcz RL, Belizan JM, Cifuentes JR, et al: Fetal and maternal monitoring in spontaneous labors and in elective inductions. *Am J Obstet Gynecol* 120:356, 1974.

59. Seitchek J: Measure of contraction strength in labor: Area and amplitude. *Am J Obstet Gynecol* 138:727, 1980.

60. Seitchek J: Quantitating uterine contractility in clinical context. *Obstet Gynecol* 57:453, 1981.

61. Seitchek J, Chatoff ML: Intrauterine pressure waveform characteristics in hypocontractile labor before and after oxytocin administration. *Am J Obstet Gynecol* 123:426, 1975.

62. Seitchek J, Chatoff ML: Oxytocin induced uterine hypercontractility pressure wave forms. *Obstet Gynecol* 48:436, 1976.

63. Seitchek J, Chatoff ML, Hayashi RH: Intrauterine pressure waveform characteristics of spontaneous and oxyto-cin-or prostaglandin F2-induced active labor. *Am J Obstet Gynecol* 127:223, 1977.

64. Silverman F, Hutson JM: The clinical and biological significance of the bottom line. *Clin Obstet Gynecol* 29:43, 1986.

65. Stookey RA, Sokol RJ, Rosen MG: Abnormal contraction patterns in patients monitored during labor. *Obstet Gynecol* 42:359, 1973.

66. Tabor BL, Maier JA: Polyhydramnios and elevated intrauterine pressure during amnioinfusion. *Am J Obstet Gynecol* 156:130, 1987.

67. Turnbull AC: Uterine contractions in normal and abnormal labor. *J Obstet Gynaec Brit Emp* 64:321, 1957.

68. Ulmsten U, Andersson K-E: Multichannel intrauterine pressure recording by means of microtransducers. *Acta Obstet Gynecol Scand* 58:115, 1979.

69. Viegas OAC, Arulkumaran S, Digg DMF, et al: Nipple stimulations in late pregnancy causing uterine hyperstimulation and profound fetal bradycardia. *Br J Obstet Gynecol* 91:364, 1984.

70. Weaver JB, Pearson JF, Turnbull AC: The effect upon the fetus of an oxytocin infusion in the absence of uterine hypertonus. *J Obstet Gynaecol Br Commonwealth* 81:297, 1974.

71. Weingold AB, Fert A, O'Sullivan MJ, et al: Fetal heart rate response in the pre-eclamptic hypertensive patient during spontaneous and oxytocin stimulated labor. *J Reprod Med* V:110, 1970.

72. Whittle MJ, Miller FC: The evaluation of uterine activity. *Am J Obstet Gynecol* 136:38, 1980.

73. Yeast JD, Garite TJ: What's available in EFM equipment? *Contemp Obstet Gynecol* Technology Issue 1984, p. 17.

Maternal/Fetal Activity

Maternal Respirations

*T*he external monitor and, to a lesser extent, the internal monitor, may reflect maternal activity on the uterine trace as well as uterine contraction configuration and frequency.

The respiratory activity of the mother may be seen by either method of uterine activity monitoring but is typically more pronounced with a tocodynamometer-derived signal, particularly when the mother uses abdominal breathing techniques.

The displayed maternal respiration may reflect a maternal response to pain and other stimuli and, furthermore, may document abnormal maternal respiratory patterns in disease states.

In patients with prior preparation in breathing techniques, it may be that only regularly changing patterns of maternal respiration are encountered such as the purposeful use of hyperventilation during peak contraction intensity.

Hyperventilation is routinely encouraged during the transition phase in most American delivery units and is considered safe.[11] The fetal response to maternal hyperventilation may be an indicator of fetal condition. Transient fetal tachycardia (accelerations) may occur in response to maternal hyperventilation in a pregnancy with a healthy fetus, but no response may occur when the fetus is chronically or acutely ill.[12]

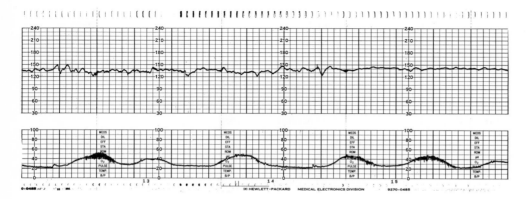

CASE INTERPRETATION: Class I

Baseline Information: normal rate, average variability with progressive smoothing to beat-to-beat variability during this segment.

Periodic or Nonperiodic Changes: small accelerations are noted.

Uterine Activity: contractions of a normal configuration every two to three minutes, as measured by an external monitor. Maternal respirations vary with the contraction phase and size.

Significance: a normal newborn outcome is predicted. The patient is exhibiting a spontaneous or trained respiratory response to labor.

CASE OUTCOME: Sixteen-year-old primigravida at 41½ weeks' gestation delivered vaginally, with unsuccessful epidural anesthesia from a vertex presentation, a 7 pound, 13 ounce (3544 gram) newborn; Apgar score 9/9. Patient and husband had attended prepared childbirth classes. The infant followed an uncomplicated newborn course.

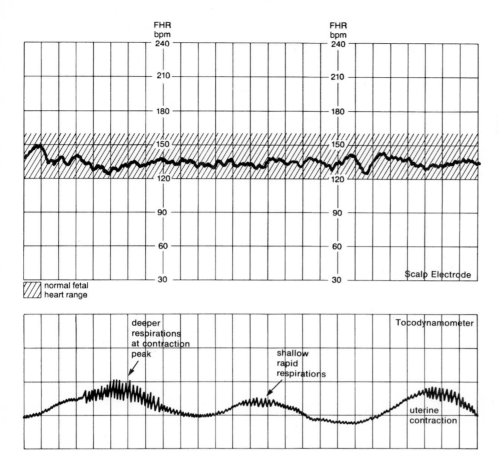

Pattern Characteristic:
Maternal Respirations

Scalp Electrode

/// normal fetal
/// heart range

deeper
respirations
at contraction
peak

shallow
rapid
respirations

Tocodynamometer

uterine
contraction

Exaggerated Maternal Respirations

*T*he Doppler transducer placement and maternal positioning affect the degree of fluctuations with the maternal respiratory activity. The deflections produced by maternal respirations are increased if the abdominal wall has an increased freedom of movement during breathing, if the mother is using an abdominal breathing technique, and if the Doppler transducer is placed loosely at the point of maximum abdominal wall deflection. The deflections will also be increased with the depth of maternal respirations.

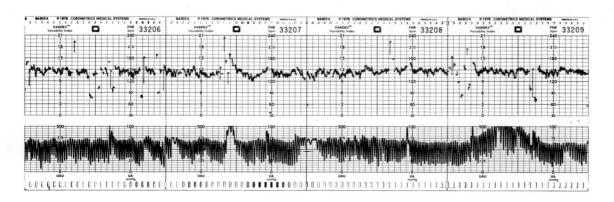

CASE INTERPRETATION: Class I

Baseline Information: a normal rate, intermittently poorly recorded fetal heart trace suggests a good beat-to-beat variability, but this is an unreliable interpretation based on measurement by an external monitor without autocorrelation.

Periodic or Nonperiodic Changes: this pattern suggests occasional accelerations that are poorly recorded.

Uterine Activity: excessive pen deflections are consistent with the maternal respiratory activity; the pattern obscures uterine contractions.

Significance: although wide fluctuations suggest excessive respiratory movements, as with hyperventilation, this sustained unusual pattern is more often seen in a patient breathing normally while on her side or in other positions in which the abdominal wall is able to make marked excursions during breathing, as perceived by the tocodynamometer pressure sensor.

CASE OUTCOME: Twenty-three-year-old gravida 3, para 2002, at 40 weeks' gestation delivered vaginally, with pudendal anesthesia, a 6 pound, 2 ounce (2778 gram) female; Apgar score 8/9. The fetus was in a vertex presentation. The patient labored and was monitored "sitting on the commode." The infant followed a normal newborn course.

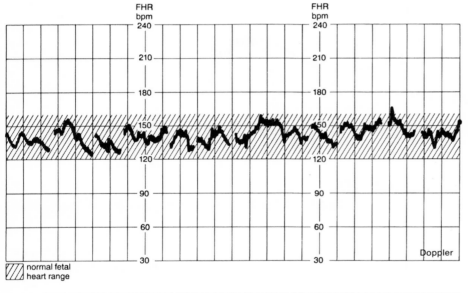

Pattern Characteristic:
Exaggerated Maternal
Respirations

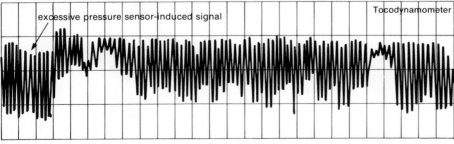

Maternal Tachypnea

*I*n addition to providing information about contraction frequency, duration, and configuration, the tocodynamometer also may reflect maternal activity superimposed on the contraction waveform. Maternal activity that has been captured on the uterine trace includes that which is associated with: crying, coughing, chills, hiccups, and straining. Variations in maternal respiration have produced many interesting patterns. These include those seen with: hyperventilation, panting, Kussmaul's respiration, sleep, obstructive sleep apnea, and tachypnea.[11,17]

Tachypnea is displayed on the uterine trace as close, choppy vertical lines, producing at a distance the appearance of a line drawn by a pen with a broad tip. The appearance is similar to that of maternal seizure activity, as recorded by a tocodynamometer, but the latter is usually transient. In the author's experience, this respiratory pattern has been seen with varicella pneumonia and the acute chest syndrome of sickle cell disease (see page 199).

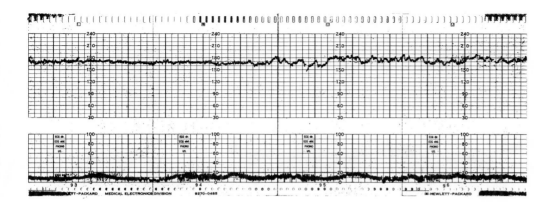

CASE INTERPRETATION: Class I

Baseline Information: moderate tachycardia, average variability.

Periodic or Nonperiodic: accelerations are present, no decelerations are recorded.

Uterine Activity: shallow uterine contractions are suggested by a tocodynamometer. Rapid parallel vertical fluctuations of the needle are superimposed on the contraction pattern.

Significance: the fetal heart rate information is consistent with a healthy fetus who is stressed by maternal fever, mild hypoxia, or drug effect. The choppy needle deflections on the maternal trace are too sustained for the usual duration of seizure activity, thus suggesting maternal respiratory activity. Such a pattern is seen with maternal tachypnea.

CASE OUTCOME: Eighteen-year-old primigravida at 34½ weeks' gestation delivered by cesarean section for a footling breech presentation, with local anesthesia, a 5 pound, 3 ounce (2353 gram) female; Apgar score 7/9. The maternal intrapartum course was complicated by severe varicella pneumonia. The mother and baby survived.

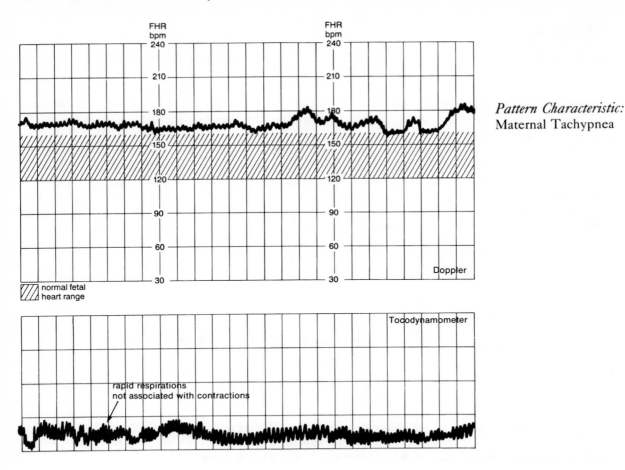

Pattern Characteristic:
Maternal Tachypnea

Maternal Kussmaul's Respirations

*T*he visual display of maternal respiratory activity may be helpful in the care of the maternal patient. Unusual respiratory patterns may be captured by the monitor and show a response to therapy. Kussmaul's respirations are typically deep and rapid, producing an external monitor-ing pattern of parallel vertical lines superimposed on the maternal activity trace. The pattern is similar to that of tachypnea that results from other causes (see pages 199 and 387). The pattern may revert to normal with treatment of the associated acidosis.

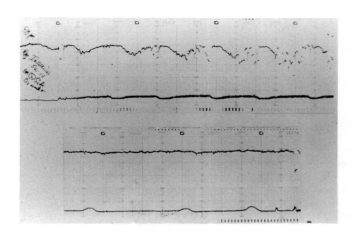

CASE INTERPRETATION:

Baseline Information: normal rate, average variability, as measured by external monitor without autocorrelation.

Periodic and Nonperiodic Changes: undulating decelerations that are possibly late or late/variable.

Uterine Activity: possible contractions "reversed." The trace has superimposed maternal activity, characterized by closely spaced, short vertical spikes.

Significance: possible fetal hypoxia; the maternal activity is probably produced by a form of tachypnea.

CASE OUTCOME: Nineteen-year-old with insulin-dependent diabetes (Class D) was monitored at 31 weeks' gestation during diabetic ketoacidosis. Her glucose was 436 mg/dl, serum acetone was positive at 1:32 dilution, and serum CO_2 5.3 meq/L. The unusual appearance of the maternal resprations on the uterine trace were produced by Kussmaul's respirations, which disappeared with insulin treatment. The patient delivered by cesarean section at 35 weeks' gestation a 4 pound, 4 ounce (1929 gram) female; Apgar score 7/8. The newborn was developmentally normal.

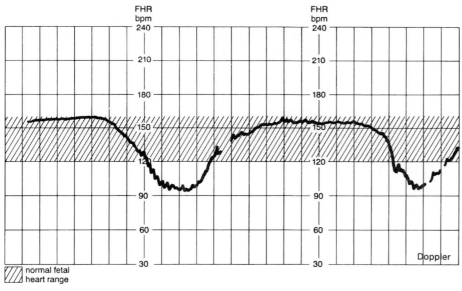

Pattern Characteristic:
Maternal Kussmaul Respirations

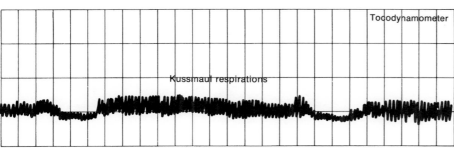

Maternal Vomiting

*B*oth the internal and external monitor record the increased maternal movements and increased uterine activity that occur with vomiting.

Transient decelerations in the fetal heart rate may accompany vomiting. This may be secondary to increased uterine activity or maternal hypoxia.[19]

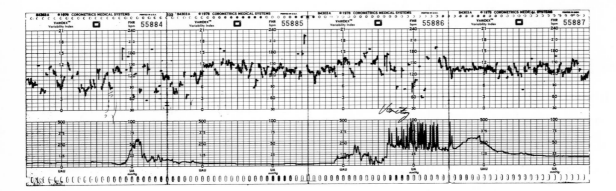

CASE INTERPRETATION: Class 0

Baseline Information: the baseline rate appears in the normal range; variability is unsatisfactory for fetal evaluation.

Periodic or Nonperiodic Changes: decelerations may be obscured during loss of a satisfactory signal.

Uterine Activity: external monitoring suggests skewed contractions. Superimposed on the contractions' waveform is a pattern of vertical spikes.

Significance: the fetal heart rate trace is unsatisfactory for evaluation of the fetal condition during this segment. This maternal activity pattern is seen with vomiting.

CASE OUTCOME: Twenty-five-year-old gravida 3, para 2002, at 42 weeks' gestation delivered vaginally, with local and pudendal anesthesia, a 5 pound, 12½ ounce (2622 gram) male; Apgar score 2/4. The newborn expired on the first day of life, secondary to persistent fetal circulation believed to be associated with meconium aspiration. Total anomalous venous return was found at the autopsy. The patient delivered shortly after this segment.

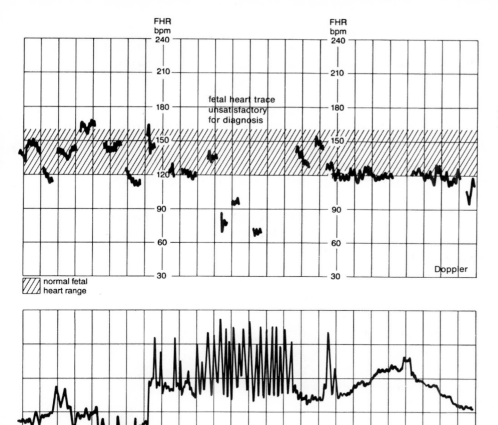

Pattern Characteristic:
Maternal Vomiting

Maternal Straining

*M*aternal straining has a similar appearance when measured by internal and external monitoring. By either method the trace typically traverses to the top of the uterine activity graph, where a horizontal line continues for the duration of the straining effort, followed by an abrupt drop at the end of the straining or pushing effort. This is repeated with a similar appearance for the number of pushing cycles per contraction. The characteristic appearance allows retrospective presumptive identification of second stage tracings, unless maternal straining takes place prior to complete cervical dilatation. The fetal hypoxia associated with the increased uterine activity and the maternal hypoxia produced during maternal straining may be sufficient to transform a normal fetal heart pattern to a stress pattern or a stress pattern into signs of decompensation.[4,5] Should such occur, temporarily discontinuing pushing or altering the pushing technique may result in an improved pattern.

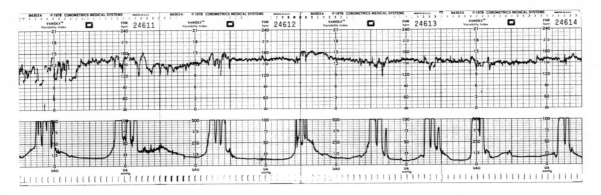

CASE INTERPRETATION: Class I-II

Baseline Information: normal rate, average variability with areas of increased variability, some instability of the baseline.

Periodic or Nonperiodic Changes: accelerations are present.

Uterine Activity: the appearance of maternal straining, as measured with an internal pressure gauge, showing polysystolic, skewed contractions.

Significance: a stressed, normal baseline tone. A healthy fetus is predicted if delivery is imminent.

CASE OUTCOME: Twenty-one-year-old primigravida at 40 weeks' gestation delivered by cesarean section, with general anesthesia for a prolonged second stage, a 6 pound, 9½ ounce (2991 gram) female; Apgar score 9/9. The fetus was in a vertex presentation. The infant followed an uncomplicated newborn course.

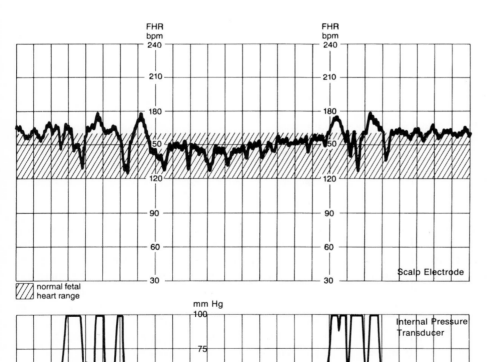

Pattern Characteristic:
Maternal Straining

Maternal Seizure

*T*he external or internal monitor captures both the increased maternal movement and the increased uterine activity that occur with seizures.

Loss of the fetal signal during the seizure is common with external monitoring. The onset of the seizure typically coincides with the onset of a contraction.[14]

The mechanism of increased uterine activity associated with a seizure is not clearly understood. Postulated factors are a decreased uterine blood flow and the release of norepinephrine.

Also common is a prolonged deceleration (see page 319) in response to the decreased oxygen exchange during the uterine activity and maternal hypoxia.[1,3,14]

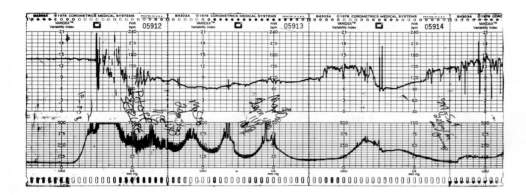

CASE INTERPRETATION: Class II

Baseline Information: moderate tachycardia, decreased variability at the onset and recovery of a prolonged deceleration.

Periodic or Nonperiodic Changes: prolonged deceleration for seven minutes, with partial recovery and a recurrence for two minutes.

Uterine Activity: tetanic contractions and superimposed maternal activity.

Significance: this pattern is compatible with maternal seizure activity. It indicates healthy fetal responses to stressful stimuli, with a potential for fetal jeopardy if the episodes are recurrent or progressive.

CASE OUTCOME: Twenty-three-year-old primigravida at 40 weeks' gestation delivered vaginally, with midforceps and local and pudendal anesthesia, a 7 pound, 5 ounce (3317 gram) male; Apgar score 6/8. The infant followed an uncomplicated newborn course. The tracing resumed a normal pattern and delivery occurred one and a quarter hours after the seizure. (See page 222 for the initial recovery pattern of this case.)

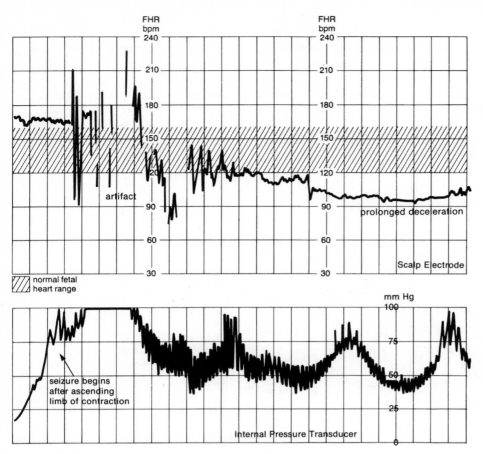

Pattern Characteristic:
Maternal Seizure

Simulated Uterine Contractions

*T*he slow development and resolution of a uterine contraction is not easily reproduced by simulated abdominal muscle activity. It is easier to gradually, voluntarily relax muscles than to gradually contract them. Simulated uter-ine activity is not a common occurrence. It may be encountered in certain anxiety states or as part of a bizarre presentation of the Munchausen syndrome. The latter is of rare occurrence in obstetrics and gynecology.[9,10]

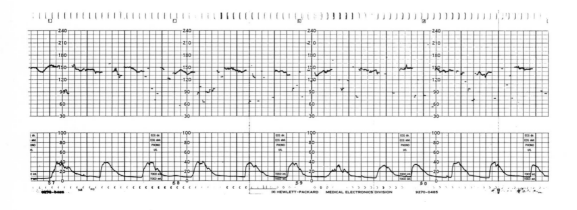

CASE INTERPRETATION: Class 0

Baseline Information: normal rate, an intermittent loss of signal, decreased variability.

Periodic or Nonperiodic Changes: it cannot be determined if decelerations are present because of the loss of a signal.

Uterine Activity: small, brief contractions with an unusual configuration, occurring every one to two minutes.

Significance: this is not the appearance of a normal labor pattern.

CASE OUTCOME: Twenty-four-year-old gravida 15, para 3384, at 31 weeks' gestation with Munchausen syndrome, repeatedly simulated uterine contractions, ruptured membranes, and vaginal bleeding, the latter produced by documented self-inflicted vaginal trauma. The patient signed out against medical advice when she was confronted with the diagnosis and given a recommendation for psychiatric help. At 33 weeks' gestation, she delivered by emergency cesarean section, performed upon her arrival at another hospital, based on only her history of a prolonged rupture of the membranes, in the setting of a breech presentation, and a previous cesarean section. The newborn was a 4 pound, 11 ounce (2120 gram) female; Apgar score 4/7. The infant survived a newborn course of hyaline membrane disease.

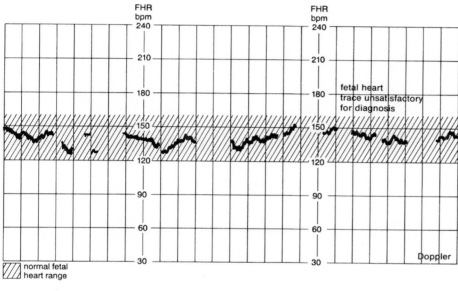

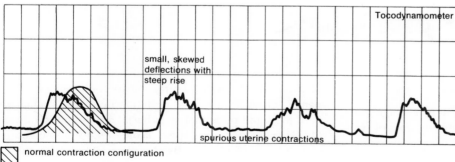

Pattern Characteristic:
Simulated Uterine Contractions

Other Maternal Activity

Any maternal activity that is accompanied by a movement of the abdominal wall against the pressure sensor of the tocodynamometer can potentially be reflected as deflections superimposed on the uterine waveform. These may be gross body movements such as turning or shivering, or may reflect abrupt diaphragm movements such as coughing, laughing, crying, and vomiting.[13]

Any maternal activity that increases intrauterine pressure may be reflected on the trace that is derived from an internal pressure transducer. Such movements also include coughing, laughing, crying, and vomiting. Awareness of the visual appearance of common maternal activities assists in "reading" information on the uterine trace and in understanding the mechanisms of signal acquisition.

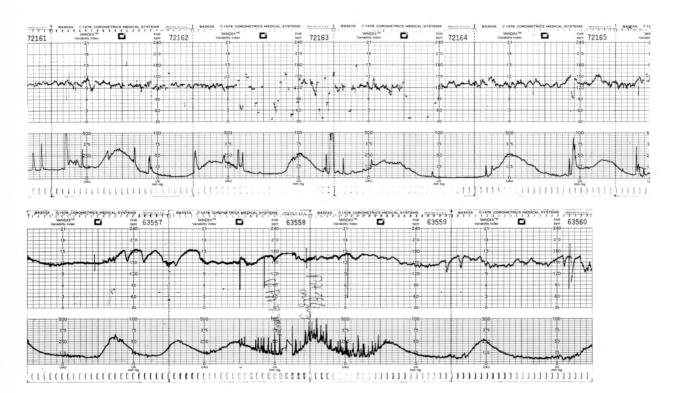

CASE #1 INTERPRETATION: Class I

Baseline Information: low normal rate, average variability, as measured by external monitoring, loss of fetal heart signal in areas.

Periodic or Nonperiodic Changes: accelerations are present; there are no decelerations during areas of satisfactory recordings.

Uterine Activity: contractions of varying configurations, with superimposed erratic spikes of maternal activity.

Significance: a good fetal condition is predicted. These are maternal activity spikes, as seen with coughing or laughing.

CASE OUTCOME: Thirty-four-year-old gravida 7, para 2223, at 38½ weeks' gestation delivered vaginally, with local and pudendal anesthesia, a 9 pound, 5 ounce (4224 gram) female; Apgar score 9/9. The newborn course was complicated by the diagnosis of a fractured clavicle, which healed without sequelae. The jovial multipara entertained friends and family members throughout her labor; her laughter was stilled intermittently by her concentration during uterine contractions.

CASE #2 INTERPRETATION: Class I

Baseline Information: normal rate, average variability; the baseline is obscured in areas by continuous accelerations.

Periodic or Nonperiodic Changes: continuous accelerations and nonperiodic accelerations, small V-shaped variable decelerations.

Uterine Activity: frequent uterine contractions without a resting phase. Spikes of maternal activity are superimposed.

Significance: the spikes do not have any regularity or increased uterine activity that is associated with patient vomiting. This pattern is seen with crying. A good fetal condition is predicted.

CASE OUTCOME: Twenty-four-year-old primigravida delivered with cesarean section for cephalopelvic disproportion, with epidural anesthesia, an 8 pound, 2 ounce (3685 gram) female; Apgar score 8/9. The infant followed an uncomplicated newborn course.

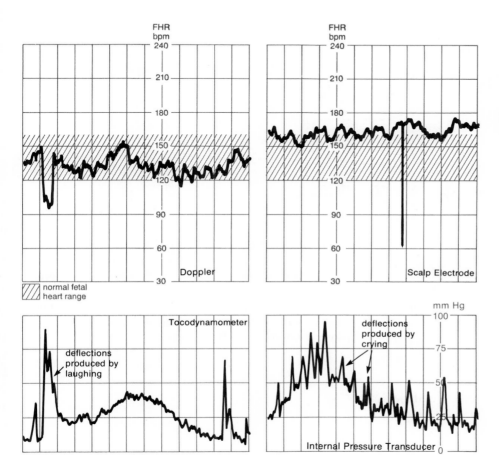

Pattern Characteristic:
Maternal: Laughing–Crying

Fetal Activity

*I*n addition to maternal activity, there is a potential for fetal activity to be superimposed on the uterine tocodynamometry-derived trace. The most common alteration of the trace attributed to the fetus is small upward deflections that are produced by fetal rolling or kicking movements.[18]

Also reported in the fetus, with potential effect on the uterine trace, are fetal seizures, tachypnea, hiccoughs, gasps, grunting (Valsalva's maneuver), and even normal respiratory movements.[2,6,7,8,15,16,18]

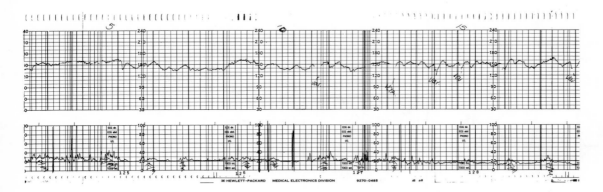

CASE INTERPRETATION: Class I

Baseline Information: normal rate, average variability.

Periodic or Nonperiodic Changes: variable accelerations associated with fetal movement. Occasional mild, small V-shaped variable declerations.

Uterine Activity: none is recorded, but the deflections of the tocodynamometer trace are consistent with fetal movement.

Significance: a healthy fetus is predicted; there is a possible vulnerable cord.

CASE OUTCOME: Twenty-five-year-old gravida 5, para 0040, delivered vaginally from a vertex presentation, with no anesthesia, a 6 pound, 9 ounce (2977 gram) female; Apgar score 8/9. This nonstress test was performed 11 days prior to delivery for an indication of possible intrauterine growth retardation. The infant followed a normal newborn course.

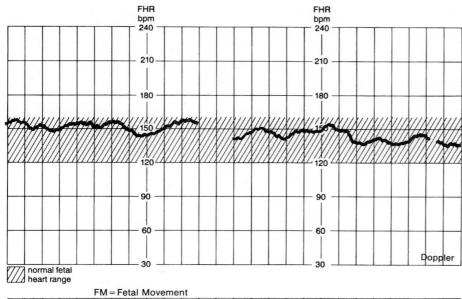

Pattern Characteristic:
Fetal Activity

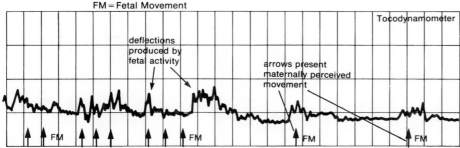

References

1. Barrett JM: Fetal resuscitation with terbutaline during eclampsia-induced uterine hypertonus. *Am J Obstet Gynecol* 150:895, 1985.

2. Boddy K, Mantell CD: Observations of fetal breathing movements transmitted through maternal abdominal wall. *Lancet* 2:1219, 1972.

3. Boehm FH, Growdon JH: The effect of eclamptic convulsions on the fetal heart rate. *Am J Obstet Gynecol* 120:851, 1974.

4. Caldeyro-Barcia R: The influence of maternal bearing-down efforts during second stage on fetal well-being. *Birth and the Family J* 6:1, 1979, p. 19.

5. Caldeyro-Barcia R, Guissi G, Storch E, et al: The bearing-down efforts and their effects on fetal heart rate. *J Perinat Med* 9:63, 1981.

6. Conover WB, Yarwood RL, Peacock MD, et al: Antenatal diagnosis of fetal seizure activity with use of realtime ultrasound. *Am J Obstet Gynecol* 155:846, 1986.

7. Duff P, Sanders RS, Hayashi RH: Intrauterine tachypnea—a sign of fetal distress? *Am J Obstet Gynecol* 142:1054, 1982.

8. Goodlin RC: Fetal cardiovascular responses to distress. *Obstet Gynecol* 49:371, 1977.

9. Goodlin RC: Pregnant women with Munchausen syndrome. *Am J Obstet Gynecol* 153:207, 1985.

10. Hustead RM, Lee RH, Maruk T: Factitious illnesses. *Obstet Gynecol* 59:214, 1982.

11. Miller FC, Petrie RH, Arce JJ, et al: Hyperventilation during labor. *Am J Obstet Gynecol* 120:489, 1974.

12. Navot D, Donchin Y, Sadovsky E: Fetal response to vol-

untary maternal hyperventilation. *Acta Obstet Gynecol Scand* 61:205, 1982.

13. Paul RH, Petrie R: *Fetal Intensive Care.* Wallingford, Connecticut, Corometrics Medical Systems, Inc., 1979, p. II 32, III 23.

14. Paul RH, Koh KS, Bernstein SC: Changes in fetal heart rate uterine contraction patterns with eclampsia. *Am J Obstet Gynecol* 130:165, 1978.

15. Romero R, Chervenak FA, Berkowitz RL, et al: Intrauterine fetal tachypnea. *Am J Obstet Gynecol* 144:356, 1982.

16. Shenker L: Fetal hiccups during labor. *Perinatology/Neonatology* March/April, p. 96, 1982.

17. Sherer DM, Caverly CB, Abramowicz JS: Severe obstructive sleep apnea and associated snoring documented during external tocography. *Am J Obstet Gynecol* 165:1300, 1991.

18. Timor-Tritsch IE, Dierker LJ, Hertz RH, et al: Fetal movement: A brief review. *Clin Obstet Gynecol* 22:583, 1979.

19. Tipton RH: Fetal heart rate monitoring in labour. *Clin in Obstet Gynaecol* 2:153, 1975.

DUAL MONITORING AND OTHER MULTIPLE BASELINES

*T*he clinician reading a fetal heart trace may encounter more than one baseline. A modern reason for the appearance of multiple baselines is that a monitor with dual heart rate channel capabilities is recording a second fetus (twin), the mother, or the same fetus by two methods (Doppler and scalp-electrode–derived signals), the latter on two different scales.

However, both modern and older models of monitors may display two baseline traces because a single fetus displays changing heart rates that are produced by various arrhythmias. Even within a single heart, it is possible to have separate atrial and ventricular rates that may be alternately captured by the monitor. In addition, a single channel may alternate between two different hearts (between twins or between the fetus and mother). A single channel trace may also produce two baselines by intermittently half counting or double counting the fetal heart rate. Due to machine logic, this is more commonly encountered when the fetal heart rate falls outside of the usual range. Since the same single channel is capable of receiving signals derived from two hearts (e.g., fetal heart motion and movement of the maternal blood vessels), as well as double counting and half counting each of those signals, it becomes apparent that there are opportunities for numerous baselines to appear intermittently on the same trace. Add dual channels and intermittent maternal or fetal arrhythmias and it almost seems that innumerable combinations of multiple baselines are possible. This section presents examples of the mechanisms of multiple baselines singly and in combination. Included also are comparisons of heart rate patterns produced or transmitted by dual instruments.

Dual Channel Monitoring

Chapter 17

Twin Monitoring Single Scale, Synchrony

*D*ual monitoring (using a single monitor) has an obvious advantage for twin gestation. Simultaneous traces are produced on the same paper strip for direct comparison of the twin heart rates with each other and in relation to uterine activity.[20] Modern advances now permit a dual Doppler-derived signal, dual electrocardiogram (ECG)-derived signals, or a combination of the two. In the absence of a monitor with dual features, two monitors may be used, allowing simultaneous data collection.[2,10] This system is also used if a dual monitoring capability is not available despite the feasibility of internal monitoring. In the latter case, the uterine waveform produced by internal monitoring may be transmitted to the second machine.[13] When a single scale is used, the two rates may be partially superimposed. Some monitors display the ECG-derived signal as a finer dotted line than the Doppler-derived signal.

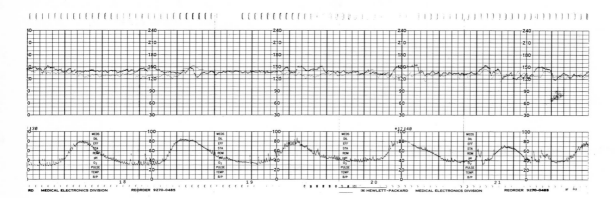

CASE INTERPRETATION: Class I-I

Baseline Information: there are two heart rates, both in a normal range with normal variability.

Periodic or Nonperiodic Changes: nonperiodic variable accelerations, usually with a synchronous occurrence.

Uterine Activity: frequent, skewed contractions.

Significance: healthy twin fetuses are predicted.

CASE OUTCOME: Twenty-seven-year-old gravida 3, para 2002, at 38 weeks' gestation delivered twin A vaginally and twin B by low transverse cesarean section for an entrapped transverse lie. Twin A, a female, was in a vertex presentation and weighed 6 pounds, 2½ ounces (2792 grams); Apgar score 9/9. Local anesthesia was used. Twin B, a female, was in a vertex presentation and weighed 6 pounds, 11½ ounces (3047 grams); Apgar score 8/9. General anesthesia was administered. The infants followed uncomplicated newborn courses.

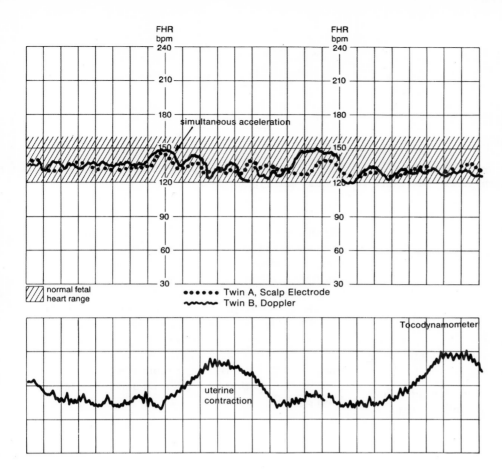

FHR bpm

240 — 210 — 180 — 150 — 120 — 90 — 60 — 30

simultaneous acceleration

FHR bpm

240 — 210 — 180 — 150 — 120 — 90 — 60 — 30

//// normal fetal heart range

●●●●●● Twin A, Scalp Electrode
〜〜〜 Twin B, Doppler

Tocodynamometer

uterine contraction

Pattern Characteristic:
Twin Monitoring Single Scale
Synchrony

Twin Monitoring Single Scale, Asynchrony

*I*n some monitors with dual monitoring, a single stylus is used rather than a hot dot matrix. The same pen traces one line and regularly traverses to the other line to place a dot at the site of the fetal heart rate and then returns to the other line. This inevitably results in loss of detail on both traces, which are displayed as dotted lines. In monitors in which twin monitoring is restricted to one ECG-derived and one Doppler-derived trace, for greatest accuracy and least potential loss of signal of internal monitoring, the stylus has been programmed to spend a greater period of time on the Doppler-derived trace. A precise display of variability is thus compromised, and the fine features of periodic changes may be lost. This may be resolved by intermittently turning off the channel to one twin, allowing full information for assessment of the other. See page 408 for further discussion of twin monitoring with asynchronous heart rate changes.

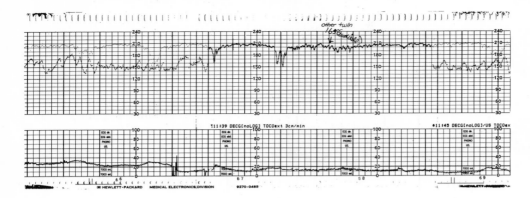

CASE INTERPRETATION: Class II-I

Baseline Information: there are two rates at the beginning and end of the segment. Only the upper rate is recorded in the midportion. The upper rate displays tachycardia, the lower rate displays a normal rate; there is an average variability on both.

Periodic or Nonperiodic Changes: the upper trace shows mild biphasic variable decelerations. The lower trace shows nonperiodic accelerations.

Uterine Activity: small tocodynamometer deflections with uterine contractions of a normal configuration.

Significance: this pattern could be asynchronous twin monitoring or fetal/maternal tachycardia. If it is twins, in view of good variability, both are reassuring, but the upper trace displays a stress pattern.

CASE OUTCOME: Twenty-two-year-old gravida 2, para 1001, delivered by cesarean section, with epidural anesthesia, twin A, 5 pounds (2268 grams), Apgar score 8/9, from a vertex presentation, and twin B, 5 pounds, 8 ounces (2495 grams), Apgar score 8/9, from a breech presentation. Both infants followed uncomplicated newborn courses.

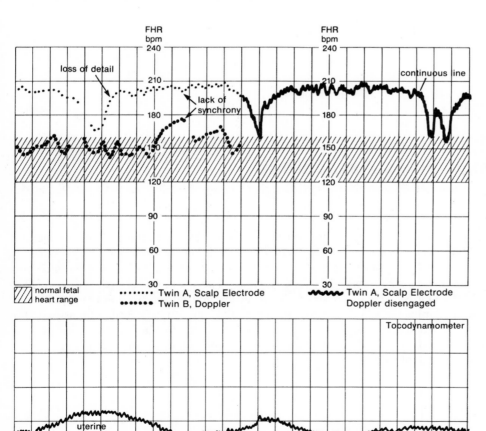

Pattern Characteristic:
Twin Monitoring Single Scale Asynchrony

Twin Monitoring Dual Scale, Synchrony

*W*hen two scales are used in the dual monitoring of twins, the similar heart rates are separated for easier distinction of cardiac responses to intrapartum events of twin A versus B. The disadvantage to this is the compression of variability in the trace on the lower scale as a fetal heart range from 1⅓ to 0.7 centimeters.

The literature is conflicting about whether a relationship exists between the presence of synchrony and the type of placenta.[4,5,15]

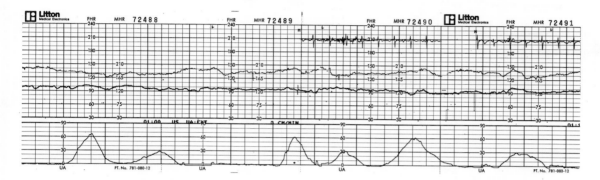

CASE INTERPRETATION: Class I-I

Baseline Information: two heart rates: the upper scale is about 130 baseline, with fair variability on the lower scale; the lower scale has a baseline of 120, with fair but further decreased variability.

Periodic or Nonperiodic Changes: the upper scale, with accelerations to 145 bpm, and the lower scale, with accelerations to 135 bpm, are simultaneously occurring.

Uterine Activity: paired, coupled contractions.

Significance: twin dual monitoring with synchrony, a reassuring pattern. The maternal ECG lead being used on the scalp electrode of twin A produces the notation M on the ECG trace.

CASE OUTCOME: Seventeen-year-old primigravida at 35 weeks' gestation delivered twins vaginally, with pudendal anesthesia. Twin A, a male, was in a vertex presentation and weighed 5 pounds, 4 ounces (2381 grams); Apgar score 9/8. Twin B, a male, in a vertex presentation and weighing 5 pounds, 2 ounces (2325 grams), was born eight minutes after twin A. The placenta was monochorionic and diamniotic. Both newborns were treated for hypoglycemia and possible sepsis. The newborns were dismissed at nine days of age.

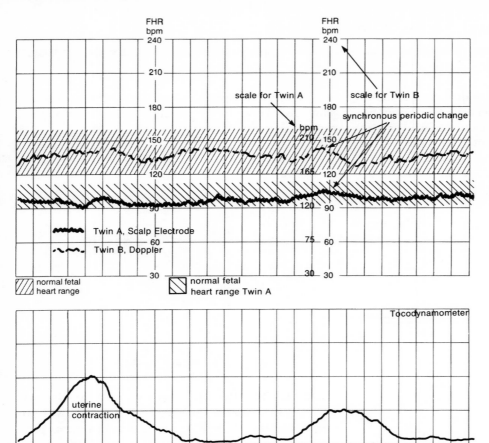

Pattern Characteristic:
Twin Monitoring Dual Scale
Synchrony

Twin Monitoring Dual Scale, Asynchrony

*L*ack of synchrony of twin heart rates during dual monitoring has been associated with significant differences in birth weight.[4] Marked differences may indicate the jeopardy of one fetus in a setting in which the other fetus is unaffected. Conditions that could jeopardize one fetus independently include a prolapsed cord and abruption of one placenta. Also, differing basal conditions (as in twin-twin transfusion syndrome) could cause one fetus to respond with a less favorable pattern to an identical stimulus. The literature is conflicting about whether a relationship exists between asynchrony and lack of shared placental tissue.[4,5,15]

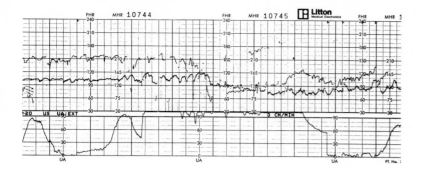

CASE INTERPRETATION: Class V-I

Baseline Information: two heart rates, the upper scale is approximately 150 bpm, the lower scale is approximately 130 bpm; average variability.

Periodic or Nonperiodic Changes: upper scale with late variable deceleration, lower scale with small acceleration.

Uterine Activity: contractions with the appearance of maternal straining.

Significance: twin dual monitoring with asynchrony, with the possibility of intrauterine growth retardation and oligohydramnios associated with the twin of the upper trace. The twin of the lower trace is not in apparent jeopardy.

CASE OUTCOME: Twin pregnancy at 37 weeks' gestation delivered vaginally by vacuum extraction. Twin A was in a vertex presentation and weighed 6 pounds, 6 ounces (2892 grams); Apgar score 8/8; Twin B was in a vertex presentation and weighed 4 pounds, 1 ounce (1843 grams); Apgar score 5/8. The umbilical pHs of twin A were 7.32 and 7.35; the umbilical pHs of twin B were 7.10 and 7.15 (artery and vein respectively).

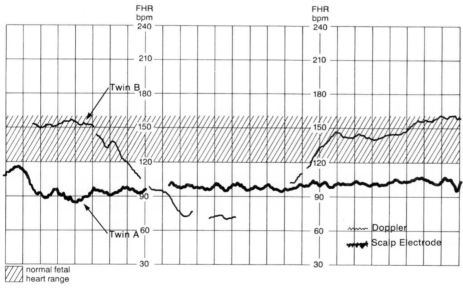

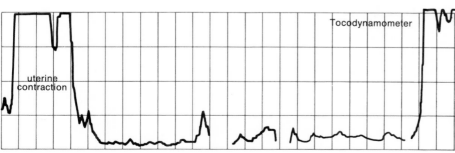

Pattern Characteristic:
Twin Monitoring Dual Scale
Asynchrony

Maternal-Fetal Monitoring Single Scale, Maternal Periodic Accelerations

*T*here are multiple reasons for simultaneous maternal-fetal monitoring: (1) maternal surveillance in a setting of maternal disease or other cardiovascular instability; (2) the distinction of maternal and fetal rates, as in the diagnosis of intrauterine fetal death or to exclude the maternal heart rate, especially in a setting of maternal and fetal tachycardia artifact; and the assessment of simultaneous fetal and maternal cardiac events in response to stressful stimuli. This is available in modern monitors. A maternal heart rate change may occur with contractions. Although accelerations are more common, decelerations have been reported.[11] Without dual monitoring and

an awareness of periodic maternal changes, maternal Doppler-derived signals may be mistaken for fetal signals, potentially resulting in clinical decisions being directed at the fetus. When the same scale is used for the fetus and the mother, the mother's rate typically appears in the fetal moderate or marked bradycardia range. Some dual monitors require that the fetal signal be Doppler-derived so that the maternal signal may be ECG-derived.[18] However, with simple modifications both maternal and fetal signals may be ECG-derived. Newer machines permit simultaneous dual Doppler traces.

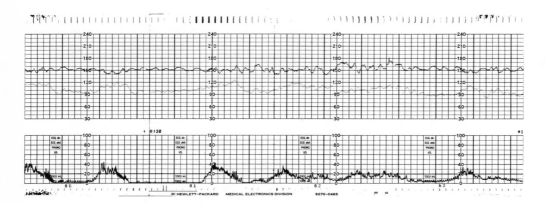

CASE INTERPRETATION: Class I-I

Baseline Information: there are two heart rates—one in the normal range with good variability, one in the moderate bradycardia range with good variability.

Periodic or Nonperiodic Changes: periodic accelerations, occurring with a lower rate.

Uterine Activity: improper placement of the tocodynamometer may underestimate contractions, which appear to be of a normal configuration.

Significance: most likely, this is an indication of simultaneous fetal-maternal monitoring rather than of discordant twins.

CASE OUTCOME: Twenty-year-old primigravida, at 41 weeks' gestation delivered by low transverse cesarean section, with general anesthesia, performed for dystocia in the presence of preeclampsia and chorioamnionitis a 7 pound, 3 ounce (3260 gram) female; Apgar score 8/9. The fetus was in a vertex presentation. Magnesium sulfate and oxytocin were administered intravenously intrapartum. The newborn course was complicated by group B streptococcal sepsis. The newborn was dismissed on the eleventh day of life.

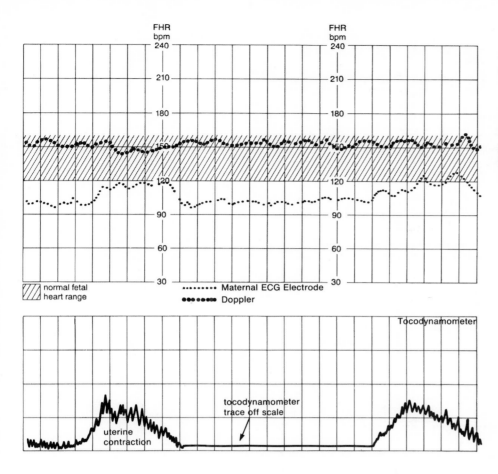

Pattern Characteristic:
Maternal-Fetal Monitoring
Single Scale Maternal Periodic
Accelerations

Maternal-Fetal Monitoring Dual Scale, Maternal Periodic Accelerations

*T*he capability of simultaneous fetal and maternal monitoring is an additional feature of modern fetal monitors. The decision to use a separate or same scale for the second heart rate trace is largely influenced by twin monitoring. Using a separate scale separates the tracings of twins with similar heart rates so that they may be less confused. When using the separate (lower) scale for maternal or fetal monitoring, it should be remembered that variability will be compressed in comparison to the upper tracing.

In addition to distinguishing between fetal and maternal heart rates, the dual monitoring provides interesting information about the maternal response to labor events and simultaneous fetal and maternal cardiac responses, for example, the disappearance of pain-triggered maternal accelerations associated with the relief of pain or the administration of epidural anesthesia, which is possibly a catecholamine-mediated phenomenon.[5,12,16]

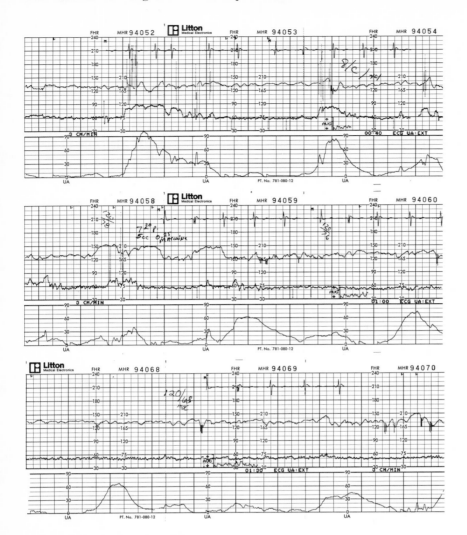

CASE INTERPRETATION: Class I-I

Baseline Information: two heart rates, one in the normal range with good variability, one in the severe bradycardic range (maternal heart rate range), on a separate scale.

Periodic or Nonperiodic Changes: the upper trace has nonperiodic accelerations near the end of the segment; the lower trace has periodic accelerations that progressively diminish.

Uterine Activity: polysystolic and skewed contractions.

Significance: simultaneous fetal-maternal monitoring; maternal accelerations may reflect a response to painful contractions.

CASE OUTCOME: Twenty-four-year-old gravida 2, para 0010, at 40 weeks' gestation delivered vaginally from a vertex presentation, with epidural anesthesia, a 7 pound, 15 ounce (3600 gram) female; Apgar score 9/9. Thin meconium was present. The infant followed an uncomplicated newborn course. The maternal accelerations diminished and disappeared after epidural anesthesia was administered.

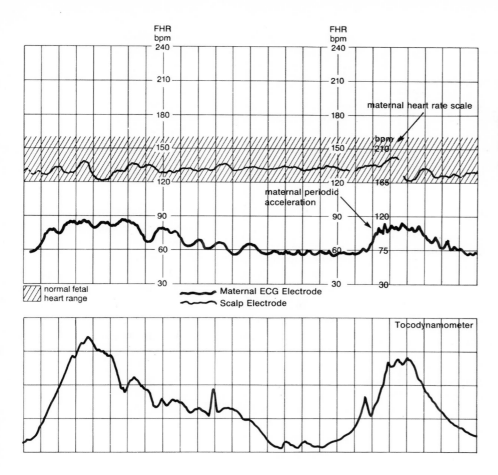

Pattern Characteristic:
Maternal-Fetal Monitoring Dual Scale Maternal Periodic Accelerations

Maternal-Fetal Monitoring Dual Scale, Maternal Hyperventilation

*B*oth fetal and maternal heart rate traces reflect the beat-to-beat changes associated with respiration. Maternal heart rate changes with respiration such as hyperventilation may be demonstrated.[17] These changes have appearances that are similar to the fetal heart rate changes associated with "respiratory" activity (see also page 462). Maternal respiratory abdominal wall movements may also be reflected on the uterine trace (see page 387).

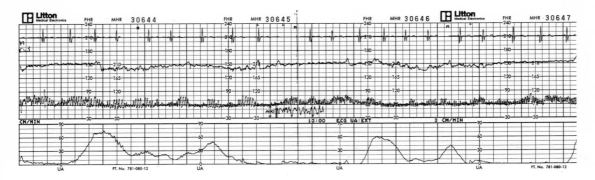

CASE INTERPRETATION: Class II-II

Baseline: there are two heart rates: the upper is in the normal fetal heart range with average variability; the lower is in the normal maternal heart range with intermittent episodes of regular increased variability.

Periodic or Nonperiodic Changes: shallow, late decelerations.

Uterine Activity: polysystalic confluent contractions.

Significance: the fetal heart rate suggests mild hypoxia, the maternal heart rate is a pattern of respiratory arrhythmia, as seen with hyperventilation.

CASE OUTCOME: Sixteen-year-old primigravida at 39 weeks' gestation delivered by cesarean section, with epidural anesthesia, performed for fetal distress and cephalopelvic disproportion an 8 pound, 3 ounce (3714 gram) male; Apgar score 8/9. Later in the labor, after the present segment was made, the fetus developed marked fetal bradycardia and decreased variability. Scalp pHs were 7.35 and 7.38 initially but 7.10, 7.21, and 7.18 in late labor. The infant followed an uncomplicated newborn course.

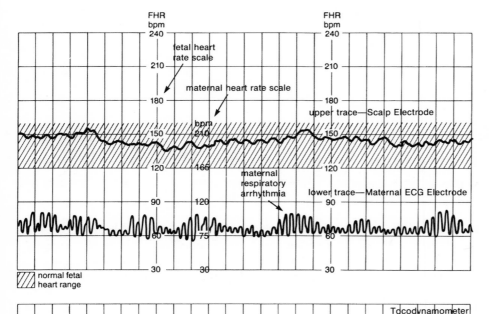

Pattern Characteristic:
Maternal-Fetal Monitoring Dual Scale Maternal Hyperventilation

Maternal-Fetal Monitoring Dual Scale, Maternal Arrhythmia

Continuous beat-to-beat monitoring and the ECG-derived maternal trace allow for the display of adult arrhythmias in a different visual form than is provided by the electrocardiogram. Visual recognition of similar patterns in the fetus may be facilitated. Also, the understanding of cycle-by-cycle changes in various arrhythmias is enhanced.

The Wenckebach phenomenon is characterized by progressive elongation of the P-R interval until a beat is dropped. This produces a beat-to-beat monitoring pattern that has a similar appearance to fetal respiratory arrhythmia (see page 462).

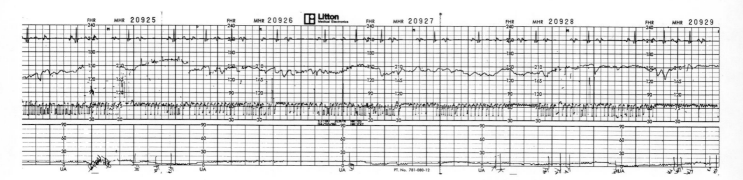

CASE INTERPRETATION: Class I-III

Baseline Information: two heart rates: one in the normal fetal range, the second in the normal maternal range. The fetal heart trace has average variability. The maternal trace demonstrates arrhythmia.

Periodic or Nonperiodic Changes: fetal accelerations are present. There are no maternal periodic changes.

Uterine Activity: possible infrequent uterine contractions, which are displayed in a "reverse" fashion.

Significance: a healthy fetus is predicted. There is a maternal arrhythmia: the Wenckebach phenomenon.

CASE OUTCOME: Sixteen-year-old primigravida at 23½ weeks' gestation delivered vaginally, with no anesthesia, a 1 pound, 8 ounce (680 gram) male; no Apgar score was assigned. The fetus was in a vertex presentation. The maternal course was complicated by an arrhythmia—the Wenckebach phenomenon—and premature labor, which was followed by premature ruptured membranes. The newborn expired on the sixth day of life with renal failure and extreme immaturity.

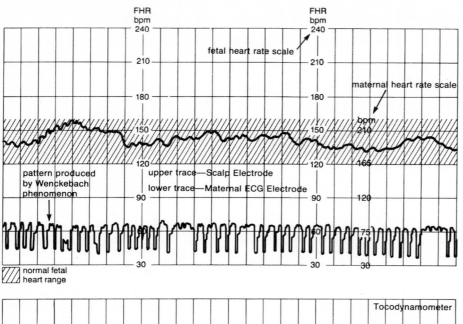

Pattern Characteristic:
Maternal-Fetal Monitoring Dual
Scale Maternal Arrhythmia

Maternal-Fetal Monitoring Single Scale, Maternal Tachycardia—"Slipping"

*T*he most frequent causes of maternal tachycardia in labor also produce simultaneous fetal tachycardia (that is, maternal fever and cardiostimulatory drugs). Occasionally, a maternal tachycardia may be produced without a change in the baseline fetal heart rate. The resulting maternal and fetal heart rates may be nearly identical. Palpation of maternal pulses or even maternal ECG monitoring may not be sufficient to distinguish fetal and maternal rates unless a continuous beat-to-beat printed mode is used, as is provided by the dual capabilities of modern fetal monitors.[9]

Simultaneous maternal (ECG-derived) and fetal (Doppler-derived) traces may demonstrate the subtle "slipping" of the Doppler signal from the fetal to maternal sources and back without a detectable gap or break in the continuity of the trace. Without dual monitoring fetal jeopardy may be undetected, while maternal signals

produce a reassuring trace. It is also possible for subtle slipping to a lower maternal rate to simulate decelerations, which may lead to untimely intervention.[1,14]

Slipping between the signals from twin hearts is rarely recognizable without dual monitoring (see insert).

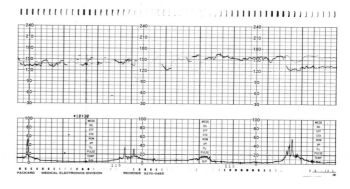

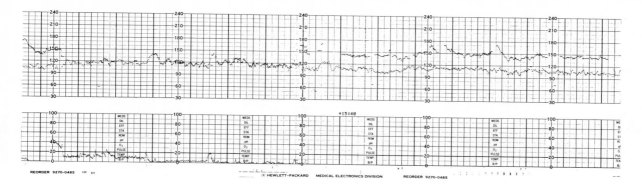

CASE INTERPRETATION: Class I-I

Baseline Information: there are two heart rates: one is in the normal fetal heart range, the other is lower in the normal to moderate bradycardia range, both with good variability. There are frequent segments in which signals from both transducers produce an identical trace.

Periodic or Nonperiodic Changes: small, nonperiodic accelerations.

Uterine Activity: none recorded.

Significance: two "hearts" are monitored, indicating either twin fetuses or maternal-fetal dual monitoring. The Doppler-derived signal frequently "slips" to a signal from the fetus or maternal vessels, as monitored also by the ECG-derived (dotted line) signal.

CASE OUTCOME: Fifteen-year-old primigravida at 40 weeks' gestation delivered vaginally, with epidural anesthesia, an 8 pound, 3 ounce (3714 gram) male; Apgar score 8/9. The fetus was in a vertex presentation. The newborn course was complicated by transient hyperbilirubinemia. The mother had unexplained sinus tachycardia without ectopy throughout the pregnancy.

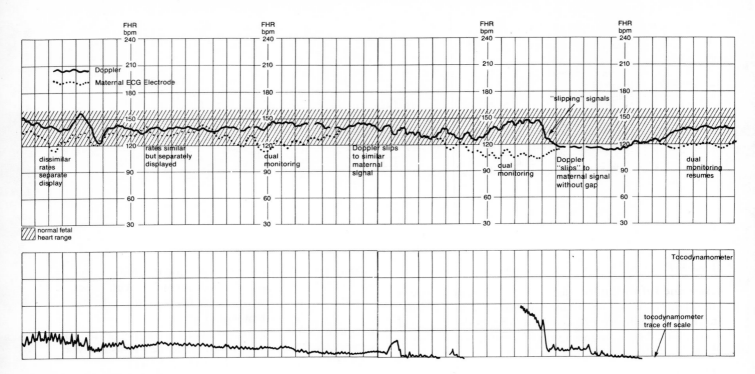

Pattern Characteristic:
Maternal Tachycardia with Slipping of Signal

Maternal-Fetal Monitoring Dual Scale, Maternal and Fetal Tachycardia

*M*aternal monitoring (with display of a signal produced by electrocardiography) clarifies those situations in which an artifact in Doppler fetal heart rate monitoring is produced by a maternal heart rate-derived signal. Use of dual scales places the maternal electrocardiographic signal at a different place on the paper than the Doppler ("fetal" transducer but maternally derived) signal. A comparison of the traces produced by two different sources then clarifies the artifact. It is maternally derived when they prove to be synchronous.[9]

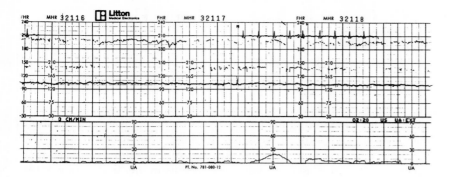

CASE INTERPRETATION: Class III-III

Baseline Information: there are four heart rates: one in the fetal marked tachycardia range with fair variability, as measured by an external monitor; one in the normal heart range on a separate scale, which is apparently synchronized with the third, also at a normal rate; the fourth shows occasional marks in the marked bradycardia range to one-half the amount of the upper heart rate.

Periodic or Nonperiodic Changes: none displayed.

Uterine Activity: occasional small contractions, as measured by a tocodynamometer.

Significance: the Doppler monitor is intermittently recording the fetal and maternal rate. The ECG-derived maternal trace provides clarification of the sources of the signals. There is rare half counting of the fetal tachycardia.

CASE OUTCOME: Thirty-one-year-old gravida 2, para 1001, at 25 weeks' gestation delivered vaginally a 1 pound, 8 ounce (680 gram) female; Apgar score 1/6. The fetus was in a vertex presentation. The pregnancy was complicated by a premature rupture of the membranes and a group B streptococcal infection. The newborn died on the fortieth day of life.

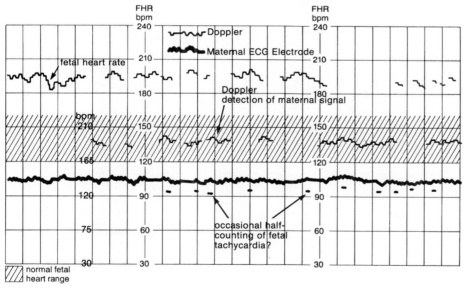

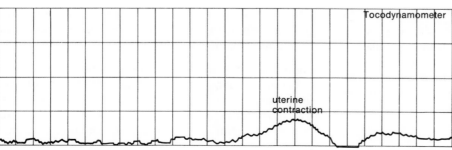

Pattern Characteristic:
Maternal and Fetal Tachycardia

Maternal-Fetal Monitoring, Single Scale, Maternal and Fetal Tachycardia, Half Counting Artifact

*H*alf counting occurs at rapid fetal heart rates when a Doppler-derived fetal heart signal occurs so close to the preceding signal that it falls within the "refractory period" of the machine.[7] The inability of the machine to accept a signal in close proximity to the preceding signal is designed to prevent counting of the second heart sound produced by diastole. It also serves under usual circumstances to reduce artifact.

Half counting by the monitor of a relatively slow heart rate cannot be explained by a refractory period concept.

This rare phenomenon is seen more often when counting the maternal heart rate that is transmitted from abdominal vessels. In these circumstances, the half counting may be the result of a weak or variable signal.

Half counting always results in the diminishing of the appearance of variability by compressing the signal in a smaller space. Smoothing of the trace also occurs because every other beat is recorded.

Dual maternal-fetal monitoring allows rapid clarification of such patterns.[9]

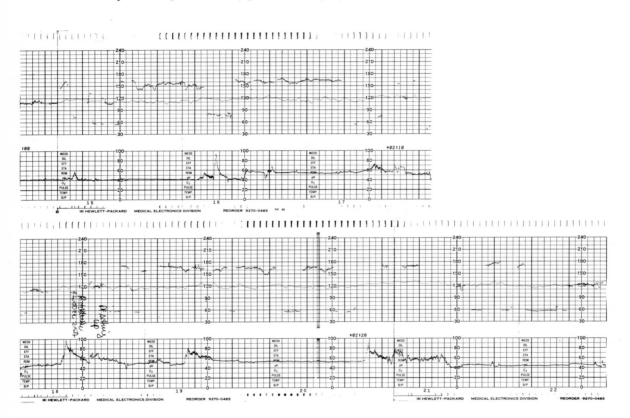

CASE INTERPRETATION: Class 1-0

Baseline Information: there are four heart rates: the top one is in the fetal moderate tachycardic range; the second is in the moderate fetal bradycardic range or maternal tachycardic range; the third is in the fetal marked bradycardic or normal maternal heart rate range; and the lowest is in the fetal and maternal bradycardic range. Variability is average on the upper two, is not discernible on the third, and is absent on the lowest.

Periodic or Nonperodic Changes: possible accelerations and small, mild variable decelerations in the upper

trace. No other periodic or nonperiodic changes are seen.

Uterine Activity: infrequent skewed contractions, suggesting a rapid rise to maximum pressure and reflecting altered maternal respirations.

Significance: this is more likely to be maternal-fetal rather than twin monitoring because of the markedly dissimilar rates. There is half counting of both heart rates. The fetus does not demonstrate a risk of acidosis at the present time, but clearer information should be sought.

CASE OUTCOME: Twenty-six-year-old primigravida, para 1001, at 29 weeks' gestation delivered vaginally, with no anesthesia, a 2 pound (900 gram) male; Apgar score 1/5. The fetus was in a vertex presentation. The newborn course was complicated by severe respiratory distress and intracranial hemorrhage. The umbilical cord pH was 7.41.

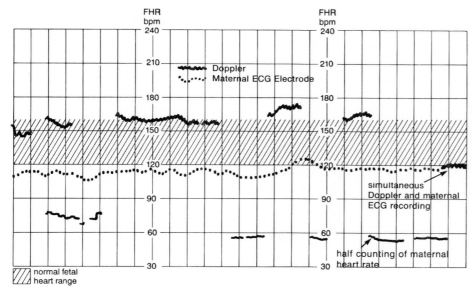

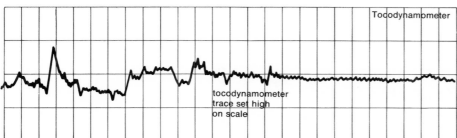

Pattern Characteristic:
Maternal-Fetal Monitoring Dual Scale Maternal and Fetal Tachycardia, Half Counting Artifact

Dual Monitoring Single Fetus, Single Scale, Internal-External Monitoring Comparison

*T*he dual channels in certain modern fetal monitors allow recording of the fetal heart by internal and external detectors simultaneously. Besides its usefulness in twin and maternal heart rate monitoring, it is also of use in demonstrating the ability of a modern external monitor to display variability without exaggeration through autocorrelation.[3,6]

Separate grids on dual scale monitor paper allow comparison on a single tracing. However, because the lower (electrocardiogram-derived signal) scale is confined to a smaller space, variability of the upper scale looks slightly better. Dual channel tracings, using the same scale, appear to be superimposed, making it impossible to assess small differences in the two monitoring techniques but emphasizing the potential loss of information with the Doppler-derived signal in comparison to the electrocardiographically derived signal.[8,19] See pages 438 and 440 for a further discussion of the comparison of autocorrelation-derived traces with Doppler- and ECG-derived traces, respectively.

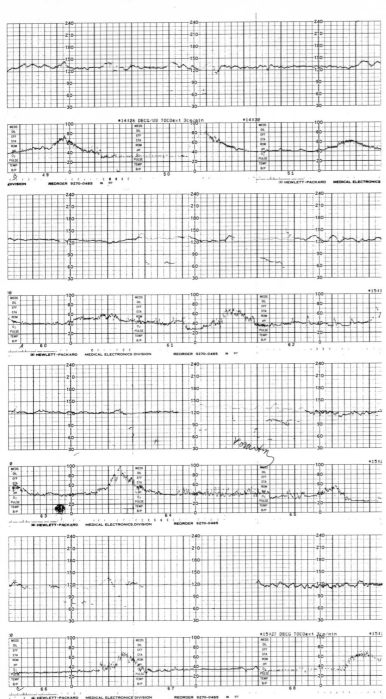

CASE INTERPRETATION: Class I-I

Baseline Information: there are two rates with a nearly identical short- and long-term variability (average).

Periodic or Nonperiodic Changes: small accelerations and mild variable decelerations.

Uterine Activity: skewed contractions of a frequency that is compatible with active labor.

Significance: the monitoring of the same heart by direct and indirect methods. A healthy fetus is predicted.

CASE OUTCOME: Twenty-year-old primigravida at 38½ weeks' gestation delivered vaginally from a vertex presentation, with local anesthesia, a 6 pound, 6 ounce (2892 gram) female; Apgar score 7/9. The infant followed an uncomplicated newborn course.

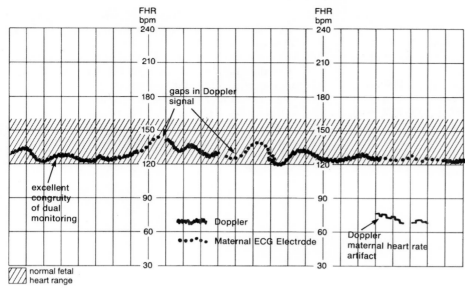

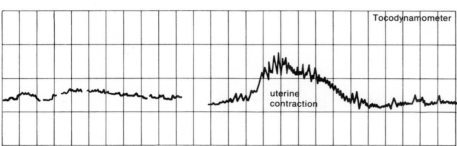

Pattern Characteristic:
Dual Monitoring Internal and
External Monitoring Comparison

References

1. Amato JC: Fetal heart rate monitoring. *Am J Obstet Gynecol* 147:967, 1983.
2. Bailey D, Flynn AM, Kelly J, et al: Antepartum fetal heart rate monitoring in multiple pregnancy. *Brit J Obstet Gynaecol* 87:561, 1980.
3. Boehm FH, Fields LM: Second-generation EFM is waiting in the wings. *Contemp Obstet Gynecol* Mar:179, 1984.
4. Devoe LD: Simultaneous antepartum testing of twin heart rates. *Southern Med J* 78:380, 1985.
5. Devoe LD, Azor H: Simultaneous nonstress fetal heart rate testing in twin pregnancy. *Obstet Gynecol* 58:450, 1981.
6. Divon MY, Torres FP, Yeh S-Y, et al: Autocorrelation techniques in fetal monitoring. *Am J Obstet Gynecol* 151:2, 1985.
7. Freeman RK, Garite TJ: *Instrumentation, Artifact, Detection*

and Fetal Arrhythmias in Fetal Heart Rate Monitoring. Baltimore, Williams & Wilkins, 1981, p. 28ff.
8. Fukushima T, Flores CA, Hon EH, et al: Limitations of autocorrelations in fetal heart rate monitoring. *Am J Obstet Gynecol* 153:685, 1985.
9. Klapholz H, Schifrin BS, Myrick R: Role of maternal artifact in fetal heart rate pattern interpretation. *Obstet Gynecol* 44:373, 1974.
10. Klaven M, Boscola MA: *A Guide to Fetal Monitoring.* Andover, MA, Hewlett-Packard, 1973, p. 100.
11. Lackritz R, Schiff I, Gibson M, et al: Decelerations on fetal electro-cardiography with fetal demise. *Obstet Gynecol* 51:367, 1978.
12. McGwier BW, Cabaniss ML: Effect of lumbar epidural anesthesia on maternal heart rate. Unpublished data.

13. Read JA, Miller FC: Technique of simultaneous direct intrauterine pressure recording for electronic monitoring of twin gestation in labor. *Am J Obstet Gynecol* 129:228, 1977.

14. Perry CP: Problem with fetal heart rate monitor (letter). *Am J Obstet Gynecol* 150:111, 1984.

15. Sherer DM, Nawrocki MN, Peco NE, et al: The occurrence of simultaneous fetal heart rate accelerations in twins during nonstress testing. *Obstet Gynecol* 76:817, 1990.

16. Shnider S, Abboud TK, Artal R, et al: Maternal catecholamines decrease during labor after lumbar epidural anesthesia. *Am J Obstet Gynecol* 147:13, 1983.

17. Souma ML, Cabaniss CD: The Valsalva maneuver: A test of autonomic nervous system function in pregnancy. *Am J Obstet Gynecol* 145:274, 1983.

18. Van Zundert AA, Vaes LE, DeWolf AM: ECG monitoring of mother and fetus during epidural anesthesia (letter). *Anesthesiology* 66:584, 1987.

19. Wagner PC: Limitations of fetal heart rate monitoring (letter). *Am J Obstet Gynecol* 156:1038, 1987.

20. Wagner PC, Cabaniss ML, Johnson TRB: What's really new in EFM equipment? *Contemp Obstet Gynecol* Technology Issue 1986, p. 91.

Single Channel Monitoring with Multiple Heart Rates

Chapter 18

Multiple Heart Rates Produced by Premature Depolarizations and Compensatory Pauses: Arrhythmia

*A*n artifact rejection system is present in most machines as a pen-lift (or heat off) feature.[6,18] The external monitor always has the pen-lift operational to minimize artifact. With internal monitoring, the pen-lift is activated when a variation greater than expected occurs between successive beats. With internal monitoring, the pen-lift may be selected as an option by using a switch on the back of the machine or inside the paper dispenser when monitoring a fetus internally with premature depolarizations.

The fetal monitor, when recording a fetal arrhythmia characterized by premature depolarizations, gives the appearance of three baseline heart rates during scalp electrode monitoring. If the logic (or pen-lift) is disengaged, vertical lines connect the three rates (see page 524). If the logic (or pen-lift) is engaged, the three rates appear as dotted lines. The upper baseline is produced by the premature beat, the middle line by the normal cardiac cycle, and the lower line by the compensatory pause.

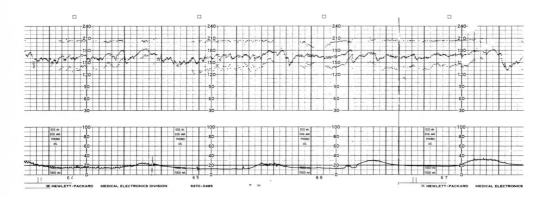

CASE INTERPRETATION: Class I

Baseline Information: there are three baselines: one in marked tachycardia range; one in high normal range; one in normal range; all with average beat-to-beat variability.

Periodic or Nonperiodic Changes: nonperiodic accelerations.

Uterine Activity: regular contractions, little deflection of the tocodynamometer.

Significance: fetal cardiac arrhythmia, the pen-lift is engaged, producing the dotted line effect. There are premature extrasystoles, which are probably ventricular in origin, requiring electrocardiography or echocardiography for confirmation.

CASE OUTCOME: Thirty-seven-year-old gravida 8, para 5025, at 38 weeks' gestation, delivered vaginally from a vertex presentation, with local anesthesia, a 6 pound, 12 ¾ ounce (3083 gram) female; Apgar score 9/9. No cardiac disease was detected in the newborn.

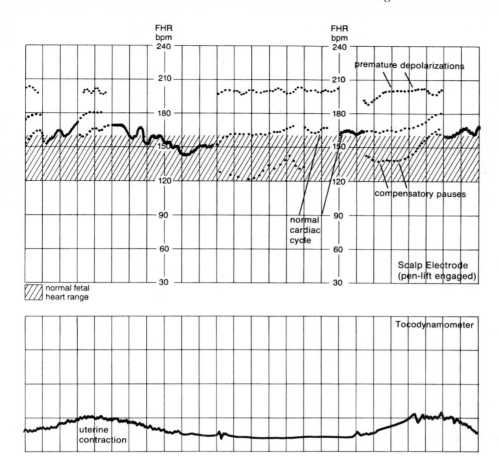

Pattern Characteristic:
Multiple Heart Rates Produced
by Fetal Arrhythmia

Multiple Heart Rates Produced by Premature Depolarizations, Conducted and Nonconducted: Arrhythmia

*T*he fetal monitor produces bizarre patterns during cardiac arrhythmias. If the pen-lift or heat off feature on the machine is disengaged, vertical lines connect rapidly changing heart rates.[6,18] If the pen-lift is engaged, multiple rates may be represented by dotted lines.

Although electrocardiography or echocardiography is most conclusive for diagnosis of each arrhythmia, analysis of the tracing alone allows certain generalizations: premature extrasystoles appear above the line that represents the normal cardiac cycle. The normal cardiac cycle usually appears in the normal fetal heart range and maintains variability. Compensatory pauses appear as spikes or dots below the normal baseline rate. Pauses produced by a single blocked supraventricular signal appear as deep spikes below the normal baseline. A continuous line in the severe bradycardia range represents either escape (e.g., junctional rhythm) or nonconduction of every other premature beat.

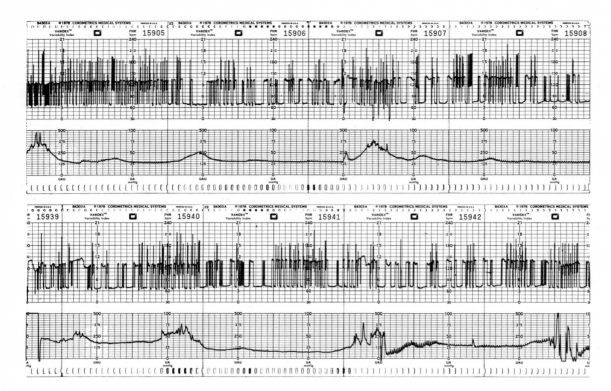

CASE INTERPRETATION: Class III

Baseline Information: there are four heart rates: one in the moderate to marked tachycardia range, indicated by single marks that are recorded as spikes; one in the normal range with decreased variability; one in the low normal to mild bradycardia range, indicated by single marks recorded as downward spikes; one in the marked bradycardia range with diminished variability.

Periodic or Nonperiodic Changes: possible small accelerations.

Uterine Activity: infrequent prolonged contractions.

Significance: this pattern occurs when the pen-lift is disengaged and arrhythmia that is caused by premature beats produces vertical parallel lines. Upward and downward spikes usually represent premature depolarizations and compensatory pauses, respectively. The normal cardiac cycle is typically recorded intermittently in the normal range. The flat rate of 70 probably represents a bradycardia that is produced when nonconducted premature beats occur in bigeminy (see page 484). An electrocardiogram or echocardiogram aids a precise diagnosis.

CASE OUTCOME: Fifteen-year-old primigravida at 40 weeks' gestation delivered vaginally, with pudendal anesthesia from a vertex presentation, a 6 pound, 14 ounce (3118 gram) female; Apgar score 7/9. There were no intrapartum pH studies or electrocardiograms done. No arrhythmia was detected in the newborn. The infant followed a normal newborn course.

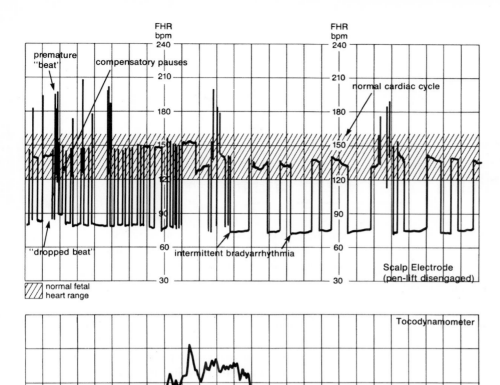

Pattern Characteristic:
Multiple Heart Rates Produced
by Fetal Arrhythmia

Maternal Heart Rate Artifact

*W*hen two heart rates appear, one in the normal fetal heart range and one in the bradycardic range, the first step in making a diagnosis is to exclude intermittent decelerations of the fetal heart. With external monitoring, the transition between a baseline rate and the rate during a deceleration may not be recorded. However, intermittent decelerations do not typically produce a flattened line consistently parallel to the fetal heart baseline as does recording of a second heart rate (usually maternal in origin). The intermittent recording of twin heart rates by a single Doppler, although theoretically a potential problem, is rarely recognizable unless dual monitoring is used (see page 416 insert). When a maternal heart rate artifact is suspected, simultaneous counting of the maternal heart rate by palpation of her pulse, cardiac auscultation, or ECG recording, promptly clarifies the issue. Relocation of the Doppler transducer, scalp electrode monitoring, or simultaneous fetal and maternal heart rate monitoring with dual channels are options that can be used to avoid further confusion.[13,18,19]

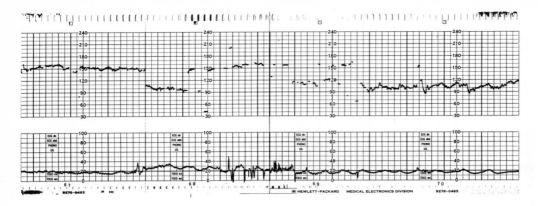

CASE INTERPRETATION: Class III-0

Baseline Information: there are two baseline heart rates: one in the high normal range with decreased variability; one in the moderate bradycardia range with variability present but not clearly recorded for diagnosis.

Periodic or Nonperiodic Changes: none (the two rates must be differentiated from intermittent decelerations).

Uterine Activity: not clearly recorded.

Significance: the most common cause of this pattern is an intermittent maternal heart rate recording. It is not confused in this case with double or half counting or with some arrhythmias because there is no mathematical association between the two rates.

CASE OUTCOME: Twenty-year-old primigravida at 26 weeks' gestation delivered by cesarean section performed for placental abruption, a 1 pound, 14 ounce (850 gram) male; Apgar score 7/7. The fetus was in a vertex presentation. The newborn expired at 26 days of age; his course was complicated by hyaline membrane disease and probable sepsis. The maternal heart rate was intermittently recorded by the fetal monitor.

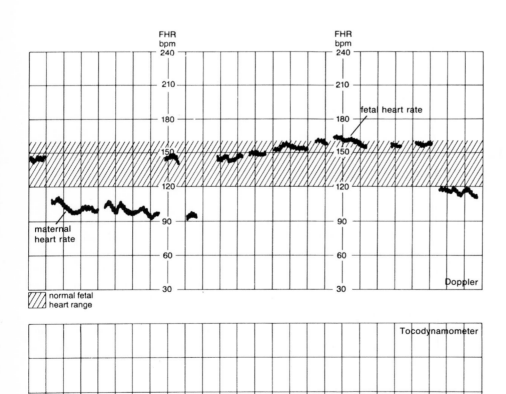

Pattern Characteristic:
Maternal Heart Rate Artifact

Maternal Heart Rate Artifact and Half Counting Artifact

*T*he fetal monitor is a computer, programmed to readily accept signals in the normal fetal heart range and more easily reject signals outside the normal fetal heart range, as a means of avoiding artifact. Maternal signal recording is therefore facilitated, even with careful Doppler placement, when simultaneous maternal and fetal tachycardia occur. In such cases, the maternal heart rate is in the normal fetal heart range and the fetal heart rate is in a tachycardic range. Simultaneously elevated rates are most commonly produced by maternal fever or the use of betamimetic agents.

The first step in making the diagnosis is recognition of a double parallel line pattern. The pattern may be confused with accelerations from a normal baseline or decelerations from a tachycardic baseline. Palpation of the maternal pulse, auscultation of the maternal heart, or direct maternal and/or fetal ECG monitoring are methods used to establish that an artifact is producing the pattern.[13,18,19] It may be important to recognize this artifact and its predisposing circumstances so that significant fetal heart rate information is not lost.[22] When both fetal and maternal heart rates are recorded intermittently by the Doppler transducer, half or double counting of either may occur (see page 437).

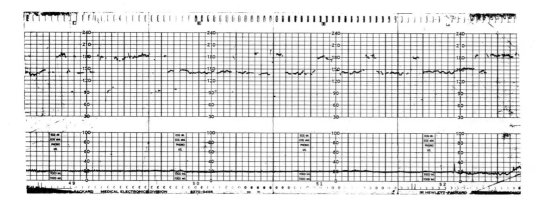

CASE INTERPRETATION: Class III-0

Baseline Information: there are three heart rates: one is in a moderate tachycardic range with decreased variability; one is in the normal range with decreased variability; one has a few marks recorded in a moderate bradycardic range.

Periodic or Nonperiodic Changes: none recorded (the pattern must be distinguished from intermittent decelerations).

Uterine Activity: none recorded.

Significance: the parallel lines are typical of alternately monitoring the maternal signal and the fetal heart with a Doppler transducer. This pattern is seen particularly in the presence of maternal fever or when using a betamimetic agent, both of which produce simultaneous fetal and maternal tachycardia.

CASE OUTCOME: Thirty-year-old gravida 3, para 2002, monitored at 28 weeks' gestation while receiving ritodrine for premature labor. The patient was readmitted at 38½ weeks' gestation and delivered vaginally, under epidural anesthesia with low elective forceps, a 6 pound, 15 ounce (3147 gram) male; Apgar score 8/9. The fetus was in a vertex presentation. The infant followed an uncomplicated newborn course.

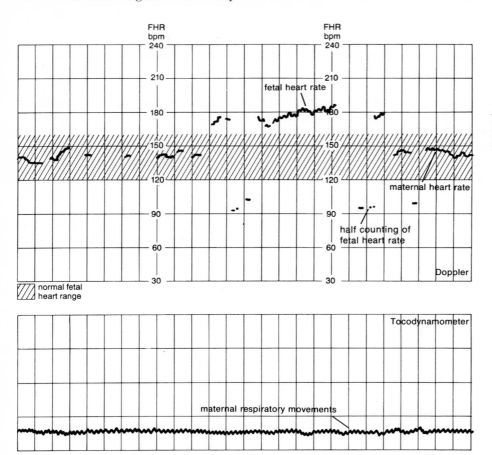

Pattern Characteristic:
Maternal Heart Rate Artifact and
Half Counting

Maternal Heart Rate Artifact and Maternal Arrhythmia

*B*ecause the external fetal monitor may capture maternal signals, it is possible to record aberrations in the maternal heart rate. Such may occur during beta sympathomimetic therapy for treatment of premature labor.[2,11] The case illustration is a maternal arrhythmia, a supraventricular tachycardia, which is displayed on the fetal heart rate trace of the monitor. During use of cardiac stimulants in pregnant patients, dual maternal-fetal monitoring provides maternal heart rate surveillance and assists in clarifying the source of abrupt or subtle baseline changes on the fetal heart trace (see dual monitoring page 418).

In the adult, supraventricular tachycardia is usually a heart rate in excess of 170 bpm; in the fetus it is usually in excess of 200 bpm.

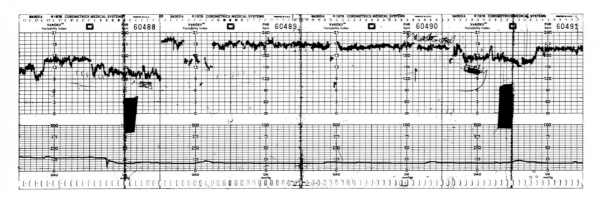

CASE INTERPRETATION: Class III-0

Baseline Information: three heart rates are detected with an external monitor: one in a marked tachycardic range; one in a moderate tachycardic range; and one in a normal fetal heart range. Variability cannot be adequately assessed by the external monitor of this machine.

Periodic or Nonperiodic Changes: possible accelerations are present from the lower of the three baselines.

Uterine Activity: small regular deflections of the tocodynamometer, suggesting mild contractions.

Significance: the lower two rates are typical of a maternal heart rate artifact associated with maternal and fetal tachycardia. Auscultation may help exclude a diagnosis of accelerations from a normal baseline or decelerations from a tachycardic baseline. The upper rate could represent a tachyarrhythmia or double counting of a moderate fetal bradycardia.

CASE OUTCOME: Twenty-five-year-old gravida 3, para 2002, was monitored at 32 weeks' gestation while receiving therapy for premature labor. A maternal and fetal tachycardia were intermittently monitored by a Doppler monitor. The mother developed a paroxysmal supraventricular tachycardia while the Doppler was recording the maternal signal. A maternal ECG documented the maternal arrhythmia as well as ST-T changes that are compatible with ischemia. The arrhythmia converted to a sinus rhythm with treatment. The same day, the patient delivered vaginally a 4 pound, 4 ounce (1928 gram) male; Apgar score 1/2. There was a 10% marginal placental abruption. The newborn course was complicated by severe respiratory distress. The newborn was dismissed on the thirty-fifth day of life.

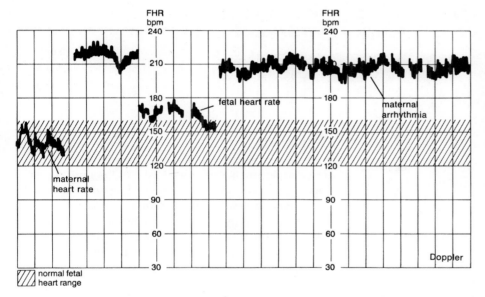

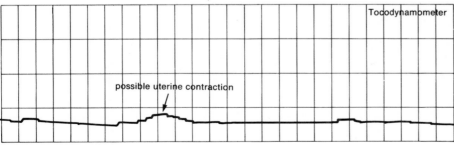

Pattern Characteristic:
Maternal Rate Artifact and
Maternal Arrhythmia

Double Counting: Artifact

*D*ouble counting is an artifact that, with rare exception, is seen only with external monitoring. It most often occurs with heart rates that fall into the fetal bradycardic range. The instrument, designed to record heart rates in the normal fetal heart range, when encountering a slow rate, may count an additional Doppler-derived motion event in the cardiac cycle.[7,12,19] The resultant doubled rate may mask significant decelerations.

When double counting occurs, the variability is always exaggerated because the resulting fetal heart rate is expanded on a wider scale.

The pattern must be distinguished from half counting of a tachycardic fetal heart rate or maternal heart rate interference with a fetal tachycardia. Auscultation clarifies the diagnosis.

Double counting is rare with internal monitoring: At very slow rates a tall peaked T wave theoretically might be counted in addition to the R wave, but usually the machine is able to distinguish characteristics (such as slope of rise), resulting in rejection of non-QRS signals.

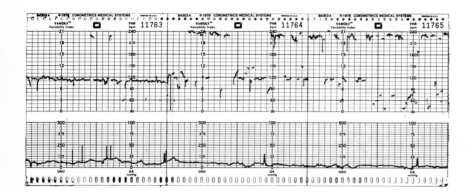

CASE INTERPRETATION: Class III

Baseline Information: there are two heart rates seen: one is in a marked fetal tachycardic range; and one is in a moderate fetal bradycardic (or maternal tachycardic) range. Variability is not interpretable.

Periodic or Nonperiodic Changes: none seen.

Uterine Activity: none clearly displayed.

Significance: the differential diagnosis is double counting of a fetal bradycardia versus half counting of a fetal tachyarrhythmia; auscultation will clarify this.

CASE OUTCOME: Twenty-six-year-old primigravida at 40 weeks' gestation delivered vaginally from a vertex presentation, with local anesthesia, a 7 pound, 8 ounce (3402 gram) male; Apgar score 9/9. The newborn course was uncomplicated. The maternal antepartum course was complicated by 12 rads of diagnostic x-ray exposure at six and a half weeks' gestation. The infant demonstrated features of a minimal brain dysfunction, which resolved at one year of age.

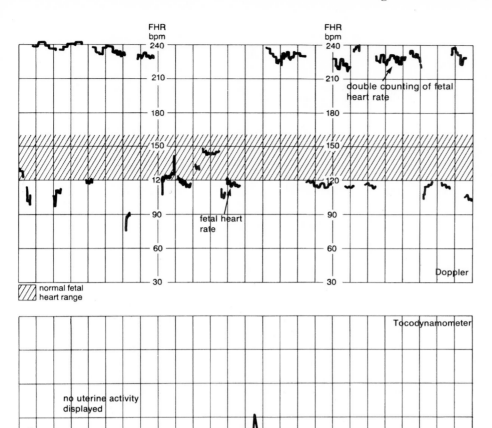

Pattern Characteristic:
Double Counting

Half Counting: Artifact

*H*alf counting is an artifact that, with rare exception, is seen only with external monitoring. It most frequently occurs with rapid heart rates. The fetal monitor, programmed to receive signals in the normal fetal heart range, receives the signal sooner than usual because of a tachycardia or tachyarrhythmia and consequently rejects the signal because of a machine refractory window.[7,12,19] The next signal is accepted. This occurs repeatedly, resulting in halving of the tachycardic rate. Occasionally, half counting occurs with normal rates or even with maternal rates below the normal fetal heart range. In the latter situations, additional mechanisms (such as alternately varying the quality of the Doppler-derived signal) may be operative.

When half counting occurs, the variability is always reduced because the resulting fetal heart rate is compressed on a smaller scale and also because a type of averaging has occurred that always produces a smoother tracing than a beat-to-beat recording.

The pattern is to be distinguished from double counting of a bradycardic fetal heart rate or maternal heart rate interference. Auscultation clarifies the diagnosis.

Half counting may occur with internal fetal monitoring with excessively rapid heart rates beyond the limits of rate of R wave signal processing.[7]

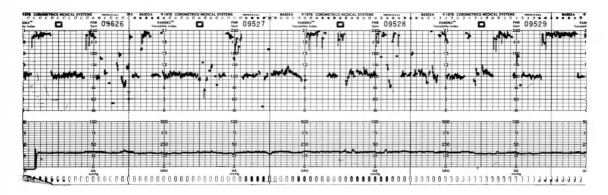

CASE INTERPRETATION: Class III

Baseline Information: there are two heart rates: the lower is in the low normal fetal heart range; the upper is in a marked fetal tachycardic range. There is decreased variability.

Periodic or Nonperiodic Changes: none displayed.

Uterine Activity: none displayed.

Significance: this pattern indicates either fetal tachyarrhythmia (with half counting) or low normal fetal heart rate with double counting. Auscultation will clarify this. Further fetal assessment is appropriate.

CASE OUTCOME: Twenty-year-old primigravida at 36 weeks' gestation delivered by low transverse cesarean section, with general anesthesia from a vertex presentation, a 7 pound, 4 ounce (3289 gram) male; Apgar score 2/6. The cesarean section was performed for failed pharmaconversion of fetal supraventricular tachycardia. The agents used were digoxin, quinidine, and verapamil. Fetal pulmonary maturity was confirmed by an amniotic fluid study done prior to the cesarean section. The newborn course was complicated by hydrops, which resolved with conversion of the supraventricular tachycardia with digoxin therapy, and hyperbilirubinemia, which responded to phototherapy.

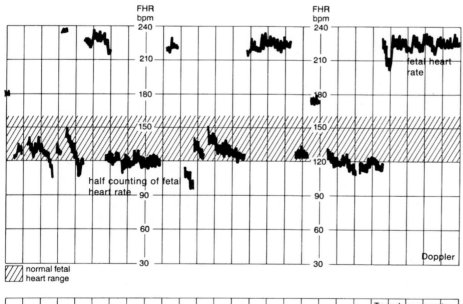

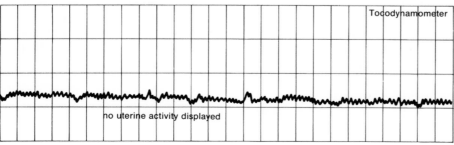

Pattern Characteristic:
Half Counting

Double Counting Maternal Heart Rate, Half Counting Fetal Heart Rate

*T*he Doppler-derived fetal monitor record is capable of displaying information from both fetal and maternal sources, even with the use of autocorrelation.[9,19] Double counting and half counting of either heart rate is then possible. This may result in multiple baseline rates that are capable of obscuring the normal fetal heart rate.

When such an artifactual tracing is encountered, auscultation and study of the entire tracing may clarify the artifact. Appropriate management is making a change in the maternal position or in the Doppler placement or changing to scalp electrode monitoring. Using dual channels for maternal and fetal heart rate recording will also clarify the artifact. See pages 418 and 420.

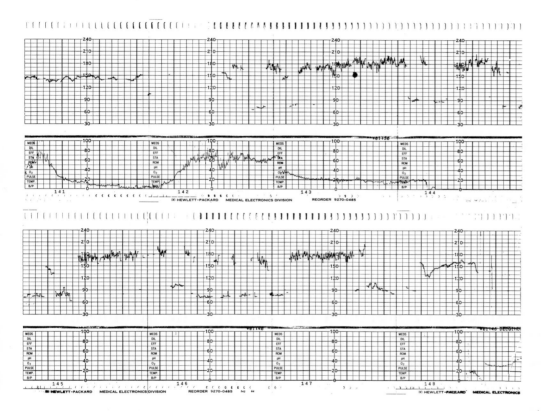

CASE INTERPRETATION: Class 0

Baseline Information: there are four heart rates: the upper rate is in a moderate fetal tachycardic range, the next is in a normal fetal heart range, and the lower two rates are in a normal maternal heart rate range (fetal marked bradycardic range). The upper trace has exaggerated variability, the next two have average variability, although they are only brief segments. The lower trace is not interpretable.

Periodic or Nonperiodic Changes: possible accelerations in the upper trace. There is a single mild atypical variable deceleration in the second trace from the top.

Uterine Activity: skewed and prolonged contractions followed by unrecorded uterine activity.

Significance: the upper trace is artifactual in appearance and most likely a double counting maternal heart rate; the second is a normal fetal heart rate; the third is a normal maternal heart rate; and the fourth appears to be a half counted fetal heart rate.

CASE OUTCOME: Fourteen-year-old primigravida at 39 weeks' gestation delivered vaginally, with low forceps and epidural anesthesia, a 7 pound, 13 ounce (3260 gram) male; Apgar score 9/9. The infant followed an uncomplicated newborn course.

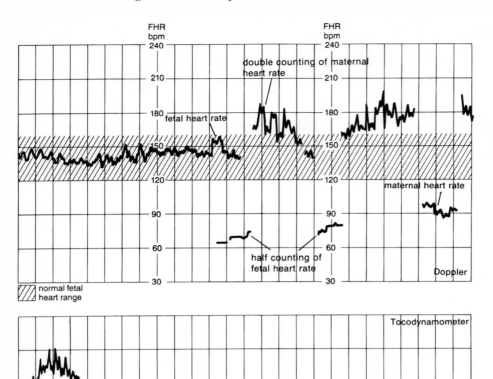

Pattern Characteristic:
Double Counting Maternal
Heart Rate Half Counting Fetal
Heart Rate

Two Instruments, Internal-External Fetal Heart Rate Monitoring Comparison—Without Autocorrelation

*I*nternal fetal heart rate monitoring is the most accurate method of obtaining beat-to-beat information because the final trace is derived from the precise electrocardiographic fetal heart signal. The fine computer of the fetal monitor is programmed to identify each R wave (or maximum deflection of the QRS complex), the interval between the two being a measure of the cardiac cycle. The signal is influenced by fetal motion, but seldom is the identification of the R wave preempted. External monitoring, prior to autocorrelation, was based on peak identification of a signal derived from fetal cardiac motion with its systolic and diastolic components. These components vary with each cycle, and the signal is altered by fetal motion so that the identified peak may vary with

each successive cardiac event. The potential result is exaggeration of "beat-to-beat" fetal heart rate variability.[12,16,17] Such exaggerated variability with external monitoring can be demonstrated by comparing external monitoring (without autocorrelation) to the internal monitoring-derived trace of another instrument.[3,5,21] Although autocorrelation minimizes exaggeration of variability, thus decreasing the need for internal monitoring, use of the scalp electrode remains an option in evaluating cases of decreased variability and in cases in which the fetal signal is lost.[1,9] For example, when the fetus moves away from the Doppler transducer, information may be erroneous.[5,20]

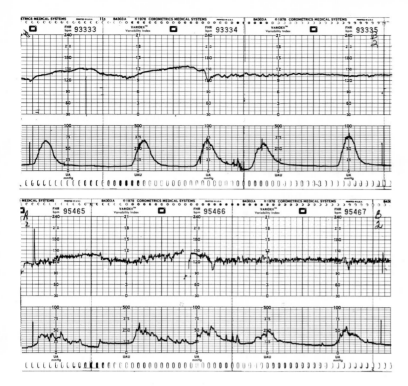

CASE INTERPRETATION: Class I-I

Baseline Information: there are two heart rates in a normal fetal heart range: the lower rate is with decreased but present beat-to-beat variability, the upper is with what appears to be average variability.

Periodic or Nonperiodic Changes: identical prolonged accelerations, the lower demonstrating decreased variability in the accelerations, single V-shaped small variable decelerations.

Uterine Activity: skewed contractions with a relatively rapid rise to maximum pressure, peaked; the frequency is consistent with active labor.

Significance: the trace with the external monitor (upper) demonstrates exaggerated variability.

CASE OUTCOME: Sixteen-year-old primigravida at 34 weeks' gestation delivered vaginally from a vertex presentation, with pudendal and local anesthesia, a 4 pound, 6 ounce (1984 gram) male; Apgar score 8/9. The maternal course was complicated by preeclampsia. The patient received magnesium sulfate intravenously intrapartum. The newborn course was complicated by hyaline membrane disease, which required respiratory therapy, and a small size for his gestational age. The newborn was dismissed at 36 days of life.

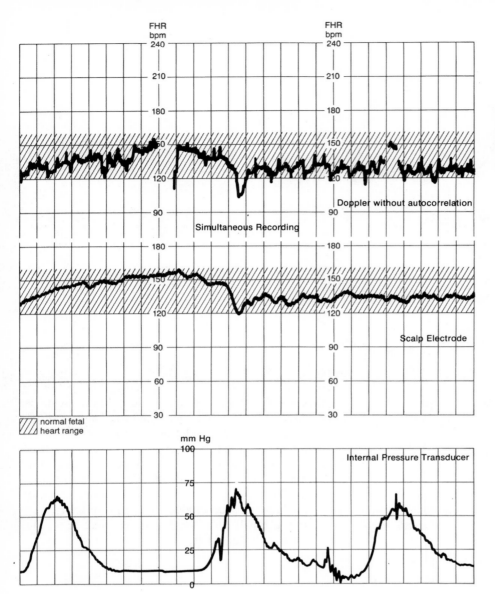

Pattern Characteristic:
Comparison of Internal Monitor and External Monitor without Autocorrelation

Two Instruments, Internal-External Monitoring Comparison— With Autocorrelation

*I*nternal fetal heart rate monitoring is the most accurate method to date of obtaining beat-to-beat fetal heart information. This is because the final trace is obtained by a computerized method of identifying and measuring fetal electrocardiographic R wave intervals. External fetal monitoring, prior to the use of autocorrelation, was po-

tentially considerably less accurate because the final trace was obtained by measuring the interval between peaks of motion-derived cardiac signals, a biologic phenomenon that is variable with each cardiac cycle.[14] Autocorrelation has enabled production of an external monitoring trace that displays beat-to-beat fetal heart rate information that approximates internal monitoring almost to precision.[4] This may be demonstrated by simultaneous comparison of external monitoring with autocorrelation of one instrument with internal monitoring of another.[3,5,15,21] This is accomplished by advanced computer technology that enables the superimposing of one motion-derived cardiac signal over another until a "best fit" is identified, thus allowing selection of a comparable event in each cardiac cycle.[3,10,21]

Neither external monitoring with autocorrelation nor internal monitoring is perfect. The former is still derived from a variable "biomechanical" event and is dependent upon the fetal heart rate remaining dominant to maternal or other signals in the field of the Doppler "inquiry."[8] The latter is dependent on an ability to distinguish R waves from other electrocardiographic events of the mother or fetus.[13,20]

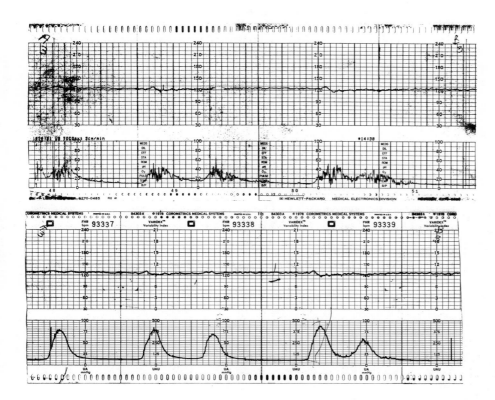

CASE INTERPRETATION: Class III-III

Baseline Information: there are two heart rates in a low normal fetal heart range, both with decreased but present short-term variability and minimal long-term variability. The lower has occasional skip areas.

Periodic or Nonperiodic Changes: none seen.

Uterine Activity: skewed and paired peaked uterine contractions of a frequency compatible with active labor; a normal baseline tone, as measured by internal monitoring.

Significance: internal and external monitoring demonstrating similar variability. Review of the entire tracing for areas of improved variability, fetal pH, or fetal stimulation may be indicated.

CASE OUTCOME: Sixteen-year-old primigravida at 34 weeks' gestation delivered vaginally from a vertex presentation, with pudendal and local anesthesia, a 4 pound, 6 ounce (1984 gram), male; Apgar score 8/9. The maternal course was complicated by preeclampsia. The patient received magnesium sulfate intravenously intrapartum. The newborn course was complicated by hyaline membrane disease, which required respiratory therapy, and a small size for his gestational age. The newborn was dismissed at 36 days of life.

Note: This special case study was performed on the same fetus as the one in the case study found on page 439.

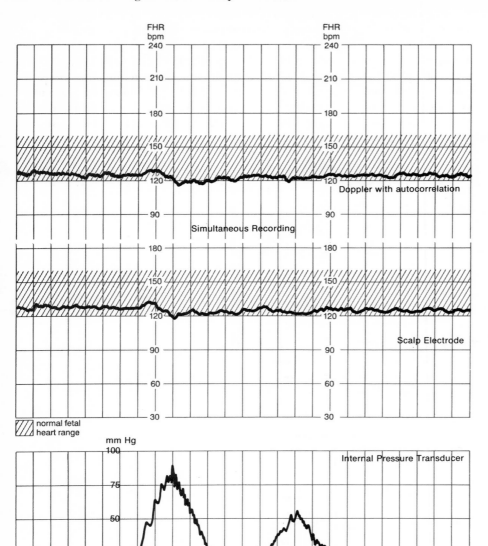

Pattern Characteristic:
Comparison of Internal Monitor and External Monitor with Autocorrelation

References

1. Amato JC: Fetal heart rate monitoring. *Am J Obstet Gynecol* 147:967, 1983.
2. Benedetti TJ: Maternal complications of parenteral beta-sympathomimetic therapy for premature labor. *Am J Obstet Gynecol* 145:1, 1983.
3. Boehm FH, Fields LM, Hutchinson JM, et al: The indirectly obtained fetal heart rate: Comparison of first and second-generation electronic fetal monitors. *Am J Obstet Gynecol* 155:10, 1986.
4. Dawes GS, Redman CWG: Fetal heart rate monitoring (letter). *Am J Obstet Gynecol* 57:513, 1987.
5. Divon MY, Torres FP, Yeh S-Y, et al: Autocorrelation techniques in fetal monitoring. *Am J Obstet Gynecol* 151:2, 1985.

6. Evans AT, Garite T: Advances in electronic fetal monitoring. *Contemp OB/GYN Technology* Issue 20:17, 1982.

7. Freeman RK, Garite TJ: *Instrumentation, Artifact Detection and Fetal Arrhythmias in Fetal Heart Rate Monitoring.* Baltimore, Williams & Wilkins, 1981, p. 28–42.

8. Fukushima T, Flores CA, Hon EH, et al: Limitations of autocorrelation in fetal heart rate monitoring. *Am J Obstet Gynecol* 153:685, 1985.

9. Fukushima T, Davidson EC, Hon EH: Limitations of fetal heart rate monitoring (letter). *Am J Obstet Gynecol* 156:1038, 1987.

10. *Hewlett-Packard Service Manual* 08040-90000, Hewlett-Packard, Andover, MA, 1983.

11. Hosenpud JD, Morton MJ, O'Grady JP: Cardiac stimulation during ritodrine hydrochloride tocolytic therapy. *Obstet Gynecol* 62:62, 1983.

12. Hutson JM, Petrie RH: Possible limitations of fetal monitoring. *Clin Obstet Gynecol* 29:104, 1986.

13. Klapholz H, Schifrin BS, Myrick R: Role of maternal artifact in fetal heart rate pattern interpretation. *Obstet Gynecol* 44:373, 1974.

14. Lauersen NH, Hochberg HM, George MED, et al: A new technique for improving the Doppler ultrasound signal for fetal heart rate monitoring. *Am J Obstet Gynecol* 128:300, 1977.

15. Lawson GW, Belcher R, Dawes GS, et al: A comparison of ultrasound (with autocorrelation) and direct electrocardiogram fetal heart rate detector systems. *Am J Obstet Gynecol* 147:721, 1983.

16. Neuman MR: The biophysical and bioengineering bases of perinatal monitoring. Part I: Fetal heart rate. *Perinatology/Neonatology* July-August, p. 16, 1978.

17. Newman J: *The Doppler Effect in Cardiac Problems in Pregnancy.* New York: Alan R. Liss, 1982, p. 463–73.

18. Parer JT: Instrumentation and techniques, in: *Handbook of Fetal Heart Rate Monitoring.* Philadelphia, W.B. Saunders, 1983, p. 55ff.

19. Paul RH, Petrie R: *Fetal Intensive Care.* Wallingford, CT. Corometrics Medical Systems, Inc., 1979.

20. Wagner PC: Limitations of fetal heart rate monitoring (letter). *Am J Obstet Gynecol* 156:1038, 1987.

21. Wagner PC, Cabaniss ML, Johnson TRB: What's really new in EFM equipment? *Contemp OB/GYN Technology* Issue 1986, p. 91.

22. Young BK, Hochberg HM, George MED: An improved data display system for fetal heart rate monitoring. *Obstet Gynecol* 47:496, 1976.

Remote Transmission

Telephone Transmission

Telemetry

Telephone Transmission

*T*elephone transmission of fetal heart data dates back to the early 1960s when the fetal electrocardiographic data was transmitted via telephone.[5] Transmission of fetal monitor tracings have several practical uses. One of the longest appreciated is the transfer of information from a labor room to a central station where the tracing receives additional surveillance and may be used for consultation and education without disturbing the private experience of the parturient and her family. This has been achieved through the use of cables.

The transfer of the tracing to the home or a more remote office of the patient's personal physician or to the office, home, or hospital of a consultant was initially achieved through the use of a Xerox telecopier functioning with phone transmission.[1] Information from the printed paper was broken into multiple signals that were transmitted through telephone wires and reassembled in a receiver unit at the destination. This method has been superseded by facsimile copiers.

Modern transmission methods also use a telephone link but these can make a printing of the actual tracing on fetal monitoring paper in the consulting or receiving unit.[23] A brief lag in transmission allows cosurveillance of the patient by the two units. Storage capabilities allow more than one patient to be followed at a time.

In some transmission systems, information may be lost in the signal processing (see page 526) and at times the baseline may not appear at precisely identical levels in comparing the original and transmitted tracings.

The uterine activity trace and fetal heart trace may be compressed on a smaller strip, requiring that some visual retraining be employed for interpretation. The modern technology available for the transmission of fetal heart rate monitor tracings enables them to be stored in a computer and retrieved with a quality of reproduction that is comparable to the original form; this is an improvement over the earlier method of microfilm storage and retrieval.[11]

Telemetered information from the patient's home regarding uterine activity is also used for surveillance, particularly for some patients who are at risk of preterm labor.[7,8,9,16,19]

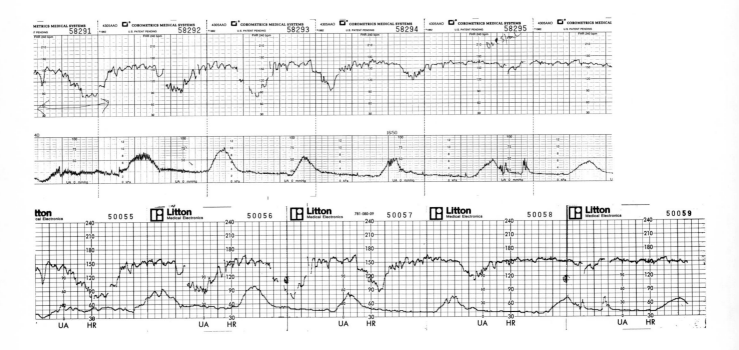

CASE INTERPRETATION: Class II-II

Baseline Information: a normal fetal heart range, original tracing at a slightly higher level than shown on the transmitted baseline. Average variability.

Periodic or Nonperiodic Changes: periodic deceleration with mixed features. These may represent late decelerations reflecting peaked contractions or may be atypical variable decelerations without primary or secondary accelerations.

Uterine Activity: peaked contractions of regular frequency. Skewing is present.

Significance: this pattern suggests a fetal response to hypoxia. Appropriate measures include improving fetal oxygenation through maternal oxygen administration, maternal position change, hydration, and a decrease in uterine activity if feasible. Delivery preparations are in order unless the pattern is corrected by the above measures.

CASE OUTCOME: Twenty-eight-year-old gravida 3, para 2002, at 40 weeks' gestation delivered by a low transverse cesarean section performed for possible fetal distress, with general anesthesia, a 6 pound, 15¼ ounce (3154 gram) female; Apgar score 9/10. A small amount of amniotic fluid was noted. The infant followed an uncomplicated newborn course.

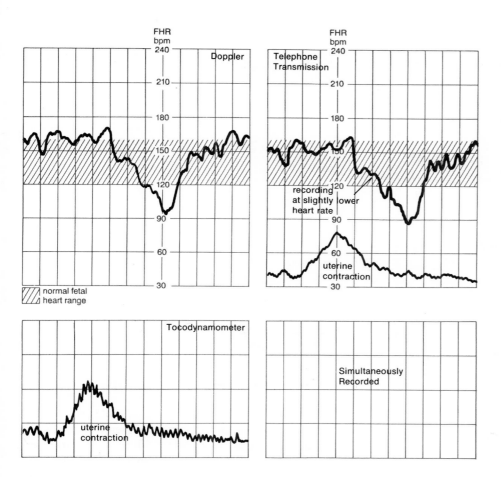

Pattern Characteristic:
Telephone Transmission

Telemetry

*R*adiotelemetry of fetal heart signals began in the early 1960s.[10] Early transmitters were placed in the vagina.[12,17] Later transmitters received signals through lead wires from scalp electrodes and intrauterine pressure transducers.[18] Because ambulatory monitoring was formerly limited to electrocardiogram-derived[13] and internal pressure transducer-derived tracings, an open amniotic sac was a necessity unless abdominal electrocardiographic signals were employed.[6,14,20,21]

Now modern technology enables Doppler signal-derived monitoring of the fetus in the ambulatory patient, a potential advantage for the intrapartum course.[2,3,4,15,22] This is achieved not with cables but with the transmission of the signal to a standard fetal monitor with telemetry reception capabilities. The quality of the trace using autocorrelation can be comparable to that of the patient who is restrained to a bed or chair by the traditional method of cable attachment to the monitor.

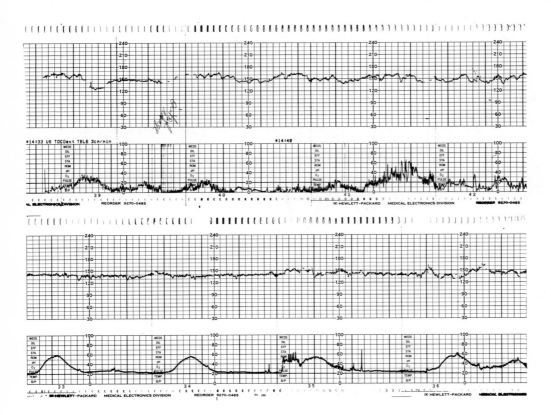

CASE INTERPRETATION: Class I-I

Baseline Information: two heart rates of similar normal rate and average variability that are not identical in recorded fluctuations.

Periodic or Nonperiodic Changes: shallow accelerations present, no decelerations seen.

Uterine Activity: occasional skewed uterine contractions, exaggerated maternal respirations.

Significance: the comparison of two fetal heart rate recording systems demonstrates comparable information for diagnosis.

CASE OUTCOME: Twenty-one-year-old gravida 2, para 1001, at 39 weeks' gestation delivered vaginally after a previous cesarean section, with pudendal anesthesia, from a vertex presentation, an 8 pound, 1 ounce (3657 gram) male; Apgar score 8/9. There was "moderate" meconium. The infant followed an uncomplicated newborn course. The upper trace was obtained traditionally, the lower by telemetry of a doppler signal from an ambulatory patient.

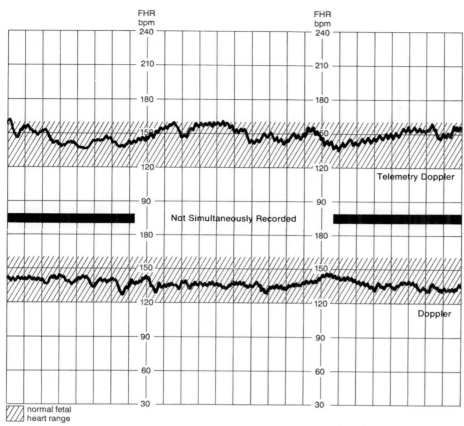

Pattern Characteristic:
Telemetry

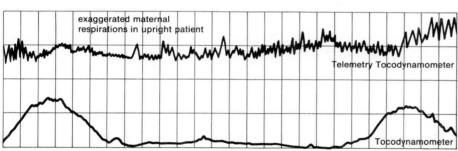

References

1. Boehm RH, Haire MF: Xerox telecopier transmission of fetal monitoring tracings: A 4-year experience. *Obstet Gynecol* 53:520, 1979.
2. Devoe LD, Arthur M, Searle N: The effects of maternal ambulation on the nonstress test. *Am J Obstet Gynecol* 157:240, 1987.
3. Diaz AG, Schwarcz R, Rescina R, et al: Vertical position during the first stage of the course of labor, and neonatal outcome. *Europ J Obstet Gynecol Reprod Biol* 11:1, 1980.
4. Flynn AM, Kelly J, Hollins G, et al: Ambulation in labour. *Brit Med J* 2:591, 1978.
5. Hagan WK, Larks SD: Long distance FM telephone transmission of fetal electrocardiogram. *Am J Med Electronics* 2:147, 1963.

6. Haukkamaa M, Purhonen M, Teramo K: The monitoring of labor by telemetry. *J Perinat Med* 10:17, 1982.

7. Iams JD, Johnson FF, O'Shaughnessy RW, et al: A prospective random trial of home uterine activity monitoring in pregnancies at increased risk of preterm labor. *Am J Obstet Gynecol* 157:638, 1987.

8. Katz M, Gill PJ: Initial evaluation of an ambulatory system for home monitoring and transmission of uterine activity data. *Obstet Gynecol* 66:273, 1985.

9. Katz M, Gill PJ, Newman RB: Detection of preterm labor by ambulatory monitoring of uterine activity: A preliminary report. *Obstet Gynecol* 68:773, 1986.

10. Kendall B, Farrell DM, Kane HA: Fetal radioelectrocardiography: a new method of fetal electrocardiography. *Am J Obstet Gynecol* 81:1629, 1962.

11. Klapholz H, Suzki K: Evaluation of the Model 78100A adult telemetry unit for use in fetal heart rate monitoring. *J Reprod Med* 18:79, 1977.

12. Lauersen NH, Hachberg HM, George MED: Microfilm storage of fetal monitoring records. *Obstet Gynecol* 51:632, 1978.

13. Lipshitz J, Wade JE, Anderson GD, et al: Evaluation of the Corometrics 315 telemetry system for fetal monitoring. *Am J Obstet Gynecol* 139:199, 1981.

14. Lupe PJ, Gross TL: Maternal upright posture and mobility in labor—a review. *Obstet Gynecol* 67:727, 1986.

15. MacRae DJ, White VGL: Further advances in radiotelemetry of the fetal heart sounds. *Int J of Gynaecol Obstet* 11:147, 1973.

16. Morrison JC, Martin JN, Martin RW, et al: Prevention of preterm birth by ambulatory assessment of uterine activity: A randomized study. *Am J Obstet Gynecol* 156:536, 1987.

17. Neuman MR, Picconnatto J, Roux JF: A wireless radiotelemetry system on monitoring fetal heart rate and intrauterine pressure during labor and delivery. *Gynecol Invest* 1:92, 1970.

18. Neuman MR, Roux JF, Patrick JE, et al: Evaluation of fetal monitoring by telemetry. *Obstet Gynecol* 54:249, 1979.

19. Newman RB, Gill PJ, Wittreech P, et al: Maternal preception of prelabor uterine activity. *Obstet Gynecol* 68:765, 1986.

20. Parer JT, Imershein SL: Clinical experience with telemetered heart rate monitoring. *J Reprod Med* 23:305, 1979.

21. Roux JF, Neuman MR, O'Gureck JE: The value and limitations of fetal monitoring by transvaginal telemetry and conventional wire systems. *Int J Gynaecol Obstet* 10:199, 1972.

22. Schwarcz R, Diaz AG, Belizan JM, et al: Influence of amniotomy and maternal position on labor, in: Proceedings of the 8th World Congress. *Gynecology and Obstetrics*, Castelazo-Ayala L, et al, (ed). Amsterdam, Excerpta Medica, 1977, p. 377–91.

23. Vintzeloes AM, Montgomery JT, Nochimson DJ, et al: Telephone transmission of fetal heart monitor data; the experience at the University of Connecticut health center. *Am J Obstet Gynecol* 155:630, 1986.

DYSRHYTHMIAS

Section VI

*T*he development and refinement of fetal electronic monitoring has brought about an increased awareness of fetal cardiac dysrhythmias. With the increasing ability to define fetal cardiac dysrhythmias there have been numerous reports of pharmacologic control of fetal dysrhythmias by administering drugs to the mother or fetus if the dysrhythmia has the potential to produce fetal jeopardy.

Basic to the understanding of the pathophysiology of cardiac dysrhythmias are the concepts of impulse formation by spontaneous diastolic depolarization ("automaticity") and the process of conduction of cardiac impulses.

Resting myocardial cells maintain a stable electrical charge across the cell membrane until an electrical impulse arrives and reduces the transmembrane charge to a threshold level, at which time the entire cell depolarizes with a propagated impulse and then actively repolarizes.

Spontaneous diastolic depolarization, or automaticity, occurs because specialized cells of the heart have the ability to rhythmically and gradually reduce their membrane charge to threshold and propagate impulses spontaneously. These cells normally reside in the sinus node, atrioventricular (AV) junction, and His-Purkinje system, but this process may occur at other sites in the heart under abnormal metabolic conditions such as hypoxia.

The rate of diastolic depolarization, or automaticity, of the sinus node is normally the fastest site of impulse formation in the heart, and the rate of impulse formation decreases decrementally from the sinus node to the AV junction to the His-Purkinje system. This provides for automatic impulse generation from the lower centers if automaticity fails or is suppressed in the higher centers and, at the same time, prevents the lower centers from usurping control of impulse formation, under normal conditions.

Conduction of these impulses that are formed by diastolic depolarization of the specialized cell takes place over defined pathways, to provide coordinated contraction and relaxation of the myocardium.

Therefore, pathophysiologically dysrhythmias result when there is disordered impulse formation (automaticity), disordered impulse conduction, or a combined disorder of formation and conduction.

A useful classification of dysrhythmias, as defined by fetal monitoring, is based upon the anatomical site of variant impulse formation, conduction, or a combination of the two.

Sinus Node Variants

Chapter 20

Sinus Bradycardia

Sinus bradycardia is defined as a heart rate under 120 bpm with the fetal electrocardiogram showing normal P waves occurring in a regular fashion preceding each QRS complex.[18]

Sinus bradycardia is produced by parasympathetic stimulation and/or the withdrawal of sympathetic stimulation. Moderate bradycardia is a normal basal rate for many healthy fetuses.

Sinus bradycardia may also occur under a limited variety of physiologic and pathologic stimuli. The most common etiology in the fetus is a response to head compression. Less frequent causes are hypothermia, hypoxia, and a response to certain drugs. "Bradycardia" is not to be confused with a transient slowing of the heart rate, which in fetal monitoring terminology is "deceleration." Bradycardia in the fetus, by definition, requires the rhythm to persist for at least 10 minutes.

See Chapter 3 for detailed discussion of fetal bradycardia.

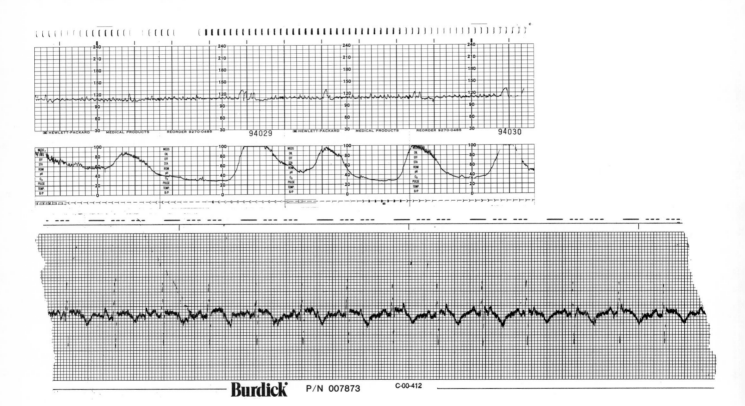

Burdick P/N 007873   C-00-412

CASE INTERPRETATION: Class I

Baseline Information: moderate bradycardia; diminished to average variability.

Periodic or Nonperiodic Changes: shallow early decelerations, small accelerations.

Uterine Activity: skewed and polysystolic contractions without a resting phase.

Significance: the most common cause of baseline bradycardia is head compression in late labor in a term or post-term fetus; it is more common in the primigravida. A normal outcome is anticipated.

Electrocardiographic Interpretation: fetal electrocardiogram. The paper speed is 25 mm/sec. The heart rate is 100 bpm. P waves, the PR interval, and QRS complexes appear to be normal and stable. This pattern is compatible with sinus bradycardia.

CASE OUTCOME: Twenty-two-year-old gravida 3, para 1011, delivered at 40½ weeks gestation vaginally from an occiput anterior position with local anesthesia an 8 pound, 5 ounce (3771 gram) male; Apgar score 8/9. The infant followed a normal newborn course. Umbilical cord gases: 7.24, PCO_2 61.1, PO_2 15.0 (arterial); 7.31, PCO_2 45.5 mmHg, PO_2 30.1 mmHg (venous).

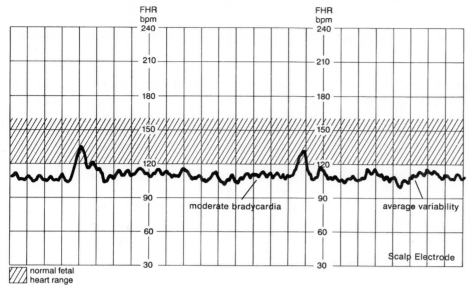

Pattern Characteristic:
Sinus Bradycardia

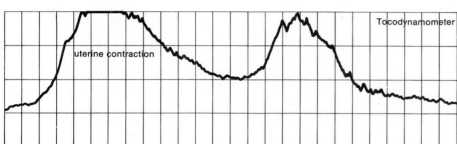

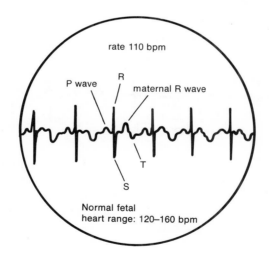

Sinus Tachycardia

Sinus tachycardia is defined as a heart rate of 160 bpm or greater, with the fetal electrocardiogram showing normal P waves occurring in a regular fashion preceding each QRS complex.[18]

Sinus tachycardia is produced by the withdrawal of parasympathetic stimulation of the sinus node and/or sympathetic stimulation.

Sinus tachycardia occurs under a wide variety of physiologic and pathologic stimuli. The most common etiologies in the fetus are responses to continuous fetal activity, maternal fever, or certain drugs. An occasional cause is a compensatory response to hypoxia.

Usually, sinus tachycardia does not exceed 200 bpm. However, occasionally this is exceeded, reaching levels where differentiation between supraventricular tachycardia and sinus tachycardia is difficult. Although the presence of beat-to-beat variability aids in differentiating sinus tachycardia from supraventricular tachycardia, variability is typically diminished at rapid heart rates because of the withdrawal of vagal tone.

See Chapter 4 for comprehensive discussion of fetal tachycardia.

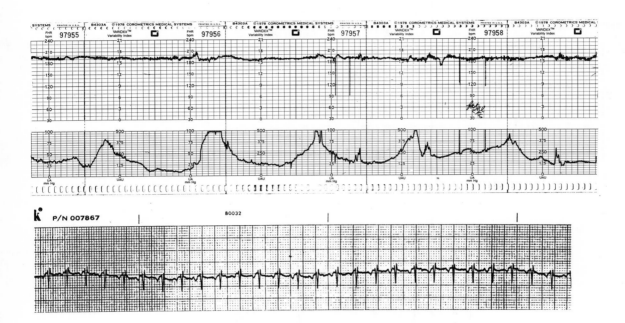

CASE INTERPRETATION: Class II

Baseline Information: moderate tachycardia. Diminished but present short- and long-term variability.

Periodic or Nonperiodic Changes: shallow accelerations and occasional small, V-shaped variable decelerations.

Uterine Activity: increased uterine activity. Peaked, skewed contractions without a resting phase.

Significance: this pattern indicates a stressed fetus with normal compensatory responses. The most common causes of fetal tachycardia are maternal fever and drug effects.

Electrocardiographic Interpretation: fetal electrocardiogram. The paper speed is 25 mm/sec. The heart rate

is 185 bpm. This is a regular, narrow QRS complex. There is a constant relationship between P waves and the QRS complex. This pattern is compatible with sinus tachycardia.

CASE OUTCOME: Fifteen-year-old primigravida at 40 weeks' gestation delivered by a low transverse cesarean section performed for cephalopelvic disproportion and chorioamnionitis, with general anesthesia from a vertex presentation, an 8 pound, 3½ ounce (3728 gram) female; Apgar score 4/6. Thick meconium was present. The infant followed an uncomplicated newborn course. The mother had a fever of 101°F intrapartum. A placental culture was positive for group B streptococcal infection.

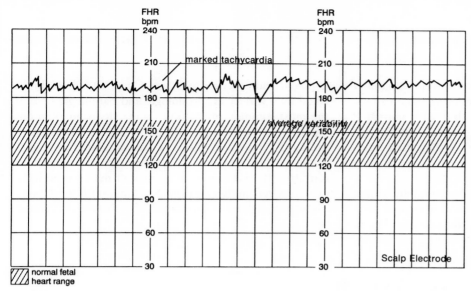

FHR
bpm
240

210

marked tachycardia

180

average variability

150

normal fetal
heart range

120

90

60

Scalp Electrode

30

FHR
bpm
240

210

180

150

120

90

60

30

Pattern Characteristic:
Sinus Tachycardia

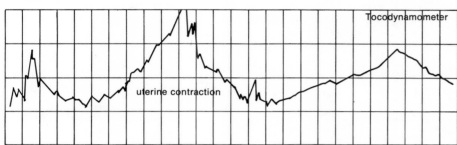

Tocodynamometer

uterine contraction

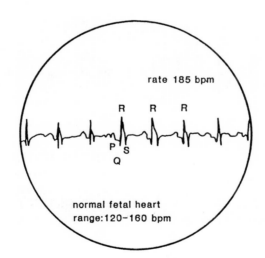

rate 185 bpm

R   R   R

P   S

Q

normal fetal heart
range: 120–160 bpm

Sinus Arrhythmia

*S*inus arrhythmia is defined as intermittent variability of the heart rate, with the fetal electrocardiogram showing variability of R to R intervals, but with normal P waves occurring in a regular fashion preceding each QRS complex.[18] (The term "arrhythmia" rather than "dysrhythmia" is retained in this instance because of long usage.)

Sinus arrhythmia is produced by varying parasympathetic stimulation. Sinus arrhythmia is a normal fetal phenomenon. It is enhanced by a limited number of physiologic and pathologic stimuli, including respiration,

hypoxia, and certain drugs (see Chap. 5).[22] It is diminished by a variety of physiologic and pathologic stimuli, the most common in the fetus being sleep, marked prematurity, certain drugs, and acidosis (see Chap. 6). In the adult, sinus arrhythmia is always related to respirations. In the fetus, however, who is breathing only intermittently, sinus arrhythmia may or may not be influenced by respiratory activity. See Chapter 6 for detailed discussion of fetal sinus arrhythmia (short-term variability).

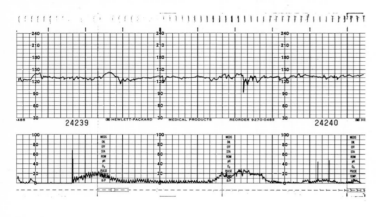

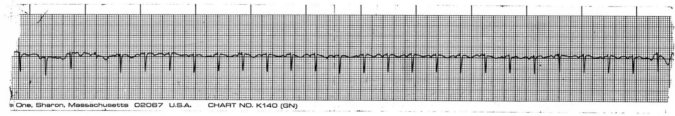

Original tracing enhanced for clarity.

CASE INTERPRETATION: Class I

Baseline Information: normal rate, variability, and stability.

Periodic or Nonperiodic Changes: small accelerations, early decelerations.

Uterine Activity: prolonged (three minute) contractions with a resting phase between.

Significance: a well fetus is anticipated; there is presumed to be head compression in active labor.

Electrocardiographic Interpretation: fetal electrocardiogram. The paper speed is 25 mm/sec. The heart rate varies between 130 to 136 bpm. P waves, PR intervals, and QRS complexes appear to be normal. This pattern is compatible with sinus arrhythmia.

CASE OUTCOME: Forty-one-year-old gravida 5, para 3013, at 42 weeks' gestation delivered vaginally, with epidural anesthesia, from a vertex presentation, a 7 pound, 11 ounce (3487 gram) male; Apgar score 9/9. The infant followed an uncomplicated newborn course.

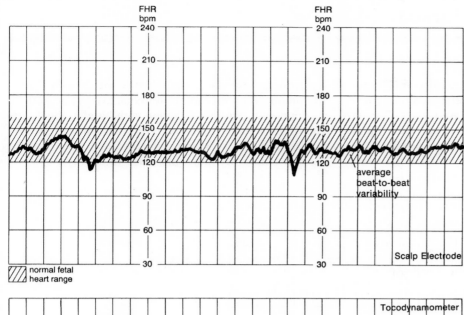

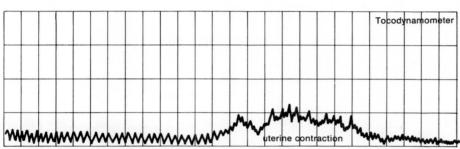

Pattern Characteristic:
Sinus Arrhythmia

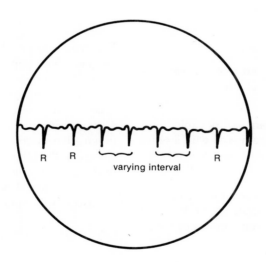

Sinus Arrhythmia—Marked

*T*he fetus demonstrates marked sinus arrhythmia in response to hypoxemia, producing in fetal monitoring terminology a saltatory pattern or increased variability. As illustrated here, the fetal heart rate may vary as much as 120 bpm within the space of five seconds, decreasing or increasing as much as 50 bpm from one beat to the next.

The most common etiology of the pattern is a parasympathetic response to fetal hypoxemia, which is usually produced by increased uterine activity. The pattern is commonly seen in association with baseline bradycardia, which is also a feature of excess parasympathetic system activity. See Chapter 5 for detailed discussion of marked sinus arrhythmia (increased variability).

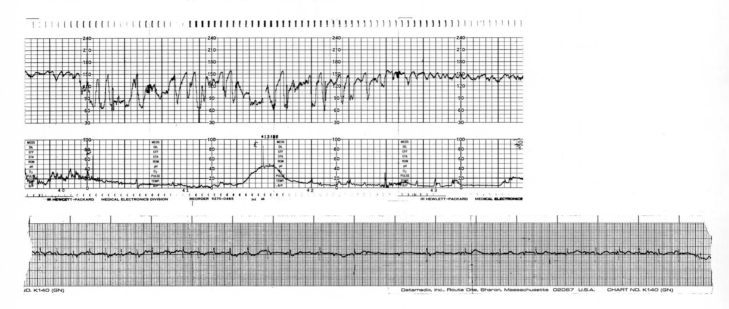

CASE INTERPRETATION: Class II

Baseline Information: normal heart rate and variability interrupted by eight minutes of saltatory pattern, which obscures the baseline.

Periodic or Nonperiodic Changes: possible prolonged or variable decelerations intermixed with a saltatory pattern with a nadir rate of 80 bpm. A single instance of a drop in the heart rate to 30 bpm or below.

Uterine Activity: there appears to be a prolonged contraction (five minutes duration) associated with the onset of a saltatory pattern, followed by contractions of a normal duration and configuration.

Significance: this pattern denotes a healthy stressed fetus who is demonstrating a compensatory response to hypoxemia that was induced by increased uterine activity. Management includes reduction of uterine activity, if feasible, and the administration of oxygen. Despite repeated rapid decreases in the heart rate, the sinus node appears to remain dominant without an escape rhythm.

Electrocardiographic Interpretation: fetal electrocardiogram. The paper speed is 25 mm/sec (although the fetal monitor paper speed is 3 cm/min, a computer prints the electrocardiogram to simulate a 25 mm/sec paper speed). The heart rate is variable 34-165 bpm. There is a progressive prolongation of R-R time, followed by a progressive shortening of R-R time, without an apparent change in the QRS complex or the relation of the P wave to the QRS complex. Maternal QRS complexes are present, the maternal heart rate is 75 bpm. This pattern is consistent with sinus arrhythmia.

CASE OUTCOME: Twenty-two-year-old primigravida at 41 weeks' gestation delivered by low transverse cesarean section performed for recurrent marked fetal stress in a patient with nonprogressive labor, a 7 pound, 14 ounce (3572 gram) male; Apgar score 8/9. The fetus was in a vertex presentation. The infant followed an uncomplicated newborn course.

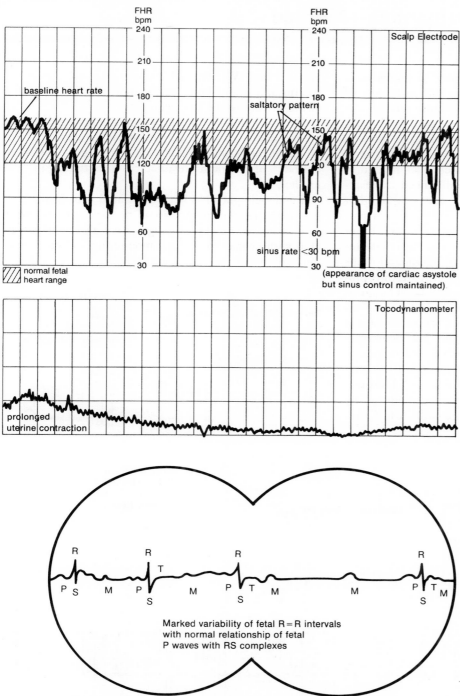

Pattern Characteristic:
Marked Sinus Arrhythmia

P = Fetal P wave; R = Fetal R wave; S = Fetal S wave; T = Fetal T wave; M = Maternal R wave

Respiratory Sinus Arrhythmia—Marked

*I*n the adult, sinus arrhythmia is related to respirations. In the fetus, who breathes only intermittently, not all sinus arrhythmia (variability) is respiratory-related. Although an increase in variability occurs with fetal respiration, most fetal respiratory activity does not produce other characteristic changes on the fetal monitor heart trace. However, exceptions have been documented.[3,4] Sinus arrhythmia, when markedly influenced by respiration, may be recognized on a fetal, newborn, or adult beat-to-beat trace by a pattern characterized by a progressively increasing heart rate followed by an abrupt drop, recurring over a narrow range. The heart rate increases in a stepwise fashion with inspiration and drops to a slower rate with expiration.[5,6,21] This pattern is produced by respiration-stimulated vagotonia. The presence of respiratory sinus arrhythmia is an indicator of autonomic nervous system integrity.[2] Correlation of the pattern with fetal respiratory motions has been performed using real time ultrasonography. The degree of respiratory arrhythmia has been demonstrated to correlate with the depth of inspiratory movements.[6] The electronic monitoring pattern is similar to that produced by Wenckebach's phenomenon (see page 415). It is distinguished from Wenckebach's phenomenon because the electrocardiogram shows no variation in the relationship of the P wave to the QRS complex.

Fetal respiratory sinus arrhythmia is believed to be a related phenomenon to certain sinusoidal patterns.[1] Fetal respiratory arrhythmia has been reported to follow an episode of marked respiratory arrhythmia in the mother.[14]

Fetal tachypnea has been associated with fetal tachycardia and regular irregularity of the baseline variability (see insert A).[12] Fetal hiccoughs have also been associated with characteristic fetal monitoring and electrocardiographic patterns (see insert B).[13,17]

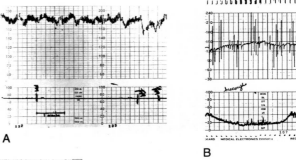

A   B

Insert above reprinted with permission from Manning FA, Heaman M, Boyce D, Carter LJ: Intrauterine Fetal Tachypnea. *Obstet Gynceol* 58:399, 1981.

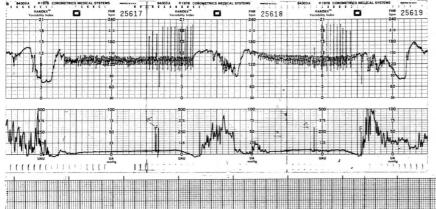

CASE INTERPRETATION: Class II

Baseline Information: a normal heart rate, unusual marked, rhythmic variability. There is also an arrhythmia characterized by a mixed pattern of upward vertical spikes and dropped beats (downward spikes). This pattern disappears with accelerations and decelerations.

Periodic or Nonperiodic Changes: accelerations are present; there are mild to moderate classic variable decelerations with contractions.

Uterine Activity: not clearly recorded because of maternal straining. Compatible with active labor.

Significance: the arrhythmia has the appearance of supraventricular premature depolarizations. These are usually benign and disappear in labor or in the newborn course. This variability pattern has a regularity that may be influenced by fetal respiratory activity. A real time ultrasonographic study was not performed simultaneously in this case.

Electrocardiographic Interpretation: fetal electrocardiogram. The paper speed is 25 mm/sec. There are normal narrow QRS complexes with a constant relationship between P waves or QRS complexes. There is a very slight variation in the R-R rate. This is characterized by a progressive shortening of the R-R time, followed by a lengthening of the R-R interval, which occurs cyclically. This pattern is compatible with sinus arrhythmia, which is similar to adult respiratory-related sinus arrhythmia.

CASE OUTCOME: Nineteen-year-old primigravida at 38 weeks' gestation delivered vaginally from a vertex presentation, with local anesthesia, a 5 pound, 10 ounce (2551 gram) male; Apgar score 9/9. The infant followed a normal newborn course and had a normal newborn electrocardiogram. There was a circumvallate placenta.

Pattern Characteristic:
Marked Respiratory Arrhythmia

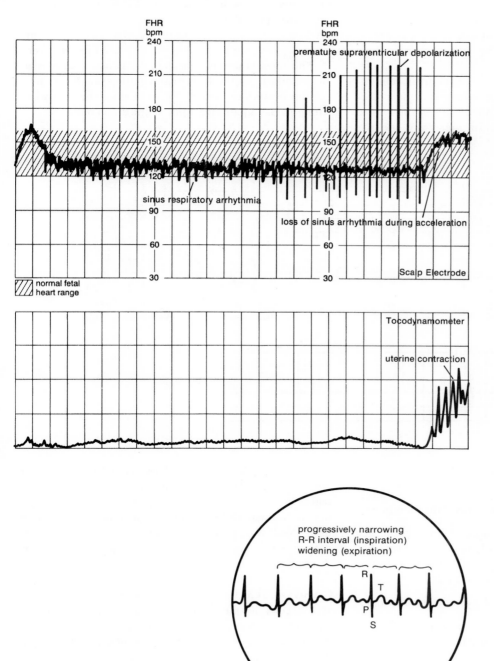

Sinus Pause with Junctional Escape

*U*nder normal circumstances, the sinoatrial node possesses the most rapid rate of spontaneous diastolic depolarization or "automaticity." Lower centers have a slower rate of automaticity and are prevented from controlling heart rate unless the sinus node rate is suppressed below the intrinsic rate of the lower center.[19]

Under strong parasympathetic influence, the sinus node depolarization may be suppressed and the atrioventricular junction (AV node) escapes at a slower intrinsic rate.[16]

The slower escape rate, because of its intrinsic regularity, presents a fetal monitoring appearance of loss of variability. This type of loss of variability is thus quite different in mechanism and significance from the flat line or "silent" patterns of the baseline heart rate. In the latter situation, pacing is still originating from the sinus node and the pattern may or may not reflect acidosis, whereas an escape pattern represents a physiologic response of a healthy fetus. This compensatory mechanism, may not be life sustaining if it is persistent over a protracted period of time. Management is directed at the primary etiology in order to insure that episodes of sinus node suppression are infrequent and brief in duration.

The most common causes of sinus node suppression are umbilical cord or fetal head compression (as with the occiput posterior position).[8,11] Both are associated with a strong parasympathetic input at the sinus node.

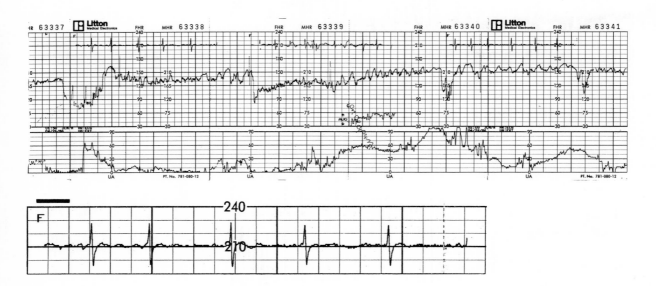

CASE INTERPRETATION: Class II

Baseline Information: normal heart rate and variability. Rebound tachycardia after prolonged decelerations.

Periodic or Nonperiodic Changes: nonperiodic accelerations are present. Classic mild to moderate variable decelerations. Shallow prolonged deceleration (three minutes duration) with rebound tachycardia.

Uterine Activity: prolonged polysystolic contractions.

Significance: this pattern denotes a healthy stressed fetus employing normal compensatory responses.

Electrocardographic Interpretation: fetal electrocardiogram. The paper speed is 25 mm/sec (computer corrected). There is a sinus bradycardia of 103 bpm. There are normal P waves. QRS complexes are followed by a pause lasting approximately 0.8 seconds, with resumption of normal QRS complexes at a slower rate of 84 bpm. No P waves are visible. This pattern is compatible with a sinus pause followed by a junctional escape rhythm.

CASE OUTCOME: Twenty-five-year-old primigravida at 40 weeks' gestation delivered vaginally, with epidural anesthesia, a 6 pound, 13½ ounce male; Apgar score 9/9. The fetus was in a vertex presentation. The infant followed an uncomplicated newborn course.

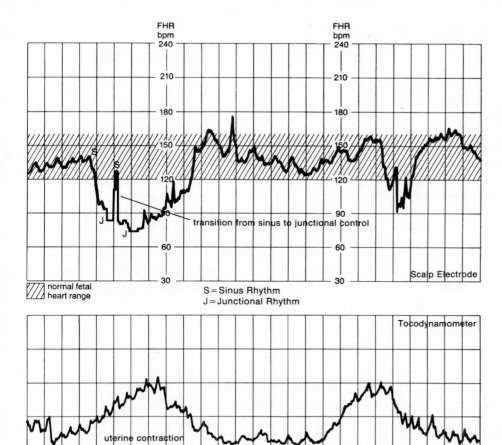

Pattern Characteristic:
Sinus Pause with Junctional
Escape

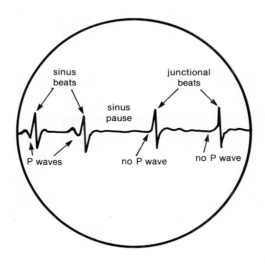

Sinus Arrest with Junctional Escape

*S*inus arrest is a unique form of sinus pause (see page 464), which is distinguished only by duration. The electrocardiogram displays cessation of P waves and QRS complexes until sinus node recovery or escape complexes ensue. The fetal monitor heart trace depicts a vertical spike to the lowest extreme of the graph, with varying duration until an upward deflection denotes escape or recovery. This is easily distinguished from a single dropped beat because the latter does not cause the fetal heart trace to fall below one-half the normal cardiac cycle. The phenomenon of sinus arrest, documented in the healthy fetus, has also been termed "fetal cardiac asystole" or "fetal cardiac arrest."[10,23] (See pages 274 and 276.) These terms would be less confusing if they were accompanied by the adjective "transient" or if they were reserved for those circumstances in which there is a failure of an escape rhythm following the sinus pause.

Because of the brief nature of sinus arrest as it is depicted here, the fetus is not considered in jeopardy.

Prolonged and recurring sinus arrest, however, may suggest excessive vagal tone, which may indicate a risk of intrauterine death.[9,10,23] Atropine may obliterate the pattern but may also modify protective vagal reflexes.[7] Its use is thus a matter of clinical controversy.

Sinoatrial block (SA block) is a form of sinus suppression that may be differentiated from sinus pause or sinus arrest by the fact that in SA block the duration of the pause is a multiple of the usual P-P cycle length.

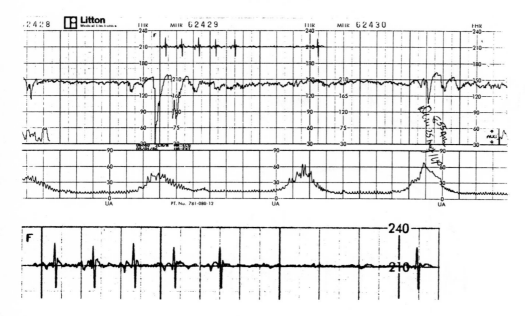

CASE INTERPRETATION: Class II

Baseline Information: normal rate, average variability. There is a slight downward trend in the baseline rate.

Periodic or Nonperiodic Changes: mild biphasic and classic variable decelerations. There is a single instance where the heart rate drops from 133 to less than 30 bpm from one beat to the next with rapid recovery to a normal basal rate.

Uterine Activity: a normal configuration, the frequency of contractions is compatible with active labor.

Significance: arrest of sinus node or asystole. A healthy fetus is predicted by the remainder of the tracing.

Electrocardiographic Interpretation: fetal electrocardiogram. The paper speed is 25 mm/sec (computer corrected). The heart rate is 150 bpm. There is a regular, narrow QRS complex. There is a sinus rhythm. Following the fifth beat displayed, there is sinus arrest lasting approximately two seconds, followed by a junctional escape that is characterized by the absence of a P wave and a narrow QRS.

CASE OUTCOME: Nineteen-year-old primigravida at 38 weeks' gestation delivered vaginally, with pudendal and local anesthesia, a 6 pound, ½ ounce (2736 gram) female; Apgar score 9/9. The fetus was in a vertex presentation. The infant followed an uncomplicated newborn course.

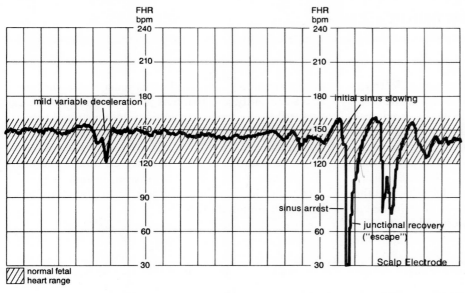

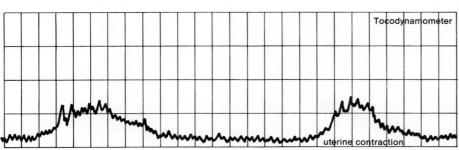

Pattern Characteristic:
Sinus Arrest with Junctional Escape

Wandering Atrial Pacemaker

*W*andering atrial pacemaker is characterized electrocardiographically by a variation in the size and shape of the P wave and a changing PR interval.[15] If the atrial pacemaker enters the atrioventricular junction, the P wave will not be visible. This may occur in an intermittent fashion, so that the pacemaker phasically is the sinus node or the atrioventricular junction. Characteristically, this occurs from a baseline of sinus bradycardia, whether it is sustained (baseline bradycardia) or brief (deceleration). The sinus node may be suppressed by a burst of parasympathetic activity. If vagotonia slows the sinus rate sufficiently, the inherent junctional rate will be expressed. In the fetus, vagotonia is demonstrated by variable decelerations such as are produced by umbilical cord impingement.[7] Thus, it is not surprising that a wandering atrial pacemaker may be observed during the nadir of variable decelerations. However, wandering atrial pacemaker has also been detected as a "baseline" fetal heart rate abnormality.[20]

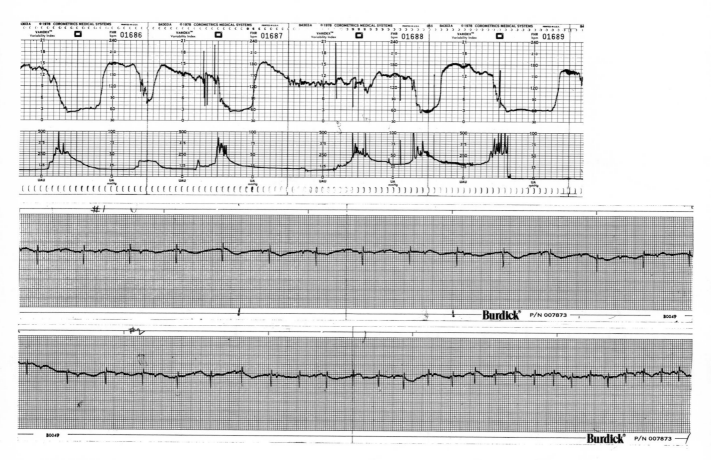

CASE INTERPRETATION: Class IV

Baseline Information: normal heart rate, average variability. There is a loss of baseline stability.

Periodic or Nonperiodic Changes: mild to severe variable decelerations with atypia, including prolonged secondary accelerations, loss of variability in the decelerations, and loss of primary accelerations. Also seen are sloping recovery limbs. One deceleration includes an S-shape but not an S-sign.

Uterine Activity: areas of elevated resting tone. Skewed contractions. Maternal straining.

Significance: there is an increased risk of a low Apgar score and acidosis, yet baseline variability is preserved at present when there is an adequate resting phase between contractions. Decisions regarding delivery timing and method of delivery are influenced by the gestation, the estimated time to delivery, and the subsequent response to measures taken to improve fetal oxygenation.

Electrocardiographic Interpretation: fetal electrocardiogram. The paper speed is 25 mm/sec. Initially, there is a junctional rate of 62 bpm, with small P waves and a PR interval of 0.08 seconds preceding the QRS complex. Toward the end of the first strip no P waves are visible.

This pattern persists in the initial portion of the second strip, followed by a gradual increase of the heart rate to 155 bpm, with the QRS preceded by a PR interval of 0.12 seconds. This pattern is consistent with a wandering atrial pacemaker.

CASE OUTCOME: Thirty-year-old primigravida at 42 weeks' gestation delivered by low transverse cesarean section performed for a fetal heart rate pattern of severe variable decelerations with progressive atypia, when delivery was not imminent, a 7 pound, 11 ounce (3487 gram) female; Apgar score 2/6. The fetus was in a vertex presentation. There was a tight nuchal cord. The newborn course was complicated by transient tachypnea.

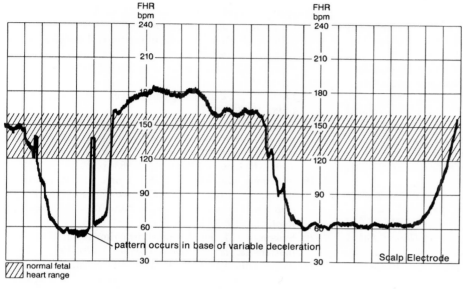

Pattern Characteristic:
Wandering Atrial Pacemaker

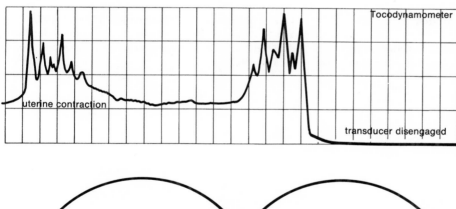

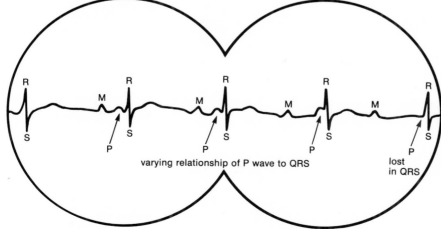

References

1. Berestha JS, Johnson TRB, Hrushosky WJ: Sinusoidal fetal heart rate pattern during breathing is related to the respiratory sinus arrhythmia: A case report. *Am J Obstet Gynecol* 160:690, 1989.

2. Divon MY, Winkler H, Yeh S-Y, et al: Diminished respiratory sinus arrhythmia in asphyxiated term infants. *Am J Obstet Gynecol* 155:1263, 1986.

3. Divon MY, Yeh S, Zimmer EZ, et al: Respiratory sinus arrhythmia in the human fetus. *Am J Obstet Gynecol* 151:425, 1985.

4. Divon MY, Zimmer EZ, Platt LD, et al: Human fetal breathing: Associated changes in heart rate and beat-to-beat variability. *Am J Obstet Gynecol* 151:403, 1985.

5. Donchin Y, Caton D, Porges SW: Spectral analysis of fetal heart rate in sheep: The occurrence of respiratory sinus arrhythmia. *Am J Obstet Gynecol* 148:1130, 1984.

6. Fouron J, Korcaz Y, Leduc B: Cardiovascular changes associated with fetal breathing. *Am J Obstet Gynecol* 123:868, 1975.

7. Gleicher N, Elkayam U: Intrauterine dysrhythmias, in: *Cardiac Problems in Pregnancy*. New York: Alan R. Liss, 1982.

8. Hon EH: *The Human Fetal Circulation in Normal Labor*. New York, Grune and Stratton, 1966.

9. Hon EH: *An Introduction to Fetal Heart Rate Monitoring*. Los Angeles, University of Southern California School of Medicine, 1973, p. 36.

10. Kates RB, Schifrin BS: Fetal cardiac asystole during labor. *Obstet Gynecol* 67:549, 1986.

11. Lipman BS, Dunn M, Massie E: Cardiac arrhythmias, in: *Clinical Electrocardiography*, 7th ed. New York, Yearbook Medical Publishers, 1984, p. 376.

12. Manning FA, Heaman M, Boyce D, et al: Intrauterine fetal tachypnea. *Obstet Gynecol* 58:398, 1981.

13. Miller FC, Gonzales F, Mueller E, et al: Fetal hiccups: An associated fetal heart rate pattern. *Obstet Gynecol* 62:253, 1983.

14. Neilsen JS, Moestrup JK: Foetal electrocardiographic studies of cardiac arrhythmias and the heart rate. *Acta Obstet Gynec Scand* 47:247, 1968.

15. Scheidt S: Basic electrocardiography: Leads, axes, arrhythmias. *Clinical Symposia* 35:2, 1983.

16. Shenker L: Fetal cardiac arrhythmias. *Obstet Gynecol Survey* 34:561, 1979.

17. Shenker L: Fetal hiccups during labor. *P-N*, March/April, p. 96, 1982.

18. Silverman ME, Myerburg RJ, Hurst JW: Variations in sinus node rhythms and atrial arrhythmias, in: *Electrocardiography. Basic Concepts and Clinical Appreciation*. New York, McGraw-Hill Book Co., 1983, p. 257.

19. Silverman ME, Myerburg RJ, Hurst JW: AV junctional rhythm disturbances, in: *Electrocardiography. Basic Concepts and Clinical Appreciation*. New York: McGraw-Hill Book Co., 1983, p. 273.

20. Symonds EM: Fetal cardiac arrhythmias and fetal acid-base status. *Aust NZJ Obstet Gynecol* 12:170, 1972.

21. Timor-Tritsch I, Zador I, Hertz RH, et al: Human fetal respiratory arrhythmia. *Am J Obstet Gynecol* 127:662, 1977.

22. Wheeler T, Murrills A: Patterns of fetal heart rate during normal pregnancy. *Br J Obstet Gynecol* 127:662, 1977.

23. Yeh S, Zanini B, Petrie RH, et al: Intrapartum fetal cardiac arrest. A preliminary observation. *Obstet Gynecol* 50:571, 1977.

Supraventricular Dysrhythmias

Chapter 21

Premature Supraventricular Depolarizations

*S*upraventricular premature depolarizations are characterized by the early discharge of an atrial focus followed by an atrioventricular nodal passage and ventricular depolarization. Electrocardiographically, a premature P wave is seen that may vary slightly from the sinus P wave and that is followed by a narrow normal appearing QRS complex (in the absence of a disturbance of intraventricular conduction).

Premature supraventricular depolarizations are frequently followed by a less than fully (incomplete) compensatory pause. The completeness of the compensatory pause may be determined by measuring the interval between the two normal beats flanking the premature beat.[53] If this distance is equal to or greater than the distance between two QRS complexes flanking a normal beat, the pause is termed "fully compensatory."

The fetal monitor heart rate trace shows vertical spikes, often creating an illusion of three parallel horizontal lines. The upper line, which is usually greater than 180 bpm, is produced by the premature beat. The lower line is produced by the incomplete compensatory pause and is usually only a short distance below the middle line, which is produced by the normal cardiac cycles. The middle line may continue to be observed for variability (although not truly beat-to-beat) and accelerations or decelerations.[13]

Premature supraventricular depolarizations occur commonly in the fetus in greater frequency than premature ventricular depolarizations and usually do not suggest underlying heart disease.[2,39,51,69,70,74,84] Enhanced atrial automaticity may be due to sympathomimetic stimuli such as maternal caffeine ingestion or to enhanced endogenous catecholamines (as might occur with alcohol or nicotine exposure).[17,18] Intrapartum arrhythmias of this nature typically disappear during labor, particularly during second stage variable decelerations at birth.[39] Therefore in utero therapy is seldom warranted.[41,81]

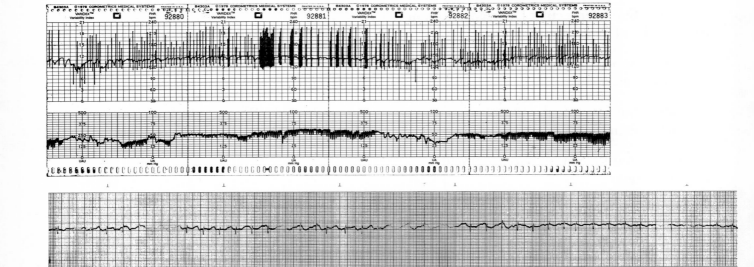

CASE INTERPRETATION: Class I

Baseline Information: normal rate and variability. Regular vertical spikes are compatible with premature beats, pauses, and occasional dropped beats.

Periodic or Nonperiodic Changes: small accelerations are present.

Uterine Activity: the uterine trace is masked by maternal respiratory activity.

Significance: the appearance of premature beats is that of a supraventricular etiology (long vertical spikes above the baseline, short spikes below the baseline), with occasional trigeminy and nonconducted beats. A healthy fetus is anticipated.

Electrocardiographic Interpretation: fetal electrocardiogram. The paper speed is 25 mm/sec. There is a normal sinus rhythm at 148 bpm. There are normal P, PR, and QRS relationships. There are premature atrial depolarizations with no discernible P waves, followed by a normal narrow QRS complex. The compensatory pause is less than fully compensatory. This pattern is compatible with premature supraventricular depolarizations, which are probably junctional in origin.

CASE OUTCOME: Twenty-seven-year-old gravida 4, para 3003, at 37 weeks' gestation delivered vaginally, with pudendal anesthesia, a 7 pound, 3 ounce (3260 gram) male; Apgar score 3/8. Thick meconium was present. Scalp pHs were 7.35 and 7.31. Endotracheal suc-

tioning contributed to the low one-minute Apgar score. Although the newborn course was complicated by transient tachypnea, the infant was dismissed on the fourth day of life.

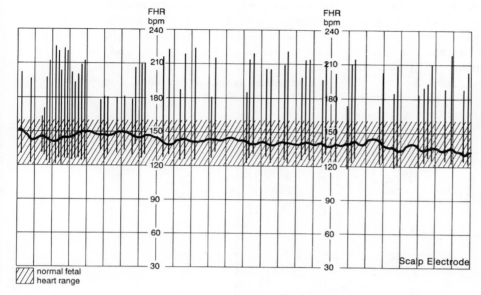

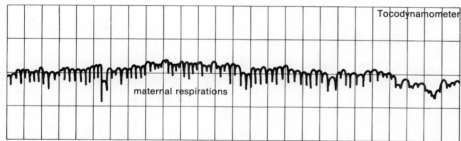

Pattern Characteristic:
Premature Supraventricular
Depolarizations

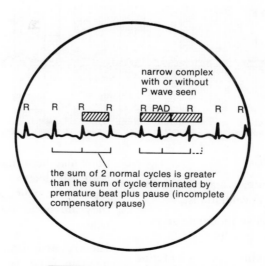

Premature Supraventricular Depolarizations in Bigeminal and Trigeminal Pattern

*P*remature atrial depolarizations occurring at fixed intervals are termed "atrial bigeminy" if every other beat is a premature atrial depolarization and "atrial trigeminy" if every third beat is a premature atrial depolarization.

The electrocardiograph appearance of premature atrial depolarizations is described on page 473.

The fetal monitor trace with bigeminy shows uninterrupted parallel vertical lines (baseline obscured). The fe-

tal monitor trace with trigeminy typically displays vertical spikes with long upward components and short downward components, in relationship to a baseline that may be observed for variability and rate identification.[13,66,85]

The pattern is usually transient, disappearing before delivery or soon after birth.

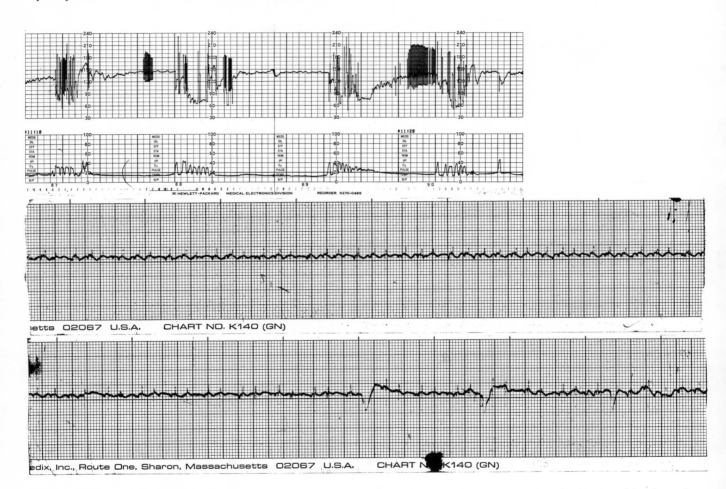

CASE INTERPRETATION: Class IV

Baseline Information: normal rate, average variability. Arrhythmia during recovery from decelerations.

Periodic or Nonperiodic Changes: moderate atypical decelerations with a slow return to baseline.

Uterine Activity: maternal straining replaces a uterine waveform.

Significance: the dysrhythmia pattern is that of bigeminy and trigeminy. Vertical excursions during decelera-

tions may be artifact or arrhythmia or a combination of both. An electrocardiogram may clarify the source of ectopic beats, which are probably supraventricular because they are occurring in a mixed pattern with dropped beats.

Electrocardiographic Interpretation: fetal electrocardiogram. The paper speed is 12.5 mm/sec. The heart rate is approximately 140 bpm. Premature atrial beats are seen occurring every other beat (bigeminy) and every third beat (trigeminy). Occasionally, there are nonconducted premature atrial depolarizations. These are consistent with premature atrial depolarizations in bigeminy and trigeminy, with occasional nonconducted premature atrial depolarizations.

CASE OUTCOME: Twenty-one-year-old primigravida at 39 weeks' gestation delivered vaginally, with pudendal anesthesia, a 9 pound, 1 ounce (4111 gram) male; Apgar score 8/8. The newborn course was uncomplicated. Premature supraventricular depolarizations with aberrant conduction persisted in the newborn period for 24 hours in a trigeminal pattern, which was both conducted and nonconducted. Rare premature ventricular depolarizations also occurred and disappeared within 48 hours of life.

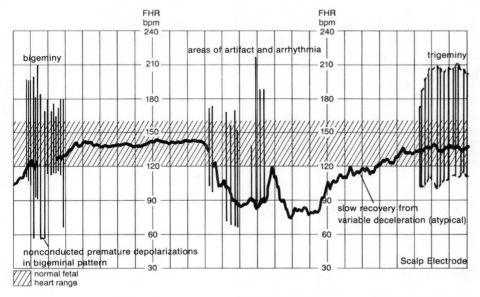

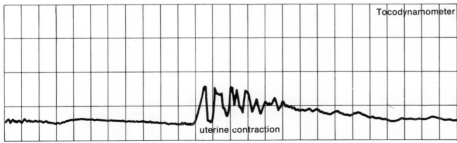

Pattern Characteristic:
Premature Supraventricular Depolarizations–Bigeminal and Trigeminal Pattern

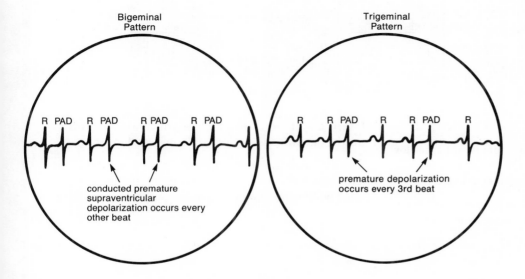

Premature Supraventricular Depolarizations in Bigeminal Pattern

Supraventricular premature depolarizations in a bigeminal pattern are produced by premature supraventricular beats that occur every other beat. It is one of the most frequently occurring intrapartum fetal dysrhythmias.[86]

The precipitating factors are similar to those for isolated supraventricular premature beats (see page 472).

The fetal monitor tracing gives the appearance of two horizontal parallel lines, the upper line representing the rate between normal and premature beats and the lower line produced by the compensatory pause.

A frequent fetal monitoring pattern is atrial bigeminy in which the occurrence of the premature beat is just before the timing of the expected normal sinus beat, producing a pattern of closely spaced horizontal lines. The electrocardiographic pattern has been termed "late cycle" premature beats. This pattern is most commonly seen in situations of slight slowing of the baseline rate or in shallow variable decelerations.

Although a similarly appearing pattern has been noted preceding fetal death and, as in the adult, the pattern may precede or herald more advanced atrial dysrhythmia, fetal atrial bigeminy is almost always benign and does not warrant in utero therapy.[10,17]

This pattern has erroneously been termed "atrial parasystole" because of the presumed presence of two independent pacemakers, both competing for ventricular response, with one presumed to be the sinus node.[21] Although two dominant pacemakers are present, coupling intervals are not variable, placing this pattern more appropriately in atrial bigeminy. The shorter the distance between the two rates, the closer the two pacemakers are in the conduction system.

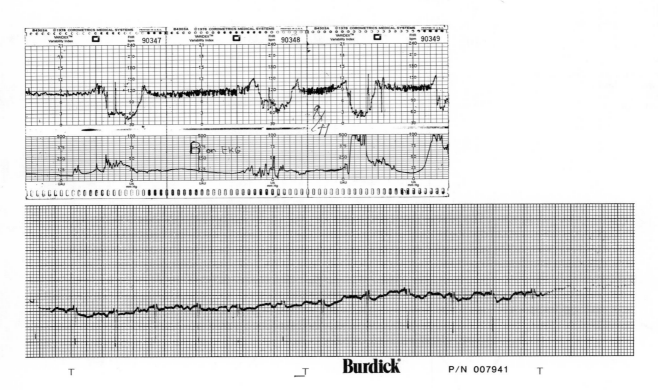

Burdick   P/N 007941

CASE INTERPRETATION: Class II

Baseline Information: moderate bradycardia to low normal rate, average variability in areas, obscured by short vertical spikes in areas between decelerations.

Periodic and Nonperiodic Changes: moderate and severe variable decelerations with classical features.

Uterine Activity: irregular pattern consistent with active labor, with areas of probable maternal straining.

Significance: this is the appearance of a bigeminal pattern, which is often seen in a healthy fetus when partial sinus node suppression occurs.

Electrocardiographic Interpretation: fetal electrocardiogram. The paper speed is 25 mm/sec. The heart rate is 108 bpm. There are normal P waves, PR intervals, and QRS complexes. There are subtle late cycle premature atrial depolarizations occurring in a bigeminal pattern.

CASE OUTCOME: Thirty-year-old gravida 5, para 4004, at 40 weeks' gestation delivered vaginally, with pudendal anesthesia, a 7 pound, 7 ounce (3374 gram) male; Apgar score 9/9. No arrhythmia was noted during the normal newborn course.

Pattern Characteristic:
Atrial Bigeminy

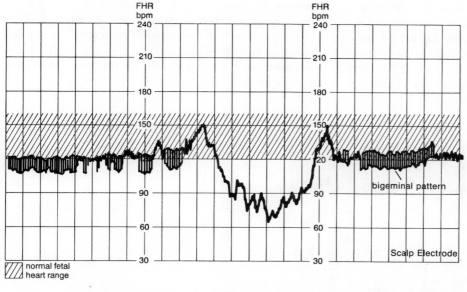

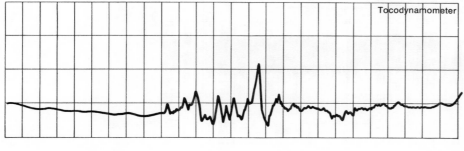

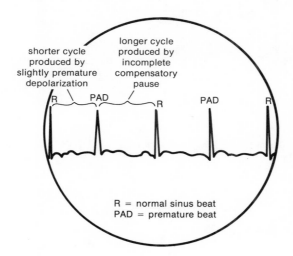

R = normal sinus beat
PAD = premature beat

Premature Supraventricular Depolarizations in Bigeminal Pattern: Marked

*W*hen atrial premature beats are very early, yet conducted, the portion of the fetal monitoring heart rate tracing representing the premature beat may exceed 200 bpm.[7] Vertical parallel lines whose maximum upward excursions represent the premature beat and whose maximum downward excursions represent the compensatory pause are not interrupted by a baseline rate. The use of M-mode echocardiography and Doppler techniques assist the assessment of the dysrhythmia.[18,19,49,50,55,72]

Interpretation of the fetal condition may require other methods of fetal assessment such as pH studies or a study of the entire tracing for segments revealing baseline data. Premature supraventricular depolarizations usually produce no serious consequences and usually disappear in late labor, particularly during contractions or soon after birth. (See page 476 for further discussion of atrial bigeminy.)

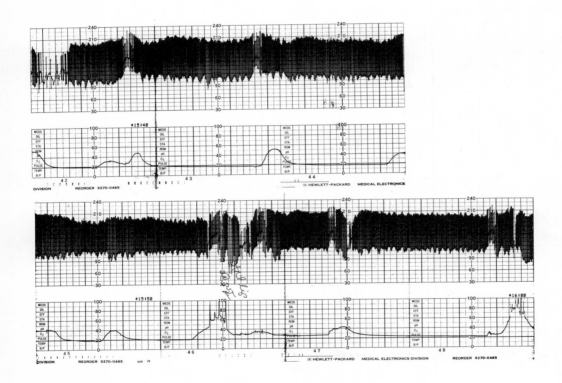

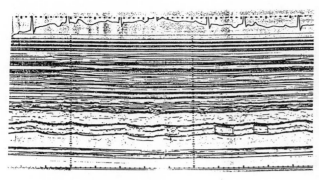

Original tracing enhanced for clarity.

Fetal Echocardiogram and Electrocardiogram

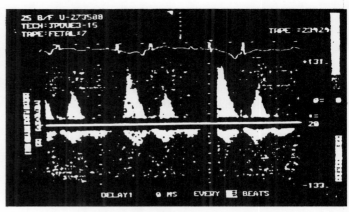

Fetal Doppler and Electrocardiogram

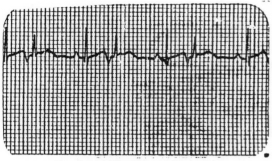

Newborn Electrocardiogram

CASE INTERPRETATION: Class I

Baseline Information: the two heart rates displayed are connected by vertical parallel lines. The upper rate is in the marked fetal tachycardic range, the lower in the moderate bradycardic range. Occasional glimpses of a widely varying baseline rate are seen with normal variability.

Periodic or Nonperiodic Changes: none are distinguishable.

Uterine Activity: infrequent, mild contractions of a varying configuration, as measured by internal monitoring. There is an elevated resting tone.

Significance: there is the appearance of a bigeminal pattern; an electrocardiogram is needed for diagnosis of a source of the ectopic beats. A probable healthy fetus is predicted, based on occasional glimpses of the baseline.

Electrocardiographic Interpretation: a scalp electrode-derived fetal electrocardiogram was done at the time of the echocardiogram. The paper speed is 100 mm/sec. The heart rate is approximately 160 bpm; premature atrial depolarizations are seen in a bigeminal pattern.

The premature complexes are narrow and closely resemble the preceding sinus beat. The premature depolarizations are preceded by ectopic P waves with an abbreviated PR interval, displaying similar features to those seen in the subsequent newborn electrocardiogram.

Newborn electrocardiogram: the paper speed is 25 mm/sec, the heart rate is 155 bpm, the basic rhythm is sinus. There are premature supraventricular depolarizations occurring in a bigeminal pattern ("atrial bigeminy").

Echocardiographic Interpretation: fetal echocardiogram of the aorta and left atrium was done, accompanied by a simultaneous electrocardiogram. The electrocardiogram shows premature depolarizations in a bigeminal pattern (see the preceding fetal electrocardiographic interpretation). The echocardiogram shows the opening of the aortic valve in a bigeminal pattern corresponding with the QRS complex of the sinus and the premature atrial depolarizations. Atrial wall motion is seen corresponding with the P waves of the sinus beat and of the premature atrial beat. Correlation of the electrocardiogram with the echocardiogram confirms premature atrial depolarization in a bigeminal pattern.

A Doppler study performed in the descending aorta with a simultaneous electrocardiogram shows paired Doppler signals corresponding to the sinus beat and to the premature atrial depolarization. The amplitude of the Doppler signal due to the premature atrial depolarization is significantly less than that of the flow following the sinus depolarization, reflecting the abbreviated diastolic filling period preceding the premature atrial depolarization.

CASE OUTCOME: Twenty-five-year-old gravida 4, para 2012, at 40 weeks' gestation delivered vaginally, with local anesthesia, a 6 pound, 4½ ounce (2850 gram) female; Apgar score 8/9. Two scalp pHs were both 7.37.

An intrapartum echocardiogram was performed with the printing of a scalp electrode-derived signal on the M-mode tracing. The newborn electrocardiogram confirmed atrial bigeminy. The frequency of premature supraventricular depolarizations progressively diminished during the nursery course. The newborn was dismissed at two days of life.

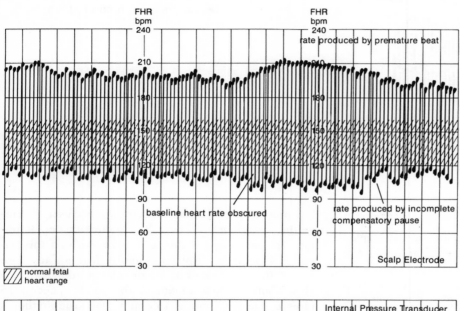

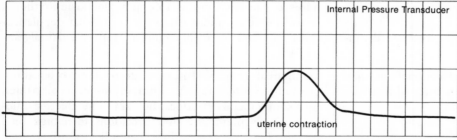

Pattern Characteristic:
Marked Atrial Bigeminy

Fetal Electrocardiogram

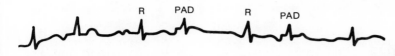

Pattern Characteristic:
Marked Atrial Bigeminy

Fetal Echocardiogram

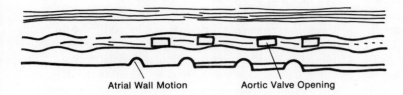

Atrial Wall Motion   Aortic Valve Opening

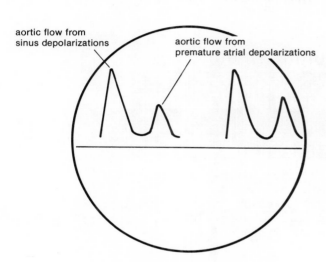

aortic flow from
sinus depolarizations

aortic flow from
premature atrial depolarizations

Fetal Doppler Study
of Descending Aorta

Nonconducted Premature Supraventricular Depolarizations

*N*onconducted premature supraventricular depolarizations occur with the discharge of an atrial focus that is sufficiently premature to be unable to traverse through the atrioventricular junctional tissue that was rendered refractory by the prior sinus beat.

The premature depolarization, because it partially penetrates the atrioventricular junction, is followed by a pause until the atrioventricular junction recovers sufficiently to admit the next sinus node discharge. Electrocardiographically, this is characterized by an early P wave, often occurring in the apex or descending limb of the previous T wave, followed by a pause that is termi-

nated by the next sinus beat. When the dysrhythmia occurs in quadrigeminy (as in the case illustrated here), the fetal monitoring pattern appears as two horizontal parallel lines that are connected by parallel vertical spikes. The upper line represents the normal cardiac cycles; the lower line represents the pause produced by the dropped beat. This pattern is usually seen to be mixed with conducted premature supraventricular depolarizations.

Fetal echocardiography may be useful in the diagnosis when atrial activity is documented without an accompanying ventricular response.[16]

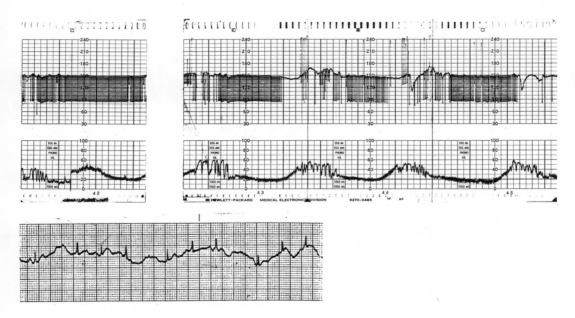

CASE INTERPRETATION: Class I

Baseline Information: there are two heart rates: one in a normal fetal heart range and one in a marked bradycardic range, connected by vertical parallel lines denoting arrhythmia. Variability appears to be diminished.

Periodic or Nonperiodic Changes: accelerations are accompanied by the disappearance of the vertical spikes.

Uterine Activity: prolonged contractions of normal frequency are accompanied by maternal straining or excessive hyperventilation. There are exaggerated respiratory movements between contractions.

Significance: this is the appearance of nonconducted premature atrial depolarizations that are usually seen in a mixed pattern with conducted premature supraventric-

ular depolarizations. These are usually benign and disappear in late labor or during the newborn period.

Electrocardiographic Interpretation: fetal electrocardiogram. The paper speed is 25 mm/sec. The heart rate is 140 bpm. The basic rhythm is sinus. Following every third beat a P wave is seen on the T wave of the preceding normal beat. This is followed by an incomplete compensatory pause that is terminated by a sinus beat. This pattern is consistent with nonconducted premature atrial depolarizations in a quadrigeminal pattern.

CASE OUTCOME: Fourteen-year-old primigravida delivered vaginally, with local and pudendal anesthesia, a 7 pound, 10 ounce (3459 gram) male; Apgar score 9/9. The fetus was in an occiput anterior position. The infant followed an uncomplicated newborn course.

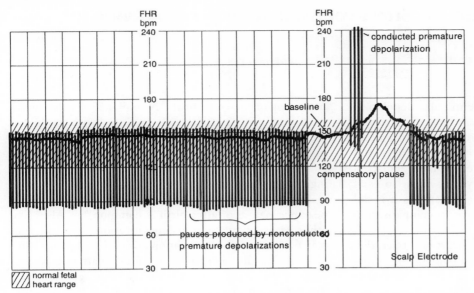

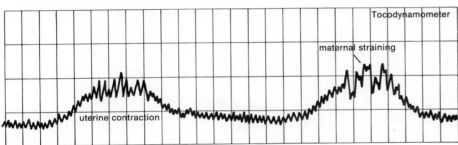

Pattern Characteristic:
Nonconducted Premature
Supraventricular Depolarizations

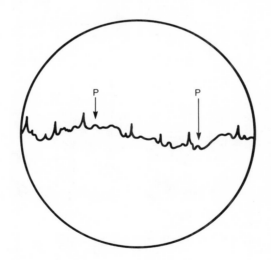

Nonconducted Premature Supraventricular Depolarizations in Bigeminal Pattern

*N*onconducted premature supraventricular depolarizations occurring every other beat result in an approximate halving of the sinus rate. Electrocardiographically, a premature atrial depolarization (P wave) is found to be unaccompanied by a corresponding ventricular depolarization.[1] This premature atrial activity may occur so early that it is identified in the T wave; sometimes it is detectable by a notching of the T wave in comparison to the "undisturbed" T waves.[20]

The arrhythmia produces a fetal heart rate trace that may be confused with severe sinus bradycardia, junctional bradycardia, atrioventricular block, or a half-counting artifact.[58] Variability (sinus arrhythmia) may be normal but is visually smoothed by the diminished frequency of the sinus beats. A similar fetal heart monitor pattern may be artifactually produced with conducted premature supraventricular depolarizations if the features of the QRS complex accompanying the atrial depolarizations do not meet the criteria for R wave counting.[30]

Like other cases of premature depolarizations, disappearance before or after birth is common.[62,80] Also, like other cases of premature depolarization, improvement may occur after discontinuation of caffeine or other stimulants. The disappearance of a fetal heart rate pattern such as the one depicted here has been reported with the correction of maternal hypokalemia.[3] (See page 42 for further discussion of this pattern.)

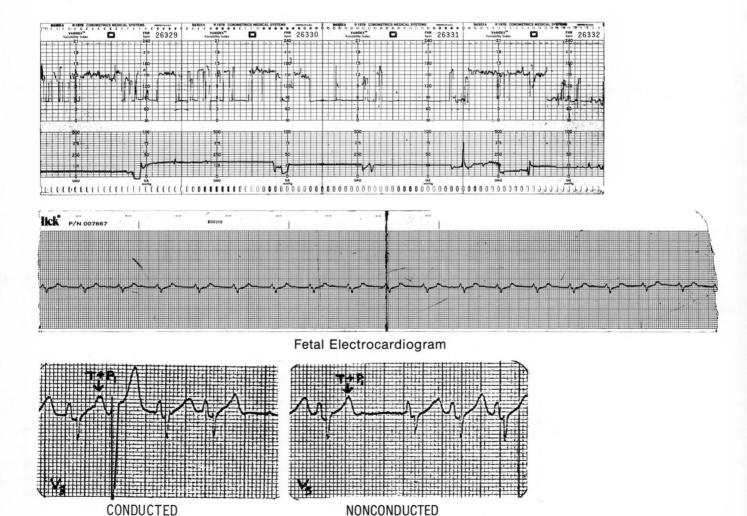

Fetal Electrocardiogram

CONDUCTED   NONCONDUCTED

Newborn Electrocardiogram

CASE INTERPRETATION: Class III

Baseline Information: the baseline alternates between a normal rate with average variability and bradycardia with decreased variability.

Periodic or Nonperiodic Changes: none seen.

Uterine Activity: not clear on the posted segment. Maternal respirations are noted.

Significance: this is a nondiagnostic pattern which may represent a bradyarrhythmia or half-counting. An electrocardiogram is needed for a diagnosis. Maternal heart rate artifact would be expected to have better variability (sinus arrhythmia).

Electrocardiographic Interpretation: Newborn electrocardiogram. The paper speed is 25 mm/sec, the heart rate is 80 bpm. PR and QRS of the conducted beat appear normal. Just before the apex of the T wave of the conducted beats, a small negative notching is noticed, representing the premature atrial depolarization that is nonconducted. This is consistent with nonconducted premature atrial depolarizations in a bigeminal pattern, producing a fetal bradycardia.

CASE OUTCOME: Thirty-seven-year-old gravida 4, para 3003, at 34 weeks' gestation delivered, with general anesthesia, a 4 pound, 4 ounce (1928 gram) female; Apgar score 2/8. Cesarean hysterectomy was performed for maternal carcinoma of the cervix uteri. Newborn diagnosis: electrocardiogram-confirmed nonconducted premature supraventricular depolarizations.

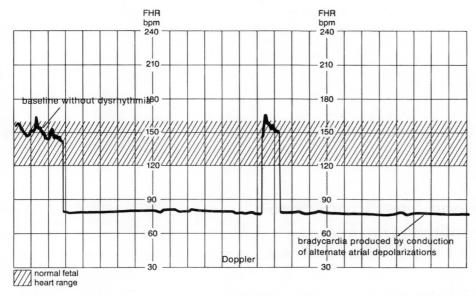

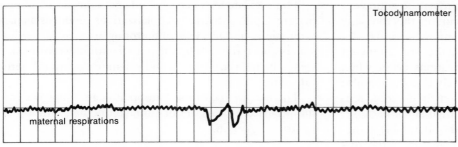

Pattern Characteristic:
Nonconducted Premature
Supraventricular Depolarizations
in Bigeminy

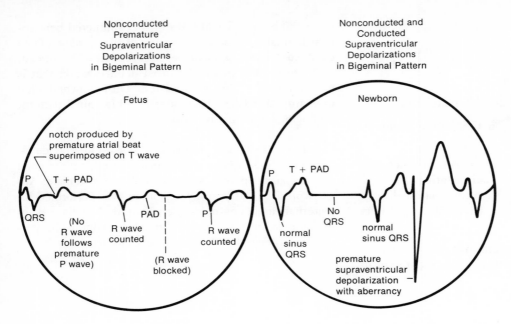

Nonconducted
Premature
Supraventricular
Depolarizations
in Bigeminal Pattern

Nonconducted and
Conducted
Supraventricular
Depolarizations
in Bigeminal Pattern

Pattern Characteristic:
Nonconducted Premature
Atrial Beats in Bigeminy

Conducted and Nonconducted Premature Supraventricular Depolarizations

*T*he occurrence of nonconducted premature supraventricular depolarizations typically occurs in the company of normally conducted premature supraventricular depolarizations. Electrophysiologically, the nonconducted premature supraventricular depolarizations occur when the atrial impulse occurs so prematurely that the impulse is unable to traverse the atrioventricular junction rendered refractory by the previous normal sinus impulse. However, since the atrioventricular junction is penetrated but not traversed by the premature atrial discharge, a further period of recovery is necessary before the next sinus depolarization, producing a pause. Conducted premature supraventricular depolarizations occur when the premature atrial discharge is able to fully traverse the atrioventricular junction and produce a QRS complex followed by a noncompensatory pause.

The coexistence of conducted and nonconducted premature supraventricular depolarizations produces a characteristic electronic fetal monitoring pattern of vertical spikes above the baseline that are continuous with small spikes below the baseline and separate downward vertical spikes.

The occurrence of the "dropped beats" suggests that the premature beats are of supraventricular, rather than ventricular, origin.

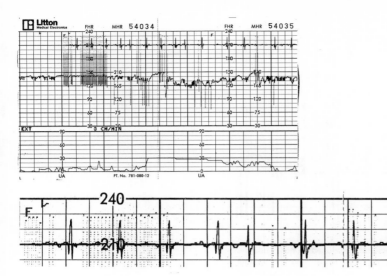

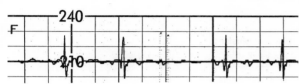

CASE INTERPRETATION: Class I

Baseline Information: normal rate and variability. Vertical spikes in a mixed pattern: some above the baseline, some below. Stable baseline rate.

Periodic or Nonperiodic Changes: small classic variable decelerations, nonperiodic variable accelerations.

Uterine Activity: not able to distinguish uterine and maternal activity.

Significance: a high degree of conformity in the appearance of the spikes is consistent with a dysrhythmia. There is the appearance of premature supraventricular depolarizations, both conducted and nonconducted. These are usually benign and disappear in late labor or during the newborn period.

Electrocardiographic Interpretation: fetal electrocardiogram. The paper speed is (computer corrected): 25 mm/sec. The heart rate is 142 bpm, with normal P waves, PR intervals, and QRS complexes. There are flat T waves. Premature supraventricular depolarizations are preceded by a P wave buried in the ST-T segments of the previous normal complex. In the second segment of the cardiogram there is a nonconducted premature atrial depolarization that is manifested by a premature P wave without a QRS complex that is followed by a pause and the resumption of a normal rhythm.

CASE OUTCOME: Twenty-five-year-old primigravida at 39½ weeks' gestation delivered by low transverse cesarean section performed for cephalopelvic disproportion, with general anesthesia, a 6 pound, 12 ounce (3062 gram) male; Apgar score 4/7. The newborn had persistent premature atrial depolarizations on the first day of life, as seen on the electrocardiogram, many of which were nonconducted. These disappeared by the time of the newborn's dismissal at three days of life.

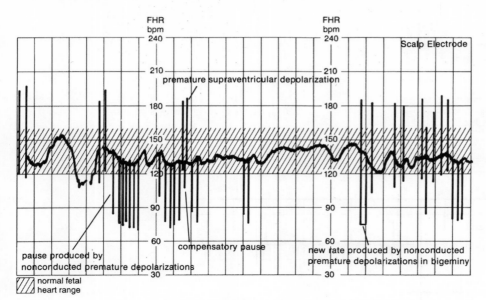

FHR bpm

premature supraventricular depolarization

compensatory pause

pause produced by nonconducted premature depolarizations

new rate produced by nonconducted premature depolarizations in bigeminy

normal fetal heart range

Scalp Electrode

Pattern Characteristic:
Premature Supraventricular
Depolarizations Conducted and
Nonconducted

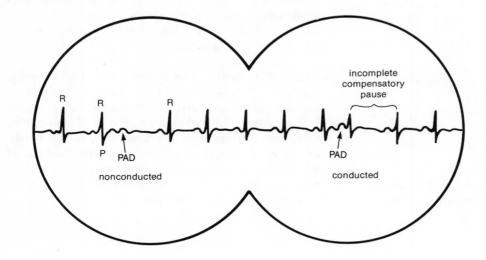

Tocodynamometer

uterine contraction

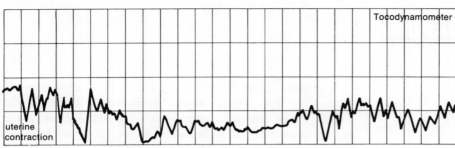

R   R   R

P   PAD

nonconducted

incomplete
compensatory
pause

PAD

conducted

Supraventricular Tachycardia

Supraventricular tachycardia is a sustained rapid regular dysrhythmia of atrial origin. The rate is by definition greater than 180 bpm and is usually in excess of 200 bpm, with rates as high as 320 bpm reported.[27,40,68] Electrophysiologically, supraventricular tachycardia is usually initiated by a premature atrial depolarization that is followed by a rapid regular dysrhythmia sustained by a mechanism termed "reentry."

There are two mechanisms of sustained tachyarrhythmias: automaticity and reentry. Reentry is by far the most common. Reentry requires that there be dual conducting pathways terminating in a final common pathway. An antegrade block in one of the conducting pathways permits antegrade passage over only the other pathway, which also characteristically has slow conduction. After passage over the unblocked pathway, the impulse may return in a retrograde fashion over the pathway that previously had antegrade block but is now recovered sufficiently to allow the impulse to return to its point of origin. There it again enters the original pathway, producing a reciprocating or reentrant tachycardia.[28] Reentry may occur anywhere in the cardiac tissue in which conduction is possible.[29] In the case of supraventricular tachycardia, the dual pathways usually exist in the atrioventricular node or via an anatomical bypass tract.[42] The majority of fetuses with this type of tachyarrhythmia are found to have Wolff-Parkinson-White syndrome with a bypass tract confirmed in the neonatal period.[83]

Electrocardiographically, there is a regular tachycardia with typically narrow QRS complexes, and usually P waves are not visible.[9]

The fetal monitor heart rate trace shows loss of variability and usually half counting of the excessive rate.

Echocardiography is useful in differentiating supraventricular tachycardia from atrial flutter (see page 492) and may provide information about structural abnormalities, which are present in 12% to 20% of cases.[65]

The undelivered or untreated fetus may develop cardiac failure and ischemic cerebral disease as a consequence of the rapid heart rate.[14,15,22,33,34,37,44,52,61,63,73,77,82] In the presence of supraventricular tachycardia, pharmacologic cardioversion is often successful in preventing or correcting fetal hydrops that is produced by congestive heart failure.[6,11,12,23,26,31,32,43,46,47,54,59,64,71,75] Such treatment may be transplacental. Direct fetal therapy may offer an advantage in certain cases.[48] Conversion by umbilical cord compression and by fetal cephalic compression under ultrasonic visualization have also been reported.[24,57]

Supraventricular tachycardia may be paroxysmal (see insert).[38,45,76] It may be induced in either the fetus or the mother by betamimetic therapy.[35] See page 61 for further discussion of supraventricular tachycardia.

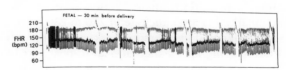

Reprinted with permission from Klapholz H, Schfrin B, Rivo E: Paroxysmal supraventricular tachycardia in the fetus. *Obstet Gynecol* 43:719; 1974.

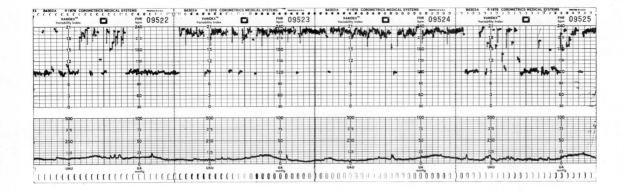

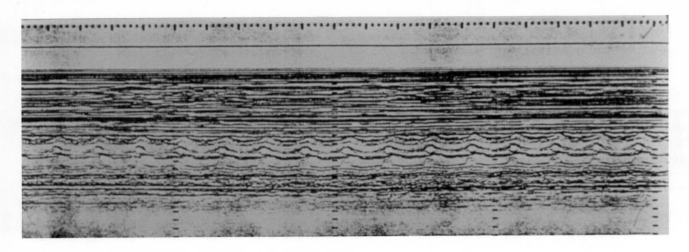

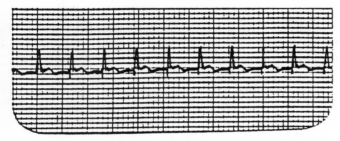

CASE INTERPRETATION: Class II

Baseline Information: there are two heart rates seen: one at a marked tachycardic rate of 220 to 230 bpm, and the second denoted by sporadic marks at 120 bpm. The rapid rate has the appearance of beat-to-beat variability but it is more "choppy" (less continuous than that seen in a usual trace).

Periodic or Nonperiodic Changes: none displayed.

Uterine Activity: shallow, infrequent contractions.

Significance: this is a pattern most consistent with tachyarrhythmia. An echocardiogram assists with making a diagnosis of the fetal cardiac status and the type of tachyarrhythmia. Also able to produce this pattern is double counting—auscultation clarifies such an artifact.

Electrocardiographic Interpretation: newborn electrocardiogram: paper speed is 25 mm/sec, heart rate is 240 bpm, QRS complexes are narrow, and no definite P waves are seen. The tachycardia is regular. This pattern is compatible with narrow-QRS or supraventricular tachycardia.

Echocardiographic Interpretation: fetal echocardiogram showing the aorta, aortic valve, and left atrium. The paper speed is 50 mm/sec. The aortic valve opening is regular at a rate of 230 bpm. The atrial wall motion is clearly seen to be associated with the aortic valve opening, which is at the same rate. This is consistent with fetal supraventricular tachycardia.

CASE OUTCOME: Twenty-year-old primigravida at 36 weeks' gestation delivered by low transverse cesarean section, with general anesthesia from a vertex presentation, a 7 pound, 4 ounce (3289 gram) male; Apgar score 2/6. The cesarean section was performed for failed pharmacoversion of fetal supraventricular tachycardia, using the agents digoxin, quinidine, and verapamil. The fetal pulmonary maturity was confirmed by an amniotic fluid study done prior to the cesarean section. The newborn course was complicated by hydrops fetalis, which resolved with the conversion of the supraventricular tachycardia with digoxin therapy. Hyperbilirubinemia responded to phototherapy.

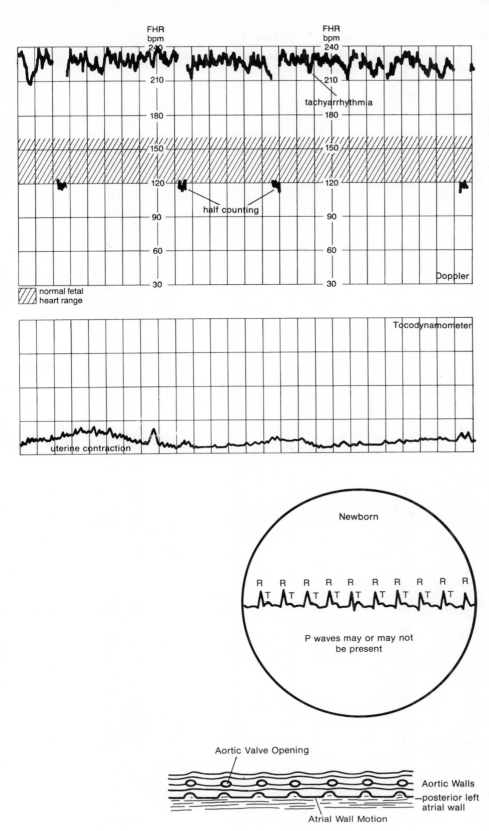

Pattern Characteristic:
Supraventricular Tachycardia

Fetal Echocardiogram

Supraventricular Tachycardia Due to Atrial Flutter

Atrial flutter is a supraventricular tachyarrhythmia that is a disorder both of impulse formation and conduction. The atrial ectopic focus produces regular impulses that vary from 300 to 460 bpm. The properties of the atrioventricular node are such that impulse conduction at such a high rate is not possible, and an at least two to one atrioventricular block is usually present.

Electrocardiographically, under ideal circumstances, flutter waves may be demonstrated. These produce a "sawtooth" appearance of the electrocardiographic baseline. The QRS complexes are narrow. Unfortunately, flutter waves may not be visible on the "single lead" fetal electrocardiogram.

The fetal monitor tracing shows loss of variability and usually half counting of the excessive rate.[36]

Two dimensional and M-mode fetal echocardiography may be of help in differentiating atrial flutter from su-

praventricular tachycardia and in diagnosing associated malformations occurring in as high as 20% of cases.[19,49, 50,56,60,67,79] If echocardiographic visualization of the fetal aorta and atrium is possible, the appearance of two atrial deflections for each aortic valve opening indicates atrial flutter with two to one block.

Atrial flutter may respond to transplacental or direct fetal pharmacotherapy when this is indicated for prevention of fetal congestive heart failure.[8,15,25,78,48]

Atrial fibrillation is rarely identified in the fetus but may be documented by electrocardiography or echocardiography and may, like atrial flutter, be associated with fetomaternal hemorrhage as well as Wolff-Parkinson-White syndrome.[4,5] See page 62 for further discussion of atrial flutter.

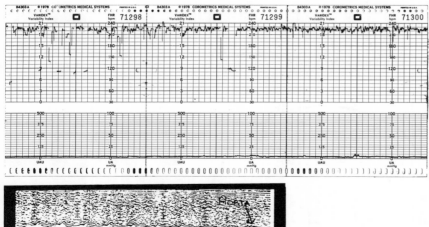

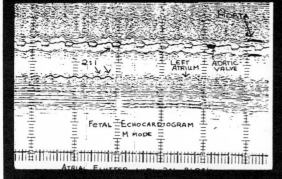

Original enhanced at time of patient care.

CASE INTERPRETATION: Class III

Baseline Information: marked tachycardia with a suggestion of decreased variability, as measured by external monitoring, as seen with tachyarrhythmia.

Periodic or Nonperiodic Changes: no reactivity or decelerations.

Uterine Activity: none recorded.

Significance: needs an echocardiogram or scalp electrode-electrocardiogram for diagnosis of the tachyarrhythmia.

Echocardiographic Interpretation: fetal echocardiogram demonstrating the aorta, aortic valve, and left atrium. The aortic valve opening occurs regularly at a rate of approximately 210 bpm. The posterior left atrial wall shows atrial motion at a rate of approximately 420 bpm, producing a two to one relation between atrial motion and aortic valve opening. This is consistent with atrial flutter with a two to one atrioventricular block.

CASE OUTCOME: Twenty-seven-year-old gravida 3, para 1011, at 32 weeks' gestation. There was an echo-cardiography diagnosis of atrial flutter with a two to one atrioventricular block in the fetus who had ascites. Maternal treatment with digoxin and verapamil was unsuccessful for fetal cardioversion. The patient delivered by repeat cesarean section a 5 pound, 5½ ounce (2420 gram) hydropic male stillborn. The fetus had trisomy 13 and multiple cardiac anomalies, including an atrioventricular canal.

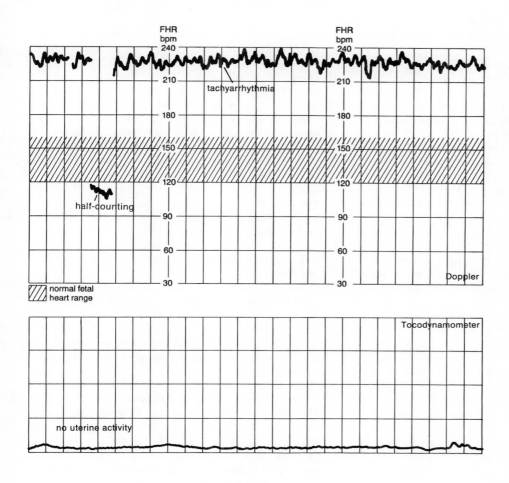

Pattern Characteristic:
Atrial Flutter

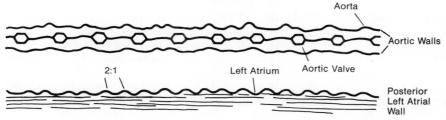

Fetal Echocardiogram
M = Mode
Atrial Flutter with 2:1 Block

References

1. Abinader EG, Dlain A, Eibschitz I, et al: The significance of fetal electrocardiography in the diagnosis of intrauterine bradyarrhythmia. *Am J Obstet Gynecol* 126:266, 1976.

2. Allan LD, Anderson RH, Sullivan ID, et al: Evaluation of fetal arrhythmias by echocardiography. *Br Heart J* 50:240, 1983.

3. Anderson GG, Hanson TM: Chronic fetal bradycardia. Possible association with hypokalemia. *Obstet Gynecol* 44:896, 1974.

4. Bacevice AE, Dierker LJ, Wolfson RN: Intrauterine atrial fibrillation associated with fetomaternal hemorrhage. *Am J Obstet Gynecol* 153:81, 1985.

5. Belhassen B, Pauzner D, Blieden L, et al: Intrauterine and postnatal atrial fibrillation in the Wolff-Parkinson-White syndrome. *Circulation* 66:1124, 1982.

6. Bergmans MGM, Jonker GJ, Kock HCLV: Fetal supraventricular tachycardia. Review of the literature. *Obstet Gynecol Survey* 40:61, 1985.

7. Bernstine RL, Winker JE, Callagan DA: Fetal bigeminy and tachycardia. *Am J Obstet Gynecol* 101:856, 1968.

8. Blumenthal S, Jacobs JC, Steer CM, et al: Congenital atrial flutter: Report of a case documented by intra-uterine electrocardiogram. *Pediatrics* 41:659, 1968.

9. Carreti NG, Galli PA, Pellegrino P: Fetal paroxysmal supraventricular tachycardia. Report of a case documented by trans-vaginal electrocardiogram during fetal distress in labour. *Acta Obstet Gynecol Scand* 63:275, 1974.

10. Cetrulo CL, Schifrin BS: Fetal heart rate patterns preceding death in utero. *Obstet Gynecol* 48:521, 1976.

11. Chelliah BP, Cabatu E, Chitklara U, et al: Polyhydramnios and elevated amniotic fluid alpha-fetoprotein caused by fetal supraventricular tachycardia. *J Reprod Med* 26:45, 1981.

12. Chitkara U, Gergely RZ, Gleicher N, et al: Persistent supraventricular tachycardia in utero. *Diagnostic Gynecology and Obstetrics* 2:291, 1980.

13. Clements J, Sobotka-Ploihar M, Exalto N, et al: A connective tissue membrane in the right atrium (Chiari's network) as a cause of fetal cardiac arrhythmia. *Am J Obstet Gynecol* 142:709, 1982.

14. Cowan RH, Waldo AL, Harris HB, et al: Neonatal paroxysmal supraventricular tachycardia with hydrops. *Pediatrics* 55:420, 1975.

15. Crawford CS: Antenatal diagnosis of fetal cardiac abnormalities. *Annals of Clinical and Laboratory Science* 12:99, 1982.

16. Crowley DC, Dick M, Rayburn WF, et al: Two-dimensional and M-mode echocardiographic evaluation of fetal arrhythmia. *Clin Cardiol* 8:1, 1985.

17. DeVore G: Case report #5, in: *Clinical Pathological Conferences in Obstetrics and Gynecology*, Roy S (ed). Excerpta Medica, 1985.

18. DeVore GR: Fetal echocardiography—a new frontier. *Clinic Obstetrics and Gynecology* 27:359, 1984.

19. DeVore GR, Siassi B, Platt L: Fetal echocardiography. III. The diagnosis of cardiac arrhythmias using real time—directed M-mode ultrasound. *Am J Obstet Gynecol* 146:792, 1983.

20. DiGani R, Borenstein R, Levani E, et al: Prenatally diagnosed blocked atrial premature beats. *Obstet Gynecol* 51:507, 1978.

21. DiLieto A, Chiariello M, Meglio D, et al: An unusual case of intermittent atrial parasystole in the fetus during labor. *Clin Exp Obst Gyn* 7:135, 1980.

22. Donn SM, Bowerman RA: Association of paroxysmal supraventricular tachycardia and periventricular leukomalacia. *Am J Perinatology* 3:50, 1986.

23. Dumesnic DA, Silverman NH, Tobias S, et al: Transplacental cardioversion of fetal supraventricular tachycardia with procainamide. *N Engl J Med* 307:1128, 1982.

24. Fernandez C, DeRosa GE, Guevara E, et al: Reversion by vagal reflex of a fetal paroxysmal atrial tachycardia detected by echocardiography. *Am J Obstet Gynecol* 159:860, 1988.

25. Funk M, Buerkle L: Intrauterine treatment of fetal tachycardia. *JOGNN* July/August, p. 290, 1986.

26. Garvin JA, Kline EM: Congenital paroxysmal tachycardia. Report of case recognized ante partum. *Am Heart J* 33:362, 1974.

27. Gleicher N, Elkayam U: Intrauterine dysrhythmias, in: *Cardiac Problems in Pregnancy*. New York, Alan R. Liss, 1982, p. 535.

28. Guntheroth WG, Cyr DR, Mack LA, et al: Hydrops from reciprocating atrioventricular tachycardia in a 27-week fetus requiring quinidine for conversion. *Obstet Gynecol* 66:29, 1985.

29. Han J: The mechanism of paroxysmal atrial tachycardia. Sustained reciprocation. *Am J Cardiology* 26:329, 1970.

30. Harrigan JT, Acerra D, LaMagra R, et al: Fetal cardiac arrhythmia during labor. *Am J Obstet Gynecol* 128:693, 1977.

31. Harrigan JT, Kangos JJ, Sikka A, et al: Successful treatment of fetal congestive heart failure secondary to tachycardia. *N Engl J Med* 304:1527, 1981.

32. Heaton FC, Vaughan R: Intrauterine supraventricular tachycardia: Cardioversion with maternal digoxin. *Obstet Gynecol* 60:749, 1982.

33. Hedvall HG: Congenital paroxysmal tachycardia—a report of three cases. *Acta Paediat Scand* 62:550, 1973.

34. Herin P, Thoren C: Congenital arrhythmias with supraventricular tachycardia in the perinatal period. *Acta Obstet Gynec Scand* 52:381, 1973.

35. Hermansen MC, Johnson GL: Neonatal supraventricular tachycardia following prolonged maternal ritodrine administration. *Am J Obstet Gynecol* 149:798, 1984.

36. Hertogs K: Supraventricular tachycardia in utero with two-to-one block in fetal monitor. *Lancet* 1:1158, 1981.

37. Hilrich NM, Evrard JR: Supraventricular tachycardia in

the newborn with onset in utero. *Am J Obstet Gynecol* 70:1139, 1955.

38. Hochberg HM, Poppers PJ: Fetal paroxysmal supraventricular tachycardia recorded by intrauterine scalp electrocardiography. *J Perinatal Med* 4:51, 1976.

39. Hon EH, Huang HS: The electronic evaluation of fetal heart rate. VII. Premature and missed beats. *Obstet Gynecol* 20:81, 1962.

40. Hughey M, Elesh R: Profound atrial tachycardia in utero. *Am J Obstet Gynecol* 120:463, 1977.

41. Itkovitz J, Timor-Tritsch I, Brandes JM: Intrauterine fetal arrhythmia: Atrial premature beats. *Int J Gynaecol Obstet* 16:419, 1979.

42. Jones JB: Accelerated rhythm causing intrapartum fetal tachycardia. *Brit J Obstet Gynaecol* 83:986, 1976.

43. Kerenyi TD, Meller J, Steinfeld L, et al: Transplacental cardioversion of intrauterine supraventricular tachycardia with digitalis. *Lancet* August 23:393, 1980.

44. Kesson CW: Foetal Paroxysmal Auricular Tachycardia. *Br Heart J* 20:552, 1958.

45. Klapholz H, Schifrin BS, Rivo E, et al: Paroxysmal supraventricular tachycardia in the fetus. *Obstet Gynecol* 43:718, 1974.

46. Klein AM, Holzman IR, Austin EM: Fetal tachycardia prior to the development of hydrops—attempted pharmacologic cardioversion: Case report. *Am J Obstet Gynecol* 134:347, 1979.

47. Klein V, Repke JT: Supraventricular tachycardia in pregnancy: Cardioversion with verapamil. *Obstet Gyecol* 63:162, 1984.

48. Kleinman CS, Copel JA: Opinion: Direct fetal therapy for cardiac arrhythmias: Who, what, when, where, why and how? Ultrasound. *Obstet Gynecol* 1:158, 1991.

49. Kleinman CS, Donnerstein RL, Jaffe CC, et al: Fetal echocardiography. A tool for evaluation of in utero cardiac arrhythmias and monitoring of in utero therapy: Analysis of 71 patients. *Am J Cardiology* 51:237, 1983.

50. Kleinman CS, Hobbins JC, Jaffe CC, et al: Echocardiographic studies of the human fetus: Prenatal diagnosis of congenital heart disease and cardiac dysrhythmias. *Pediatrics* 65:1059, 1980.

51. Komaromy B, Gaal J, Lampe L: Fetal arrhythmia during pregnancy and labour. *Br J Obstet Gynaecol* 84:492, 1977.

52. Levkoff AH: Perinatal outcome of paroxysmal tachycardia of the newborn with onset in utero. *Am J Obstet Gynecol* 104:73, 1969.

53. Lipman BS, Dunn M, Massie E: *Cardiac arrhythmias in clinical electrocardiography*, 7th ed. Chicago, Yearbook Medical Publishers, 1984, p. 376.

54. Lingman G, Ohrlander S, Ohlin P: Intrauterine digoxin treatment of fetal paroxysmal tachycardia case report. *Br J Obstet Gynaecol* 87:340, 1980.

55. Lodeiro JG, Feinstein SJ, Lodeiro SB: Fetal premature contractions associated with hydralazine. *Am J Obstet Gynecol* 160:105, 1989.

56. Losure TA, Roberts NS: In utero diagnosis of atrial flutter by means of real-time-directed M-mode echocardiography. *Am J Obstet Gynecol* 149:903, 1984.

57. Martin CB, Niihuis JG, Weiier AA: Correction of fetal supraventricular tachycardia by compression of the umbilical cord: Report of a case. *Am J Obstet Gynecol* 150:324, 1984.

58. Minagawa Y, Akauva A, Hidaka T, et al: Severe supraventricular bradyarrhythmia without fetal hypoxia. *Obstet Gynecol* 70:454, 1987.

59. Newburger JW, Keane JF: Intrauterine supraventricular tachycardia. *J Pediatrics* 95:780, 1979.

60. Pearl W: Cardiac malformations presenting as congenital atrial flutter. *Southern Med J* 70:622, 1977.

61. Radford DJ, Izukawa T, Rowe RD: Congenital paroxysmal atrial tachycardia. *Archives of Disease in Childhood* 51:613, 1976.

62. Redman TF: The significance of some unusual foetal cardiac arrhythmias. *J Obstet Gynaecol Brit Empire* 65:304, 1958.

63. Rees L, Vlies PR, Adams J: Hydrops fetalis, an unusual cause, presentation and method of diagnosis. *Br J Obstet Gynaecol* 87:1169, 1980.

64. Rey E, Duperron L, Cauthier R, et al. Transplacental treatment of tachycardia induced fetal heart failure with verapamil and amiodarone: A case report. *Am J Obstet Gynecol* 153:311, 1985.

65. Scagliotti D, Deal BJ: Arrhythmias in the tiny, premature infant. *Clinics in Perinatology* 13:339, 1986.

66. Schneider H, Weinstein HM, Young BK: Fetal trigeminal rhythm. *Obstet Gynecol* (Suppl.) 50:58s, 1977.

67. Shenker L: Fetal cardiac arrhythmias. *Obstet Gynecol Surv* 34:561, 1979.

68. Silber D, Durnin RE: Intrauterine atrial tachycardia. *Am J Dis Child* 117:722, 1969.

69. Silverman ME, Myerburg RJ, Hurst JW: The differential diagnosis of a tachycardia, in: *Electrocardiography. Basic Concepts and Clinical Appreciation*. New York, McGraw-Hill, 1983, p. 291.

70. Southall DP, Richards J, Hardwick R, et al. Prospective study of fetal heart rate and rhythm patterns. *Arch Dis Child* 55:506, 1980.

71. Spinnato JA, Shaver DC, Flinn GS, et al: Fetal supraventricular tachycardia: In utero therapy with digoxin and quinidine. *Obstet Gynecol* 64:730, 1984.

72. Steinfeld L, Rappaport HL, Rossbach HC, et al: Diagnosis of fetal arrhythmias using electrocardiographic and Doppler techniques. *J Am Coll Cardiol* 8:1425, 1986.

73. Stevens DC, Hilliard JK, Schreiner RL, et al: Supraventricular tachycardia with edema, ascites, and hydrops in fetal sleep. *Am J Obstet Gynecol* 142:316, 1982.

74. Sugarman RG, Rawlinson KF, Schifrin BS: Fetal arrhythmia. *Obstet Gynecol* 52:301, 1978.

75. Teuscher A, Bossi E, Imhof P, et al: Effect of propranolol on fetal tachycardia in diabetic pregnancy. *Am J Cardiology* 42:304, 1978.

76. Tuxen P, Kaplan EL, Veland K: Intrauterine paroxysmal atrial tachycardia. *Am J Obstet Gynecol* 109:958, 1971.

77. Valerius NH, Jacobsen JR: Intrauterine supraventricular tachycardia. *Acta Obstet Gynecol Scand* 57:407, 1978.

78. Van Der Horst RL: Congenital atrial flutter and cardiac failure. *South African Medical Journal* 12:1037, 1970.

79. Vintzileos AM, Campbell WA, Soberman SM, et al: Fetal

atrial flutter and X-linked dominant vitamin D-resistant rickets. *Obstet Gynecol* 65:39s, 1985.

80. Webster RD, Cudmore DW, Gray J: Fetal bradycardia without fetal distress. *Obstet Gynecol* 50:50s, 1977.

81. Weiner CP, Thompson MIB: Direct treatment of supraventricular tachycardia after failed transplacentai therapy. *Am J Obstet Gynecol* 158:570, 1988.

82. Wells DH, Shaw CG, McNeal RM, et al: Neonatal paroxysmal supraventricular tachycardia. *Clin Pediat* 17:581, 1978.

83. Wolff CS, Han J, Curran J: Wolff-Parkinson-White syndrome in the neonate. *Am J Cardiology* 41:559, 1978.

84. Wolff F, Dreuker KH, Schlensker KH, et al: Prenatal diagnosis and therapy of fetal heart rate anomalies: With a contribution on the placental transfer of verapamil. *J Perinat Med* 8:203, 1980.

85. Young BK: Fetal cardiac arrhythmia in labor. *Perinatal Care* 2:40, 1978.

86. Young BK: Intrapartum fetal cardiac arrhythmias. *Obstet Gynecol* 54:427, 1979.

Ventricular Dysrhythmias

Chapter 22

Premature Ventricular Depolarizations Including Bigeminal Pattern

Ventricular premature depolarizations are produced by premature discharges from a focus below the atrioventricular junction occurring either in the bundle branches, His-Purkinje system, or ventricular myocardium. They occur less frequently than supraventricular depolarizations.[3,16,19,23]

Electrocardiographically, no P wave is seen, and the premature QRS is bizarre and wide, with the T wave usually directed opposite to the polarity of the QRS complex.[13] The ventricular premature depolarization is followed by a fully compensatory pause, meaning that the interval between two normal complexes flanking the premature ventricular depolarization is equal to or greater than the interval produced by the sum of two cardiac cycles.[21]

Occasionally, the compensatory pause may be absent (interpolated beat). Typically, the interval between the normal beat and premature ventricular depolarization is fixed.[10]

The fetal monitor heart trace shows vertical spikes fairly equidistant above and below the normal fetal heart rate. This produces the appearance of three parallel horizontal lines, the upper representing the rate produced by the premature beat and the lower produced by the compensatory pause. The middle line representing the rate produced by normal cardiac cycles gives some reflection of variability, although not beat-to-beat.

When the premature depolarizations occur in a bigeminal pattern, there is no "middle" line. Therefore, baseline fetal heart rate and variability is obscured. Ventricular bigeminy may also be displayed as a bradycardia if the R wave of the ventricular premature depolarization does not have characteristics that qualify it for counting by the monitor.[1] (See page 528 for a discussion of masked premature ventricular depolarizations.)

When three premature ventricular depolarizations occur in succession, ventricular tachycardia is diagnosed.[12,24] This has rarely been documented in the fetus and is not a common finding in the newborn.[20] Ventricular fibrillation has not been documented in the fetus.[12]

Echocardiographically, the distinction between atrial or ventricular premature depolarizations is not consistently reliable. However, if the echocardiogram beam is traversing the aortic root and the atrium, atrial contraction can be inferred from the motion of the atrial wall toward the posterior wall of the aorta. Ventricular contraction is associated with the opening of the aortic valve, as seen within the aortic root. Therefore, if opening of the aortic valve is seen to occur prematurely, and no evidence of atrial wall motion is seen preceding this, a ventricular premature beat is likely.[2,7] Measurement of a fully compensatory pause after a premature beat (as calculated echocardiographically from recurring cardiac events) is an additional presumptive, but not diagnostic, indication of premature ventricular depolarizations.[5,15]

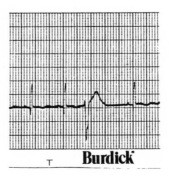

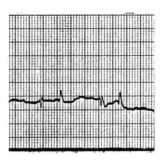

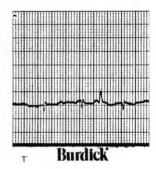

CASE INTERPRETATION: Class I-III

Baseline Information: a normal rate is indicated by a heavy dotted line with apparently average variability. Arrhythmia is characterized by a parallel vertical line extending from the marked tachycardic to the moderate bradycardic range. Some areas have totally obscured the baseline, and others demonstrate an interspersed baseline rate for one or more beats (dots). There are rare downward vertical excursions to a 70 bpm heart rate.

Uterine Activity: irregular contractions in shape and frequency, as measured by external monitoring, with a superimposed maternal respiratory pattern.

Significance: premature supraventricular or ventricular depolarizations are consistent with a bigeminal and trigeminal pattern. An electrocardiogram or echocardiogram is needed for a diagnosis. Downward spikes may be machine-rejected premature beats.

Electrocardiographic Interpretation: fetal electrocardiogram. The paper speed is 25 mm/sec. The heart rate is 135 bpm. The basic rhythm is sinus. There are premature beats occurring in a dominantly bigeminal pattern. The QRS complex of the premature depolarizations is wider than the preceding sinus beat, and the polarity of the QRS is opposite to that of the preceding sinus beat. The compensatory pause is complete. This is compatible with ventricular premature depolarizations in a bigeminal pattern. Also seen in this strip is a similar premature ventricular depolarization which, however, occurs in the interval between two sinus beats, and there is no compensatory pause. This is compatible with an interpolated ventricular premature depolarization.

Newborn electrocardiogram: There is a single premature depolarization that is illustrated as the fourth beat. This interrupts the T wave of the preceding sinus beat. The polarity of the premature beat is opposite in direction to the sinus beat. There is a fully compensatory pause.

CASE OUTCOME: Eighteen-year-old primigravida at 39 weeks' gestation delivered vaginally from a vertex presentation, with pudendal and local anesthesia, a 7 pound, 6 ounce (3345 gram) female; Apgar score 8/8. The newborn had persistent premature ventricular depolarizations. No heart disease was diagnosed.

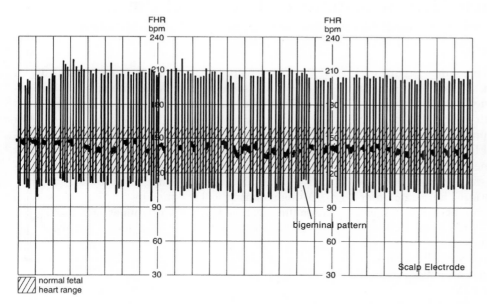

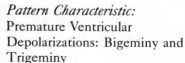

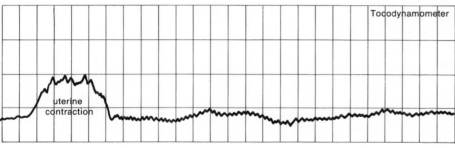

Pattern Characteristic:
Premature Ventricular Depolarizations: Bigeminy and Trigeminy

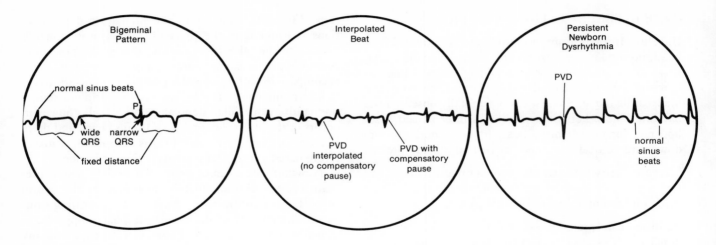

Pattern Characteristic:
Premature Ventricular Depolarizations

Premature Ventricular Depolarizations in Trigeminal Pattern

*P*remature ventricular depolarizations may occur in an automatic and repetitive fashion. If this occurs every other beat, it is termed "bigeminy"; every third beat, "trigeminy"; and so on.[13,24] With trigeminy, the fetal monitor heart rate pattern that is produced is a dramatic, regular pattern of vertical parallel lines. The rate at the upper extremes of the vertical lines is produced by the premature beat, and the rate at the lower end is produced by the compensatory pause. The single interspersed normal cardiac cycle beat is reflected by a single dot at the normal fetal heart rate. The resulting effect is three nearly parallel horizontal lines. Some assessment of variability may be made by observing the middle of the three lines, but because it represents only every third beat, it is not true beat-to-beat variability.[11] If the R wave is not counted by the monitor, the ventricular premature beats may be displayed as pauses[9] (see page 528). Ventricular premature depolarizations usually form vertical spikes fairly equidistant above and below the baseline, whereas the spikes of supraventricular depolarizations are predominately above the baseline in a pattern often mixed with "dropped beats."

Premature ventricular depolarizations are usually of no serious consequence.[15,16] As is true of premature supraventricular depolarizations, they tend to disappear in late labor, particularly during contractions or soon after birth.[18] Presumably, the frequency of premature ventricular depolarizations may be increased by the same factors that increase the frequency of premature atrial depolarizations (e.g., caffeine, nicotine, and alcohol).[6]

Although pharmacologic therapy may be successful in controlling fetal ventricular arrhythmias, it is usually not warranted because there is seldom fetal jeopardy.[4,8]

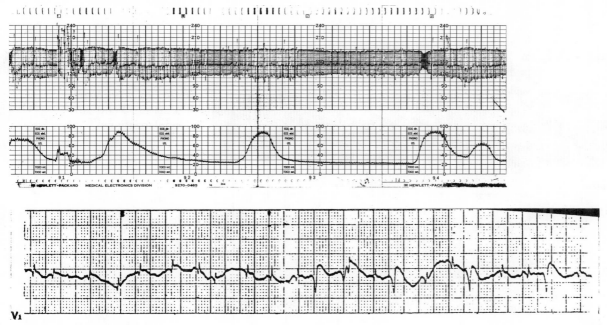

Original enhanced at time of patient care.

CASE INTERPRETATION: Class IV

Baseline Information: three heart rates are displayed: one in the moderate to marked tachycardic range, one in the normal range, and one in the low normal to moderate bradycardic range. All have decreased short- and long-term variability. Vertical parallel spikes connect the three lines. The upper and lower lines are a similar distance from the middle horizontal line. Fluctuation in long-term variability, especially during uterine contractions, is accompanied by a converging of the three lines. Disappearance of the pattern is seen during contractions in the second stage of labor.

Periodic and Nonperiodic Changes: moderate variable decelerations with slight atypia, characterized by slow recovery, appear in the second segment.

Uterine Activity: there are skewed contractions every three minutes. There is maternal straining in the second segment.

Significance: there is the appearance of premature ventricular depolarizations in a trigeminal pattern. (A normal heart rate is identified for one beat between the rates produced by premature beats and the compensatory pauses.)

Electrocardiographic Interpretation: fetal electrocardiogram. The paper speed is 25 mm/sec. The heart rate is 180 bpm. There are premature depolarizations seen every third beat. The QRS complex of the premature depolarizations is wider than the QRS complex of the two preceding sinus beats. The polarity is opposite from the polarity of the sinus beats, and the configuration of the QRS in the premature depolarizations is bizarre. This is compatible with ventricular premature depolarizations in a trigeminal pattern.

CASE OUTCOME: Sixteen-year-old gravida 2, para 1001, delivered vaginally, with low forceps and epidural anesthesia, a 7 pound, 4 ounce (3289 gram) male; Apgar score 8/9. The fetus was in a persistent occiput posterior position. The fetal electrocardiogram demonstrated premature ventricular depolarizations. These became infrequent in the second stage of labor. The infant followed an uncomplicated newborn course. There was no evidence of heart disease.

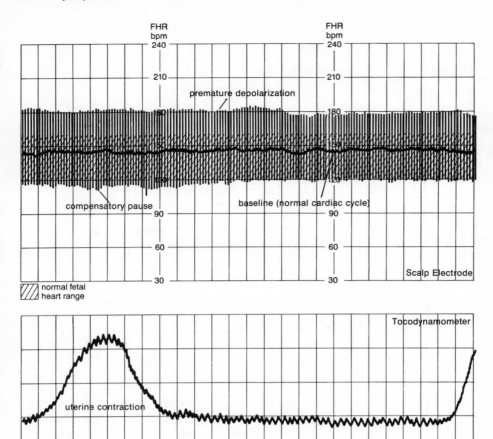

Pattern Characteristic:
Premature Ventricular
Depolarizations

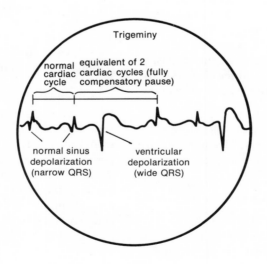

Premature Ventricular Depolarizations as Fusion Beats

*P*remature ventricular depolarizations may occur as fusion beats in the fetus.[24] This is diagnosed when a ventricular premature depolarization occurs simultaneously with atrial depolarization, resulting in a hybrid depolarization. It is recognized by a wide, bizarre beat that is preceded by a normal P wave with normal timing.[17]

The fusion beat, because it occurs at the time normal depolarizations would be seen, does not produce a compensatory pause.

Although there is no compensatory pause, the fetal monitor is able to detect the very slight difference in timing of the fusion QRS compared to the expected normal QRS, and a pattern consistent with a premature beat followed by a pause is created. The fetal monitor tracing, therefore, presents a pattern that is unlike usual premature ventricular depolarizations in that the vertical spikes do not occur at a regular distance above and below the line produced by the normal fetal heart. Therefore, three parallel horizontal lines are not produced.

The pattern may be misdiagnosed as maternal QRS interference because auscultation may not identify an irregular rate. An electrocardiogram is required for diagnosis.

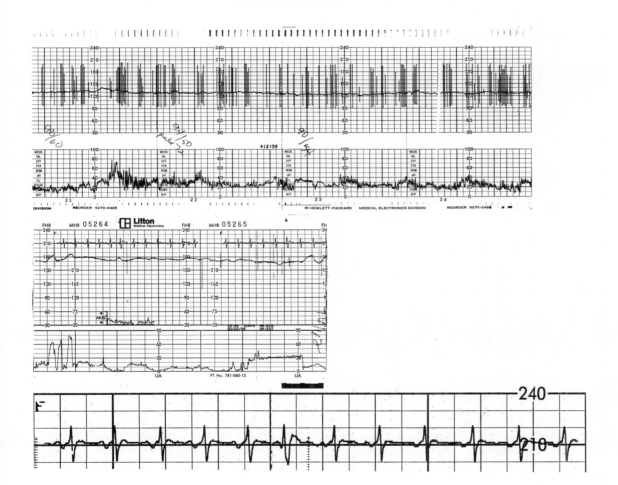

CASE INTERPRETATION: Class I

Baseline Information: normal heart rate, average to decreased short- and long-term variability. There are vertical spikes of varying length above and below fetal heart trace.

Periodic or Nonperiodic Changes: rare, shallow acceleration.

Uterine Activity: there appear to be irregular contractions with superimposed maternal respirations or other activity.

Significance: there is the appearance of premature depolarizations with compensatory pauses. The premature beats are occurring at varying intervals from the normal beats. An electrocardiogram is needed for a diagnosis. This pattern needs to be distinguished from a maternal QRS-counting artifact.

Electrocardiographic Interpretation: fetal electrocardiogram. The paper speed is 25 mm/sec (computer corrected). The heart rate is 165 bpm. The basic rhythm is sinus tachycardia. There are occasional QRS complexes that are wider than the QRS complexes of the sinus beats but of the same general configuration. These beats are

preceded by a normal P wave and the rhythm is not interrupted by these aberrant depolarizations. These are compatible with ventricular premature depolarizations that occur as fusion beats.

CASE OUTCOME: Nineteen-year-old gravida 2, para 0010, at 40 weeks' gestation delivered vaginally from a vertex presentation, with epidural anesthesia, a 7 pound, 6 ounce (3345 gram) female; Apgar score 8/10. A newborn electrocardiogram was not performed. The newborn's heart rate was monitored, with no abnormal findings.

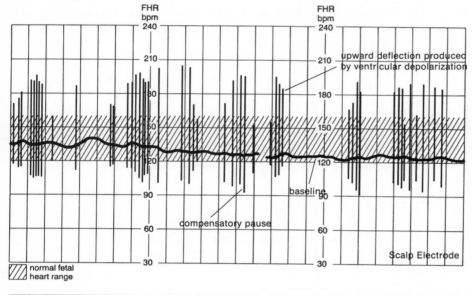

Pattern Characteristic:
Fusion Beats

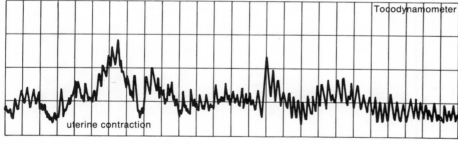

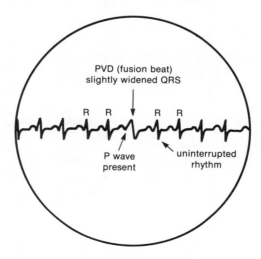

Premature Ventricular Depolarizations Demonstrating Parasystole

*P*arasystole is a variant of premature ventricular depolarizations. Electrophysiologically, there is an automatic focus of ventricular ectopic activity that is protected from depolarization by the normal depolarization process. This automatic focus is discharging locally but may only exit and produce a depolarization when the ventricle is not refractory.[17] This is a random occurrence that depends on the interaction of the two rates. This produces the electrocardiographic pattern of ventricular premature depolarizations occurring with no fixed relationship to the prior normal beats, and because of this fusion beats are frequently seen in parasystole. Because of the automaticity of the protected focus (which can only emerge when the ventricle is nonrefractory), this dysrhythmia can be recognized by the fact that all interectopic intervals are multiples of the shortest interectopic interval.[22]

In the adult, the pattern of parasystole carries a benign prognosis. This appears to be a rare dysrhythmia in the fetus.

The fetal heart monitor pattern is similar to that of fusion beats (see page 503), with vertical deflections of varying lengths. An electrocardiogram is necessary to distinguish the fusion beat pattern from maternal QRS interference and to diagnose the presence of parasystole. However, the presence of parasystole may be suspected by the peculiar spacing of the vertical spikes produced by the premature beats.

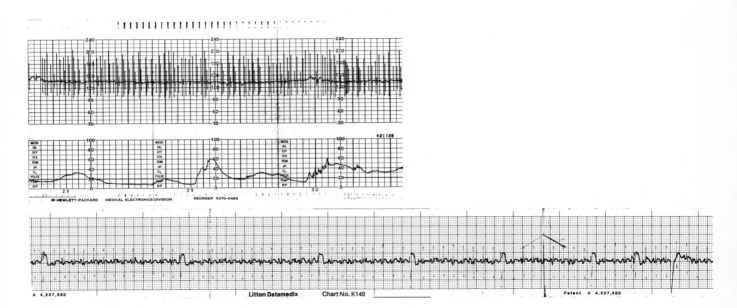

CASE INTERPRETATION: Class I

Baseline Information: a normal heart rate, average to decreased variability, vertical spikes above and below the fetal heart trace.

Periodic or Nonperiodic Changes: rare, shallow accelerations.

Uterine Activity: frequent contractions of a varying configuration and with a varying resting interval.

Significance: there is the appearance of premature depolarizations (probably ventricular) and compensatory pauses. There is an unusual variation in the distances of the premature beat from the normal beats. An electrocardiogram is needed for diagnosis and to exclude maternal QRS-counting artifact.

Electrocardiographic Interpretation: fetal electrocardiogram. The paper speed is 12.5 mm/sec. The heart rate is 140 bpm. The basic rhythm is sinus. There are premature depolarizations with a slightly widened QRS complex. The configuration is bizarre. The coupling interval of the premature depolarizations is not constant in relation to the preceding sinus complex. An occasional fusion beat is seen. By measuring the interval between the two closest of these premature depolarizations, the intervals between the other premature depolarizations are seen to be multiples of the shortest interectopic interval. This is compatible with ventricular premature depolarizations from a parasystolic focus or "ventricular parasystole."

CASE OUTCOME: Twenty-six-year-old primigravida at 38 weeks' gestation delivered by low transverse cesarean section performed for cephalopelvic disproportion an 8 pound, 5 ounce (3771 gram) female; Apgar score 9/9.

The fetus was in a vertex presentation. Oxytocin was administered for premature ruptured membranes at term gestation. The infant followed a normal newborn course with no cardiac disease identified.

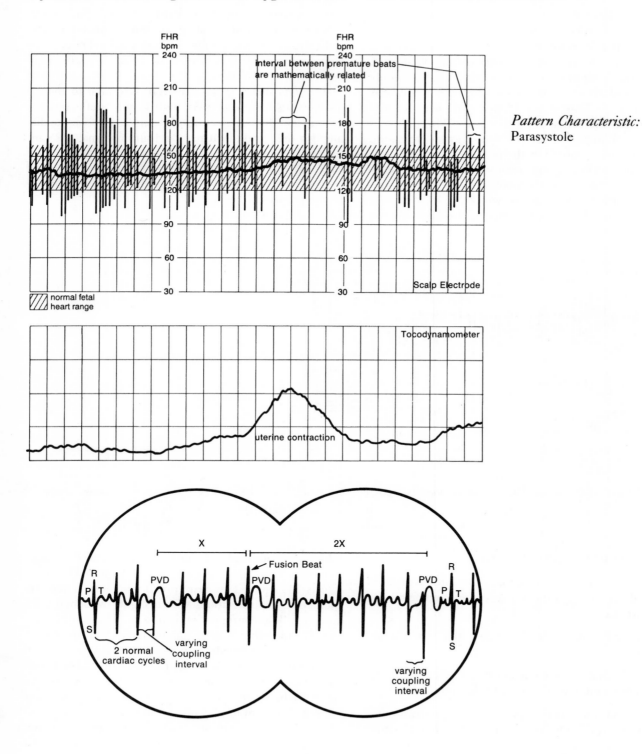

Pattern Characteristic:
Parasystole

Accelerated Idioventricular Rhythm

*I*dioventricular rhythm is a dysrhythmia generated by independent ventricular beating that occurs at a slower rate and is more stable than a usual ventricular tachycardia. Electrophysiologically, there is a rhythmic, spontaneously depolarizing focus in the ventricle that is not allowed to exit and capture ventricular control until the normal sinus mechanism slows below the intrinsic rate of the idioventricular focus.[17]

It often begins with a fusion beat as the normal sinus mechanism slows and the first beat of the accelerated idioventricular rhythm fuses with the normal sinus beat. It is characteristic that, although the accelerated focus cannot gain control of the ventricle until the sinus rate falls below that of the idioventricular focus, neither can the normal sinus beat completely depolarize the accelerated idioventricular focus. In long electrocardiogram strips, accelerated idioventricular rhythm and the normal sinus rhythm can be seen alternating with each other, depending on the phasic slowing of the sinus node.

The QRS complexes are typically wide and characteristic of a ventricular origin.

The fetal monitor pattern displayed in this case enters the dysrhythmia with an upward spike occurring amid a deceleration, which reflects the initial sinus slowing. The trace is then sustained at the apex of the spike until the accelerated idioventricular rhythm is resolved.

This dysrhythmia is seen frequently in the adult with acute myocardial infarction which produces slowing of the sinus mechanism that is due to ischemia of the sinus and atrioventricular nodes. In light of this information, this dysrhythmia may not be reassuring when seen in the fetus. However, the in utero electrocardiographic diagnosis of a sick fetus is, as yet, an undeveloped scientific field.[14]

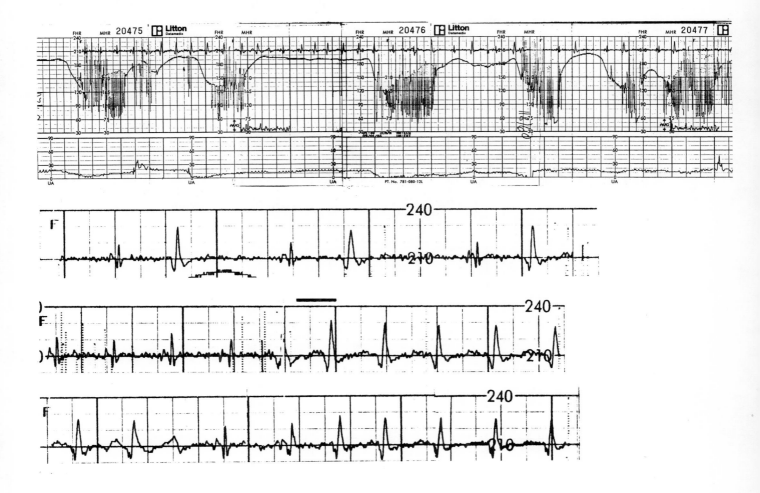

CASE INTERPRETATION: Class V

Baseline Information: severe tachycardia, absent variability, loss of stability.

Periodic or Nonperiodic Changes: atypical, severe variable decelerations, with loss of variability in the descending and ascending limbs and prolonged secondary accelerations. The nadir of the decelerations are obscured by an unusual pattern, suggesting a dysrhythmia in a bigeminal pattern or artifact.

Uterine Activity: infrequent contractions are recorded in some areas, no uterine activity is identified by the tocodynamometer in others.

Significance: there is a high risk of a low Apgar score, and acidosis. An electrocardiogram is needed for a diagnosis of the possible dysrhythmia.

Electrocardiographic Interpretation: fetal electrocardiogram. The paper speed is 25 mm/sec (computer corrected). The heart rate is 175 bpm. The basic rhythm is sinus tachycardia. There are obvious ventricular premature depolarizations, many of which occur as a bigeminal pattern, as seen on the electrocardiogram. At intervals, there is a run of these with a regular rhythm at a rate slightly faster than the basic sinus rhythm. These runs are interrupted by the intermittent nature of the electrocardiogram acquisition. No P waves are visible preceding the beats, and the QRS configuration is identical to the configuration of the ventricular premature depolarizations. This rhythm is seen to be initiated by a QRS complex intermediate between the sinus depolarization and the ventricular premature depolarizations. This constitutes a fusion beat. This regular wide QRS rhythm that occurs in competition with the basic sinus rhythm is compatible with an accelerated idioventricular rhythm.

CASE OUTCOME: Thirty-five-year-old gravida 2, para 1001, at 26 weeks' gestation delivered vaginally, with epidural anesthesia, a 2 pound, 8½ ounce (1148 gram) male; Apgar score 0/0. The fetus was grossly malformed. Anomalies included hypertelorism, ear deformities, a compressed nose, clinodactyly, equinus varus, pulmonary hypoplasia, fetal edema, and pleural and pericardial effusion.

The pregnancy had been complicated by oligohydramnios. A laparotomy was required in the second trimester for an incarcerated retroverted uterus.

Although newborn congestive heart failure was noted on the autopsy, there were no structural cardiac lesions. Multiple cerebral hemorrhages were present.

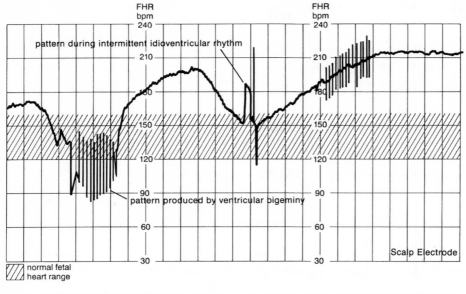

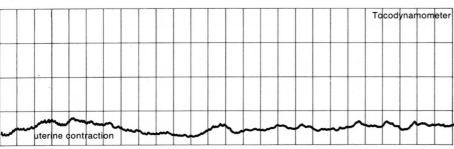

Pattern Characteristic:
Accelerated Idioventricular
Rhythm

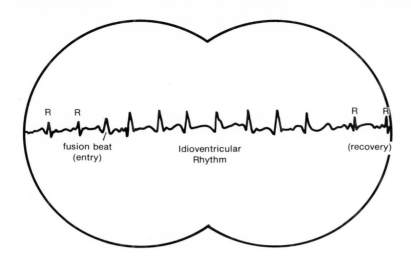

fusion beat
(entry)

Idioventricular
Rhythm

(recovery)

References

1. Abinader EG, Klein A, Eibschitz I, et al: The significance of fetal electrocardiography in the diagnosis of intrauterine bradyarrhythmia. *Am J Obstet Gynecol* 126:266, 1976.
2. Allan LD, Anderson RH, Sullivan ID, et al: Evaluation of fetal arrhythmias by echocardiography. *Br Heart J* 50:240, 1983.
3. Cabaniss ML, Wagner PC, Cabaniss CD: Fetal ventricular arrhythmias. *Proceedings of the Society of Perinatal Obstetricians*, Orlando, FL, February 1987, no. 222.
4. Clement D, Schifrin BS: Diagnosis and management of fetal arrhythmias. *Perinatology/Neonatology* March/April, p. 9, 1987.
5. Crowley DC, Dick M, Rayburn WF, et al: Two-dimensional and M-mode echocardiographic evaluation of fetal arrhythmias. *Clin Cardiol* 8:1, 1985.
6. DeVore GR: Fetal echocardiography—a new frontier. *Clin Obstet Gynecol* 27:359, 1984.
7. DeVore GR, Siassi B, Platt LD: Fetal echocardiography. III. The diagnosis of cardiac arrhythmias using real-time–directed M-mode ultrasound. *Am J Obstet Gynecol* 146:792, 1983.
8. Eibshitz I, Abinader EG, Klein A, et al: Intrauterine diagnosis and control of fetal ventricular arrhythmia during labor. *Am J Obstet Gynecol* 122:597, 1975.
9. Freeman RK, Garite TJ: Instrumentation artifact detection and fetal arrhythmias, in: *Fetal Heart Rate Monitoring*. Baltimore, Williams & Wilkins, 1981, p. 42.
10. Freistadt H: Fetal bigeminal rhythm. Report of a case. *Am J Obstet Gynecol* 84:13, 1962.
11. Garite TJ, Freeman RK: Case 2—Interpreting another arrhythmia. *Contemporary Obstet Gynecol* September, p. 25, 1984.
12. Gleicher N, Elkayam U: Intrauterine dysrhythmias, in: *Cardiac Problems in Pregnancy*, Elkayam and Gleicher, eds. New York, Alan R. Liss, 1982, p. 535.
13. Hon EH, Hauang HS: The electronic evaluation of fetal heart rate. VII. Premature and missed beats. *Obstet Gynecol* 20:81, 1962.
14. Jenkins HML, Symonds EM: Can fetal electrocardiography improve the prediction of intrapartum fetal acidosis. *Br J Obstet Gynaecol* 93:6, 1986.
15. Kleinman CS, Donnerstein RL, Jaffe CC, et al: Fetal echocardiography. A tool for evaluation of in utero cardiac arrhythmias and monitoring of in utero therapy: Analysis of 71 patients. *Am J Cardiol* 51:237, 1983.
16. Komaromy B, Gaal J, Lampe L: Fetal arrhythmia during pregnancy and labour. *Br J Obstet Gynaecol* 84:492, 1977.
17. Lipman BS, Dunn M, Massie E: *Cardiac Arrhythmias in Clinical Electrocardiography.* 7th ed. New York, Year Book Medical Publishers, 1984, p. 376.
18. Paul RH, Petrie R: *Fetal Intensive Care.* Wallingford, CT, Corometrics Medical Systems, 1979.
19. Scagliotti D, Deal BJ: Arrhythmias in the tiny, premature infant. *Clin Perinatol* 13:339, 1986.
20. Shenker L: Fetal cardiac arrhythmias. *Obstet Gynecol Surv* 34:561, 1979.
21. Silverman ME, Myerburg RJ, Hurst WJ: Arrhythmic patterns due to various interacting mechanisms, in: *Electrocardiography, Basic Concepts and Clinical Application.* New York, McGraw-Hill, 1983, p. 309.
22. Silverman ME, Myerburg RJ, Hurst WJ: Ventricular arrhythmias, in: *Electrocardiography, Basic Concepts and Clinical Application.* New York, McGraw-Hill, 1983, p. 281.
23. Southall DP, Richards J, Hardwick R, et al: Prospective study of fetal heart rate and rhythm patterns. *Arch Dis Child* 55:506, 1980.
24. Young BK, Katz M, Klein SA: Intrapartum fetal cardiac arrhythmias. *Obstet Gynecol* 54:427, 1979.

Atrioventricular Block

Chapter 23

Complete Atrioventricular Block: Fetal Monitoring with Echocardiographic Diagnosis

Atrioventricular block may be defined by the severity of the degree of interference with the passage of the depolarization impulse from the atria to the ventricles. First, second, and third degree blocks are recognized.

First degree atrioventricular block is diagnosed when prolongation of the PR interval is above acceptable limits for the patient's age. Prolongation of the PR interval is difficult to recognize in fetal electrocardiograms, and since pathophysiology has not been associated with this entity in the fetus, it is not discussed further here.

Second degree atrioventricular block is divided into Mobitz type I and type II blocks. Wenckebach's phenomenon is synonymous with Mobitz type I atrioventricular block.

Mobitz type I atrioventricular block (Wenckebach's phenomenon) is recognized by progressive prolongation of the PR interval until a ventricular depolarization is dropped. This produces a pause and may occur in a 2:1, 3:2, etc. pattern.[53] Beat-to-beat monitoring produces a characteristic pattern of parallel close short vertical lines, the lower created by the dropped beat, the upper with the appearance of a sinus or respiratory arrhythmia. See page 416 for the electronic heart rate monitoring appearance of Wenckebach's phenomenon in the adult. This pattern has not been described in the fetus.

Mobitz type II atrioventricular block is recognized by the sudden failure of atrial depolarization to produce ventricular depolarization, resulting in a dropped beat without an antecedent prolongation of the PR interval. This may occur in 2:1, 3:1, 4:1, etc. combinations.[2,8,11,22] This diagnosis is difficult to make in the fetus because at times, even with complete heart block, atrial and ventricular rates may appear to be mathematically related.

Third degree atrioventricular block is synonymous with complete heart block (discussed on pages 41 and 515).

The fetal monitoring trace shows the ventricular heart rate if it is derived from an electrocardiogram, but it may display either ventricular or atrial rates or both if it is Doppler-derived.[21]

Fetal echocardiography that is taken in the aortoatrial plane may demonstrate atrial excursions at multiples of aortic valve opening, for example, atrial contractions at 140 bpm and an aortic valve opening at 70 bpm, confirming a 2:1 atrioventricular block.[15] With complete heart block, independent atrial and ventricular beating may be recognized on real time studies and in the M-mode.[16,17,18,29,30]

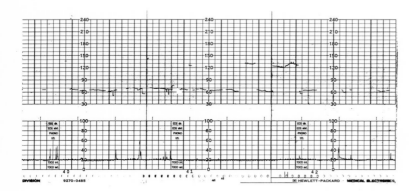

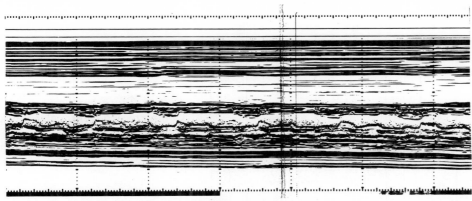

Fetal Echocardiogram

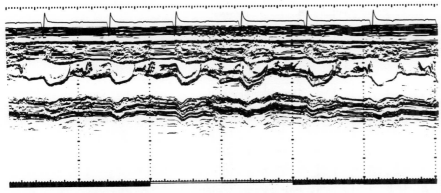

Newborn Echocardiogram

CASE INTERPRETATION: Class III

Baseline Information: there are two heart rates seen: one is in the normal fetal heart rate range, and the other is at one-half that rate in the marked bradycardic range. Variability appears to be decreased in both.

Periodic and Nonperiodic Changes: no accelerations or decelerations are seen.

Uterine Activity: no uterine activity displayed.

Significance: this pattern is seen with half-counting, arrhythmia (atrioventricular block), nonconducted premature supraventricular depolarizations in bigeminy, or a maternal heart rate artifact. Auscultation and a fetal echocardiogram (or electrocardiogram) are needed for further clarification.

Echocardiographic Interpretation: fetal echocardiogram displays an M mode recorded in an unused plane in which the mitral valve and the posterior atrial wall are recorded simultaneously. Motion of the atrial wall is seen at a regular rate in excess of and without relation to the opening of the mitral valve demonstrating that the atrial and ventricular activity are independent.

Newborn Echocardiogram: The accompanying electrocardiogram shows obvious complete heart block with no relationship of the P waves to the QRS. The M mode representation of the mitral valve shows abnormal A waves superimposed on the open mitral valve. These abnormal A waves correspond in timing to the P waves seen on the electrocardiogram.

CASE OUTCOME: Twenty-four-year-old primigravida at 34 weeks' gestation delivered by low transverse cesarean section that was performed for an indication of type I diabetes mellitus, Class F, from a vertex presentation with epidural anesthesia, a 5 pound, 15½ ounce (2707 gram) female; Apgar score 8/9. The newborn had a single ventricle. There was no evidence of maternal collagen vascular disease. The newborn survived until age 3 having undergone numerous cardiac surgical procedures. A fetal echocardiogram and newborn echocardiograms and electrocardiograms revealed a complete atrioventricular block.

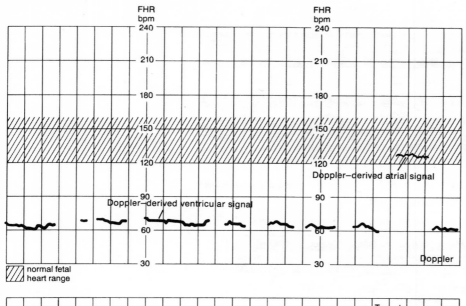

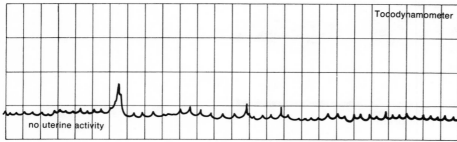

Pattern Characteristic:
Complete Atrioventricular Block

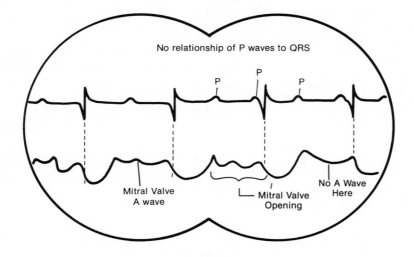

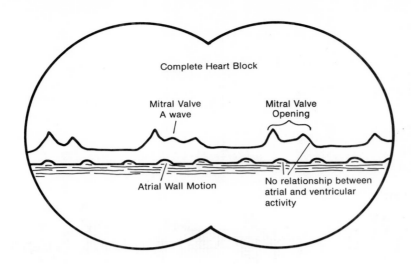

Complete Atrioventricular Block: Fetal Monitoring with Electrocardiographic Diagnosis

*C*omplete (third degree) atrioventricular block is recognized by the failure of any atrial depolarizations to produce ventricular depolarizations. The ventricle is controlled by an escape focus that is either located in the atrioventricular junction or in the ventricle below the atrioventricular junction. The result is that there are independent atrial and ventricular rates, with the ventricular rate typically being slower than the atrial.[35]

If the escape focus controlling the ventricle is junctional, the QRS complex will be narrow and normal. If the focus is ventricular, the QRS complex will be wide and bizarre. Electrocardiographically, this produces a regular ventricular complex at a rate consistent with its junctional or ventricular origin and an independent atrial depolarization rate with no relationship between the P waves and QRS complexes.[4]

The case presented here was studied with abdominal electrocardiography, a technique no longer used. When studied by abdominal electrocardiography, maternal signals are large, whereas they are small or absent when measured by scalp electrode-derived tracings.[18,24,43,44,57] P waves are not distinguishable with abdominal electrocardiography, unlike the case with scalp electrode-derived electrocardiograms.[45,55] Therefore, abdominal electrocardiography is inconclusive for this diagnosis.

Doppler auscultation reveals a bizarre, variable slow ventricular sound, and with repositioning of a Doppler, the more rapid atrial rate.[20,28,39] The external fetal monitor prints the ventricular rate or the atrial rate, depending on the Doppler placement.[21]

The abdominal electrocardiogram or scalp electrode electrocardiogram-derived fetal monitor signal produces a trace of the slower ventricular rate.[19,36] Although usually very regular, it is possible for this rate to vary.

Fetal complete heart block is associated with maternal collagen vascular disease, the conduction defect produced by transplacental antibodies (e.g., anti-Ro [SSA]), directed against fetal cardiac antigens. This produces cardiac tissue damage.[6,9,10,14,19,26,27,32,33,36,37,40,41,46,47,56,58,59] Fetal hydrops may result from the effects of low tissue perfusion, but may also be produced by an immune mechanism that is responsive to maternally administered steroid therapy.[5,7,31,48] Congenital complete atrioventricular block has a 30% to 50% risk of associated cardiac structural defects.[1,12,13,23,25,42,49,51] When accompanied by collagen vascular disease, the risk of cardiac malformations is approximately 23%, but these are usually not complex or fatal.[52] Complex lesions with atrioventricular canal defects and isomerism have been reported in cases without maternal connective tissue disease. These are usually fatal.[5,38,50,52]

Fetal heart block has also been reported with fetal cytomegalovirus infection.[34]

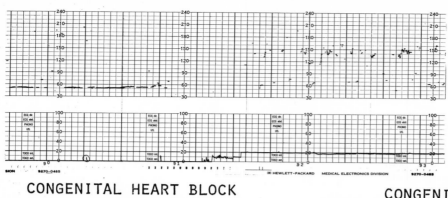

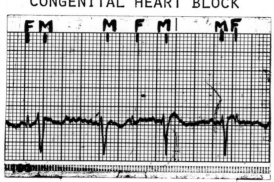

CONGENITAL HEART BLOCK

ABDOMINAL EKG

Original enhanced at time of patient care.

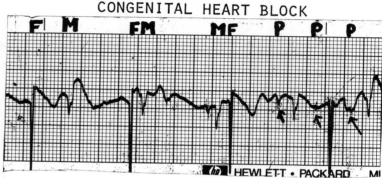

CONGENITAL HEART BLOCK

SCALP ELECTRODE EKG

CASE INTERPRETATION: Class III

Baseline Information: there are two heart rates seen: one in the normal fetal heart range, with a suggestion of normal variability; and one with absent (flat-line) short- and long-term variability in the marked fetal heart range.

Periodic or Nonperiodic Changes: none displayed.

Uterine Activity: no uterine activity displayed, no recording in some areas.

Significance: this pattern is seen with maternal heart rate half counting or arrhythmia (atrioventricular block). The lower trace is not one-half the upper trace so half counting fetal heart rate and nonconducted premature supraventricular depolarizations in bigeminy are not appropriate considerations in this differential diagnosis.

Electrocardiographic Interpretation: abdominal electrocardiogram. The paper speed is 25 mm/sec. Small, narrow fetal QRS complexes are seen at a regular rate of 55 bpm; the P waves are not recognizable. The maternal electrocardiogram shows a heart rate of 92 bpm. On the basis of the extremely slow fetal rate, complete atrioventricular block is suspected.

Fetal (scalp electrode) electrocardiogram: paper speed is 25 mm/sec. There is a fetal heart rate of 57 bpm. Random P waves are seen. Maternal QRS complexes are recognized at a rate of 75 bpm. This is compatible with a diagnosis of congenital complete atrioventricular block (complete heart block). The fetal QRS is significantly narrower than the maternal QRS on this tracing, as on the abdominal electrocardiogram. However, the amplitude of the QRS deflection is greater on the fetal complexes in this electrocardiogram, whereas it is greater on the maternal complexes on the abdominal electrocardiogram.

CASE OUTCOME: Eighteen-year-old gravida 4, para 3003, at 40 weeks' gestation delivered vaginally, with low forceps and epidural anesthesia, a 7 pound, 13 ounce (3544 gram) female; Apgar score 9/9. The newborn heart rate was greater than 70 bpm. The newborn did not require a pacemaker. Maternal evaluation for collagen vascular disease was negative. The tracing was obtained by an abdominal electrocardiographic recording of the ventricular rate, followed by a Doppler recording of the atrial rate. See page 41 for the scalp electrode-derived fetal monitoring pattern of the same patient.

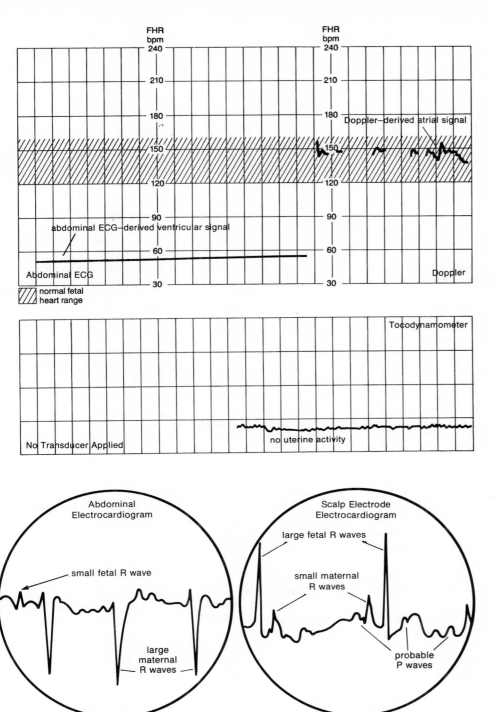

Pattern Characteristic:
Complete Atrioventricular Block

References

1. Abdulla U, Charters DW: Congenital heart block diagnosed antenatally associated with multiple fetal abnormality. *Br Med J* 4:263, 1975.
2. Allan LD, Anderson RH, Sullivan ID, et al: Evaluation of fetal arrhythmias by echocardiography. *Br Heart J* 50:240, 1983.
3. Altenburger KM, Jedziniak M, Roper WL, et al: Congenital complete heart block associated with hydrops fetalis. *J Ped* 91:618, 1977.
4. Armstrong DH, Murata Y, Martin CB, et al: Antepartum detection of congenital complete fetal heart block: A case report. *Am J Obstet Gynecol* 126:291, 1976.
5. Baxi L, Bierman F, Ursell P: Evaluation of complete heart block in a fetus and its perinatal management. *Am J Perinat* 4:348, 1987.
6. Berube S, Lister G, Toews WH, et al: Congenital heart block and maternal systemic lupus erythematosus. *Am J Obstet Gynecol* 130:595, 1978.
7. Bierman FZ, Baxi L, Jaffe I, et al: Fetal hydrops and congenital complete heart block: Response to maternal steroid therapy. *J Ped* 112:646, 1988.
8. Boos R, Auer L, Ruttgers H, et al: A contribution to the monitoring of fetal arrhythmias. *J Perinat Med* 10:85, 1982.
9. Carter JB, Dlieden LC, Edwards JE: Congenital heart block. Anatomic correlations and review of the literature. *Arch Pathol* 97:51, 1974.
10. Chameides L, Truex RC, Vetter V, et al: Association of maternal systemic lupus erythematosus with congenital complete heart block. *N Engl J Med* 297:1204, 1977.
11. Chan T-S, Potter RT, Liu L: Congenital intraventricular tri fascicular block. *Am J Dis Child* 125:82, 1973.
12. Chatterjee MS, Kenel-Pierre C, Sekar S, et al: Prenatal diagnosis of complete heart block. *Am J Obstet Gynecol* 151:1082, 1985.
13. Crawford CS: Antenatal diagnosis of fetal cardiac abnormalities. *Annals of Clinical and Laboratory Science* 12:99, 1982.
14. Crawford D, Chapman M, Allan L: The assessment of persistent bradycardia in prenatal life. *Br J Obstet Gynaecol* 92:941, 1985.
15. Crowley DC, Dick M, Rayburn WF, et al: Two-dimensional and M-mode echocardiographic evaluation of fetal arrhythmia. *Clin Cardiol* 8:1, 1985.
16. DeVore GR: Fetal echocardiography—a new frontier. *Clin Obstet Gynecol* 27:359, 1984.
17. DeVore GR, Siassi B, Platt LD: Fetal echocardiography. III. The diagnosis of cardiac arrhythmias using real-time-directed M-mode ultrasound. *Am J Obstet Gynecol* 146:792, 1983.
18. Dunn HP: Antenatal diagnosis of congenital heart block. *J Obstet Gynecol Brit Empire* 67:1006, 1960.
19. Esscher E, Scott JS: Congenital heart block and maternal systemic lupus erythematosus. *Brit Med J* 1:1235, 1979.
20. Freeman RK, Garite TJ: Instrumentation, artifact detection and arrhythmias, in: *Fetal Heart Rate Monitoring*, Freeman RK, Garite TJ (eds.). Baltimore, Williams & Wilkins, 1981, p. 28.
21. Garite TJ, Freeman RK: Case 2. Intermittent complete heart block unusual. *Contemporary OB/GYN* February: 15, 1983.
22. Gleicher N, Elkayam U: Intrauterine dysrhythmias, in: *Cardiac Problems in Pregnancy*, Liss AR (ed.), New York, 1982, p. 535.
23. Gochberg SH: Congenital heart block. *Am J Obstet Gynecol* 88:238, 1964.
24. Hamilton LA, Fisher E, Horn C, et al: A new prenatal cardiac diagnostic device for congenital heart disease. *Obstet Gynecol* 50:491, 1977.
25. Hawrylyshyn PA, Miskin M, Gilbert BW, et al: The role of echocardiography in fetal cardiac arrhythmias. *Am J Obstet Gynecol* 141:223, 1981.
26. Ho SY, Esscher E, Anderson RH, et al: Anatomy of congenital complete heart block and relation to maternal anti-Ro antibodies. *Am J Cardiol* 58:291, 1986.
27. Hull D, Binns BAD, Joyce D: Congenital heart block and widespread fibrosis due to maternal lupus erythematosus. *Arch Dis Child* 41:688, 1966.
28. Iverson O, Lossius P, Lovset T, et al: Case report: Complete fetal heart block diagnosed by ultrasound. *Acta Obstet Gynecol Scand* 64:533, 1985.
29. Kleinman CS, Donnerstein RL, Jaffe CC, et al: Fetal echocardiography. A tool for evaluation of in utero cardiac arrhythmias and monitoring of in utero therapy: Analysis of 71 patients. *Am J Cardiology* 51:237, 1983.
30. Kleinman CS, Hobbins JC, Jaffer CC, et al: Echocardiographic studies of the human fetus: Prenatal diagnosis of congenital heart disease and cardiac dysrhythmias. *Pediatrics* 65:1059, 1980.
31. Komaromy B, Gaal J, Lampe L: Fetal arrhythmia during pregnancy and labour. *Brit J Obstet Gynaecol* 84:492, 1977.
32. Kosmetatos N, Blackman MS, Elrad H, et al: Congenital complete heart block in the infant of a woman with collagen vascular disease. *J Reprod Med* 22:213, 1979.
33. Lee LA, Bias WB, Arnett FC, et al: Immunogenetics of the neonatal lupus syndrome. *Ann Intern Med* 99:592, 1983.
34. Lewis PE, Cefalo RC, Zaritsky AL: Fetal heart block caused by cytomegalovirus. *Am J Obstet Gynecol* 136:967, 1980.
35. Lipman BS, Dunn M, Massie E: *Cardiac Arrhythmias in Clinical Electrocardiography*, 7th ed. Chicago, Year Book Medical Publishers, 1984. p. 376.
36. Litsey SE, Noonan JA, O'Conoor WN, et al: Maternal connective tissue disease and congenital heart block. Demonstration of immunoglobulin in cardiac tissue. *N Engl J Med* 312:98, 1985.

37. Lumpkin LR, Hall J, Hogan JD, et al: Neonatal lupus erythematosus: A report of three cases associated with anti-Ro/SSA antibodies. *Arch Dermatol* 121:377, 1985.

38. Maehad MVZ, Tynan MJ, Corry PVL, et al: Fetal complete heart block. *Br Heart J* 60:512, 1988.

39. Madison JR, Sukhum P, Williamson DP, et al: Echocardiography and fetal heart sounds in the diagnosis of fetal heart block. *Am Heart J* 98:505, 1979.

40. McCue CM, Mantakas ME, Tinglestad JB, et al: Congenital heart block in newborns of mothers with connective tissue disease. *Circulation* 56:82, 1977.

41. Moore PJ: Maternal systemic lupus erythematosus associated with fetal congenital heart block. *SA Med J*, 60:285, 1981.

42. Nakamura FF, Nadas AS: Complete heart block in infants and children. *N Engl J Med* 270:1261, 1964.

43. Oldenburg JT, Macklin M: Changes in the conduction of the fetal electrocardiogram to the maternal abdominal surface during gestation. *Am J Obstet Gynecol* 129:425, 1977.

44. Plant RK, Steven RA: Complete A-V block in a fetus. *Am Heart J* 30:615, 1945.

45. Platt LD, Manning FA, Gray C, et al: Antenatal detection of fetal A-V dissociation utilizing real-time B-mode ultrasound. *Obstet Gynecol* 53:595, 1979.

46. Provost TT, Watson R, Gammon WR, et al: The neonatal lupus syndrome associated with U.RNP (nRNP) antibodies. *N Engl J Med* 316:1135, 1987.

47. Reid RL, Pancham SR, Kean WF, et al: Maternal and neonatal implications of congenital complete heart block in the fetus. *Obstet Gynecol* 54:470, 1979.

48. Richards DSV, Cabaniss ML, Wagman AJ: Fetal ascites not due to congestive heart failure in a fetus with lupus-induced heart block. *Obstet Gynecol* 76:957, 1990.

49. Scagliotti D, Deal BJ: Arrhythmias in the tiny, premature infant. *Clinics in Perinatology* 13:339, 1986.

50. Schmidt KG, Ulmer HE, Silverman NH, et al: Perinatal outcome of complete atrioventricular block. *J Am Coll Cardiol* 17:1360, 1991.

51. Shenker L: Fetal cardiac arrhythmias. *Obstet Gynecol Survey* 34:561, 1979.

52. Shenker L, Reed KL, Anderson CF, et al: Congenital heart block and cardiac anomalies in the absence of maternal connective tissue disease. *Am J Obstet Gynecol* 157:248, 1987.

53. Silverman ME, Myerburg RJ, Hurst JW: Abnormalities of conduction and heart block in electrocardiography. Basic concepts and clinical appreciation. New York, McGraw Hill Book, 1984, p. 299.

54. Singsen BH, Akhter JE, Weinstein MM, et al: Congenital complete heart block and SSA antibodies: Obstetric implications. *Am J Obstet Gynecol* 152:655, 1985.

55. Sokol RJ, Hutchison P, Krouskop RW, et al: Congenital complete heart block diagnosed during intrauterine fetal monitoring. *Am J Obstet Gynecol* 120:1115, 1974.

56. Taylor PV, Scott JS, Gerlis LM, et al: Maternal antibodies against fetal cardiac antigens in congenital complete heart block. *N Engl J Med* 315:667, 1986.

57. Teteris NJ, Chisholm JW, Ullery JC: Antenatal diagnosis of congenital heart block. *Obstet Gynecol* 32:851, 1968.

58. Veille JC, Sunderland C, Bennete RM: Complete heart block in a fetus associated with maternal Sjögren's syndrome. *Am J Obstet Gynecol* 151:660, 1985.

59. Watson R: Neonatal lupus syndrome. *Ped Annals* 15:605, 1986.

Dysrhythmias Masked by Instrument Characteristics

Chapter 24

Dysrhythmia Masked by Doppler Signal Processing

*A*ll external fetal heart rate monitors have artifact rejection logic. This is necessary to present a clean fetal heart rate trace that is free of extraneous signals produced by innumerable sources of motion such as fetal motion, intestinal motion, and maternal vessel motion. This signal rejection exists at the expense of the loss of cardiac signals during dysrhythmias, specifically the loss of the beats produced by premature depolarizations and the beats following compensatory pauses.[1,2,6]

Due to the fact that the scalp electrode presents an electrocardiogram-derived signal, there is less extraneous "noise" produced by maternal and fetal motion and,

therefore, artifact-rejection logic for that purpose is not mandatory. However, artifacts may be produced by electrical signals simulating or masking the fetal R wave, so that use of artifact rejection logic is an option with internal monitoring. Again, this logic is at the expense of the loss of dysrhythmia-produced beats, which are outside the rate of the normal cardiac cycles of the monitored fetus. When such logic is not engaged, the scalp electrode presents the full dysrhythmia pattern.[1]

Auscultation identifies the irregular heart rate that is not "seen" by the external monitoring.

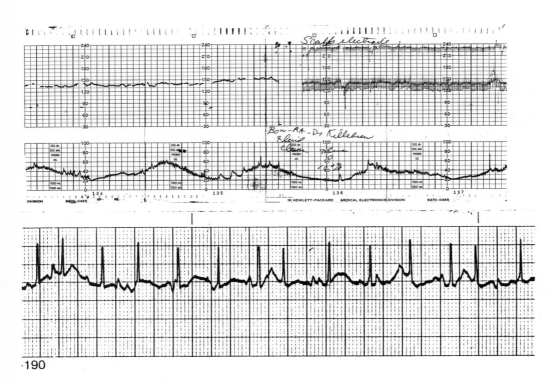

·190

CASE INTERPRETATION: Class I-III

Baseline Information: a normal heart rate, decreased to average variability. Vertical spikes appear at the onset of internal monitoring. Horizontal parallel lines are produced.

Periodic or Nonperiodic Changes: none displayed.

Uterine Activity: prolonged contractions with a minimal resting phase.

Significance: there is the appearance of premature supraventricular depolarizations occurring in a regular pattern, every fourth beat. An electrocardiogram is needed for confirmation. A dysrhythmia is not displayed until the scalp electrode presents signals without the logic operative.

Electrocardiographic Interpretation: fetal electrocardiogram. The paper speed is 25 mm/sec. The heart rate is 145 bpm. The basic rhythm is sinus. Every fourth beat is a premature atrial depolarization. This is recognized by the premature occurrence of a normal narrow QRS complex preceded by a P wave, which deforms the downslope of the T wave of the preceding normal sinus complex. The compensatory pause following these premature depolarizations is not complete. This pattern is compatible with premature atrial depolarizations, which occur every fourth beat.

CASE OUTCOME: Fourteen-year-old primigravida at term delivered vaginally, with local and pudendal anesthesia, a 7 pound, 10 ounce (3459 gram) male; Apgar score 9/9. The fetus was in an occiput anterior position. The infant followed an uncomplicated newborn course, with no cardiac disease detected.

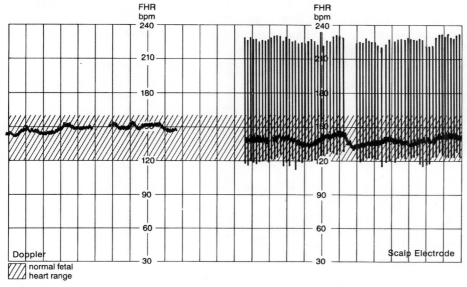

Pattern Characteristic:
Masked Arrhythmia: Doppler Signal Processing

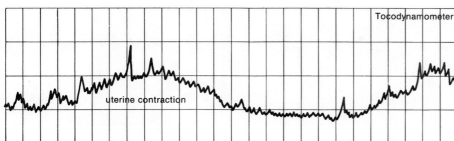

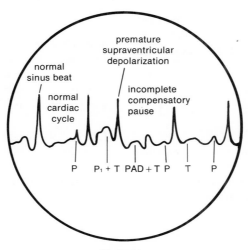

Masked by
Doppler Signal Processing

Dysrhythmia Masked by Engagement of Instrument Logic

*I*nternal fetal monitoring using the scalp electrode has an option of artifact-rejection logic. The advantage of such logic is to clean the R wave-derived signal from erroneous vertical spikes that are produced by such artifacts as maternal QRS interference, displacement of the electrode by the uterine cervix, and inconsistent identification of the fetal R wave. The disadvantage to using the instrument logic is that vertical spikes produced by dysrhythmias are also discarded.[1,6] Often, the stylus places a dot at the point of maximum excursion of what

would have been a vertical spike, but the pen-lift feature produced by engaging the logic prevents the pen from traversing the fetal monitor paper. The dysrhythmia is suspected by the auscultation of an irregular heart rate, the "dotted line" appearance of the fetal heart trace, and the regularity of unconnected dots appearing parallel to the fetal heart trace.

Disengagement of the logic allows the dysrhythmia to be demonstrated.[2,7]

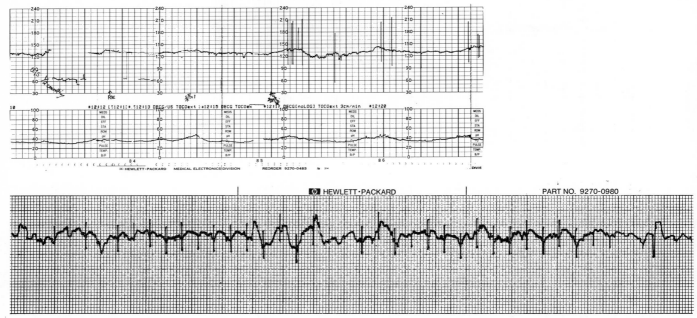

Original tracing enhanced for clarity.

CASE INTERPRETATION: Class I

Baseline Information: a normal heart rate, decreased to average variability. Vertical spikes above and below the baseline appear after onset of the logic adjustment.

Periodic or Nonperiodic Changes: a single, small V-shaped variable deceleration. Accelerations are present.

Uterine Activity: small contractions of normal frequency, as measured by a tocodynamometer.

Significance: there is the appearance of either premature supraventricular or ventricular depolarizations or artifact. An electrocardiogram and auscultation are needed for clarification. Spikes appear when the logic is not operative ("pen-lift" is disengaged).

Electrocardiographic Interpretation: fetal electrocardiogram. The paper speed is 12.5 mm/sec. There are narrow QRS complexes at a regular rate of 138 bpm, which are presumed to be sinus rhythm. Two wide and bizarre premature complexes are noted. The polarity of these premature complexes is negative. The compensatory pause is complete. The premature complexes are compatible with premature ventricular depolarizations.

CASE OUTCOME: Twenty-three-year-old gravida 3, para 2002, at 40 weeks' gestation delivered vaginally, with local anesthesia, a 6 pound, 12 ounce (3062 gram) female; Apgar score 8/9. The infant followed a normal newborn course.

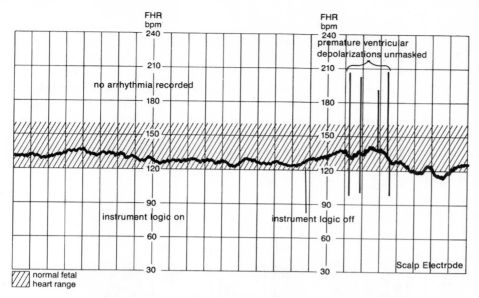

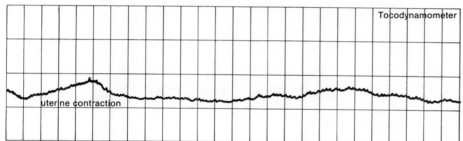

Pattern Characteristic:
Masked Arrhythmia: Instrument Logic

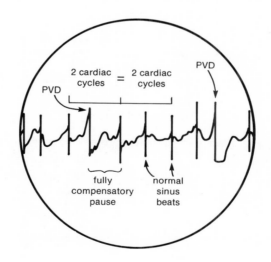

Dysrhythmia Masked by Transmission Logic

*R*emote transmission of both externally (Doppler) and internally (R wave) derived fetal heart signals is possible. Doppler signal processing always includes use of the artifact rejection logic to exclude extraneous signals produced by various maternal and fetal motion other than fetal heart activity. With scalp electrode usage, artifact-rejection logic is optional. It is usually desirable not to engage the logic when obtaining R-wave derived signals so as not to lose important information allowing identification of cardiac arrhythmias.[1]

However, remote transmission, because it must transfer information from both external and internal monitoring, includes logic.[4] Therefore, dysrhythmias may be masked in transmission.

The dysrhythmia is suspected because of the dotted-line appearance of the fetal heart trace and the unconnected dots appearing parallel to the fetal heart trace.

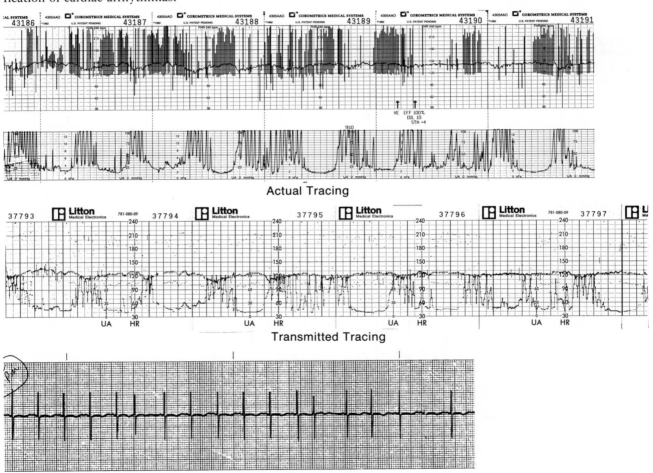

Actual Tracing

Transmitted Tracing

Original tracing enhanced for clarity.

OHIO MEDICAL PRODUCTS   RECORDER PAPER   309-3215-3(

CASE INTERPRETATION: Class I

Baseline Information: the first tracing displays a normal heart rate and average variability. There are vertical spikes above and below the fetal heart trace, with occasionally interspersed downward vertical spikes. These are not seen on the second tracing, although dots appear at the extremes of the pen excursions.

Periodic or Nonperiodic Changes: accelerations are present.

Uterine Activity: frequent, skewed contractions, with maternal activity superimposed.

Significance: there is the appeearence of premature supraventricular depolarizations that are intermittently nonconducted, producing "dropped beats." An electrocardiogram is needed for diagnosis. The logic is operative in the production of the second tracing.

Electrocardiographic Interpretation: Newborn electrocardiogram: the paper speed is 25 mm/sec, the heart rate is 125 bpm. The basic rhythm is sinus. The fourth beat is premature, it resembles the dominant sinus beat. The compensatory pause is not complete. This represents a premature atrial depolarization. After the tenth beat, there is a pause followed by resumption of the sinus rhythm. This pattern is compatible with nonconducted premature supraventricular depolarization (although a sinus pause is not excluded).

CASE OUTCOME: Twenty-four-year-old primigravida at 40 weeks' gestation delivered vaginally from a vertex presentation, with pudendal anesthesia, a 7 pound, 13½ ounce (3099 gram) male; Apgar score 9/10. The newborn electrocardiogram showed transient premature supraventricular depolarizations; there was no structural heart disease.

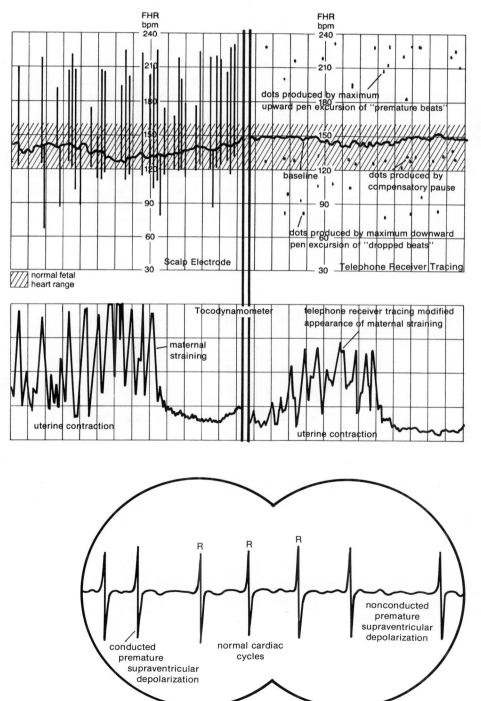

Pattern Characteristic:
Masked Arrhythmia:
Transmission Logic

Premature Supraventricular and Ventricular Depolarizations Rejected as Artifact

*E*ach fetal monitor has a template for identification of R waves. It is carefully designed to exclude fetal P and T waves and maternal QRS signals if at all possible. This template recognizes certain physical characteristics of a depolarization, including the rate of rise of the deflection as well as the absolute size of the deflection. If a premature or ectopic beat does not meet recognition characteristics of this template, the ectopic activity is simply rejected and the resultant compensatory pause recorded.[3,4] This may occur because of the bizarre configuration of ventricular depolarizations or with aberrant conduction, which may occur in supraventricular beats. Aberration implies that depolarization of the ventricle takes place over pathways that differ from the usual depolarization pathways. These are recognized by premature depolarizations that grossly resemble the normal dominant beat. They may or may not be preceded by a P wave which, when present, may deform the T wave of the preceding normal beat. These often appear at "splintered" ventricular complexes, and the QRS duration may be slightly greater than the QRS duration of the normal beats.

An aberration may occur because of the prematurity of the atrial depolarization. The impulse finds the conduction pathways not sufficiently recovered from the prior normal beat, so that the impulse preferentially follows abnormal depolarizing routes.

An electrocardiogram is needed to identify aberrance. If the QRS of the premature beat retains a sufficient number of characteristics of the dominant beat for machine recognition, the beat is usually printed. If the aberrance is marked, the beat may be rejected as artifact, with only a downward vertical deflection appearing in the trace.

This machine characteristic cannot be altered by the machine user but is dependent on characteristics built in by the manufacturer.[4]

A second circumstance under which a premature depolarization is rejected is if the depolarization occurs too soon after the preceding normal QRS—by less than 250 milliseconds—which is the "refractory period" of the instrument.[5]

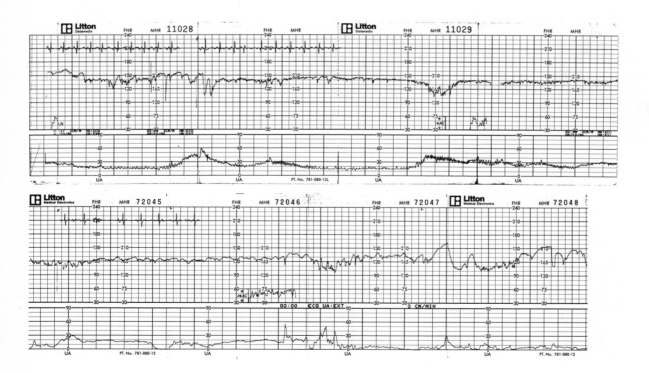

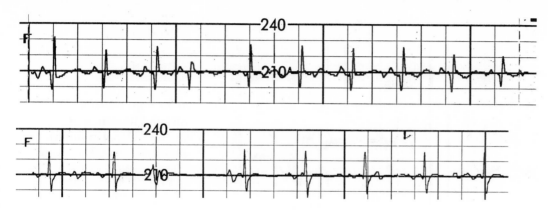

SUPRAVENTRICULAR CASE INTERPRETATION: Class I-II

Baseline Information: a normal heart rate, average variability, and occasional vertical spikes, suggest artifact or an arrhythmia.

Periodic or Nonperiodic Changes: possible late deceleration associated with a prolonged contraction.

Uterine Activity: discordant pattern.

Significance: a mildly stressed fetus; an electrocardiogram is needed to distinguish artifact from arrhythmia (automatically triggered in this case). There is a vertical spike configuration such as that of premature supraventricular depolarizations, both conducted and nonconducted.

Electrocardiographic Interpretation: fetal electrocardiogram. The paper speed is 25 mm/sec (computer corrected), the heart rate is 143 bpm. Premature QRS complexes are seen. These are narrow and closely resemble QRS complexes of the sinus beats. There is, however, diminution of amplitude in the terminal portion of the QRS complex, and this probably represents a minor degree of aberration. These premature QRS complexes are preceded by a P wave and the compensatory pause is not complete. This pattern is compatible with premature atrial depolarizations with a minor degree of aberration.

SUPRAVENTRICULAR CASE OUTCOME: Nineteen-year-old primigravida at 42 weeks' gestation delivered vaginally, with local anesthesia, a 7 pound, 3 ounce (1559 gram) female; Apgar score 9/10. The infant followed an uncomplicated newborn course. No cardiac irregularity was noted.

VENTRICULAR CASE INTERPRETATION: Class I

Baseline Information: a normal heart rate and average variability. A single downward vertical deflection to 55 bpm triggers a recording of the arrhythmia/artifact detector.

Periodic or Nonperiodic Changes: shallow accelerations, mild variable decelerations.

Uterine Activity: irregular deflections seen on the tocodynamometer trace are not interpretable.

Significance: a healthy fetus is predicted. The "dropped beat" may be nonconducted premature supraventricular depolarizations, a weak signal, or unrecognized QRS complexes. An electrocardiographic interpretation clarifies the etiology in this instance.

Electrocardiographic Interpretation: fetal electrocardiogram. The paper speed is 25 mm/sec. The heart rate is 118 bpm. After the second sinus depolarization there is a wide and bizarre biphasic depolarization that occurs prematurely. No P wave is recognized preceding this complex. The compensatory pause is complete. This is probably a ventricular premature depolarization, although the possibility of artifact cannot be excluded.

VENTRICULAR CASE OUTCOME: Twenty-seven-year-old gravida 3, para 1001, at term delivered vaginally from a vertex presentation, with pudendal anesthesia, a 7 pound, 6 ounce (3345 gram) male; Apgar score 6/9. The infant followed an uncomplicated newborn course. Premature depolarizations of an identical appearance were recorded sporadically by the artifact/arrhythmia detector electrocardiogram throughout labor, although only one premature beat is displayed here, making a random artifact a possibility.

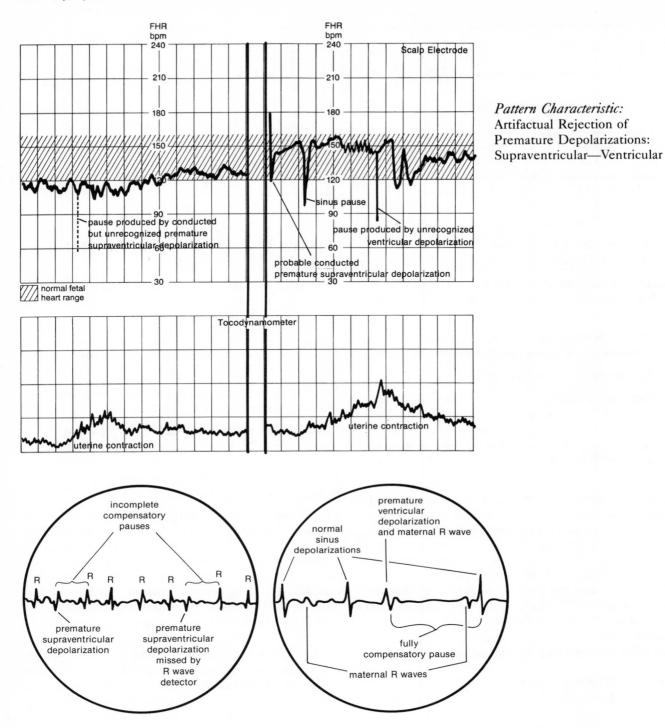

Pattern Characteristic:
Artifactual Rejection of
Premature Depolarizations:
Supraventricular—Ventricular

Artifactual Rejection of the Sinus R Wave
(In Favor of a Premature Depolarization)

*T*he fetal monitor is a computer programmed to identify and "count" the fetal R wave of the QRS electrical signal. The interval between R waves is then translated via computer to a beat-to-beat rate that forms the basis of the heart rate printed trace. The monitor is programmed to not "look for" the next fetal QRS signal for a period of time (usually 250 milliseconds) after counting an R wave. During this "window" of time, the tallest signal with features most like the usual fetal R wave is selected. The purpose of this feature is to reduce artifact (e.g., avoid counting maternal R waves or electrical "noise"). It has the disadvantage of masking an arrhyth-

mia when the premature beat occurs very close to the normal cycle beat.

A rare artifact produced by this programming is rejection of the normal cycle beat in favor of the premature beat when the latter "looks more like" a normal fetal R wave than the actual sinus beat. The end effect in the case demonstrated here is reminiscent of the fetal monitoring trace of the Wenckebach phenomenon (see page 415) and respiratory arrhythmia (see page 462), both characterized by a downward vertical spike and intervening upward undulations.

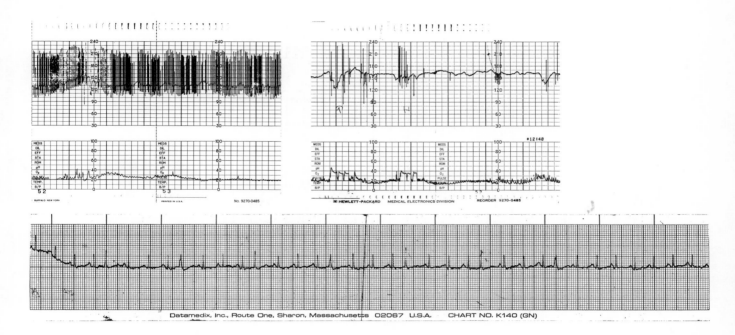

CASE INTERPRETATION: Class I

Baseline Information: normal rate, average variability. In early labor, the baseline is almost obscured by vertical spikes that are predominantly above the baseline with continuous brief downward excursions. These are rare in late labor. An unusual pattern is seen of short, downward vertical spikes separated by a stepwise trend back to baseline over the next two beats.

Periodic or Nonperiodic Changes: accelerations in early labor, mild variable decelerations in late labor.

Uterine Activity: maternal straining is seen with some contractions in late labor.

Significance: premature depolarizations are most likely supraventricular in origin, with bigeminal, trigeminal,

and quadrageminal patterns. Both premature beats and the short, downward vertical spikes need electrocardiographic (or echocardiographic) study for a precise diagnosis.

Electrocardiographic Interpretation: fetal electrocardiogram. The paper speed is 25 mm/sec. The heart rate is 165 bpm. The basic rhythm is sinus tachycardia. Following every third sinus depolarization, a premature depolarization is seen. This complex has greater amplitude and a slightly widened form, as compared to the preceding sinus complex. Definite P waves cannot be identified preceding these complexes. These are compatible with supraventricular depolarizations, with a slight aberration occurring every fourth beat.

CASE OUTCOME: Twenty-eight-year-old gravida 2, para 0010, at 41 weeks' gestation delivered vaginally, with epidural anesthesia, a 9 pound, 4 ounce female; Apgar score 9/9. The infant followed an uncomplicated newborn course. The dysrhythmia that was detected several weeks prior to delivery disappeared during the second stage of labor and was not detected in the healthy newborn.

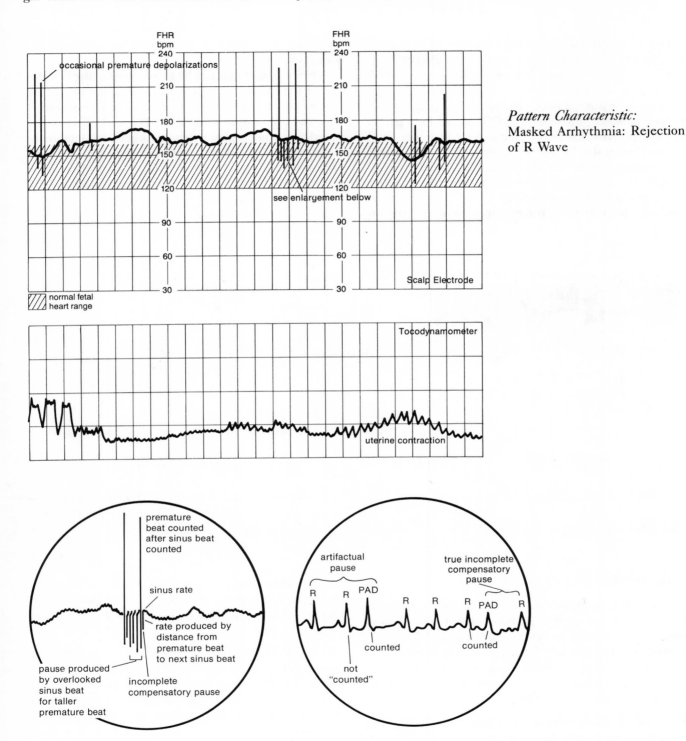

Pattern Characteristic:
Masked Arrhythmia: Rejection of R Wave

References

1. Beall MH, Paul RH: Artifacts, blocks, and arrhythmias: Confusing nonclassical heart rate tracings. *Clinical Obstet Gynecol* 29:83, 1986.
2. Boos R, Ruttgers H, Kubli F, et al: A contribution to the monitoring of fetal arrhythmias. *J Perinat Med* 10:85, 1982.
3. Crawford CS: Antenatal diagnosis of fetal cardiac abnormalities. *Annals of Clinic and Laboratory Science* 12:99, 1982.
4. Fisher T, Litton Datametrix: Personal communication.
5. Freeman RK, Garite TJ: Instrumentation, artifact detection, and fetal arrhythmias, in: *Fetal Heart Rate Monitoring.* Baltimore, Williams & Wilkins, 1981, p. 28.
6. Newman J: Intrauterine electrocardiography, in: *Cardiac Problems in Pregnancy.* Alan R. Liss, 1982, p. 475.
7. Miller FC, Paul RH: Intrapartum fetal heart rate monitoring. *Clin Obstet Gynecol* 21:561, 1978.

Artifacts

Chapter 25

Factitious Pause Produced by Indistinct Fetal QRS Signal

*T*he scalp electrode transmits fetal QRS signals to a computer in the fetal monitor. The signals are processed in various ways. The R wave (or point of maximum deflection of the QRS complex) is identified. The interval between successive R waves is measured and is converted to a heart rate, the heart rate is updated for each beat-to-beat interval.

The measurement of beat-to-beat variability depends upon a QRS deflection size that is sufficient for instrument recognition.[2] When orientation of the single lead recorded in fetal electrocardiography is altered (as by fetal movement), a marked diminution in the QRS signal may occur with the failure of the instrument to recognize the QRS, and a pause is recorded.

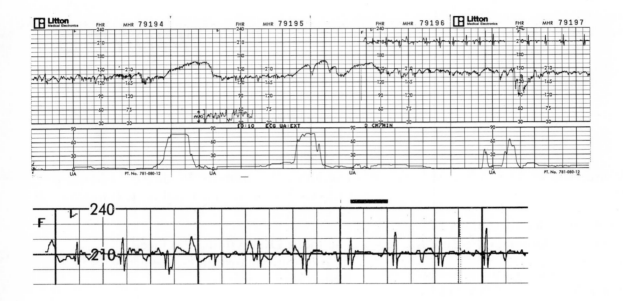

CASE INTERPRETATION: Class I

Baseline Information: normal fetal heart rate and average variability. A single downward vertical spike to 80 bpm triggers a recording of the arrhythmia/artifact detector.

Periodic or Nonperiodic Changes: nonperiodic accelerations and mild variable decelerations.

Uterine Activity: infrequent contractions of varying configurations, as measured with an external monitor.

Significance: a healthy fetus is anticipated. A downward vertical spike or "dropped beat" may be produced by a nonconducted premature supraventricular depolarization, a weak QRS signal, or failure of the machine to recognize the QRS signal. The electrocardiogram clarifies the diagnosis in this instance.

Electrocardiographic Interpretation: fetal electrocardiogram. The paper speed is 25 mm/sec (computer corrected), and the heart rate is 155 bpm. The basic rhythm is sinus. Following the second sinus beat, the next sinus beat fails to display an upright R wave. This is followed by an obvious artifact, and the next sinus depolarization is minute (almost obscured).

CASE OUTCOME: Thirty-one-year-old gravida 5, para 4004, at 42 weeks' gestation delivered vaginally, precipitously, from a vertex presentation, an 8 pound, 9 ounce (3884 gram) female; Apgar score 9/10. The infant followed an uncomplicated newborn course.

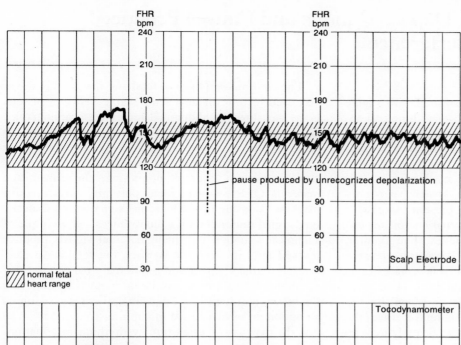

pause produced by unrecognized depolarization

Scalp Electrode

/// normal fetal heart range

Pattern Characteristic:
Factitious Pause Produced by
Indistinct Fetal QRS Signal

Tocodynamometer

deflection possibly produced by fetal movement

uterine contraction

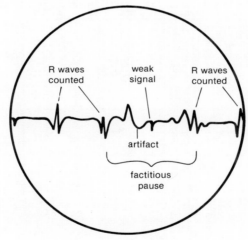

R waves counted

weak signal

R waves counted

artifact

factitious pause

Factitious Premature Depolarizations and Pauses Produced by Maternal QRS Interference

*T*he maternal QRS is typically transmitted with a large R wave in relation to the fetal QRS signal during an abdominal fetal electrocardiogram, a technique no longer used. A fetal heart rate trace is produced by electronically obliterating maternal signals.[11] The maternal QRS is transmitted to varying degrees, if at all, via the fetus to the scalp electrode-derived trace. Usually, it is one-fifth the size of the fetal QRS, if it is present.[7] Occasionally, for unknown reasons, the maternal complexes can approach the size of the fetal complexes. The monitor, programmed to count the prominent R waves, counts the maternal signal, too. Since the maternal heart rate has no relationship to the fetal heart rate, the interval between the dually derived R waves is random.[2] When the maternal R wave is close to the preceding fetal R wave, the machine assumes it to be a premature beat. It may record a fast rate for one beat (upward spike). The machine also may drop beats or pause because of its own refractory period (downward spike). An electrocardiogram is needed to verify the diagnosis of maternal R wave interference. The maternal QRS can be distinguished from the fetal QRS (0.04 seconds) on the electrocardiogram because it is wider (0.08 milliseconds or greater).[10]

The transmission of both fetal and maternal R waves was used historically as a semireliable indicator of fetal lie as measured by abdominal fetal electrocardiography. Concordant R waves correlated most often with breech presentations, and discordant R waves occurred more commonly with vertex presentations.[3,8]

With modern internal monitoring, the transmitted maternal QRS produces an opportunity for artifactual machine counting of the maternal signal rather than the fetal signal under certain circumstances. An example of a clinical situation in which maternal signals produce marked fetal interference is when the fetal scalp electrode is partially embedded in the maternal cervix.[9,10]

Although this artifact can be obliterated by engaging the instrument logic (e.g., pen-lift), which is available as an option on most interval monitoring systems, to do so is at the expense of losing true dysrhythmia information.

The audible sound produced during internal monitoring reproduces the irregularity since it is an artificial sound also derived from the R wave. Doppler or stethoscope auscultation clarifies this pattern, in that no irregularity is heard.

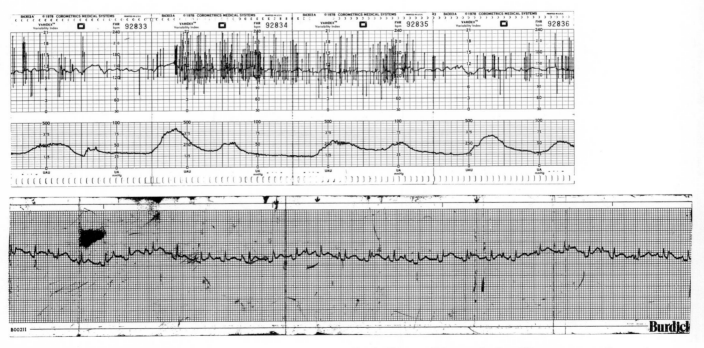

CASE INTERPRETATION: Class I

Baseline Information: a normal heart rate, average variability. Patterns of vertical spikes with an erratic association to the baseline. This may be an artifact or a dysrhythmia.

Periodic or Nonperiodic Changes: small accelerations are present.

Uterine Activity: long contractions with a minimal resting phase.

Significance: needs electrocardiogram for diagnosis. Probable maternal QRS counting because of bizarre pattern.

Electrocardiographic Interpretation: fetal electrocardiogram. The paper speed is 25 mm/sec. The fetal heart rate is 140 bpm. The maternal heart rate is 105 bpm. The maternal QRS is wider than the fetal QRS. However, the amplitude is comparable to that of the fetal QRS. Because of the varying rates, varying relationships of the maternal and fetal complexes occur.

CASE OUTCOME: Nineteen-year-old primigravida, at term delivered vaginally from a vertex presentation, with pudendal anesthesia, a 6 pound, 10 ounce (3005 gram) male; Apgar score 8/9. The infant followed an uncomplicated newborn course.

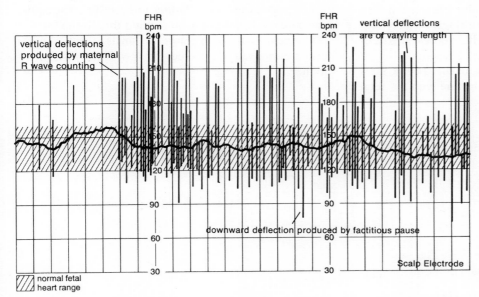

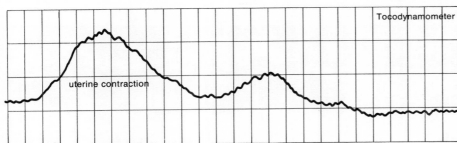

Pattern Characteristic:
Maternal R Wave Interference

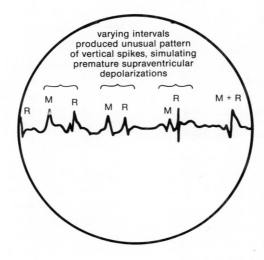

Simulation of Premature Supraventricular Depolarizations Produced by Maternal QRS Interference

*M*aternal heart rate interference during internal monitoring is usually suspected when the appearance of the resulting vertical spikes is very erratic. In contrast, with the exception of fusion beats, most types of premature depolarizations present a fairly reproducible relationship, with the normal depolarizations resulting in a very regular fetal monitoring pattern of parallel vertical spikes of a similar size (reminiscent of a picket fence).

Under certain conditions, because of the specific rates involved, the maternal QRS may interfere with the fetal QRS in a regular fashion that simulates a trigeminal rhythm or other dysrhythmia.

Atypical features of the fetal heart trace, an electrocardiogram identifying prominent maternal QRS complexes, and auscultation failing to identify an irregular heart rate are key findings in making the diagnosis.

The degree to which maternal signals as well as other noise are counted or rejected varies with the instrumentation.[12]

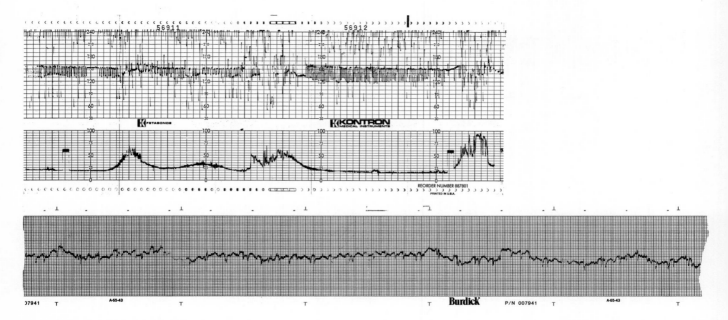

CASE INTERPRETATION: Class III

Baseline Information: four heart rates are identifiable. The upper one is produced by vertical spikes to a level above the 240 bpm limit of the paper. The next one, with reduced variability, occurs at the upper normal fetal heart range. The following one, with some variability suggested, occurs in the normal fetal heart range. The lower one is produced by downward vertical spikes to varying levels below the "normal" fetal heart trace.

Periodic or Nonperiodic Changes: none displayed.

Uterine Activity: increased uterine activity characterized by three contractions occurring in succession without a resting phase. Superimposed maternal activity.

Significance: this looks on the surface like premature supraventricular depolarizations, which occasionally are nonconducted. However, there are some features that are atypical. The upward spikes occur above the usual limits of the instrument. Not all of the upward spikes return immediately to a point below the normal fetal heart trace, as would ordinarily be produced by incomplete compensatory pauses. A similar lack of usual chronologic events is seen throughout the erratic upper trace. An electrocardiogram is needed for clarification.

Electrocardiographic Interpretation: fetal electrocardiogram. The paper speed is 25 mm/sec. The fetal heart rate is 103 bpm. Although wider, the amplitude of the maternal QRS signal is similar to that of the fetal QRS and at times coalesces with the fetal signal. There is no fetal dysrhythmia.

CASE OUTCOME: Seventeen-year-old primigravida at 40 weeks' gestation delivered by low elective forceps, with pudendal and local anesthesia, a 7 pound, 3 ounce (3260 gram) female; Apgar score 8/9. The fetus was in a vertex presentation. The infant followed an uncomplicated newborn course.

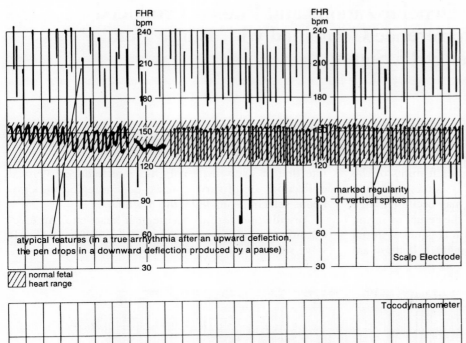

Pattern Characteristic:
Maternal R Wave Interference

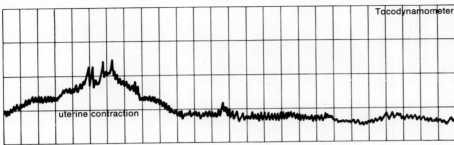

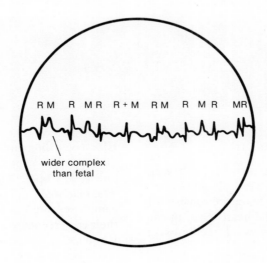

Factitious Premature Depolarizations and Pauses Produced by Maternal QRS Interference Combined with Large Fetal P Waves and Small Fetal QRS Signal

*W*hen the alignment of the single lead vector of the fetal QRS produces a small signal, automatic gain occurs as a computer-directed machine characteristic. This may increase the maternal signal, and other features of the fetal cardiac cycle such as the P or T wave, such that artifactual counting by the machine may occur. (A large fetal P wave has been identified in the fetus, as in the neonate and adult, in association with congenital mitral valve disease with left atrial enlargement.)[5] If these are already prominent, the instrument, programmed to count R waves, now has multiple sources of conflicting information. The resultant fetal monitoring trace is unlike that of solely maternal QRS interference.[2] Vertical deflections are of varying sizes, depending on the erroneous selections made by the machine.

Auscultation verifies no irregular heart rate. An electrocardiogram shows the processed signals from which R wave selections are made.

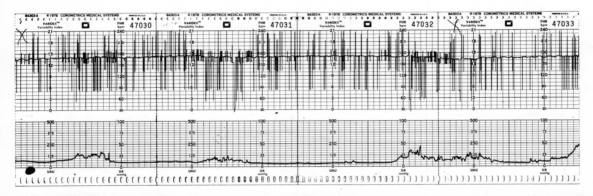

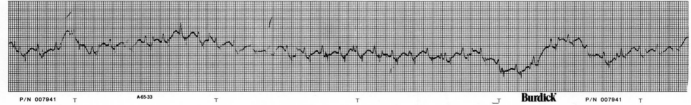

CASE INTERPRETATION: Class III

Baseline Information: moderate tachycardia, average to decreased variability. There are vertical spikes above and below the fetal heart baseline. Some are consistently short and equidistant from the fetal heart trace, in contrast to the other upward and downward needle excursions.

Periodic or Nonperiodic Changes: none displayed.

Uterine Activity: infrequent, prolonged contractions are suggested.

Significance: short vertical spikes are most often seen with atypical features of a QRS configuration. The erratic nature of the remaining spikes favors maternal QRS interference rather than dysrhythmia, but an electrocardiogram is needed for diagnosis.

Electrocardiographic Interpretation: fetal electrocardiogram. The paper speed is 25 mm/sec. The fetal heart rate is 135 bpm. The maternal heart rate is 117 bpm. The maternal QRS complexes, although wider than fetal complexes, are taller in amplitude and are magnified by their coalescence with the large fetal P or the small fetal R waves.

CASE OUTCOME: Twenty-seven-year-old primigravida at 43 weeks' gestation delivered by low transverse cesarean section performed for cephalopelvic disproportion a 9 pound, 3 ounce (4167 gram) male; Apgar score 3/7. The three scalp pHs were each 7.27. There was "moderate" meconium at delivery. The fetus was in a vertex presentation. The newborn electrocardiogram demonstrated no dysrhythmia; there were normal P waves.

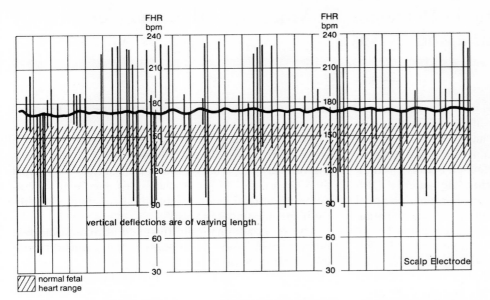

FHR
bpm

FHR
bpm

vertical deflections are of varying length

Scalp Electrode

▨ normal fetal
▨ heart range

Pattern Characteristic:
Factitious Premature
Depolarizations and Pauses
Produced by Maternal QRS
Interference Combined with
Large Fetal P Waves and Small
Fetal QRS Signal

Tocodynamometer

uterine contraction

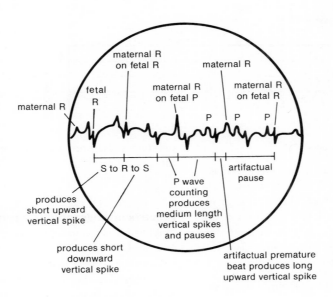

Factitious Dysrhythmia Produced by Maternal QRS Interference with Fetal R, R Prime and P Wave

*I*t is possible for the machine to correctly exclude maternal R wave counting because of its wider shape and shorter height. Likewise, the P and T waves that may be prominent in a variety of circumstances are typically rejected by the R wave signal detection because of their contour and height. However, when the maternal QRS complex coincides with a P wave or a portion of the fetal QRS complex not regularly counted, the combination may produce the prerequisites of the machine for R wave identification. The result produces a vertical spike followed by a compensatory pause.[1]

Irregularities produced by a combination of maternal QRS with a fetal signal present only sporadic deflections since the simultaneous occurrence of the two phenomena involved is infrequent.

When the event of the fetal cardiac cycle counted is antecedent to, but close to, the true R wave, the resulting vertical spike is only a short distance from the normal fetal heart trace. This observation, coupled with auscultation of no fetal heart irregularity, predicts the electrocardiographic findings.

Use of an automatically triggered arrhythmia/artifact detector permits the direct study of the events that produce fetal monitoring trace deflections.

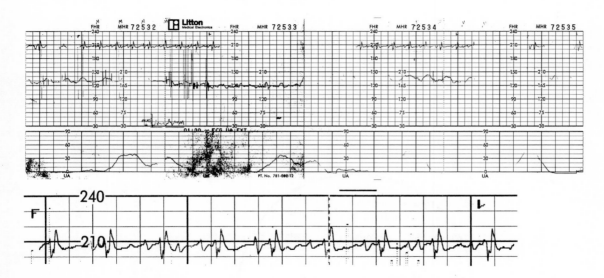

CASE INTERPRETATION: Class I

Baseline Information: a normal heart rate; average variability; short vertical spikes, which are equidistant above and below the fetal heart trace. These trigger recordings of the arrhythmia/artifact detector. Also seen are more pronounced upward vertical spikes that are followed by a short downward spike, the former also triggering the arrhythmia/artifact detector.

Periodic or Nonperiodic Changes: shallow, small accelerations, an obscure baseline in areas.

Uterine Activity: polysystolic contractions.

Significance: a healthy fetus is anticipated. Short, vertical spikes are usually seen with QRS complex variants. Since the upward spike occurs before the downward spike, an R R′ variant or prominent Q wave is predicted. Prominent upward spikes may also be produced by supraventricular premature depolarizations with an incomplete compensatory pause or maternal QRS interference. An electrocardiogram makes a clarification in this instance.

Electrocardiographic Interpretation: fetal electrocardiogram. The paper speed is 25 mm/sec. The fetal heart rate is 130 bpm. The QRS complex is widened and splintered with an RSR′ configuration. The R′ is wider and taller than the R wave. Occasionally, the narrower R wave, particularly if coalesced with a maternal R wave, achieves a competitive height.

CASE OUTCOME: Twenty-six-year-old primigravida, at term delivered by low elective forceps, with epidural anesthesia from an occiput anterior position, a 7 pound, 6 ounce (3345 gram) male; Apgar score 7/8. The infant followed an uncomplicated newborn course.

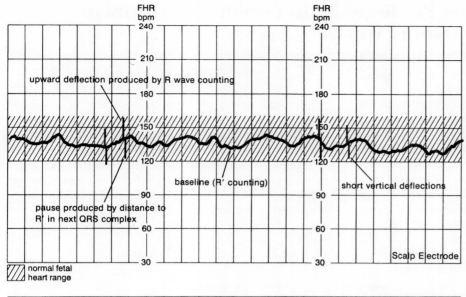

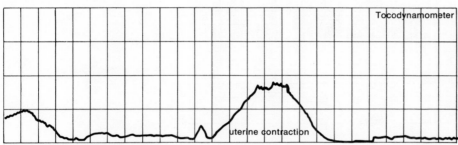

Pattern Characteristic:
Artifactual Arrhythmia:
R′ Counting

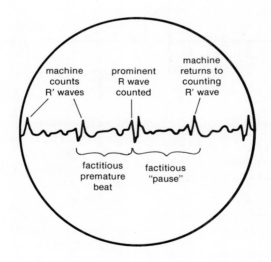

Factitious Dysrhythmia Produced by Intermittent Instrument Selection of Q Rather than R Wave

*C*hoppy looking traces produced by short vertical deflections above and below the normal rate are usually produced by an error in R wave identification that is caused by an atypical shape in the QRS complex. The trace has a similar appearance to 60 Hz power-line interference and to reversed polarity patterns in early fetal monitors when the monitor counted from the "wrong side" of the QRS signal, an artifact corrected by reversing leads of the scalp electrode.[2,6]

Although newer monitors reverse polarity automatically if the major QRS deflection is downward, variations in one QRS compared to the next may result in inconsistent machine selection of R wave versus Q or S wave or R prime.[4] It is possible to predict whether the erroneously counted event in the cardiac cycle occurs before or after the R wave by whether the initial vertical spike is upward or downward.

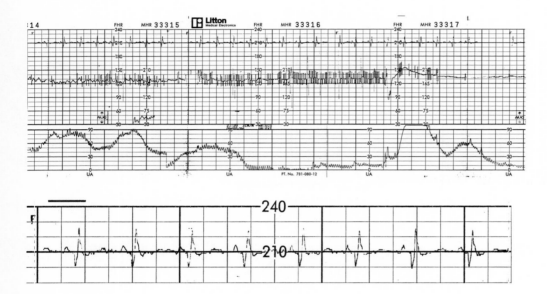

CASE INTERPRETATION: Class I-IV

Baseline Information: normal heart rate and variability. Short, vertical spikes are seen equidistant above and below the fetal heart trace. These trigger recordings of the arrhythmia/artifact detector.

Periodic or Nonperiodic Changes: single, nonperiodic variable deceleration with mild atypia.

Uterine Activity: irregular uterine contractions of varying configuration and superimposed maternal respirations.

Significance: the appearance of artifact produced by QRS configuration. Because the upward deflection occurs before the downward deflection, an event prior to the R wave such as a prominent Q wave is most likely being counted. The electrocardiogram is used for clarification in this instance.

Electrocardiographic Interpretation: fetal electrocardiogram. The paper speed is 25 mm/sec (computer corrected). The fetal heart rate is 127 bpm. There is a QR complex, with the Q of slightly lower amplitude than the R wave. On occasion, the R wave presents a broader configuration.

CASE OUTCOME: Twenty-two-year-old gravida 3, para 1011, at 32½ weeks' gestation, delivered vaginally from a vertex presentation, with pudendal and local anesthesia, a 5 pound, 3½ ounce (2367 gram) male; Apgar score 8/9. A 20% placental abruption was noted at delivery. The maternal course was complicated by AE hemoglobin. The newborn followed an uncomplicated newborn course.

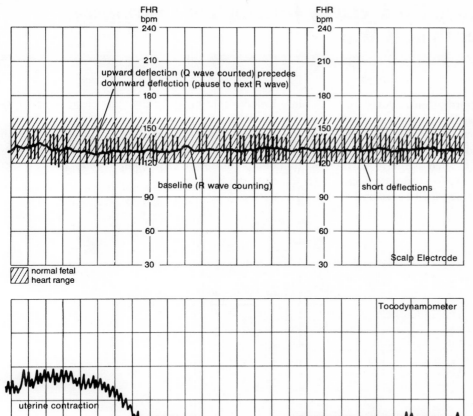

Pattern Characteristic:
Artifactual Arrhythmia: Q Wave Counting

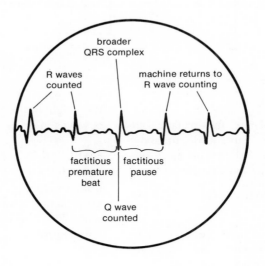

Factitious Dysrhythmia Produced by Intermittent Instrument Selection of S Rather than R Wave

*A*utomatically triggered artifact/arrhythmia detectors permit the study of single events that produce vertical deflections. Short deflections above and below the normal fetal heart trace are usually produced by errors in the selection of a consistent QRS event such as the R wave for counting. The upward vertical spike and its associated downward deflection (pause) are small because the counted electrocardiographic event is close in relationship to the R wave.

A downward deflection *preceding* an upward deflection is not typical of a fetal heart dysrhythmia. It implies selection of a point on the QRS complex *after* the R wave, for example, an S wave.

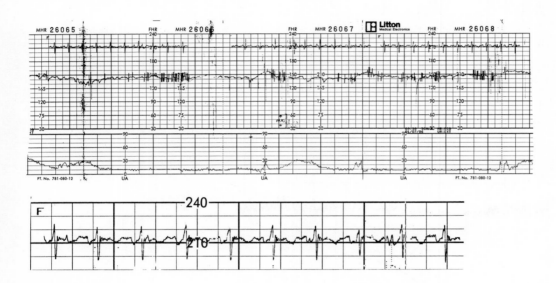

CASE INTERPRETATION: Class I

Baseline Information: normal rate and average variability. Very short vertical spikes occur equidistant above and below the fetal heart trace. Erratic and more pronounced vertical spikes also occur sporadically.

Periodic or Nonperiodic Changes: accelerations and mild variable decelerations.

Uterine Activity: shallow, infrequent uterine contractions, as measured by external monitor, and occasional bursts of fetal or maternal activity are suggested.

Significance: short, vertical spikes suggest an artifact produced by the QRS configuration. Since the downward spike precedes the upward spike, a prominent S wave is most likely.

Electrocardiographic Interpretation: fetal electrocardiogram. The paper speed is 25 mm/sec (computer corrected). The fetal heart rate is 142 bpm. The fetal complexes have an RS configuration, with the S exceeding the height of the R in some segments and with dominant R waves in other segments.

CASE OUTCOME: Twenty-five-year-old gravida 3, para 2002, at 42 weeks' gestation delivered vaginally from a vertex presentation, with pudendal and local anesthesia, a 6 pound, 13 ounce (3090 gram) male; Apgar score 7/9. The infant followed an uncomplicated newborn course.

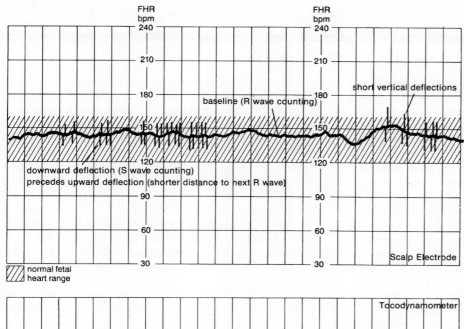

FHR
bpm

baseline (R wave counting)

short vertical deflections

Pattern Characteristic:
Artifactual Arrhythmia: S Wave
Counting

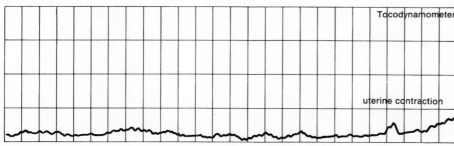

downward deflection (S wave counting)
precedes upward deflection (shorter distance to next R wave)

Scalp Electrode

normal fetal
heart range

Tocodynamometer

uterine contraction

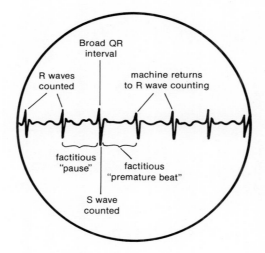

Broad QR
interval

R waves
counted

machine returns
to R wave counting

factitious
"pause"

factitious
"premature beat"

S wave
counted

References

1. Cabaniss ML, Wagner PC, Cabaniss CD: Fetal and maternal heart rate monitoring: Mechanisms for vertical spike deflections in fetal and maternal heart rate traces. *Abstract Soc Perin Obstet.* San Antonio, 1986, #208.

2. Freeman RK, Garite TJ: Instrumentation, artifact detection, and fetal arrhythmias, in: *Fetal Heart Rate Monitoring.* Baltimore, Williams & Wilkins, 1981, p. 28.

3. Hon EH, Hess DW: The clinical value of fetal electrocardiography. *Am J Obstet Gynecol* 79:1012, 1960.

4. Hutson JM, Petrie RH: Possible limitations of fetal monitoring. *Clin Obstet Gynecol* 29:104, 1986.

5. Katz M, Valdes-Cruz LM, Creco MA, et al: Diagnosis of congenital mitral and aortic stenosis from the fetal electrocardiogram. *Obstet Gynecol* 54:372, 1979.

6. Klapholz H: Artifactual fetal heart rate recording secondary to 60-Hz power-line interference. *Obstet Gynecol* 53:245, 1979.

7. Klapholz H, Schifrin BS, Myrick R: Role of maternal artifact in fetal heart rate pattern interpretation. *Obstet Gynecol* 53:245, 1979.

8. Larks SD, Webster A, Larks GG: Quantitative studies in fetal electrocardiography. III. Comparison of breech and cephalic presentation data; endocrine basis for fetal rotation, a hypothesis. *Am J Obstet Gynecol* 103:282, 1969.

9. Parer JT: The fetal heart rate monitor, in: *Handbook of Fetal Heart Rate Monitoring.* Philadelphia, W.B. Saunders, 1983, p. 55.

10. Shenker L: Fetal cardiac arrhythmias. *Obstet Gynecol Survey* 34:561, 1979.

11. van Bemmel JH, Peeters L, Hengeveld SJ: Influence of the maternal ECG on the abdominal fetal ECG complex. *Am J Obstet Gynecol* 102:556, 1968.

12. Westin B, Soderberg G: Equipment for direct FHR monitoring during labour. A comparative artifact study. *Acta Obstet Gynaec Scand* 52:41, 1973.

13. Zilianti M: Fetal electrocardiogram changes related to heart patterns during labor. *Am J Obstet Gynecol* 122:536, 1975.

Index

Page numbers followed by f indicate figures

ISBN 0-397-50824-7

90000